Dietary Fibers and Human Health

Special Issue Editor

Megan A. McCrory

MDPI • Basel • Beijing • Wuhan • Barcelona • Belgrade

Special Issue Editor
Megan A. McCrory
Boston University
USA

Editorial Office
MDPI AG
St. Alban-Anlage 66
Basel, Switzerland

This edition is a reprint of the Special Issue published online in the open access journal *Nutrients* (ISSN 2072-6643) from 2016–2017/ (available at: http://www.mdpi.com/journal/nutrients/special_issues/dietary_fibers).

For citation purposes, cite each article independently as indicated on the article page online and as indicated below:

Author 1; Author 2. Article title. *Journal Name* **Year**, *Article number*, page range.

First Edition 2017

ISBN 978-3-03842-581-6 (Pbk)
ISBN 978-3-03842-582-3 (PDF)

Table of Contents

About the Special Issue Editor

Megan A. McCrory is a research associate professor in the Sargent College of Health and Rehabilitation Sciences in Boston University, USA. Prof. McCrory's research and scholarly interests include: (1) Roles of eating patterns, dietary composition and their interaction effects on energy regulation; (2) Physiological and psychological factors influencing energy balance; (3) Improvement in dietary intake, physical activity and body composition assessment methods.

Preface to "Dietary Fibers and Human Health"

Research on the role dietary fibers in a vast array of health issues continues to evolve. This book contains some of the latest, cutting-edge research on dietary fiber in colon health; prevention and treatment of chronic diseases such as cancer, cardiovascular disease, and type 2 diabetes; weight management; dietary fiber intake and methodology is also covered. I would like to take the time to acknowledge the excellent work of the author contributors, and the people who contributed their time to review each paper, without whom this book would not be possible.

Megan A. McCrory
Special Issue Editor

nutrients

MDPI

Article

Efficacy of Synbiotics in Patients with Slow Transit Constipation: A Prospective Randomized Trial

Chao Ding [1,†], Xiaolong Ge [1,†], Xueying Zhang [1], Hongliang Tian [1], Hongkan Wang [2], Lili Gu [1], Jianfeng Gong [1,*], Weiming Zhu [1] and Ning Li [1,*]

1 Department of General Surgery, Jinling Hospital, Medical School of Nanjing University, Nanjing 210002, China; jinlingh_dc@163.com (C.D.); xiaolongge9118@126.com (X.G.); 15996282291@163.com (X.Z.); kevin_thl@163.com (H.T.); njumedgll@126.com (L.G.); jinlingh_zwm@sina.com (W.Z.)
2 First Affiliated Hospital, School of Medicine, Zhejiang University, Hangzhou 310003, China; njumedcy@126.com
* Correspondence: jinlingh_gongjf@163.com (J.G.); jinlingh_lining@163.com (N.L.); Tel.: +86-25-8086-0036 (J.G.); +86-25-8086-0045 (N.L.)
† These authors contributed equally to this work.

Received: 27 August 2016; Accepted: 22 September 2016; Published: 28 September 2016

Abstract: Synbiotic intake may efficiently restore the balance of gut microbiota and improve gastrointestinal functions. The aim of the study was to evaluate the efficacy of a synbiotic in patients with slow transit constipation. A total of 100 patients with slow transit constipation were randomized to receive either a synbiotic or placebo twice daily for 12 weeks. The primary efficacy endpoints were the clinical remission and improvement rates at weeks 4 and 12. Stool frequency and consistency, colonic transit time (CTT), evacuation and abdominal symptoms, patient assessment of constipation symptoms, gastrointestinal quality-of-life index scores, satisfaction scores, and adverse events were also monitored. The clinical remission rates reached 37.5% at week 4 and 45.8% at week 12 in the treatment group, compared to 13.3% at week 4 and 16.7% at week 12 in the placebo group ($p < 0.01$ for both comparisons). Over 12 weeks, 64.6% of the patients who received the synbiotic experienced clinical improvement, compared to 29.2% of the patients in the placebo group ($p < 0.01$). During the intervention period, patients who were treated with the synbiotic exhibited increased stool frequency, improved stool consistency, decreased CTT, and improved constipation-related symptoms. This randomized, placebo-controlled trial suggested that dietary supplementation with a synbiotic improved evacuation-parameters-associated symptoms and colonic motility in patients with slow transit constipation (STC).

Keywords: synbiotic; soluble dietary fiber; slow transit constipation; microbiota

1. Introduction

Chronic constipation has become a common, often long-term, functional gastrointestinal disease that influences the quality of life in patients worldwide [1]. According to the Rome III criteria for chronic constipation [2], almost 16% of all adults are affected by chronic constipation worldwide, and it is more prevalent and symptomatic in women and elderly people [3]. Constipation is defined as difficult or infrequent passage of stool, hardness of stool, or a feeling of incomplete evacuation [4]. Clinically, constipation can always be categorized as normal transit constipation (NTC), slow transit constipation (STC), pelvic floor dysfunction, or a defecatory disorder due to assessments of anorectal function and colonic transit time [5]. Among these, STC is the major category and is characterized by a decreased rate of colonic transit [5].

The treatments for chronic constipation are varied, but remain challenging [6]. Most patients with chronic constipation have used laxatives (osmotic or stimulant) or prokinetic agents to alleviate symptoms empirically [7]. Although there is a wide range of medications, many patients are still dissatisfied with their current treatments, according to the results of a long-term survey, due to insufficient efficacy and some adverse effects [8]. Sajid et al. [9] reported that adverse events or side effects such as abdominal cramps, rash, excessive flatulence, and dizziness have occurred in constipated patients who used prucalopride, which is a new pharmacotherapy for chronic constipation. From our clinical experience in constipation, laxatives or other agents could be efficient at the beginning of chronic constipation, but they gradually become largely ineffective. Therefore, novel effective therapies are still needed.

Probiotics are live microorganisms that may benefit human health, and are now used widely to treat some diseases. Cui et al. [10] reported that *Bifidobacteria* intake could play a role in the remission of ulcerative colitis (UC) and that prebiotics, such as dietary fiber, are ingredients in food that may increase the functions of probiotics in the human body. Previous research has suggested that a sufficient intake of dietary fiber with prebiotic effects is necessary for patients with chronic constipation [11–13]. Pectin, one typical kind of dietary fiber, is usually present in the cell walls of fruits, vegetables, and legumes [14]. It is fermented by the intestinal microbiota in the gut and can strongly stimulate the growth and activity of some bacteria, such as *Bifidobacterium* and *Lactobacillus* [14]. Some reports have also shown that therapy with increasing dietary fiber intake, especially soluble fibers, was beneficial for individuals with chronic constipation [15]. Soluble dietary fiber, which includes pectin, is physiologically important [16]. Pectin can be digested into short-chain fatty acids (SCFAs) by intestinal microbiota, which may have effects on motility [17]. Fukumoto et al. [18] reported that SCFAs could stimulate the colon to release serotonin, which is an important factor in colonic motility. In addition, butyrate is used in treating various gastrointestinal motility disorders that are associated with the inhibition of colonic transit [17].

Currently, the combination of prebiotics and probiotics is called synbiotics, and it may have synergistic effects [19]. Morelli et al. [20] suggested that microbiota composition could be modified by synbiotics, which might play a role in gastrointestinal functions. This prospective, randomized study was designed to measure the effects of a symbiotic consisting of *Enterococci*, *Bifidobacteria*, and *Lactobacilli* triple viable bacteria (BIFICO) and pectin on slow transit constipation [10]. This was the first study to assess a specific synbiotic containing triple viable bacteria and pectin in individuals with constipation.

Our objective was to evaluate the clinical efficacy of synbiotic treatment in individuals with slow transit constipation. The primary aim was to assess clinical improvement and remission at weeks 4 and 12. The secondary aim was to assess the frequency of bowel movements, stool consistency, and colonic transit time. Other aims included the assessment of constipation-related symptoms, and the gastrointestinal quality-of-life index.

2. Materials and Methods

2.1. Ethical Issues

This study was registered in the Clinical Trials Database (ID: NCT02844426) and conducted at Jinling Hospital, a teaching hospital of Nanjing University. The current study was approved by the Ethical Committee of Jinling Hospital. All participants provided written informed consent.

2.2. Patients

- Patients were eligible if they fulfilled the following criteria:

Inclusion criteria: age ≥18 years; body mass index 18.5–25 kg/m^2; chronic constipation was diagnosed according to the Rome III criteria with two or fewer spontaneous, complete bowel movements (SCBMs) per week for a minimum of 6 months [21]; colonic transit time (CTT) >48 h [22]; mild-to-moderate constipation with a Wexner constipation scale score between 16 and 25 [23,24].

Exclusion criteria: Megacolon, intestinal obstruction, inflammatory bowel disease, and cancer; secondary constipation (i.e., due to drugs, endocrine disorders, neurological disorders, metabolic disorders, psychological disorders or abdominal surgery); severe anterior rectocele or full thickness rectorectal intussusception according to defecography; pregnant or lactating women; infection with an enteric pathogen; usage of antibiotics or proton pump inhibitors (PPIs); hepatic, renal, cardiovascular, respiratory or psychiatric disease; and other diseases or factors evaluated by the investigator which could influence intestinal transit or intestinal microbiota [24].

2.3. Study Design

A total of 100 patients were screened for eligibility to participate in our study. The sealed envelope method was used to randomize the participants into either the treatment group or the placebo group. After a week of non-interventional clinical observation, the treatment or placebo group blindly received the synbiotic or placebo twice daily for 12 weeks. The synbiotic (BIFICOPEC) contained 0.63 g of bifid triple viable capsules (BIFICO) [10] and 8 g of soluble dietary fiber (Pectin, provided by Ander Group in Yantai, China) [24]. The placebo group was treated with digestible maltodextrin (CTFH pharmaceutical company, Nanjing, China) by an experienced doctor. These constipated patients were advised to participate in a healthy lifestyle, including proper diet and exercise, and to avoid any other probiotics and dietary fiber during the study period. If patients did not have a bowel movement for 3 or more consecutive days, they were permitted to take up to 20 g of Macrogol 4000 powder (Forlax®, Ipsen, Paris, France). If ineffective, an enema could be used.

During the follow-up, patients were asked to keep daily diaries of their bowel symptoms, including stool consistency, as rated by the Bristol Stool Form Scale (BSFS). The trained physicians, who were blinded to the treatments, assessed the quality of life and constipation-related symptoms of all of the participants at weeks 4 and 12 via phone or e-mail. Adverse events were also monitored during follow-up.

2.4. Outcomes

The primary efficacy endpoints were as follows: (1) Clinical remission rate: the proportion of patients having an average of three or more spontaneous complete bowel movements (SCBMs) per week during the observation period of weeks 4 and 12; and (2) Clinical improvement rate: the proportion of patients with an average increase of one or more SCBMs per week compared with baseline at weeks 4 and 12.

The secondary efficacy endpoints were as follows: (1) Number of bowel movements within one week [24]; (2) Stool consistency according to the BSFS: stool types 1 and 2 indicated constipation, types 3, 4, and 5 indicated a normal consistency, and types 6 and 7 indicated diarrhea [24]; and (3) Colonic transit time (CTT), which was measured at baseline and at weeks 4 and 12 by the Metcalf method [22].

Other endpoints included the following: (1) The Patient Assessment of Constipation Symptoms (PAC-SYM) questionnaire was administered at baseline and at weeks 4 and 12. The questionnaire contained 12 symptoms that were grouped into three subscales for stool, abdominal, and rectal symptoms. For the overall scale and each subscale, the scores ranged from 0 (symptoms absent) to 4 (symptoms very severe) [25]; (2) The Gastrointestinal Quality-of-Life Index (GIQLI) assessment, which was used to evaluate the quality of life in patients with gastrointestinal diseases, comprised 36 questions using a 5-point Likert-type scale ranging from 0 to 4 (0, worst; 4, best) [26]; (3) The satisfaction scoresof constipated patients, which used a 5-point ordinal scale. The score ranged from 1 (extremely unsatisfied) to 5 (extremely satisfied); (4) For evacuation symptoms, patients recorded their perception of straining, lumpy hard stools, the sensation of incomplete evacuation, and the sensation of anorectal blockage according to a 5-point ordinal scale (1, none; 2, mild; 3, moderate; 4, severe; or 5, very severe); (5) Finally, abdominal symptoms were categorized, patients recorded their symptoms of abdominal pain or cramps and bloating or flatulence according to five classifications (1, none; 2, mild; 3, moderate; 4, severe; or 5, very severe).

2.5. Safety Assessments

During treatment and follow-up, patients were advised to record adverse events in daily diaries and to report adverse events immediately. Adverse events could include abdominal pain, flatulence, borborygmus, and other gastrointestinal symptoms.

2.6. Sample Size

The sample size was calculated based on the frequency of evacuation and the standard deviation of the difference as 0.8 between the groups [27]. Therefore, a total sample size of 100 (50 in each group) was sufficient to expect a 95% power with a two-sided significance level of 0.05.

2.7. Statistical Analysis

The results were analyzed with SPSS 19.0 (SPSS, Inc., Chicago, IL, USA). Continuous data were presented as the mean ± standard deviation and categorical data were presented as *n* (%). Paired *t* tests or a repeated measures ANOVA were performed for continuous variables, and for categorical variables; Pearson's chi-square test or the Fisher exact test was performed as appropriate. p values < 0.05 were considered statistically significant for all comparisons.

3. Results

3.1. Baseline Characteristics

In our study, a total of 100 patients were enrolled and randomized into two groups, with 50 participants per group. Seven patients did not complete the study protocol. Therefore, a total of 93 patients, including 48 patients who had received the synbiotic and 45 patients who had received placebo, were included in the final analysis. The patient flow is detailed in Figure 1. The baseline characteristics of patients in the treatment or placebo group are shown in Table 1. Most enrolled patients were females (63.44%) compared to males (36.56%). The disease durations of 7.1 ± 4.2 years and 7.4 ± 3.9 years in the placebo and treatment groups, respectively, were not significantly different. There were also no differences in gender, age, BMI, Wexner score, stool consistency, or colonic transit time.

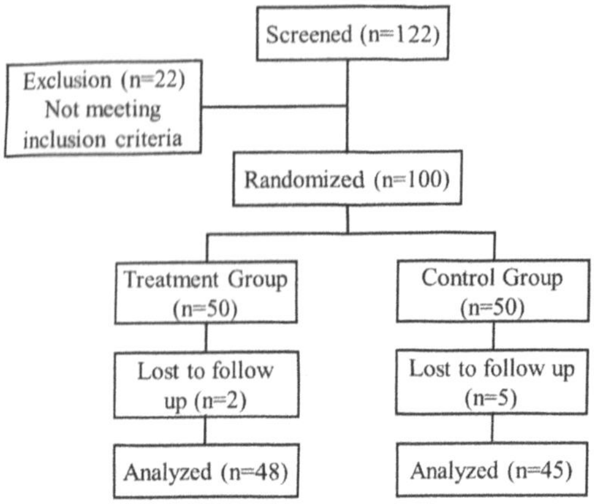

Figure 1. Consolidated standards of reporting trials (CONSORT) flow diagram of patients recruitment and analysis.

Table 1. Baseline demographics in patients received treatment or placebo.

Characteristics	Placebo (n = 45)	Treatment (n = 48)	p Value
Sex (male/female) *	16 (35.6)/29 (64.4)	18 (37.5)/30 (62.5)	0.846
Age (year) †	48.3 ± 11.3	47.2 ± 10.7	0.638
BMI (kg/m^2) †	22.8 ± 1.1	22.6 ± 1.1	0.305
Disease duration (year) †	7.1 ± 4.2	7.4 ± 3.9	0.695
Wexner score †	19.8 ± 2.0	20.0 ± 2.2	0.797
No. of BMs/week †	2.1 ± 0.6	2.2 ± 0.7	0.615
Stool consistency †	2.0 ± 0.6	2.1 ± 0.5	0.366
CTT (h) †	73.0 ± 10.3	71.7 ± 10.8	0.567
Smoker *	3 (6.7)	4 (8.3)	0.761
Alcohol consumer *	6 (13.3)	5 (10.4)	0.663
Regular exercise *	12 (26.7)	14 (29.2)	0.788

BMI, body mass index; BM, bowel movement; CTT, colonic transit time. * Values are expressed as n (%), † values are expressed as the mean ± standard deviation.

3.2. Primary and Secondary Efficacy Endpoints

During the follow-up period, more patients in the synbiotic group achieved a mean of three or more bowel movements per week than in the placebo group at both weeks 4 and 12, and the clinical remission rate in the synbiotic group reached 18% at week 4 and 22% at week 12. There were significant differences in clinical improvement in the synbiotic and the placebo groups at weeks 4 and 12 ($p < 0.01$). After treatment, compared to the placebo group, the number of bowel movements in the synbiotic group improved significantly within one week and reached 4.5 ± 1.6 and 5.1 ± 2.0 at weeks 4 and 12 ($p < 0.001$). In addition, the stool consistency score was statistically significantly increased in the treatment group compared to the placebo group (week 4, 3.2 ± 1.2 vs. 2.5 ± 0.8, $p < 0.001$; week 12, 3.5 ± 1.1 vs. 2.4 ± 0.8, $p < 0.001$). The results of CTT showed that patients who had received the synbiotic treatment had a shorter transit time than did patients in the placebo group at weeks 4 and 12, which could reflect improved intestinal motility. The detailed data are shown in Table 2.

Table 2. Clinical outcomes of treatment vs. placebo groups.

Endpoint	4 Week		12 Week	
	Placebo	Synbiotic	Placebo	Synbiotic
Clinical remission rate (%) †	6 (13.3)	18 (37.5) **	8 (16.7)	22 (45.8) **
Clinical improvement rate (%) †	11 (24.4)	25 (52.1) **	14 (29.2)	31 (64.6) **
No. of BMs/week ‡	2.9 ± 1.1	4.5 ± 1.6 ***	3.1 ± 1.4	5.1 ± 2.0 ***
Stool consistency ‡	2.5 ± 0.8	3.2 ± 1.2 ***	2.4 ± 0.8	3.5 ± 1.1 ***
CTT (h) ‡	68.2 ± 11.3	53.8 ± 10.9 **	70.5 ± 12.1	49.3 ± 11.7 ***

BM, bowel movement; CTT, colonic transit time. † Values are expressed as n (%), ‡ values are expressed as the mean ± SD. ** p value < 0.01; *** p value < 0.001.

3.3. Other Efficacy Results

Treatment with the synbiotic relieved the symptoms of constipated patients. Compared with baseline, the PAC-SYM score significantly decreased in the treatment group at weeks 4 and 12 ($p < 0.001$). However, there was no statistically significant decrease in the PAC-SYM score in the placebo group (Table 3). As shown in Table 3, the GIQLI score in the synbiotic group was 83.5 ± 12.6 before treatment, and it increased to 117.8 ± 15.8 at week 4 ($p < 0.01$) and 126.9 ± 16.5 at week 12 ($p < 0.001$). Although the GIQLI score in the placebo group also improved from 86.3 ± 11.2 to 91.7 ± 12.8 at week 4 and 95.5 ± 15.3 at week 12, no significant difference was found. We also recorded the satisfaction scores of constipated patients during follow-up. Similarly, satisfaction scores in the placebo and treatment groups were analyzed. Our results showed that the score in the treatment group was significantly higher than in the placebo group, not only at week 4, but also at week 12—which indicates that more patients were satisfied with the treatment (Table 3).

In terms of evacuation symptoms, patients in the treatment group reported significantly less straining and fewer lumpy hard stools (Figure 2). No significant improvement was found in the sensation of incomplete evacuation at week 4, but a significantly higher proportion of patients in the treatment group at week 12 reported an improvement in this sensation ($p < 0.05$) (Figure 2). However, there was no significant difference in the sensation of anorectal blockage between groups (Figure 2). For abdominal symptoms, a trend toward improvement was found in the treatment group, but there were no significant differences between the groups (Figure 2). No significant adverse events associated with treatment were reported.

Table 3. Efficacy endpoints.

Week	PAC-SYM †		GIQLI †		Satisfaction Score †	
	Placebo	Synbiotic	Placebo	Synbiotic	Placebo	Synbiotic
Baseline	1.9 ± 0.3	1.9 ± 0.2	86.3 ± 11.2	83.5 ± 12.6	—	—
4 weeks	1.8 ± 0.3	1.4 ± 0.5 **	91.7 ± 12.8	117.8 ± 15.8 **	2.8 ± 1.2	3.5 ± 1.4 *
12 weeks	1.7 ± 0.4	1.2 ± 0.6 ***	95.5 ± 15.3	126.9 ± 16.5 ***	2.9 ± 1.3	3.8 ± 1.4 **

GIQLI, Gastrointestinal Quality-of-Life Index; PAC-SYM, Patient Assessment of Constipation Symptoms. † Values are expressed as the mean ± SD; — indicates not applicable. * p value < 0.05; ** p value < 0.01; *** p value < 0.001.

(1) Improvement of evacuation symptoms (score ≤2).

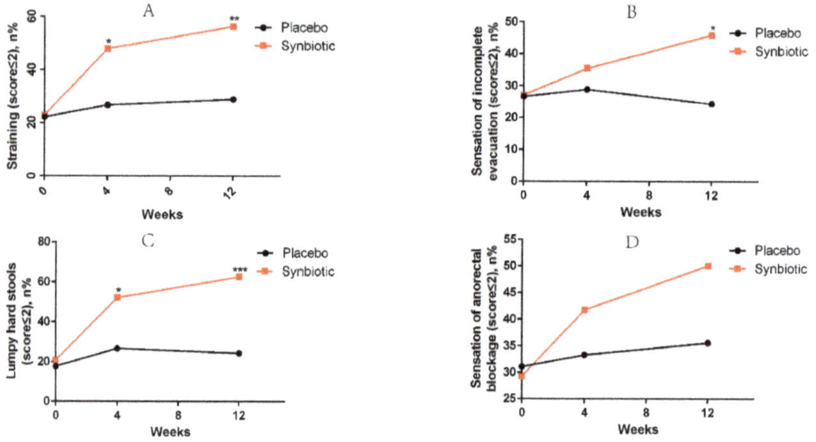

(2) Improvement of abdominal symptoms (score ≥4).

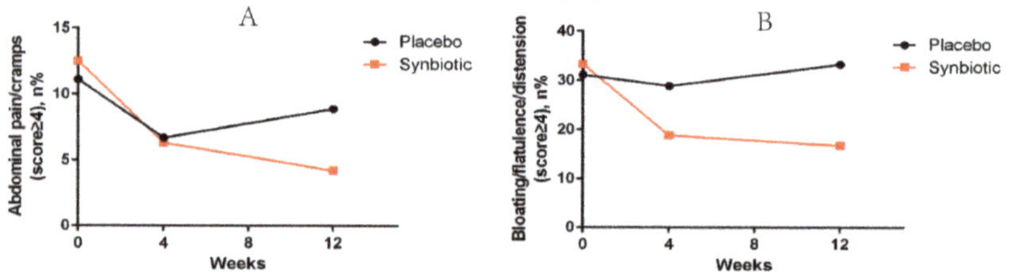

Figure 2. Improvement of constipation-ralated symptoms in the treatment vs. placebo groups. 5-point ordinal scale, 1 indicates none, 2 mild, 3 moderate, 4 severe, and 5 very severe. * p value < 0.05; ** p value < 0.01; *** p value < 0.001. (1) Improvement of evacuation symptoms in treatment vs. placebo groups at baseline, week 4, and week 12; (2) Improvement of abdominal symptoms in treatment vs. placebo groups at baseline, week 4, and week 12.

4. Discussion

This was a prospective randomized trial to evaluate the efficacy of a synbiotic (BIFICOPEC) comprised of probiotics (BIFICO) [10] and soluble dietary fiber (Pectin) in patients with slow transit constipation who met the Rome III criteria. Our study found that 12 weeks of supplementation with probiotics and soluble dietary fiber increased bowel movements, improved the PAC-SYM and GIQLI scores, relieved constipation-related symptoms, and decreased CTT. Finally, the clinical remission and clinical improvement rates reached 45.8% and 64.6%, respectively, at week 12 among patients with mild-to-moderate constipation. No serious treatment-related adverse events were observed during the follow-up period.

Slow transit constipation, which is one type of chronic idiopathic constipation, has an important pathophysiological feature of decreased colonic motility, which could be diagnosed by using radiopaque markers, as occurred in this study [28]. Recently, many researchers have focused on the relationship between intestinal microbiota and constipation and have demonstrated that intestinal microbiota contribute to the pathophysiology of functional gastrointestinal disorders [29]. Parthasarathy et al. [30] suggested that the profile of microbiota in the intestine was associated with colonic transit, and genera from *Firmicutes* was related with faster colonic transit. Zhu et al. [31] reported that, compared with a control group, individuals in a constipation group had a distinct microbiome in the gut. Moreover, the Bristol Stool Scale classification has been widely used to reflect intestinal colon transit time in constipated patients. Vandeputte et al. [32] advised that stool consistency, as evaluated using the Bristol Stool Scale, was strongly correlated with intestinal microbiota. These studies all suggest that gut microbiota contribute to the etiology in constipation. Our previous study [33] reported that the reestablishment of the whole intestinal flora with fecal microbiota transplantation could alleviate the symptoms of slow transit constipation, which might provide a basis for the considerable role of gut microbiota in constipation from the perspective of clinical treatment.

Recently, emerging studies on the individual benefits of probiotics and prebiotics in the treatment of chronic constipation have been reported. Ford et al. [19] reported a systematic review and meta-analysis and showed that probiotics appeared to have beneficial effects in chronic idiopathic constipation (CIC), but only a few RCTs were available for the analysis. Data from RCTs for prebiotics and synbiotics in individuals with CIC are also sparse. Some studies found that prebiotics had a positive effect in constipated patients. Christodoulides et al. [34] suggested that fiber was moderately effective for chronic idiopathic constipation in adults. Suares et al. [35] also reported that soluble fiber might be more beneficial than insoluble fiber in constipated patients in alleviating straining, pain on defecation, improving stool consistency, and other constipation-related symptoms. In addition, research on the changes in intestinal microbiota in individuals with constipation indicated that microbiota other than *Lactobacillus* and *Bifidobacteria* also changed, which might indicate the importance of stability and integration of intestinal microbiota. Therefore, supplementation with both probiotics and prebiotics is better than treatment with probiotics or prebiotics alone.

Pectin is an important soluble dietary fiber that can be fermented by gut microbiota. The most familiar and predominant structural element in pectin is formed by the "smooth" homogalacturonan regions and is composed predominantly of a homopolymer of partially methyl esterified (1–4)-linked α-D-galacturonic acid (GalA) units [12]. The health benefits of pectin might include alterations in the composition of intestinal microbiota and the production of short-chain fatty acids [36,37]. Onumpai et al. [37] reported that pectin could stimulate the activity of *Bifidobacterium* and *Lactobacillus*. Recently, our team also found that fecal microbiota transplantation, in combination with soluble dietary fiber, could improve the symptoms of patients with slow transit constipation, indicating that the regulation of intestinal microecology was associated with constipation [24]. The addition of pectin to the treatment regimen further improved the symptoms in constipated patients. Therefore, pectin may play a beneficial role in constipation.

In contrast, butyrate, which is a byproduct of pectin fermentation by certain microbiota, is necessary for colonic homeostasis and provides energy for intestinal epithelial cells [38]. We chose maltodextrin as a placebo control because maltodextrin is an easily digested carbohydrate, but it is not fermented by intestinal microbiota; thus, it would not affect gut metabolism and microbial ecology [27].

In our study, we provided constipated patients with bifid triple viable capsules and pectin for 12 weeks. Our results revealed an improvement in the number of bowel movements per week, stool consistency, and colonic transit time in constipated patients, which are related to intestinal motility. Intestinal microbiota analysis has already shown that microbiota are associated with colonic transit, stool frequency, and stool consistency in humans [30,32]. During the follow-up, we found that the improvement in stool consistency was the most obvious effect, but a significant improvement in the sensation of incomplete evacuation did not appear until three months after treatment initiation. Harder stools and decreased frequency are associated with a slower colonic transit time, while increased incomplete evacuation is related to outlet obstructive constipation [22]. So the efficacy of synbiotics in constipation might depend on the improvement of intestinal motility through regulating intestinal microecology.

Because pharmacological interventions have limited efficacy and more side effects, traditional treatments have not been able to fully satisfy constipated patients [39]. Prucalopride is a widely used prokinetic agent, but adverse events such as abdominal cramps, headache, skin disorders, and drug dependence have been reported with its use [9]. During our treatment and follow-up, no serious adverse events occurred in the patients. It is found that constipated patients at our hospital prefer to use prebiotics, probiotics, or synbiotics rather than some laxatives.

However, our pilot study does have several limitations. First, this was a single-center study, and the sample size of our trial was relatively small. A multicenter randomized controlled study should be performed to verify these findings. Second, our follow-up period was restricted to 12 weeks. The clinical efficacy of treatment for chronic constipation should be examined in a study with a longer follow-up. Finally, we did not analyze the structural changes in the gut microbiota in constipated patients before and after treatment. Intestinal microbiota analysis might provide us a new perspective to explain the therapeutic mechanism underlying synbiotic treatment.

5. Conclusions

In conclusion, we found that 12 weeks of treatment with a synbiotic that contained pectin as a prebiotic and bifid triple viable capsule (BIFICO) as a probiotic was effective in increasing stool frequency, improving stool consistency, decreasing colonic transit time, and relieving constipation-related symptoms. In addition, synbiotic treatment effectively improved the quality of life in patients with mild-to-moderate constipation. Therefore, additional multicenter randomized clinical trials are needed to confirm these results and assess the role of the regulation of gut microbiota in treatment of constipation.

Acknowledgments: This study was funded by the National Natural Science Foundation of China (81270006) and the National Gastroenterology Research Project (2015BAI13B07). The authors thank Huatong Liu from the Australian National University for checking the entire manuscript for grammar and typographical errors.

Author Contributions: Ning Li, Weiming Zhu and Jianfeng Gong conceived and designed the study; Chao Ding, Xiaolong Ge, Xueying Zhang, and Hongliang Tian performed all required data collection for the study experiment; Hongkan Wang and Lili Gu analyzed the data; Xiaolong Ge and Chao Ding wrote the paper.

Conflicts of Interest: The authors declare no conflicts of interest.

References

1. Nelson, A.D.; Camilleri, M.; Chirapongsathorn, S.; Vijayvargiya, P.; Valentin, N.; Shin, A.; Erwin, P.J.; Wang, Z.; Murad, M.H. Comparison of efficacy of pharmacological treatments for chronic idiopathic constipation: A systematic review and network meta-analysis. *Gut* **2016**. [CrossRef] [PubMed]

2. Higgins, P.D.; Johanson, J.F. Epidemiology of constipation in north america: A systematic review. *Am. J. Gastroenterol.* **2004**, *99*, 750–759. [CrossRef] [PubMed]
3. Mugie, S.M.; Benninga, M.A.; Di Lorenzo, C. Epidemiology of constipation in children and adults: A systematic review. *Best Pract. Res. Clin. Gastroenterol.* **2011**, *25*, 3–18. [CrossRef] [PubMed]
4. Rao, S.S.; Rattanakovit, K.; Patcharatrakul, T. Diagnosis and management of chronic constipation in adults. *Nat. Rev. Gastroenterol. Hepatol.* **2016**, *13*, 295–305. [CrossRef] [PubMed]
5. Bharucha, A.E.; Pemberton, J.H.; Locke, G.R., III. American gastroenterological association technical review on constipation. *Gastroenterology* **2013**, *144*, 218–238. [CrossRef] [PubMed]
6. American Gastroenterological Association; Bharucha, A.E.; Dorn, S.D.; Lembo, A.; Pressman, A. American gastroenterological association medical position statement on constipation. *Gastroenterology* **2013**, *144*, 211–217. [CrossRef] [PubMed]
7. Ford, A.C.; Suares, N.C. Effect of laxatives and pharmacological therapies in chronic idiopathic constipation: Systematic review and meta-analysis. *Gut* **2011**, *60*, 209–218. [CrossRef] [PubMed]
8. Camilleri, M.; Kerstens, R.; Rykx, A.; Vandeplassche, L. A placebo-controlled trial of prucalopride for severe chronic constipation. *N. Engl. J. Med.* **2008**, *358*, 2344–2354. [CrossRef] [PubMed]
9. Sajid, M.S.; Hebbar, M.; Baig, M.K.; Li, A.; Philipose, Z. Use of prucalopride for chronic constipation: A systematic review and meta-analysis of published randomized, controlled trials. *J. Neurogastroenterol. Motil.* **2016**, *22*, 412–422. [CrossRef] [PubMed]
10. Cui, H.H.; Chen, C.L.; Wang, J.D.; Yang, Y.J.; Cun, Y.; Wu, J.B.; Liu, Y.H.; Dan, H.L.; Jian, Y.T.; Chen, X.Q. Effects of probiotic on intestinal mucosa of patients with ulcerative colitis. *World J. Gastroenterol.* **2004**, *10*, 1521–1525. [CrossRef] [PubMed]
11. Kaczmarczyk, M.M.; Miller, M.J.; Freund, G.G. The health benefits of dietary fiber: Beyond the usual suspects of type 2 diabetes mellitus, cardiovascular disease and colon cancer. *Metabolism* **2012**, *61*, 1058–1066. [CrossRef] [PubMed]
12. Tian, L.; Bruggeman, G.; van den Berg, M.; Borewicz, K.; Scheurink, A.J.; Bruininx, E.; de Vos, P.; Smidt, H.; Schols, H.A.; Gruppen, H. Effects of pectin on fermentation characteristics, carbohydrate utilization and microbial community composition in the gastrointestinal tract of weaning pigs. *Mol. Nutr. Food Res.* **2016**. [CrossRef] [PubMed]
13. Voderholzer, W.A.; Schatke, W.; Muhldorfer, B.E.; Klauser, A.G.; Birkner, B.; Muller-Lissner, S.A. Clinical response to dietary fiber treatment of chronic constipation. *Am. J. Gastroenterol.* **1997**, *92*, 95–98. [PubMed]
14. Tian, L.; Scholte, J.; Borewicz, K.; Bogert, B.V.; Smidt, H.; Scheurink, A.J.; Gruppen, H.; Schols, H.A. Effects of pectin supplementation on the fermentation patterns of different structural carbohydrates in rats. *Mol. Nutr. Food Res.* **2016**. [CrossRef] [PubMed]
15. Chan, A.O.; Leung, G.; Tong, T.; Wong, N.Y. Increasing dietary fiber intake in terms of kiwifruit improves constipation in chinese patients. *World J. Gastroenterol.* **2007**, *13*, 4771–4775. [CrossRef] [PubMed]
16. Eswaran, S.; Muir, J.; Chey, W.D. Fiber and functional gastrointestinal disorders. *Am. J. Gastroenterol.* **2013**, *108*, 718–727. [CrossRef] [PubMed]
17. Soret, R.; Chevalier, J.; De Coppet, P.; Poupeau, G.; Derkinderen, P.; Segain, J.P.; Neunlist, M. Short-chain fatty acids regulate the enteric neurons and control gastrointestinal motility in rats. *Gastroenterology* **2010**, *138*, 1772–1782. [CrossRef] [PubMed]
18. Fukumoto, S.; Tatewaki, M.; Yamada, T.; Fujimiya, M.; Mantyh, C.; Voss, M.; Eubanks, S.; Harris, M.; Pappas, T.N.; Takahashi, T. Short-chain fatty acids stimulate colonic transit via intraluminal 5-ht release in rats. *Am. J. Physiol. Regul. Integr. Comp. Physiol.* **2003**, *284*, R1269–R1276. [CrossRef] [PubMed]
19. Ford, A.C.; Quigley, E.M.; Lacy, B.E.; Lembo, A.J.; Saito, Y.A.; Schiller, L.R.; Soffer, E.E.; Spiegel, B.M.; Moayyedi, P. Efficacy of prebiotics, probiotics, and synbiotics in irritable bowel syndrome and chronic idiopathic constipation: Systematic review and meta-analysis. *Am. J. Gastroenterol.* **2014**, *109*, 1547–1561. [CrossRef] [PubMed]
20. Morelli, L.; Zonenschain, D.; Callegari, M.L.; Grossi, E.; Maisano, F.; Fusillo, M. Assessment of a new synbiotic preparation in healthy volunteers: Survival, persistence of probiotic strains and its effect on the indigenous flora. *Nutr. J.* **2003**, *2*, 11. [CrossRef] [PubMed]
21. Drossman, D.A. The functional gastrointestinal disorders and the rome iii process. *Gastroenterology* **2006**, *130*, 1377–1390. [CrossRef] [PubMed]

22. Emmanuel, A.; Cools, M.; Vandeplassche, L.; Kerstens, R. Prucalopride improves bowel function and colonic transit time in patients with chronic constipation: An integrated analysis. *Am. J. Gastroenterol.* **2014**, *109*, 887–894. [CrossRef] [PubMed]
23. Agachan, F.; Chen, T.; Pfeifer, J.; Reissman, P.; Wexner, S.D. A constipation scoring system to simplify evaluation and management of constipated patients. *Dis. Colon Rectum* **1996**, *39*, 681–685. [CrossRef] [PubMed]
24. Ge, X.; Tian, H.; Ding, C.; Gu, L.; Wei, Y.; Gong, J.; Zhu, W.; Li, N.; Li, J. Fecal microbiota transplantation in combination with soluble dietary fiber for treatment of slow transit constipation: A pilot study. *Arch. Med. Res.* **2016**, *47*, 236–242. [CrossRef] [PubMed]
25. Frank, L.; Kleinman, L.; Farup, C.; Taylor, L.; Miner, P., Jr. Psychometric validation of a constipation symptom assessment questionnaire. *Scand. J. Gastroenterol.* **1999**, *34*, 870–877. [PubMed]
26. Eypasch, E.; Williams, J.I.; Wood-Dauphinee, S.; Ure, B.M.; Schmulling, C.; Neugebauer, E.; Troidl, H. Gastrointestinal quality of life index: Development, validation and application of a new instrument. *Br. J. Surg.* **1995**, *82*, 216–222. [CrossRef] [PubMed]
27. Waitzberg, D.L.; Logullo, L.C.; Bittencourt, A.F.; Torrinhas, R.S.; Shiroma, G.M.; Paulino, N.P.; Teixeira-da-Silva, M.L. Effect of synbiotic in constipated adult women—A randomized, double-blind, placebo-controlled study of clinical response. *Clin. Nutr.* **2013**, *32*, 27–33. [CrossRef] [PubMed]
28. Li, N.; Jiang, J.; Feng, X.; Ding, W.; Liu, J.; Li, J. Long-term follow-up of the jinling procedure for combined slow-transit constipation and obstructive defecation. *Dis. Colon Rectum* **2013**, *56*, 103–112. [CrossRef] [PubMed]
29. Drossman, D.A. Functional gastrointestinal disorders: History, pathophysiology, clinical features and Rome IV. *Gastroenterology* **2016**, *150*, 1262–1279. [CrossRef] [PubMed]
30. Parthasarathy, G.; Chen, J.; Chen, X.F.; Chia, N.; O'Connor, H.M.; Wolf, P.G.; Gaskins, H.R.; Bharucha, A.E. Relationship between microbiota of the colonic mucosa vs feces and symptoms, colonic transit, and methane production in female patients with chronic constipation. *Gastroenterology* **2016**, *150*, 367–379. [CrossRef] [PubMed]
31. Zhu, L.; Liu, W.; Alkhouri, R.; Baker, R.D.; Bard, J.E.; Quigley, E.M.; Baker, S.S. Structural changes in the gut microbiome of constipated patients. *Physiol. Genom.* **2014**, *46*, 679–686. [CrossRef] [PubMed]
32. Vandeputte, D.; Falony, G.; Vieira-Silva, S.; Tito, R.Y.; Joossens, M.; Raes, J. Stool consistency is strongly associated with gut microbiota richness and composition, enterotypes and bacterial growth rates. *Gut* **2016**, *65*, 57–62. [CrossRef] [PubMed]
33. Tian, H.; Ding, C.; Gong, J.; Ge, X.; McFarland, L.V.; Gu, L.; Wei, Y.; Chen, Q.; Zhu, W.; Li, J.; et al. Treatment of slow transit constipation with fecal microbiota transplantation: A pilot study. *J. Clin. Gastroenterol.* **2016**. [CrossRef] [PubMed]
34. Christodoulides, S.; Dimidi, E.; Fragkos, K.C.; Farmer, A.D.; Whelan, K.; Scott, S.M. Systematic review with meta-analysis: Effect of fibre supplementation on chronic idiopathic constipation in adults. *Aliment. Pharmacol. Ther.* **2016**, *44*, 103–116. [CrossRef] [PubMed]
35. Suares, N.C.; Ford, A.C. Systematic review: The effects of fibre in the management of chronic idiopathic constipation. *Aliment. Pharmacol. Ther.* **2011**, *33*, 895–901. [CrossRef] [PubMed]
36. Dongowski, G.; Lorenz, A.; Proll, J. The degree of methylation influences the degradation of pectin in the intestinal tract of rats and in vitro. *J. Nutr.* **2002**, *132*, 1935–1944. [PubMed]
37. Onumpai, C.; Kolida, S.; Bonnin, E.; Rastall, R.A. Microbial utilization and selectivity of pectin fractions with various structures. *Appl. Environ. Microbiol.* **2011**, *77*, 5747–5754. [CrossRef] [PubMed]
38. Wong, J.M.; de Souza, R.; Kendall, C.W.; Emam, A.; Jenkins, D.J. Colonic health: Fermentation and short chain fatty acids. *J. Clin. Gastroenterol.* **2006**, *40*, 235–243. [CrossRef] [PubMed]
39. Muller-Lissner, S.; Tack, J.; Feng, Y.; Schenck, F.; Specht Gryp, R. Levels of satisfaction with current chronic constipation treatment options in europe - an internet survey. *Aliment. Pharmacol. Ther.* **2013**, *37*, 137–145. [CrossRef] [PubMed]

nutrients

MDPI

Review

Role of Fiber in Symptomatic Uncomplicated Diverticular Disease: A Systematic Review

Marilia Carabotti [1,2,*], Bruno Annibale [1], Carola Severi [2] and Edith Lahner [1]

1 Medical-Surgical Department of Clinical Sciences and Translational Medicine, University Sapienza, Via di Grottarossa 1035, 00189 Rome, Italy; bruno.annibale@uniroma1.it (B.A.); edith.lahner@uniroma1.it (E.L.)

2 Department of Internal Medicine and Medical Specialties, University Sapienza, Viale del Policlinico 155, 00161 Rome, Italy; carola.severi@uniroma1.it

* Correspondence: mariliacarabotti@gmail.com; Tel.: +39-06-49978377

Received: 23 December 2016; Accepted: 14 February 2017; Published: 20 February 2017

Abstract: Symptomatic uncomplicated diverticular disease (SUDD) is a syndrome characterized by recurrent abdominal symptoms in patients with colonic diverticula. There is some evidence that a high-fiber diet or supplemental fibers may reduce symptoms in SUDD patients and a high-fiber diet is commonly suggested for these patients. This systematic review aims to update the evidence on the efficacy of fiber treatment in SUDD, in terms of a reduction in symptoms and the prevention of acute diverticulitis. According to PRISMA, we identified studies on SUDD patients treated with fibers (PubMed and Scopus). The quality of these studies was evaluated by the Jadad scale. The main outcome measures were a reduction of abdominal symptoms and the prevention of acute diverticulitis. Nineteen studies were included, nine with dietary fiber and 10 with supplemental fiber, with a high heterogeneity concerning the quantity and quality of fibers employed. Single studies suggest that fibers, both dietary and supplemental, could be beneficial in SUDD, even if the quality is very low, with just one study yielding an optimal score. The presence of substantial methodological limitations, the heterogeneity of the therapeutic regimens employed, and the lack of ad hoc designed studies, did not permit a summary of the outcome measure. Thus, the benefit of dietary or supplemental fiber in SUDD patients still needs to be established.

Keywords: diverticular disease; dietary fiber; supplemental fiber; symptomatic uncomplicated diverticular disease

1. Introduction

Colonic diverticula are common in Western countries, affecting up to 60% of subjects over 70 years of age [1]. In about 80% of patients, colonic diverticula remain asymptomatic (diverticulosis), while approximately 20% of patients may develop abdominal symptoms (symptomatic uncomplicated diverticular disease, SUDD) and, eventually, complications such as bouts of diverticulitis or bleeding [2]. SUDD has been defined as a syndrome which is characterized by recurrent abdominal symptoms (i.e., abdominal pain and bloating resembling or overlapping those present in irritable bowel syndrome), attributed to diverticula in the absence of macroscopically evident alterations, other than the presence of diverticula [3,4]. The impact of these complaints is variable, and the severity and frequency of symptoms may range from mild and rare episodes, to a severe, chronic, recurrent disorder, impacting daily activities and the quality of life of patients [5,6]. About 4% of patients develop acute diverticulitis, an inflammatory process that may result in complications in about 15% of patients, with the development of abscesses, perforation, fistula, obstruction, or peritonitis [7]. A recurrence of diverticulitis after the first episode has been reported to occur in 15%–30% of patients [8,9].

The main goals of managing SUDD are both the reduction of abdominal symptoms and the prevention of acute diverticulitis. Even if recommendations for the treatment of SUDD have been issued by the medical societies of various countries [3,10–13], a standard therapeutic approach still remains to be defined. Fibers have been suggested for the treatment of SUDD patients, but the therapeutic benefit is not yet fully understood. Fibers might confer benefits by increasing fecal mass and regularizing bowel movements, as well as acting as prebiotics in the colon, favoring health-promoting species of the intestinal microbiota [14]. Fibers are defined as the edible parts of plants or the analogous carbohydrates that are resistant to digestion and absorption in the human small intestine, with complete or partial fermentation in the colon [15]. Fiber intake may be achieved by consuming fruits, vegetables, and cereal grains (dietary fibers), and/or by diet supplementation with specific commercial preparations containing fibers (supplemental fibers).

A previous systematic review assessed whether a high-fiber diet can improve symptoms or prevent complications of diverticular disease. Few studies were identified, and the authors concluded that evidence for a therapeutic benefit of a high-fiber diet in the treatment of diverticular disease is poor [16].

This systematic review aims to update the evidence on the efficacy of treatment with fiber in SUDD, in terms of the reduction of symptoms and the prevention of acute diverticulitis.

2. Methods

2.1. Study Selection

The search was conducted according to the PRISMA (Preferred Reporting Items for Systematic Reviews and Meta-Analyses) guidelines [17]. The electronic databases PubMed MEDLINE (U.S. National Library of Medicine, Bethesda, MD, USA) and Scopus were systematically searched according to the following search strategy, using the following MesH terms:

((("diverticulum" [MeSH Terms] OR "diverticulum" [All Fields] OR "diverticulosis" [All Fields]) OR diverticular [All Fields] OR ("diverticulum" [MeSH Terms] OR "diverticulum" [All Fields] OR "diverticula" [All Fields]) OR ("diverticulitis" [MeSH Terms] OR "diverticulitis" [All Fields])) AND (("colon" [MeSH Terms] OR "colon" [All Fields]) OR ("colon" [MeSH Terms] OR "colon" [All Fields] OR "colonic" [All Fields]) OR ("colon, sigmoid" [MeSH Terms] OR ("colon" [All Fields] AND "sigmoid" [All Fields]) OR "sigmoid colon" [All Fields] OR "sigmoid" [All Fields])) AND (("dietary fiber" [MeSH Terms] OR ("dietary" [All Fields] AND "fiber" [All Fields]) OR "dietary fiber" [All Fields] OR "fiber" [All Fields]) OR fibre [All Fields] OR ("diet" [MeSH Terms] OR "diet" [All Fields] OR "dietary" [All Fields]) OR insoluble [All Fields] OR soluble [All Fields] OR ("fruit" [MeSH Terms] OR "fruit" [All Fields]) OR ("vegetables" [MeSH Terms] OR "vegetables" [All Fields] OR "vegetable" [All Fields]) OR ("(1-6)-alpha-glucomannan" [Supplement *] OR "(1-6)-alpha-glucomannan" [All Fields] OR "glucomannan" [All Fields]) OR ("starch" [MeSH Terms] OR "starch" [All Fields]) OR fructooligosaccharides [All Fields] OR bran [All Fields] OR ("inulin" [MeSH Terms] OR "inulin" [All Fields]) OR ("psyllium" [MeSH Terms] OR "psyllium" [All Fields]))) AND ("humans" [MeSH Terms] AND (English [lang] OR French [lang] OR German [lang] OR Italian [lang] OR Spanish [lang]) AND "adult" [MeSH Terms]) AND ("therapy" [Subheading] OR "therapy" [All Fields] OR "treatment" [All Fields] OR "therapeutics" [MeSH Terms] OR "therapeutics" [All Fields]) AND ("humans" [MeSH Terms] AND (English [lang] OR French [lang] OR German [lang] OR Italian [lang] OR Spanish [lang]) AND "adult" [MeSH Terms]).

The search strategy excluded reviews, meta-analyses, case reports, and animal studies. The following study types were included: randomized controlled trials (blinded and/or placebo-controlled), open randomized clinical trials, and non-randomized open studies. Pediatric subjects were excluded from this review. No publication data restriction was imposed. Reports published in English, German, French, Italian, and Spanish were considered.

Clinical studies published up to 7 October 2016 were considered for inclusion in this review, if they described in adults (>18 years) with SUDD, the efficacy of fiber treatment with respect to the baseline (i) on reduction or remission of abdominal symptoms; and/or (ii) on prevention of acute diverticulitis.

Potentially relevant articles were independently screened for eligibility in an un-blinded standardized manner by the two reviewers (M.C., E.L.), initially by abstract, and then by full text when necessary, in order to determine whether they met the inclusion criteria. Reviews, letters, books, and/or editorials were excluded on the basis of the abstract and/or title; in other cases, the judgement of inclusion/exclusion was based on an evaluation of the full-text. Disagreement between reviewers was resolved by discussion. The reference lists of the identified articles, as well as of the identified relevant reviews, were manually searched for additional studies that may have been overlooked using a computer-assisted search strategy.

2.2. Data Extraction

We developed a data extraction sheet, pilot-tested it on three randomly-selected included studies, and refined it accordingly. One review author (M.C.) extracted the data from the included studies and the second author (E.L.) checked the extracted data. Disagreements were resolved by discussion between the two review authors. The following information was extracted from each included paper: (1) author and year of publication; (2) characteristics of fibers; (3) characteristics of study participants (number, mean age, and gender); (4) diagnosis of SUDD; (5) study type and treatment arms; (6) type of intervention; (7) follow-up; (8) outcome measure (reduction of abdominal symptoms; occurrence of acute diverticulitis); (9) efficacy of intervention; (10) adverse effects of fiber arms; (11) single or multiple centers.

The diagnosis of SUDD was considered appropriate when patients with colonic diverticula had recurrent abdominal symptoms such as abdominal pain, which were eventually associated with bloating or bowel habit alteration [3]. Studies which did not completely fulfill this definition were not excluded a priori, but the specific clinical settings were singularly extracted and described in detail.

For the purpose of this paper, dietary fibers were defined as the intake of food fibers in fruits, vegetables, and cereal grains. A high-fiber diet has been defined as at least a 30 g daily intake of dietary fibers [18]. When indicated, the amount of daily fiber intake was extracted from each paper. Supplemental fibers were defined as diet supplementation with specific commercial preparations containing one or more types of fiber.

2.3. Statistical Analysis

Originally, a meta-analysis was planned in order to provide a numerical estimate of the overall effect of interest, for which the outcome measure (effect size) comprised the proportion of patients who showed a positive response to fiber treatment with respect to the baseline, or with respect to controls, defined as the reduction of abdominal symptoms and prevention of acute diverticulitis. Due to the heterogeneity of the retrieved studies and their low quality, a meta-analysis was not considered applicable. The efficacy of the interventions reported in the retrieved studies was described in a qualitative manner.

2.4. Quality Assessment

The two reviewers evaluated the quality of all of the included studies, using the Jadad scale for randomized controlled trials [19]. This scale awards a maximum of five points to each study. The considered categories are randomization, blinding of outcome assessment, description of withdrawals and dropouts, and description and appropriateness of randomization and blinding. A study can be awarded a maximum of one point for each category (Table S1). Discrepancies in the quality assessment were discussed and resolved by the two reviewers.

3. Results

3.1. Search Results

The electronic search study identified a total of 374 records from electronic databases, 351 of which were unique (Figure 1).

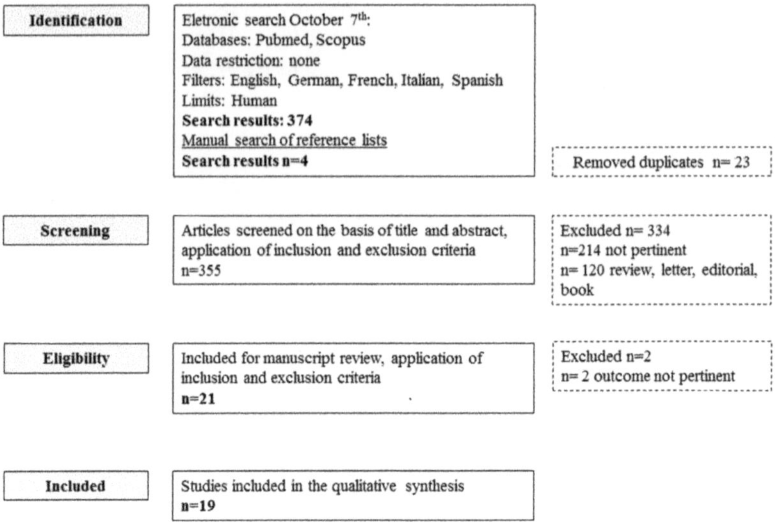

Identification
Eletronic search October 7th:
Databases: Pubmed, Scopus
Data restriction: none
Filters: English, German, French, Italian, Spanish
Limits: Human
Search results: 374
Manual search of reference lists
Search results n=4
Removed duplicates n= 23
Screening
Articles screened on the basis of title and abstract, application of inclusion and exclusion criteria
n=355
Excluded n= 334
n=214 not pertinent
n= 120 review, letter, editorial, book
Eligibility
Included for manuscript review, application of inclusion and exclusion criteria
n=21
Excluded n=2
n= 2 outcome not pertinent
Included
Studies included in the qualitative synthesis
n=19

Figure 1. Flow-chart of study selection.

Manual searching of a reference list of potentially relevant papers contributed another four articles. The articles were screened on the basis of the title and abstract and, after application of the inclusion and exclusion criteria, 21 articles were retrieved for a full-paper evaluation. Of these 21 papers, 19 met the eligibility criteria and were subjected to data extraction. Two studies were excluded because the outcome was not pertinent to the present study purpose, since it only evaluated constipated patients [20,21]. Thus, 19 articles were included for qualitative synthesis (Table 1).

Table 1. Type of fibers and dosage used in the included studies.

Author, Year (Reference)	Type of Fibers and Dosage
	Dietary
Lahner E., 2012 [22]	Dietary fiber (at least 30 gr/day)
Annibale B., 2011 [23]	Dietary fiber (at least 30 gr/day)
Colecchia A., 2007 [24]	Dietary fiber (at least 20 gr/day)
Smits B.J., 1990 [25]	Dietary fiber (30–40 gr/day)
Leahy A.L., 1985 [26]	Dietary fiber (>25 gr/day)
Hyland J.M.P., 1980 [27]	Dietary fiber (37.9 gr/day)
Brodribb A.J.M., 1977 [28]	Bran crispbread (6.7 gr/day) Wheat crispbread (0.6 gr/day)
Plumley P.F., 1973 [29]	High-fiber crispbread (96 gr/day total unavailable fraction)
Painter N.S., 1972 [30]	High-residue, low sugar diet with unprocessed bran (12–14 gr/day)

Table 1. *Cont.*

Author, Year (Reference)	Type of Fibers and Dosage
	Supplemental
Lanas A., 2013 [31]	Plantago ovata (7 gr/day)
Latella G., 2003 [32]	Glucomannan (4 gr/day)
Papi C., 1995 [33]	Glucomannan (2 gr/day)
Papi C., 1992 [34]	Glucomannan (2 gr/day)
Thorburn H.A., 1992 [35]	Ispaghula husk (7 gr/day)
Ornstein M.H., 1981 [36]	Bran (6.99 g/day) Ispaghula (9.04 gr/day)
Eastwood M.A., 1978 [37]	Bran (20 g/day) Isphaghula (2 sachets/day)
Hodgson W.J.B., 1977 [38]	Methylcellulose (1000 mg/day)
Brodribb A.J.M., 1976 [39]	Wheat bran (24 gr/day)
Taylor I., 1976 [40]	High roughage diet with bran supplement Bran (18 gr/day)

3.2. *Quality Assessment*

Details of the quality assessment of the included studies are given in Supplementary Table S1 (see Supplementary material). Of the 19 studies included, six achieved 0 points [26,27,35,36,39,40], three achieved 1 point [25,29,30], two achieved 2 points [28,38], seven achieved 3 points [22–24,31,33,34,36], and only one achieved 5 points [33], according to Jadad scale.

3.3. *Characteristics of Included Studies*

The main characteristics of the 19 included studies are summarized in Table 2. Considering the high heterogeneity of the fibers used, studies are grouped on the basis of dietary (nine articles) or supplemental fibers (ten articles).

Table 2. Main characteristics of the 19 selected studies on fibers in symptomatic uncomplicated diverticular disease (SUDD).

Author, Year (Reference)	N/F/Mean Age	Diagnosis of SUDD	Study Type/Arms	Single Center Yes/No
Dietary				
Lahner E., 2012 [22]	44/35/66	App	Open RCT/2	No
Annibale B., 2011 [23]	50/32/65	App	Open RCT/3	No
Colecchia A., 2007 [24]	307/189/62	App	Open RCT/2	No
Smits B.J., 1990 [25]	43/28/59	App	Open RCT/2	Yes
Leahy A.L., 1985 [26]	56/-/-	App	Retrospective study/2	Yes
Hyland J.M.P., 1980 [27]	100/73/67	NcApp [1]	Retrospective study/1	Yes
Brodribb A.J.M., 1977 [28]	18/9/60	App	Double-blind RCT	Yes
Plumley P.F., 1973 [29]	48/-/71	NcApp [2]	Prospective interventional, partly cross-over study/2	Yes
Painter N.S., 1972 [30]	70/25/60	App	Prospective interventional study, not controlled/1	Yes
Supplemental				
Lanas A., 2013 [31]	165/59/54	NcApp [3]	Open RCT/2	No
Latella G., 2003 [32]	968/501/63	App	Open RCT/2	No
Papi C., 1995 [33]	168/100/62	App	Double-blind placebo controlled/2	No
Papi C., 1992 [34]	217/112/65	App	Open RCT/2	No
Thorburn H.A., 1992 [35]	10/4/66	NcApp [4]	Open/1	Yes
Ornstein M.H., 1981 [36]	58/36/64	App	Double-blind, cross-over, RCT/3	No
Eastwood M.A., 1978 [37]	31/-/60	NcApp [5]	Prospective, not randomized/3	Yes
Hodgson W.J.B., 1977 [38]	30/18/60	App	Double-blind, cross-over RCT/2	Yes
Brodribb A.J.M., 1976 [39]	40/-/-	App	Prospective, not controlled/1	Yes
Taylor I., 1976 [40]	20/-/-	NcApp [6]	Cross-over RCT	Yes

App: appropriate; NcApp: not completely appropriate; F: female gender; N: number of patients; RCT: randomized controlled trial; [1] an unspecified number of pts with acute diverticulitis were included; [2] 4 pts with diverticulosis were included; [3] pts with a recent episode of colonic diverticulitis, current in remission were included, [4] 3 pts with diverticulosis were included; [5] an unspecified number of pts with diverticulosis were included; [6] 8 pts with acute diverticulitis were included.

In thirteen studies, SUDD was appropriately diagnosed [22–26,28,30,32–34,36,38,39], while in six studies, the diagnosis was not completely appropriated [27,29,35,37,40] (see Table 2). The latter studies include three in which SUDD patients with diverticulosis were included [29,35,37], and in the other two studies, SUDD patients with acute diverticulitis were included [27–40]. In one study, patients who had reported a recent episode of colonic diverticulitis, but were currently in remission, were included [31].

3.4. Dietary Fiber

Articles concerning dietary fibers were performed over a period of 40 years, from 1972 to 2012, and only three of them were published in the last 10 years [22–24]. Six of these were single center studies and three were multicenter studies [22–24]. Six studies were conducted in the United Kingdom [25–30] and three were completed in Italy [22–24].

An overall number of 736 patients with SUDD were investigated, for which the female gender was slightly prevalent (n = 391), but in two articles [26–29], the gender of the patients was lacking. Patients had a mean age of 64 years, ranging from 59 to 71 years. In one study, the age of patients was lacking [26].

With regard to the study type, four were randomized controlled open trials [22–25], two were retrospective studies [26,27], one was a double-blind RCT [28], one was a prospective partly cross-over study [29], and the remaining one was an un-controlled study [30].

With regard to the fibers used, in the majority of the studies, patients were treated with dietary fibers [22–27], in two articles crispbread was used [28,29], and in the last study, a high residue, low sugar with unprocessed bran was utilized [30]. In addition, the amount of dietary fiber utilized was variable, ranging from 20 [24] to 96 gr/day [29]. In five studies, a high-fiber diet was employed [22,23,25,27,29], but in the other studies, the dosage of fiber seemed to be lower than 30 gr daily [24,26,28,30]. Unfortunately, it was not possible to assess the proportion of soluble or insoluble fibers for each dietary regimen, since its exact composition was not reported.

The follow-up protocol was very variable between studies, ranging from three [25–28] to 65 months [27]. Also, the interventions were variable between studies: in four studies, the dietary fiber was a control arm and was compared in two articles to symbiotic preparations [22,23], in another it was compared to rifaximin [24], and in the last it was compared to lactulose [25]. In one study, a high-fiber diet was compared to one which was not high in fiber [26], and in two studies, high-fiber crispbread was compared to lower fiber crispbread [28,29]. One study used a high-fiber diet without a control arm [27], and the other study used a high-residue, low sugar diet with unprocessed bran [30]. With regard to the outcome measures, seven articles assessed the reduction of abdominal symptoms [22,23,25,27–30], and two assessed the reduction of symptoms and/or complications.

Two of the most recent open RCT studies compared a high-fiber diet with the combined treatment of a high-fiber diet and a symbiotic preparation [22,23]. In the first study, both treatments significantly reduced abdominal pain [22], whereas in the second, the high-fiber diet alone did not improve abdominal symptoms, compared to the baseline [23]. Another open RCT study compared a high-fiber diet with the combination of a high-fiber diet and rifaximin, and showed that both treatments significantly improved abdominal symptoms, compared to the baseline [24]. The occurrence of diverticulitis was reduced during the administration of a high-fiber diet in comparison to one which was not high in fiber, at a follow-up of 65 months [26]. Another study showed a similar frequency of diverticulitis occurrence in both treatment arms, for both dietary fiber and dietary fiber plus rifaximin, after 24 months [24]. Table 3 summarizes the type of intervention, follow-up protocols, the outcome measure, and the efficacy of each intervention included in the selected studies.

Table 3. Intervention and follow-up protocol in the selected studies of dietary fiber treatment in symptomatic uncomplicated diverticular disease (SUDD).

Author, Year (Reference)	Intervention	FU (Months)	Outcome Measure	Efficacy of Intervention	Adverse Effects
Lahner E., 2012 [22]	T1: High-fiber diet T2: Symbiotic preparation + high-fiber diet	6	Reduction of abdominal symptoms	T1 and T2: decrease of abdominal pain <24 h and >24 h in T1 and T2 ($p < 0.05$); T1 and T2: decrease of intensity of abdominal pain <24 h and bloating ($p < 0.05$)	None
Annibale B., 2011 [23]	T1: High-fiber diet T2: Symbiotic (1 sachet bid) + high-fiber diet for 14 days/months T3: Symbiotic (2 sachets bid) + high-fiber diet for 14 day/months	6	Reduction of abdominal symptoms	T1: no significant efficacy; T2 and T3: decrease of bloating VAS ($p < 0.05$), and abdominal pain >24 h ($p = 0.016$)	T3: 1 pt diarrhea
Colecchia A., 2007 [24]	T1: Dietary fiber T2: Dietary fiber + Rifaximin 400 mg bid for 7 days/months	24	Reduction of abdominal symptoms and diverticulitis	T1 and T2: significant reduction of symptomatic score compared to baseline; T1 has similar frequency of diverticulitis of T2 (4 pts in T1 vs. 2 pts in T2; $p = 1$)	Nausea, headache and weakness, T1: 3 pts, T2: 4 pts (p = ns)
Smits B.J., 1990 [25]	T1: High-fiber diet T2: Lactulose 15 mL bid	3	Reduction of abdominal symptoms	T1 and T2: reduction of abdominal pain frequency (T1: $p = 0.022$ and T2 $p = 0.0015$) and severity (T1: $p = 0.028$ and T2 $p = 0.009$) in comparison to baseline	T1: none, T2 :4 pts drops out for abdominal pain, nausea, vomiting
Leahy A.L., 1985 [26]	T1: High-fiber diet T2: Non High-fiber diet	65	Occurrence of symptoms and diverticulitis	T1 reported fewer symptoms and surgery or complications in comparison to T2 (19.3% vs. 44% and 6.4% vs. 32%; $p < 0.05$)	Not reported
Hyland J.M.P., 1980 [27]	T1: High dietary fiber	60	Reduction of abdominal symptoms	T1: 91% (91/100) were symptoms free at 5 years	Not reported
Brodribb A.J.M., 1977 [28]	T1: Bran crispbread T2: Wheat crispbread	3	Reduction of symptoms	T1 reduction of total symptom score in comparison to T2 (from 34.3 to 8.1 and from 42.0 to 35.1 respectively $p < 0.002$)	Not reported
Plumley P.F., 1973 [29]	T1: High fiber crispbread T2: Standard crispbread for at least 2 months	21	Reduction of abdominal symptoms	T1: 29/42 (69%) pts with pain were controlled satisfactory. Only 14 pts took part in the cross over trial (taking T2), but no results are available	Not reported
Painter N.S., 1972 [30]	T1: High-residue, low sugar diet with unprocessed bran	22	Reduction of abdominal symptoms	T1: 88.6% of symptoms relieved or resolved	8 pts did not tolerate bran diet

FU: follow-up; pts: patients; T1: treatment arm 1; T2: treatment arm 2; T3: treatment arm 3.

Due to the poor quality of the studies and the heterogeneity of the study design (mean Jadad score 1.5 $\pm$ 1.2 points), a meta-analysis could not be performed to provide a pooled estimate of the outcome measure. With regard to adverse effects, data were not reported in four studies [26–29], no adverse effect was observed in two studies [22–25], and in three studies, some minor effects were reported [23,24,30].

3.5. Supplemental Fiber

These studies were performed over a range of 37 years, from 1976 to 2013, and just one article was published in the last 10 years. Five studies were single center in nature [35,37–40] and five were multicenter studies [31–34,36]. Five studies were conducted in the United Kingdom [35–37,39,40], three in Italy [32–34], one in Spain [31], and one in the USA [38]. The ten included studies investigated an overall total number of 1707 patients, of which 830 were female, but in three studies, the gender of the patients was lacking [37–39]. Patients had a median age of 62 years, ranging from 54 to 66 years, but in two studies, the age of patients was lacking [39,40].

With regard to the study type, three were open randomized controlled trials [31,32,34], two were double blind-cross over studies [36,38], one was a double-blind randomized placebo controlled study [33], two were open un-controlled studies [35,39], and the last was a cross-over RCT [40].

With regard to the type of supplementation, patients were treated with glucomannan [32,34], ispaghula [35–37], bran [36–38,40], plantago ovata [31], and methylcellulose [38]. None of the studies achieved a high dosage of fiber intake with the prescribed supplementation regimen. Because the fiber intake of the diet was not reported, it may be that the total amount of the daily fiber intake is higher than that reported. With regard to fiber solubility, soluble fibers were used in five studies [31–35], both insoluble and soluble fibers were used in two studies [36,37], and in three studies, insoluble fibers were used [38–40].

With regard to the follow-up protocol, the studies were variable, ranging from one to 12 months. Five studies observed patients for a period of less than six months [35–38,40]. In addition, the interventions were very variable: in four studies, fibers were administrated together with a drug (rifaximin) and compared with the efficacy of the fiber alone [32–34]; in two studies, the efficacy of ispaghula and bran was respectively compared to a placebo [36] or lactulose [37], or were administrated as a unique arm of treatment in open un-controlled studies [35,39]. In another study, the efficacy of bran was compared to a high roughage diet or bulk laxative [40], or methylcellulose was compared to a placebo [38]. With regard to the outcome measures, the majority of studies evaluated the reduction of abdominal symptoms [33,35–40], two evaluated the reduction of symptoms and the occurrence of diverticulitis [32,34], and another study only considered the recurrence of diverticulitis [31]. In three open RCTs, the efficacy of glucomannan (2 or 4 gr/day) was compared to glucomannan, together with cyclic rifaximin, analysing the improvement of abdominal symptoms in SUDD patients [32–34]. In all three studies, a significant reduction of abdominal symptoms in the treatment arm with just glucomannan was achieved. In two of these three studies, the glucomannan treatment arm had a similar occurrence of diverticulitis to the antibiotic arm [33,34], while in the Latella study, the glucomannan arm treatment reported more complications ($p < 0.05$) [32]. Table 4 summarizes the type of intervention, follow-up protocols, outcome measures, and efficacy of interventions.

Table 4. Intervention and follow-up protocol in the selected studies of supplemental fiber treatment in symptomatic uncomplicated diverticular disease (SUDD).

Author, Year (Reference)	Intervention	FU (Months)	Outcome Measure	Efficacy of Intervention	Adverse Effects
Lanas A., 2013 [31]	T1: Plantago ovata 3.5 gr bid T2: Plantago ovata 3.5 gr bid + Rifaximin 400 mg bid for 7 days/months	12	Recurrence of diverticulitis	T1: recurrences in 17/88 pts (19.3%) T2: recurrences in 8/77 (10.4%) T1 had a significant higher risk of recurrence $p = 0.025$; OR 3.2 (95% CI: 1.16–8.82)	T1: 13/88 (14.8%) T2: 17/77 (22.1%) ($p = 0.225$)
Latella G., 2003 [32]	T1: Glucomannan 4 gr/day T2: Glucomannan 4 gr/day + Rifaximin 400 mg bid for 7 days/months	12	Reduction of abdominal symptoms and occurrence of diverticulitis	T1 and T2: significant reduction of global symptomatic score in comparison to baseline; T2 had more asymptomatic pts in comparison to T1: 29.2% vs. 56.5% pts at 12 months ($p < 0.001$); T1 reported more diverticulitis in comparison to T2: 11 pts vs. 6 pts ($p < 0.05$).	Nausea, headache, and asthenia: T1: 5 (1.34%) T2: 10 (1.68%) ($p = 0.7932$)
Papi C., 1995 [33]	T1: Glucomannan 2 gr/die + placebo T2: Glucomannan 2 gr/die + Rifaximin 400 mg bid for 7 days/month	12	Reduction of abdominal symptoms	T1 and T2: reduction of global symptom score in comparison to baseline; T2 had more asymptomatic pts in comparison to T1: 68.9% vs. 39.5% pts at 12 month ($p = 0.001$); No differences in preventing diverticulitis.	None
Papi C., 1992 [34]	T1: Glucomannan 2 gr/die T2: Glucomannan 2 gr/die + Rifaximin 400 mg bid for 7 days/months	12	Reduction of abdominal symptoms and occurrence of diverticulitis	T1 and T2: reduction of global symptom score in comparison to baseline. T2 had a marked reduction of score in comparison to T1 (47.6% vs. 63.9%: $p <$ 0.001); No differences in preventing diverticulitis (T1: 3 vs. T2: 0, $p = 0.2467$)	Not reported
Thorburn H.A., 1992 [35]	T1: Ispaghula husk	1	Reduction of abdominal symptoms	Improvement of abdominal pain in 71.4% (5/7); Bowel habit improves in 66.6% (6/9)	Not reported
Ornstein M.H., 1981 [36]	T1: Bran (6.99 gr/day) T2: Ispaghula (9.04 gr/day) T3: Placebo (2.34 gr/die)	4	Reduction of abdominal symptoms	No change in pain. T1 and T2: improvement of straining ($p < 0.01$)	T2: 2 pts diarrhea T3: 1 pt constipation
Eastwood M.A., 1978 [37]	T1: Bran (20 gr/die) T2: Ispaghula (2 sachets/day) T3: Lactuose (20–40 mL/day)	1	Reduction of abdominal symptoms	T1, T2 and T3 alleviated symptoms	Not reported
Hodgson W.J.B., 1977 [38]	T1: Methylcellulose 500 mg bid T2: Placebo	3	Reduction of abdominal symptoms	Symptoms score decrease significantly in T1 (from 19 ± 6, to 13 ± 4 $p < 0.01$) but not in T2 (from 21 ± 7 to 17 ± 9, p = ns)	Not reported
Brodribb A.J.M., 1976 [39]	T1:Wheat bran 24 gr/die	6	Reduction of abdominal symptoms	60% of symptoms were abolished and 28% relieved	Not reported
Taylor I., 1976 [40]	T1: High roughage diet with bran supplement T2: Bulk laxative plus antispasmodic T3: Bran tablets (18 gr/day)	2	Reduction of abdominal symptoms	T3 was most effective in reduce symptoms. Asymptomatics pts were: T1 = 20%; T2 = 40%; T3 = 60%	Not reported

FU: follow-up; pts: patients; T1: treatment arm 1; T2: treatment arm 2; T3: treatment arm 3.

Also, due to the poor quality of the studies and their heterogeneity (mean Jadad score 1.9 ± 1.8 points), a meta-analysis could not be performed.

On the basis of the heterogeneity of these papers, it was not possible to perform a sub-analysis assessing the differences between dietary and supplemental fibers, the effects of high- or low fiber diet/supplementation, or the differences between soluble and insoluble fibers.

With regard to adverse effects, data were not reported in six studies [34,35,37–40], some minor adverse effects were reported in the fiber arm in three studies [31,32,36], and in another study, the only double-blind randomized placebo controlled report, no adverse effects were observed [33].

4. Discussion

Dietary fibers are defined as the edible parts of plants or the analogous carbohydrates that are resistant to digestion and absorption in the human small intestine, with complete or partial fermentation in the colon [15]. Dietary fibers include non-starch polysaccharides, resistant oligosaccharides, and other carbohydrates, such as resistant starch and dextrins, and lignin [41,42]. Non-starch polysaccharides can be further subdivided into soluble and insoluble fibers: soluble fibers dissolve in water-forming viscous gels, bypass the digestion of the small intestine, and are easily fermented by the gut microbiota (i.e., pectins, gums, inulin-type fructans, and some hemicelluloses). In contrast, insoluble fibers are not water soluble, they do not form gels due to their water insolubility, and fermentation is severely limited (i.e., lignin, cellulose, and some hemicelluloses). The Academy of Nutrition and Dietetics declared that the adequate intake of fiber is 14 gr total per 1000 kcal, or 25 gr for adult women and 38 gr for adult men [18]. In Western countries, the daily fiber intake can change from region to region, and may change over the years. The mean intake of dietary fiber in the United States is 17 gr/day, with only 5% of the general population meeting the adequate intake [18]. In contrast, in a recent study evaluating the changes in food consumption and nutrient intake in a Mediterranean cohort, it has been observed that fiber intake has a baseline of 24.3 ± 9.4 gr/day; after 10 years, it was observed that fiber intake increased by 1.8 gr/day, thus augmenting over time [43]. Even if the health benefits of dietary fibers have long been appreciated, especially for their effect on cardiovascular diseases, type II diabetes, glycemic control, and gastrointestinal conditions [14], these data underline that dietary habits in Western countries may be far from the recommended adequate intake.

With regard to the risk of developing colonic diverticula, it has been proposed that "fiber deficiency", caused by the spreading of refined carbohydrates in the Western diet, may play an important role. However, little evidence is available to substantiate this hypothesis [44,45], and more recently, this concept has been reviewed. A colonoscopy-based, cross-sectional study on the dietary risk factors for diverticulosis found that a high fiber diet was even associated with a higher prevalence of colonic diverticula [46]. The association with dietary fiber intake was dose-dependent and stronger when limited to cases with multiple diverticula. Although it has been suggested that a high-fiber diet does not protect against the development of colonic diverticulosis, it may reduce the abdominal symptoms related to diverticular disease.

Patients with SUDD may complain of chronic recurrent abdominal symptoms, and fibers might confer benefits by increasing fecal mass and promoting the regularity of bowel movements. Another beneficial effect of fibers in the treatment of SUDD may be ascribed to their capability to act as prebiotics in the colon, by favoring health-promoting species of the intestinal microbiota, especially bifidobacteria and lactobacilli [14].

Diverticular disease is a complex, multifactorial disorder, in which the gut microbiota could play a key role. Recently, Barbara et al. reported that patients with diverticular disease showed depletion of microbiota members with anti-inflammatory properties, including Clostridium cluster IV, Clostridium cluster IX, Fusobacterium, and Lactobacillaceae, with microbiota changes being correlated with mucosal immune activation [47]. The gut microbiota, indeed, shifts rapidly in response to dietary changes, particularly with fiber intake [48]. For this reason, high-fiber intake represents a promising treatment option in diverticular disease. In this condition, a high-fiber diet based on fruits, vegetables, and cereal grains may be difficult to achieve and should be supported with an adequate dietary counseling, and in a subset of patients, the use of supplemental fibers might be useful.

The beneficial effect on potential microbiota changes achieved with dietary fibers, based on different amounts of soluble and insoluble fibers, or the supplementation of commercial fibers of the same type, may be different and not necessarily comparable. However, it was not possible to perform a sub-analysis assessing the differences between dietary or supplemental fibers, or between high- or low-fiber diet/supplementation. Unfortunately, on the basis of these studies, it was not possible to assess differences between the effect of soluble or insoluble fibers, even if the relative amount might have influenced the outcome of treatment. In patients with irritable bowel syndrome, a condition that might be considered similar to SUDD, the effect of fibers appears to be limited to the soluble type [49].

In clinical practice, a high-fiber diet or fiber supplementation are commonly used in patients affected by diverticular disease, even if most recommendations are based on poor evidence. A previous systematic review, performed in 2012, was restricted to the use of a high-fiber diet in diverticular disease and only included controlled studies in the English language, reporting that high-quality evidence for a high-fiber diet in the treatment of this condition is scarce [16].

The present systematic review represents an attempt to provide an updated measure of evidence on the efficacy of dietary and supplemental fibers in SUDD, in terms of the reduction of abdominal symptoms and the prevention of acute diverticulitis.

The research was updated until October 2016, considering randomized controlled trials (blinded and/or placebo-controlled), open randomized clinical trials, non-randomized open studies, and also taking into consideration papers in German, French, Italian, and Spanish. The selected studies, all of which came from Western countries with just one study from the USA, presented a high heterogeneity concerning the quantity and quality of the fibers employed, notwithstanding dietary and supplemental fibers, which were evaluated separately. However, the quality of the studies was very low, with just one study yielding an optimal score [33]. Based on the available studies, it was not possible to draw conclusions regarding the efficacy of fiber treatment in SUDD patients, neither in terms of the reduction of abdominal symptoms, nor for the prevention of acute diverticulitis.

5. Conclusions

Single low quality studies suggest that fibers, both dietary and supplemental, could be beneficial in the treatment of SUDD. The presence of substantial methodological limitations, the heterogeneity of therapeutic regimens employed, and the lack of ad hoc designed studies, do not permit a summary of the outcome measures. Up to now, high-quality evidence on the efficacy of fiber treatment for the reduction of symptoms in SUDD and for the prevention of acute diverticulitis, is lacking. Thus, further, well-designed studies, specifically focusing on the efficacy of fibers in SUDD, dietary or supplemental, are needed.

Supplementary Materials: The following are available online at http://www.mdpi.com/2072-6643/9/2/161/s1.

Acknowledgments: This study was in part supported by a Grant of University Sapienza, Roma 2014.

Author Contributions: Marilia Carabotti performed the data extraction and collection, and wrote the manuscript. Edith Lahner performed the data extraction, collection, and contributed to final revision of the manuscript. Carola Severi contributed to the critical revision of the manuscript. Bruno Annibale contributed to the conception and design of the study and to the final revision of the manuscript. All authors approved the final draft submitted.

Conflicts of Interest: The authors declare no conflict of interest.

References

1. Parra-Blanco, A. Colonic diverticular disease: Pathophysiology and clinical picture. *Digestion* **2006**, *73* (Suppl. 1), 47–57. [CrossRef] [PubMed]
2. Stollman, N.; Raskin, J.B. Diverticular disease of the colon. *Lancet* **2004**, *363*, 631–639. [CrossRef]

3. Cuomo, R.; Barbara, G.; Pace, F.; Annese, V.; Bassotti, G.; Binda, G.A.; Casetti, T.; Colecchia, A.; Festi, D.; Fiocca, R.; et al. Italian consensus conference for colonic diverticulosis and diverticular disease. *United Eur. Gastroenterol. J.* **2014**, *2*, 413–442. [CrossRef] [PubMed]
4. Annibale, B.; Lahner, E.; Maconi, G.; Usai, P.; Marchi, S.; Bassotti, G.; Barbara, G.; Cuomo, R. Clinical features of symptomatic uncomplicated diverticular disease: A multicenter Italian survey. *Int. J. Colorectal Dis.* **2012**, *27*, 1151–1159. [CrossRef] [PubMed]
5. Bolster, L.T.; Papagrigoriadis, S. Diverticular disease has an impact on quality of life-results of a preliminary study. *Colorectal Dis.* **2003**, *5*, 320–323. [CrossRef] [PubMed]
6. Comparato, G.; Fanigliulo, L.; Aragona, G.; Cavestro, G.M.; Cavallaro, L.G.; Leandro, G.; Pilotto, A.; Nervi, G.; Soliani, P.; Sianesi, M.; et al. Quality of life in uncomplicated symptomatic diverticular disease: Is it another good reason for treatment? *Dig. Dis.* **2007**, *25*, 252–259. [CrossRef] [PubMed]
7. Shahedi, K.; Fuller, G.; Bolus, R.; Cohen, E.; Vu, M.; Shah, R.; Agarwal, N.; Kaneshiro, M.; Atia, M.; Sheen, V.; et al. Long-term risk of acute diverticulitis among patients with incidental diverticulosis found during colonoscopy. *Clin. Gastroenterol. Hepatol.* **2013**, *11*, 1609–1613. [CrossRef] [PubMed]
8. Anaya, D.A.; Flum, D.R. Risk of emergency colectomy and colostomy in patients with diverticular disease. *Arch. Surg.* **2005**, *140*, 681–685. [CrossRef] [PubMed]
9. Broderick-Villa, G.; Burchette, R.J.; Collins, J.C.; Abbas, M.A.; Haigh, P.I. Hospitalization for acute diverticulitis does not mandate routine elective colectomy. *Arch. Surg.* **2005**, *140*, 576–581. [CrossRef] [PubMed]
10. Binda, G.A.; Cuomo, R.; Laghi, A.; Nascimbeni, R.; Serventi, A.; Bellini, D.; Gervaz, P.; Annibale, B.; Italian society of colon and rectal surgery. Practice parameters for the treatment of colonic diverticular disease: Italian society of colon and rectal surgery (SICCR) guidelines. *Tech. Coloproctol.* **2015**, *19*, 615–626. [CrossRef] [PubMed]
11. Andersen, J.C.; Bundgaard, L.; Elbrønd, H.; Laurberg, S.; Walker, L.R.; Støvring, J.; Danish Surgical Society. Danish national guidelines for treatment of diverticular disease. *Dan. Med. J.* **2012**, *59*, C4453. [PubMed]
12. Pietrzak, A.; Bartnik, W.; Szczepkowski, M.; Krokowicz, P.; Dziki, A.; Reguła, J.; Wallner, G. Polish interdisciplinary consensus on diagnostics and treatment of colonic diverticulosis (2015). *Pol. Przegl. Chir.* **2015**, *87*, 203–220. [CrossRef] [PubMed]
13. Strate, L.L.; Peery, A.F.; Neumann, I. American gastroenterological association institute technical review on the management of acute diverticulitis. *Gastroenterology* **2015**, *149*, 1950–1976. [CrossRef] [PubMed]
14. Slavin, J. Fiber and prebiotics: Mechanisms and health benefits. *Nutrients* **2013**, *5*, 1417–1435. [CrossRef] [PubMed]
15. The Definition of Dietary Fiber. Available online: http://www.aaccnet.org/initiatives/definitions/documents/dietaryfiber/dfdef.pdf (accessed on 16 February 2017).
16. Ünlü, C.; Daniels, L.; Vrouenraets, B.C.; Boermeester, M.A. A systematic review of high-fibre dietary therapy in diverticular disease. *Int. J. Colorectal Dis.* **2012**, *27*, 419–427. [CrossRef] [PubMed]
17. Moher, D.; Liberati, A.; Tetzlaff, J.; Altman, D.G.; PRISMA Group. Preferred reporting items for systematic reviews and meta-analyses: The PRISMA statement. *PLoS Med.* **2009**, *6*, e1000097. [CrossRef] [PubMed]
18. Dahl, W.J.; Stewart, M.L. Position of the academy of nutrition and dietetics: Health implications of dietary fiber. *J. Acad. Nutr. Diet.* **2015**, *115*, 1861–1870. [CrossRef] [PubMed]
19. Jadad, A.R.; Moore, R.A.; Carroll, D.; Jenkinson, C.; Reynolds, D.J.; Gavaghan, D.J.; McQuay, H.J. Assessing the quality of reports of randomized clinical trials: Is blinding necessary? *Control Clin. Trials* **1996**, *17*, 1–12. [CrossRef]
20. Coste, T.; Rautureau, J.; Paraf, A. Treatment of constipation and colonic diverticulosis by bran. *Med. Chir. Dig.* **1978**, *7*, 631–634. [PubMed]
21. Ewerth, S.; Ahlberg, J.; Holmström, B.; Persson, U.; Udén, R. Influence on symptoms and transit-time of Vi-SiblinR in diverticular disease. *Acta Chir. Scand. Suppl.* **1980**, *500*, 49–50. [PubMed]
22. Lahner, E.; Esposito, G.; Zullo, A.; Hassan, C.; Cannaviello, C.; Di Paolo, M.C.; Pallotta, L.; Garbagna, N.; Grossi, E.; Annibale, B. High-fibre diet and *Lactobacillus paracasei* B21060 in symptomatic uncomplicated diverticular disease. *World J. Gastroenterol.* **2012**, *18*, 5918–5924. [CrossRef] [PubMed]
23. Annibale, B.; Maconi, G.; Lahner, E.; De Giorgi, F.; Cuomo, R. Efficacy of *Lactobacillus paracasei* sub. *paracasei* F19 on abdominal symptoms in patients with symptomatic uncomplicated diverticular disease: A pilot study. *Minerva Gastroenterol. Dietol.* **2011**, *57*, 13–22. [PubMed]

24. Colecchia, A.; Vestito, A.; Pasqui, F.; Mazzella, G.; Roda, E.; Pistoia, F.; Brandimarte, G.; Festi, D. Efficacy of long term cyclic administration of the poorly absorbed antibiotic Rifaximin in symptomatic, uncomplicated colonic diverticular disease. *World J. Gastroenterol.* **2007**, *13*, 264–269. [CrossRef] [PubMed]
25. Smits, B.J.; Whitehead, A.M.; Prescott, P. Lactulose in the treatment of symptomatic diverticular disease: A comparative study with high-fibre diet. *Br. J. Clin. Pract.* **1990**, *4*, 314–318.
26. Leahy, A.L.; Ellis, R.M.; Quill, D.S.; Peel, A.L. High fibre diet in symptomatic diverticular disease of the colon. *Ann. R. Coll. Surg. Engl.* **1985**, *67*, 173–174. [PubMed]
27. Hyland, J.M.; Taylor, I. Does a high fibre diet prevent the complications of diverticular disease? *Br. J. Surg.* **1980**, *67*, 77–79. [CrossRef] [PubMed]
28. Brodribb, A.J. Treatment of symptomatic diverticular disease with a high-fibre diet. *Lancet* **1977**, *1*, 664–666. [CrossRef]
29. Plumley, P.F.; Francis, B. Dietary management of diverticular disease. *J. Am. Diet. Assoc.* **1973**, *63*, 527–530. [PubMed]
30. Painter, N.S.; Almeida, A.Z.; Colebourne, K.W. Unprocessed bran in treatment of diverticular disease of the colon. *Br. Med. J.* **1972**, *2*, 137–140. [CrossRef] [PubMed]
31. Lanas, A.; Ponce, J.; Bignamini, A.; Mearin, F. One year intermittent rifaximin plus fibre supplementation vs. fibre supplementation alone to prevent diverticulitis recurrence: A proof-of-concept study. *Dig. Liver Dis.* **2013**, *45*, 104–109. [CrossRef] [PubMed]
32. Latella, G.; Pimpo, M.T.; Sottili, S.; Zippi, M.; Viscido, A.; Chiaramonte, M.; Frieri, G. Rifaximin improves symptoms of acquired uncomplicated diverticular disease of the colon. *Int. J. Colorectal Dis.* **2003**, *18*, 55–62. [CrossRef] [PubMed]
33. Papi, C.; Ciaco, A.; Koch, M.; Capurso, L. Efficacy of rifaximin in the treatment of symptomatic diverticular disease of the colon. A multicentre double-blind placebo-controlled trial. *Aliment. Pharmacol. Ther.* **1995**, *9*, 33–39. [CrossRef] [PubMed]
34. Papi, C.; Ciaco, A.; Koch, M.; Capurso, L. Efficacy of rifaximin on symptoms of uncomplicated diverticular disease of the colon. A pilot multicentre open trial. Diverticular Disease Study Group. *Ital. J. Gastroenterol.* **1992**, *24*, 452–456. [PubMed]
35. Thorburn, H.A.; Carter, K.B.; Goldberg, J.A.; Finlay, I.G. Does ispaghula husk stimulate the entire colon in diverticular disease? *Gut* **1992**, *33*, 352–356. [CrossRef] [PubMed]
36. Ornstein, M.H.; Littlewood, E.R.; Baird, I.M.; Fowler, J.; North, W.R.; Cox, A.G. Are fibre supplements really necessary in diverticular disease of the colon? A controlled clinical trial. *Br. Med. J.* **1981**, *282*, 1353–1356. [CrossRef]
37. Eastwood, M.A.; Smith, A.N.; Brydon, W.G.; Pritchard, J. Comparison of bran, ispaghula, and lactulose on colon function in diverticular disease. *Gut* **1978**, *19*, 1144–1147. [CrossRef] [PubMed]
38. Hodgson, W.J. The placebo effect. Is it important in diverticular disease? *Am. J. Gastroenterol.* **1977**, *67*, 157–162. [PubMed]
39. Brodribb, A.J.; Humphreys, D.M. Diverticular disease: Threee studies. Part II—Treatment with bran. *Br. Med. J.* **1976**, *1*, 425–428. [CrossRef] [PubMed]
40. Taylor, I.; Duthie, H.L. Bran tablets and diverticular disease. *Br. Med. J.* **1976**, *1*, 988–990. [CrossRef] [PubMed]
41. Hamaker, B.R.; Tuncil, Y.E. A perspective on the complexity of dietary fiber structures and their potential effect on the gut microbiota. *J. Mol. Biol.* **2014**, *426*, 3838–3850. [CrossRef] [PubMed]
42. Jones, J.M. CODEX-aligned dietary fiber definitions help to bridge the 'fiber gap'. *Nutr. J.* **2014**, *13*, 34. [CrossRef] [PubMed]
43. De la Fuente-Arrillaga, C.; Zazpe, I.; Santiago, S.; Bes-Rastrollo, M.; Ruiz-Canela, M.; Gea, A.; Martinez-Gonzalez, M.A. Beneficial changes in food consumption and nutrient intake after 10 years of follow-up in a Mediterranean cohort: The SUN project. *BMC Public Health* **2016**, *16*, 203. [CrossRef] [PubMed]
44. Painter, N.S.; Burkitt, D.P. Diverticular disease of the colon: A deficiency disease of Western civilization. *Br. Med. J.* **1971**, *2*, 450–454. [CrossRef] [PubMed]
45. Korzenik, J.R. Case closed? Diverticulitis: Epidemiology and fiber. *J. Clin. Gastroenterol.* **2006**, *40* (Suppl. 3), S112–S116. [CrossRef] [PubMed]

46. Peery, A.F.; Barrett, P.R.; Park, D.; Rogers, A.J.; Galanko, J.A.; Martin, C.F.; Sandler, R.S. A high-fiber diet does not protect against asymptomatic diverticulosis. *Gastroenterology* **2012**, *142*, 266–272. [CrossRef] [PubMed]
47. Barbara, G.; Scaioli, E.; Barbaro, M.R.; Biagi, E.; Laghi, L.; Cremon, C.; Marasco, G.; Colecchia, A.; Picone, G.; Salfi, N.; et al. Gut microbiota, metabolome and immune signatures in patients with uncomplicated diverticular disease. *Gut* **2016**. [CrossRef] [PubMed]
48. David, L.A.; Maurice, C.F.; Carmody, R.N.; Gootenberg, D.B.; Button, J.E.; Wolfe, B.E.; Ling, A.V.; Devlin, A.S.; Varma, Y.; Fischbach, M.A.; et al. Diet rapidly and reproducibly alters the human gut microbiome. *Nature* **2014**, *505*, 559–563. [CrossRef] [PubMed]
49. Moayyedi, P.; Quigley, E.M.; Lacy, B.E.; Lembo, A.J.; Saito, Y.A.; Schiller, L.R.; Soffer, E.E.; Spiegel, B.M.; Ford, A.C. The effect of fiber supplementation on irritable bowel syndrome: A systematic review and meta-analysis. *Am. J. Gastroenterol.* **2014**, *109*, 1367–1374. [CrossRef] [PubMed]

nutrients

MDPI

Article

The Effects of Moderate Whole Grain Consumption on Fasting Glucose and Lipids, Gastrointestinal Symptoms, and Microbiota

Danielle N. Cooper [1], Mary E. Kable [2], Maria L. Marco [3], Angela De Leon [1], Bret Rust [1,2], Julita E. Baker [1], William Horn [2], Dustin Burnett [2] and Nancy L. Keim [1,2,*]

[1] Department of Nutrition, University of California at Davis, 1 Shields Ave, Davis, CA 95616, USA; dncooper@ucdavis.edu (D.N.C.); adeleon@ucdavis.edu (A.D.L.); brust@ucdavis.edu (B.R.); jemadejska@ucdavis.edu (J.E.B.)

[2] Western Human Nutrition Research Center, USDA-ARS, 430 West Health Sciences Drive, Davis, CA 95616, USA; Mary.Kable@ars.usda.gov (M.E.K.); William.Horn@ars.usda.gov (W.H.); Dustin.Burnett@ars.usda.gov (D.B.)

[3] Food Science and Technology, University of California at Davis, 1 Shields Ave, Davis, CA 95616, USA; mmarco@ucdavis.edu

* Correspondence: Nancy.Keim@ars.usda.gov; Tel.: +1-530-752-4163

Received: 29 December 2016; Accepted: 16 February 2017; Published: 21 February 2017

Abstract: This study was designed to determine if providing wheat, corn, and rice as whole (WG) or refined grains (RG) under free-living conditions will change parameters of health over a six-week intervention in healthy, habitual non-WG consumers. Measurements of body composition, fecal microbiota, fasting blood glucose, total cholesterol, high density lipoprotein (HDL), low density lipoprotein (LDL), and triglycerides were made at baseline and post intervention. Subjects were given adequate servings of either WG or RG products based on their caloric need and asked to keep records of grain consumption, bowel movements, and GI symptoms weekly. After six weeks, subjects repeated baseline testing. Significant decreases in total, LDL, and non-HDL cholesterol were seen after the WG treatments but were not observed in the RG treatment. During Week 6, bowel movement frequency increased with increased WG consumption. No significant differences in microbiota were seen between baseline and post intervention, although, abundance of order *Erysipelotrichales* increased in RG subjects who ate more than 50% of the RG market basket products. Increasing consumption of WGs can alter parameters of health, but more research is needed to better elucidate the relationship between the amount consumed and the health-related outcome.

Keywords: whole grains; maize; brown rice; whole wheat; fasting glucose; fasting blood lipids; microbiota; bowel movement frequency; gastrointestinal symptoms

1. Introduction

Grains are a staple of the average American diet and therefore changes to grain products, especially the level of refinement, can have a notable effect on Americans' consumption of fiber, minerals, and vitamins [1]. The topic of whole grains has come to wider public attention since the publication of the 2005 Dietary Guidelines for Americans, which recommends half of one's daily grain intake (3–5 servings or 48–80 g for adults) should be in the form of whole grains [2]. However, there is still a huge disparity between the recommended level of whole grain consumption and the actual amount of consumption in the US with most adults only consuming on average 9.76 g of whole grains daily, as reported by the 2009–2010 National Health and Nutrition Examination Survey (NHANES) [3].

Botanically, grains are defined as the caryopsis or dried fruit (also called corn) of a cereal plant [4]. True cereals include wheat (*Triticum* spp.), corn/maize (*Zea mays*), rice (*Oryza* spp.), oats (*Avena* spp.), and barley (*Hordeum* spp.), whereas the pseudocereals include foods such as amaranth (*Amaranthus* spp.), buckwheat (*Fagopyrum esculentum*) and quinoa (*Chenopodium quinoa*) [5]. Grains are made up of three distinct components: the fibrous bran, the starchy endosperm, and the lipid containing germ. In addition to these three components, some grains, such as oats, grow within an inedible husk which is removed prior to human consumption. Whole grains are defined as the intact edible portion of the fruit of the cereal plant or the ground, cracked, flaked, or rolled fruit so long as the original proportions of the bran, endosperm, and germ are present in nearly the same proportions in the processed grain as were found in the intact grain [5,6].

Refined grains are grains that have been altered so that they are devoid of some, or all, of their naturally occurring germ and/or bran. In removing the germ, the shelf life of the grain is generally improved due to the absence of the lipid component of the germ that can become rancid [5]. Removal of the bran is often done to remove fibrous and potentially bitter components of the grain to improve the hedonic experience of the consumer and lighten the color of the resulting grain product [7]. Unfortunately, the removal of the bran and germ removes many bioactive components including vitamins, minerals, antioxidants, phenolics, flavonoids, carotenoids and critically fiber, particularly insoluble fiber [4,8]. To ameliorate some of the losses in the refining process and increase consumption of vitamins and minerals, enrichment or fortification is done with riboflavin, niacin, thiamin, folate, iron, and calcium, however nothing is done to increase the fiber level of refined grains [9].

In addition to not consuming enough whole grains, Americans are also not consuming enough fiber. The 2009–2010 NHANES data reported adults were only consuming on average 17 g of fiber per day despite the recommendation to consume 25 to 38 g per day [3]. Consumption of more whole grains has been suggested as an excellent way for Americans to bridge the fiber gap because many palatability studies have shown that in moderate proportions substituting whole grains for refined grains does not change the "liking" of grain based foods [3,10].

Consumption of whole grains is associated with decreased risk of type 2 diabetes and major chronic diseases, such as cardiovascular disease, and may even decrease the risk for some types of cancers, such as colorectal cancer [4,11,12]. Alteration of glucose homeostasis [13–16] and reduction of total cholesterol and low density lipoprotein (LDL) have been somewhat inconsistently reported in connection with increased whole grain consumption [12,13,17,18]. Beneficial alteration of the gut microbiota is often cited as a possible reason for health improvements seen with increased whole grain consumption, although a relationship between the two is not always observed [8,13,14,19]. Fiber can be mechanistically linked to all these health improvements and the content of fiber varies from grain to grain, which might explain some of the mixed reports. Another potential confounding variable is how much fiber subjects are consuming either prior to the dietary interventions or as part of their background diet [20,21].

Our study was conducted to document biological changes that occur with increased whole grain consumption. We hypothesized that compared to the subjects consuming refined grains the whole grain consumers would have lower concentrations of fasting blood glucose, total cholesterol and LDL, increased bowel movement frequency, a shift to midrange fecal firmness, and increased abundance of *Bacteroidetes*. The three grains most commonly consumed in the United States, wheat, maize, and rice [1] were used in the grain interventions, which were provided in weekly "market baskets" containing an array of either whole or refined grain foods. The number of servings per day provided to each subject was intended to be ~100% of the total grain recommendations for their maintenance calorie level.

We found that measures of fasting blood cholesterol significantly improved with the whole grain intervention. We also found that bowel movement frequency was significantly improved relative to percent consumption of the whole grains, and blood glucose tended to decrease as well with increased percent consumption of whole grains. Additionally, we observed increased abundance of order *Erysipelotrichales*, with greater amounts of refined grain consumption.

2. Materials and Methods

Prior to initiating the study, the study plan and consent form were reviewed by the Institutional Review Board (IRB) of the University of California-Davis and approved (IRB ID 235561). The study is registered with clinicaltrials.gov (NCT01403857).

2.1. Subjects and Study Design

This study was a six-week intervention trial that was preceded by a screening period to determine eligibility and a pre-intervention baseline test visit (Table 1).

Table 1. Study design and procedures.

Screening	Baseline Test Day	Six Week Intervention (Each Event Occurred Weekly)	Post-Intervention Test Day

• Consent to participate
• Determine eligibility
	• Fasted blood draw
	• Fecal sample collected
	• Body composition testing
		• Pick up the market basket and dropping off the last week's unconsumed food
		• Complete and return logs of:
		  ◦ market basket consumption
		  ◦ bowel movements
		  ◦ gastrointestinal symptoms
			• Fasted blood draw
			• Fecal sample collected
			• Body composition testing

Subjects were consented and went through a screening process to determine if they were eligible to participate based on inclusion and exclusion criteria. To be included, subjects needed to be healthy adults, between the ages of 19 to 46 years with body mass index (BMI) 20 to 28 kg/m^2. They had to be "low whole grain consumers" consuming not more than 1 serving of whole grains/whole grain products per day, on average. This was evaluated using a screener that probed 81 different grain products including food items like breads, pastas, cereals, and snack bars. Subjects were asked to report how often they consumed these products by circling the option most appropriate to their consumption habits from consuming a serving of the product "never or less than once per month", "1–3 per month" then one through seven times per week, to the greatest frequency queried "2 per day". Subjects were disqualified for the study if they reported consuming seven or more servings of whole grain products per week. They also reported that their body weight had remained stable (within $\pm$3 kg) for the past 6 months and they were not currently dieting to lose weight. It was also necessary that subjects be able to prepare and eat the majority of their meals at home.

Potential subjects were excluded if they reported having a diagnosis of type 1 or 2 diabetes mellitus, gastrointestinal diseases including malabsorption syndromes, chronic inflammatory bowel disease, colorectal cancer, celiac disease (gluten sensitivity), diverticulitis, Crohn's disease; regular use of colonics and/or laxatives; recent (within 3 months) use of antibiotics, appetite suppressants, mood altering medications, and/or regular use of tobacco/tobacco products. Females were excluded if they were currently pregnant or were pregnant within the last six months. Eating habits were also queried, and subjects were excluded if the majority of meals were eaten away from home, in restaurants, or from fast food establishments. If qualified based on these criteria, a fasting blood sample was sent to a certified clinical chemistry lab at the University of California at Davis for a comprehensive clinical chemistry panel and a complete blood count to rule-out existing health problems, of which the subject may be unaware.

Eligible subjects were randomly assigned in blocks to the control (refined grain market basket) or treatment (whole grain market basket) groups to achieve a 1:2 ratio of those receiving refined grain to whole grain. Overall 46 subjects enrolled in the study. Results from the analysis of fasting blood samples are based on 45 subjects due to a missing post intervention sample; body composition data were available for only for 43 subjects due to equipment malfunction; gastrointestinal (GI) symptoms were assessed for 37 subjects due to incomplete record keeping by subjects, microbial analysis was performed on 28 subjects due to fecal sample loss or poor reading depth resulting from sequencing. Table 2 contains information about the subjects.

Table 2. Demographic information of subjects who received refined grain (RG) or whole grain (WG) market baskets [1].

Subjects	Sex F = Female M = Male	Age (Years)	BMI (kg/m^2)	Calculated Daily Calorie Needs (kcal/day)	Percent of Market Basket Consumed
			All Subjects in Sample		
Total (n = 46)	25 F, 21 M	25.8 ± 0.9	23.4 ± 0.6	2247.8 ± 48.2	47.1 ± 2.9
RG (n = 11)	3 F, 8 M	24.6 ± 1.6	25.5 ± 2.1	2363.6 ± 96.6	44.7 ± 7.8
WG (n = 35)	22 F, 13 M	26.2 ± 1	22.8 ± 0.5	2211.4 ± 55	47.9 ± 3

[1] Values are means ± standard error of the mean (SEM).

2.2. Market Baskets and Consumption Log

The market baskets consisted of foods made of either refined or whole wheat (representing ~75% of the products), corn (~15%), or rice (~10%). Three grain products were developed for the study: cookies, muffins and baking mixes; the others were commercially prepared items: bread, ready to eat cereals, couscous, crackers, pastas, rice, and tortillas (Table 3).

Table 3. Products contained in the market baskets. For reference the 2000 kcal portions are provided. All products were packaged by the metabolic kitchen, and no original labels or brand names were attached to the products given to the subjects.

Consumable	Refined Grain Products		Whole Grain Products		Servings/Week
Food Item	Description	Brand	Description	Brand	At 2000 kcal
Wheat bread	White, slices	Sysco Classic	100% whole wheat, slices	Hi Vibe	7 slices
Cereal	Cornflakes	Kellogg's	Wheaties	General Mills	5 cups
Cookie	Chocolate chip with white enriched flour	Recipe developed for study	Chocolate chip with whole wheat flour	Recipe developed for study	2 cookies, 2 $\frac{1}{2}$ inch diameter
Couscous	Refined Wheat	Giusto	Whole Wheat	Woodland Farms	$\frac{1}{2}$ cup prepared + 3 oz. dry
Crackers	Goldfish, cheddar, original	Pepperidge Farms	Goldfish, cheddar, whole wheat	Pepperidge Farms	26 crackers
Corn Muffin	Made with finely ground cornmeal	Recipe developed for study	Made with whole kernel cornmeal	Recipe developed for study	2 muffins
Penne Pasta	Semolina Wheat	La Bella	Semolina Whole Wheat	La Bella	$\frac{1}{2}$ cup prepared + 2 oz. dry
Rice	Long-rain, white	Sysco Classic	Long-grain, brown	Sysco Classic	$\frac{1}{2}$ cup prepared + 4 oz. dry
Spaghetti	Semolina Wheat	La Bella	Semolina, Whole Wheat	La Bella	$\frac{1}{2}$ cup prepared + 2 oz. dry
Tortilla	Wheat	Mi Rancho	Whole Wheat	Mi Rancho	1 tortilla (12-inch diameter)
Baking Mix	Based on enriched white flour	Formula developed for study	Based on whole wheat flour	Formula developed for study	1 cup

The contents of the market baskets (number of grain servings per week) were determined based on the caloric needs of the subjects, determined using the Harris-Benedict equation [22]. The calorie prescriptions were made in 200-kcal intervals. For example, a subject with an estimated energy expenditure of 1960 kcals would be provided a 2000 kcal per day basket and would receive six servings of grains per day, and a total of 42 servings of grains in their weekly market basket. All grain products were weighed prior to being given to the subjects. At the 2000 kcal level the whole grain market basket supplied 96 g of fiber, an average of 13.7 g per day whereas the refined grain market basket supplied 29.7 g of fiber, an average of 4.2 g per day. Subjects were asked to maintain their typical diet during the market basket intervention. We had planned to monitor dietary intake using unannounced multi-pass 24-h recalls collected by phone interview. However, we were unable to obtain a sufficient number of recalls, and between-interviewer variation was problematic. Thus, we have deemed the 24-h recall data of poor quality and have chosen not to present those data.

Subjects were asked to record the type, amount, preparation, as well as date and time of the grains used from the market basket. The grain products were pre-portioned for the subjects to increase convenience and help with record keeping in the log books (Figure A1). Subjects were not required to consume all grain products but where encouraged to replace what they would normally consume with products from the provided market baskets whenever possible. The log data were compared with the disappearance data generated by weighing back the returned market basket containing the prepared or unprepared unused grain products. If there was a discrepancy between the log data and what was returned in the market basket, in absence of a note from the subject explaining the discrepancy, the weigh back data was deemed preferred and used in the consumption calculation. After the initial basket was picked up subjects returned once weekly to return their past week's unused food, return their log books, and pick up materials for the following week. The intervention period was six weeks. The post-intervention test day was scheduled during the sixth week.

2.3. Body Composition

Subject's body composition was determined using air displacement plethysmometry (BodPod, COSMED, USA, Inc., Concord, CA, USA) in conjunction with a calibrated digital scale (Scale-tronic model 6002, Wheaton, IL, USA). Height was determined by a wall-mounted stadiometer (Ayrton Stadiometer model S100, Prior Lake, MN, USA). Subjects were required to wear tight fitting clothing such as a bathing suits or compression shorts as well as swim caps prior to entering the chamber. Subjects were evaluated twice, once in the baseline period and once after the sixth week of intervention, on both occasions they were tested after an overnight fast.

2.4. Clinical Parameters

Twelve-hour fasting blood samples were obtained by a licensed phlebotomist twice during the study. Whole blood was sent to the UC Davis Medical Center's clinical laboratory for analysis of glucose, lipids, cell counts, and iron status. The first collection occurred at baseline, the second occurred post intervention.

2.5. Gastrointestinal Symptoms Log Book

GI symptom log books were distributed and collected weekly with the market baskets. The goal of the logs was to monitor GI tolerability of the market basket products. Subjects were asked to record the day and time of each bowel movement and rate the consistency of each bowel movement using the Bristol stool scale [23]. There was also a short questionnaire in the log book that asked subjects to reflect over the past week when reporting their answers. The questions regarded frequency of experiencing gas, bloating, abdominal pain, nausea, or flatulence, and responses were recorded on a 5-point Likert scale [24]. There was a query about experiencing a change in stool and, if so, how they felt about the change.

2.6. Fecal Collection

A single bowel movement was collected by the subject at baseline and then again post intervention using a feces collection kit. The kit consisted of a plastic container lined with a ziplock bag, gloves, pens for labeling, and a hard-sided cooler with dry ice to keep their samples frozen until they could be delivered to the research center (WHNRC) for immediate storage at −20 °C.

2.7. Gut Microbial Community Analysis

The composition of the fecal microbiota was determined by sequencing of bacterial 16S rRNA genes. Comparisons of the fecal microbiota at baseline and post intervention were used to determine the change in relative abundance of specific taxa. Bacterial DNA was extracted as previously described [25]. Briefly, approximately 200 mg of fecal material was placed in a 2 mL screw cap tube containing 300 mg of 0.1 mm diameter zirconia/silica beads (Biospec Products, Bartlesville, OK, USA), the mixture was treated with lysozyme from the QIAamp DNA Stool Mini Kit (QIAGEN) and held for 30 min at 37 °C. Next mechanical lysis was performed by bead beating for 1 min, twice, at 6.5 m/s (FastPrep-24, BP Biomedicals, Santa Ana, CA, USA) in 1.5 mL ASL buffer [25,26]. Finally, the suspension was heated to 95 °C for 5 min while shaking at 500 rpm. DNA was then purified using the QIAamp DNA Stool Mini Kit (QIAGEN) according to the manufacturer's instructions.

The V4 region of the 16S rRNA gene was selected for PCR amplification because it has been shown to faithfully represent the taxonomic profile of microbial communities relative to characterization of the full length 16S gene sequences [27]. Primers F515 and R806 [28] were used to amplify the 16S rRNA V4 region from each purified DNA sample. An eight base pair (bp) barcode was present on the 5′ end of primer F515 [29] to facilitate demultiplexing of pooled sequence samples during downstream analysis. The PCR products were pooled and gel purified using the Wizard SV Gel and PCR Clean-Up System (Promega, Madison, WI, USA). Amplicons were then sent to the UC Davis Genome Center (http://www.genomecenter.ucdavis.edu/) for library preparation and paired-end 250 bp sequencing using the Illumina MiSeq platform (San Diego, CA, USA).

QIIME (Quantitative Insights into Microbial Ecology) [30] was used to join paired ends [31], quality filter, and demultiplex the sequencing data. Chimeras were identified using USEARCH [32,33] and removed. Operational Taxonomic Units (OTUs) were picked from the assembled sequences using the open reference OTU picking method and a threshold of 97% pairwise identity [30]. Very low abundance (0.005% or less) OTUs were removed prior to statistical analysis [34].

2.8. Statistical Methods

Microsoft Excel (Microsoft, Redmond, WA, USA)) was used to format data. JMP (JMP ®, Version 12.1.0. SAS Institute Inc., Cary, NC, USA) and R (R, Version 3.3.2, R Foundation for Statistical Computing, Vienna, Austria) were used for analysis. Data were tested for normal distribution using the Shapiro–Wilks test of normality and if non-normally distributed transformation using Box Cox was performed, if transformation was unsuccessful (w above 0.96) nonparametric testing was used. Body composition data and fasting blood data were analyzed using linear regression and analysis of variance using baseline measures as a cofactor in the regression model. Gastrointestinal symptoms, bowel movement frequency, Bristol scores of feces, and microbial abundance could not be normalized using Box Cox transformations so non-parametric Wilcoxon Signed Ranks tests were used to determine significance following logistical regression [35]. For the microbial data, OTU counts were rarefied to a depth of 15,000 sequences per sample prior to analysis. This number was chosen because at this sequencing depth the number of unique OTUs observed was no longer exponentially increasing. Samples from two subjects on the whole grain market basket intervention had fewer than 15,000 sequences and so were discarded prior to analysis. Taxa that were present in at least 2% relative abundance in at least one sample were analyzed for differential abundance between experimental groups using LefSe [36]. For the purposes of determining fold change, sequence counts of 0, when they occurred, were replaced with a sequence count of 1. Due to the increased risk of type 1 errors with multiple comparisons, the Benjamini–Hochberg False Discovery Rate Procedure was implemented to reduce the risk of false discovery [37].

3. Results

3.1. Market Basket Consumption

There was a wide range of consumption of the market baskets products with refined grain consumption ranging from 1.1% to 95.1% and whole grain consumption ranging from 18.1% to 97.5% (Figure 1).

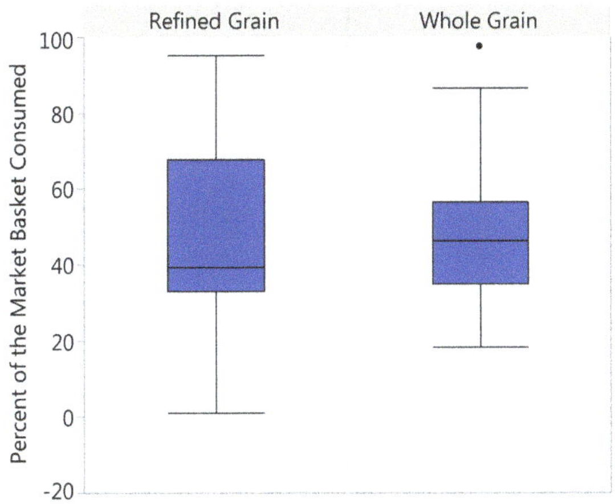

Figure 1. Range of Market Basket Consumption. Consumption of the refined grain market basket ranged from 1.1% to 95.1% with the average consumption being 44.7% and a standard error of the mean of 7.8. Consumption of the whole grain market basket ranged from 18.1% to 97.5% with the average consumption being 47.9% and a standard error of the mean of 3.0.

3.2. Changes in Body Composition from Baseline to Post-Intervention

Air displacement plethysmometry performed at baseline and post intervention was used to calculate the change in Body Mass Index (BMI), fat mass, and fat free mass between baseline and post intervention. Using baseline measures as a cofactor linear regression followed by analysis of variance were performed in the treatment groups and no significant differences were seen (Table 4). Similar analysis was performed on each treatment group relative to the percent of the market basket consumed and significant differences were still not observed (Figure 2).

Table 4. Change in body mass index and body composition over the six-week intervention for refined grain (RG) and whole grain (WG) and treatments [1,2].

Treatment	Change in BMI (kg/m^2)	Change in Fat Mass (kg)	Change in Fat Free Mass (kg)
RG	0.01 ± 0.11	1.13 ± 0.57	−0.45 ± 0.56
WG	0.05 ± 0.10	0.49 ± 0.31	−0.43 ± 0.37
p value	0.846	0.936	0.936

[1] Values are reported as the mean ± the standard error of the mean; [2] Change in BMI (RG: *n* = 11, WG: *n* = 34), change in Fat Mass and Fat Free Mass (RG: *n* = 10, WG: *n* = 33).

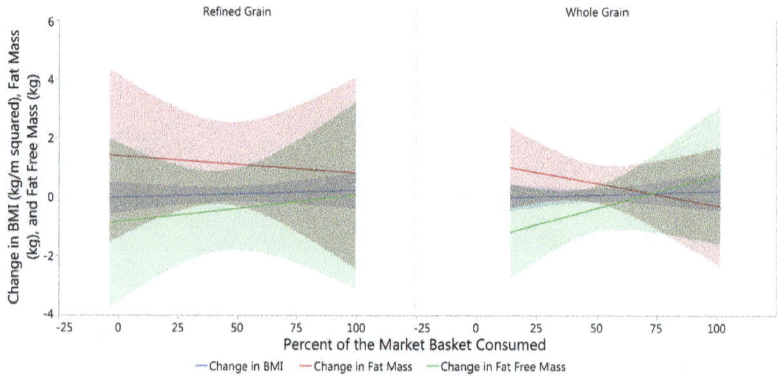

Figure 2. Changes in Body Composition with Percent Consumption of the Market Baskets. No significant differences were found using analysis of variance in the change of BMI (RG $p = 0.494$, WG $p = 0.658$), fat mass (RG $p = 0.962$, WG $p = 0.372$), or fat free mass (RG $p = 0.823$, WG $p = 0.561$) from baseline to post intervention.

3.3. Changes in Fasting Blood Glucose from Baseline to Post-Intervention

Similar to our findings with body composition, we found there was no significant impact of the type of market basket consumed on fasting blood glucose and the mean change for both treatment groups was negligible (RG = -3.00 ± 2.38 mg/dL; WG = -0.29 ± 1.62 mg/dL; $p = 0.250$). However, the percent of the WG market basket consumed trended with decreased fasting blood glucose when looking at the change in blood glucose from baseline to post intervention while controlling for baseline levels using linear regressions followed by analysis of variance ($p = 0.053$). This observation was not replicated with RG market basket consumption ($p = 0.590$), indicating that a certain quantity of whole grain consumption may be reducing fasting blood glucose (Figure 3).

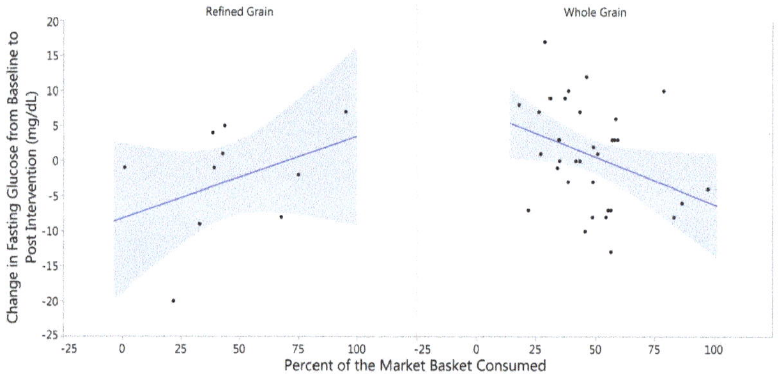

Figure 3. Percent of Market Basket Consumed Related to Change in Fasting Glucose. Increased consumption of the whole grain market basket was related to lower ($p = 0.053$) fasting blood glucose in the whole grain treatment, whereas there was a pattern of increased blood glucose with increased consumption of the refined grain market basket ($p = 0.590$).

3.4. Changes in Fasting Blood Lipids from Baseline to Post Intervention

When observing the changes in fasting blood lipids from baseline to post intervention between the RG and WG treatments, while controlling for baseline levels, significant differences were seen in total cholesterol (p = 0.018), LDL cholesterol (p = 0.035), and in non-high density lipoprotein (HDL) cholesterol (p = 0.047) (Figure 4). Negligible changes were seen in HDL cholesterol (RG = 1.55 ± 1.49 mg/dL; WG = −2.41 ± 1.31 mg/dL; p = 0.178) and triglycerides (RG = 2.73 ± 14.47 mg/dL; WG = 6.29 ± 8.97 mg/dL; p = 0.799).

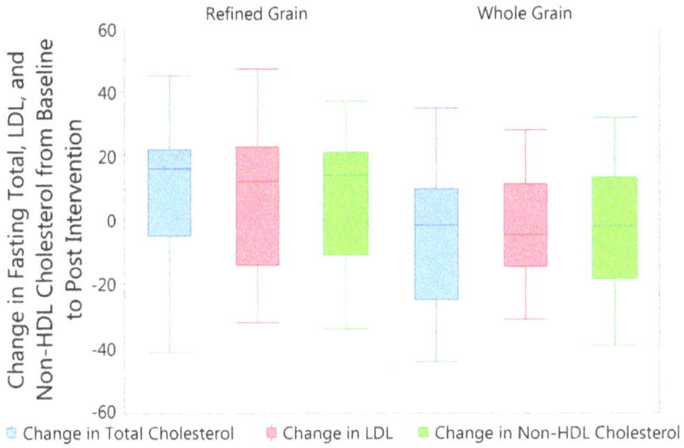

Figure 4. Consumption of the Whole or Refined Grain Market Basket Related to Change in Fasting Total, LDL, and Non-HDL Cholesterol. Consumption of the WG market basket was significantly associated with lower fasting levels of total cholesterol (p = 0.018), LDL cholesterol (p = 0.035), and non-HDL cholesterol (p = 0.047) when compared to subjects that consumed the RG market basket.

When comparing fasting lipid levels to percent consumption of the market baskets while controlling for baseline levels no significant differences were seen in the change in total (RG p = 0.179; WG p = 0.122), LDL (RG p = 0.0682; WG p = 0.265), HDL (RG p = 0.972; WG p = 0.816), or non-HDL (RG p = 0.313; WG p = 0.313) cholesterol, or triglycerides (RG p = 0.790; WG p = 0.313).

3.5. Gastrointestinal Tolerability

Gastrointestinal symptoms were reported by subjects in their weekly log books. Table 5 represents the self-reported gastrointestinal symptoms of bloating or gas, abdominal pain, nausea, flatulence, changes in stool, change in feelings about changes in stool, bowel movement frequency, and Bristol stool score for weeks one and six during the market basket intervention.

Table 5. GI symptoms reported at Weeks 1 and 6 of the refined grain (RG) (n = 10) and whole grain (WG) (n = 27) interventions [1,2].

Treatment	Bloating and Gas	Abdominal Pain	Nausea	Flatulence	Change in Stool	Feeling about Change in Stool	Bowel Movement Frequency	Average Bristol Score
				Week 1 Responses				
RG	0.80 ± 0.29	0.70 ± 0.30	0.60 ± 0.31	0.90 ± 0.38	0.8 ± 0.25	2.14 ± 0.25	7.00 ± 0.61	3.18 ± 0.23
WG	0.78 ± 0.20	0.56 ± 0.12	0.38 ± 0.12	1.04 ± 0.24	1.17 ± 0.21	2.14 ± 0.23	8.28 ± 0.65	4.16 ± 0.54
p value	0.824	0.863	0.595	0.573	0.371	0.785	0.397	0.088
				Week 6 Responses				
RG	0.40 ± 0.22	0.20 ± 0.13	0.10 ± 0.10	0.60 ± 0.31	0.90 ± 0.28	2.00± 0.19	7.00 ± 0.70	3.42 ± 0.25
WG	0.64 ± 0.14	0.44 ± 0.10	0.40 ± 0.14	0.68 ± 0.18	0.92 ± 0.20	2.18 ± 0.23	7.93 ± 0.59	3.41 ± 0.14
p value	0.307	0.198	0.187	0.774	0.952	0.518	0.535	0.959

[1] Values are means ± SEM. [2] Higher values represent increases in symptoms, frequency, changes, positive feelings, or firmness of feces while lower numbers represent decreases in symptoms, frequency, changes, positive feelings, or firmness of feces.

The average bowel movement frequency for subjects during the sixth week of the intervention was compared to the average grain product consumption (percent consumed) by rank (50% or higher consumption verses less than 50% consumption) by subject in each treatment group, respectively.

Using logistical regression and Wilcoxon Rank Sum testing, it was determined that there was a significant increase in bowel movement frequency with increased consumption of the whole grain market basket ($p = 0.046$). There was no association between increased frequency and the refined grain treatment ($p = 0.407$) (Figure 5).

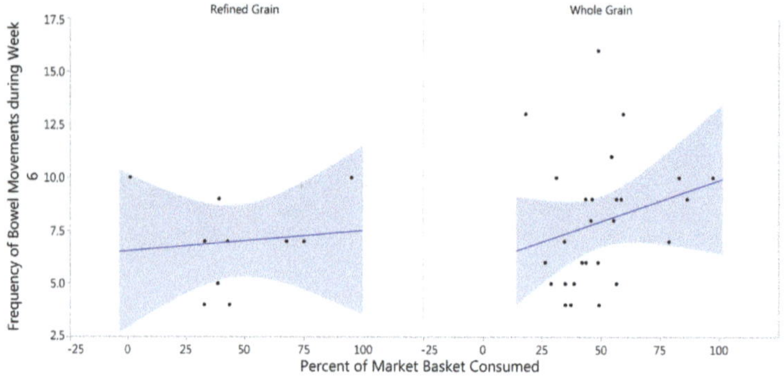

Figure 5. Percent of market basket consumed related to bowel movement frequency. The association between bowel movement frequency and percent of market basket consumed for refined grain consumers (**left** panel) and whole grain consumers (**right** panel) as determined by logistical regression and Wilcoxon Rank Sum testing. The refined grain treatment represents data from ten subjects; the whole grain treatment represents data from 27 subjects. There is a significant positive association with whole grain consumption ($p = 0.046$), but not with refined grain consumption ($p = 0.407$).

3.6. Fecal Microbiota Analysis

To determine if there were significant changes in the gut microbial community mediated by diet, which could then potentially influence changes in the health parameters observed, we sequenced the 16S rRNA V4 region of the bacterial DNA in subject stool collected at baseline and after six weeks of either WG or RG market basket consumption. A total of 2,983,060 sequences were obtained after quality filtering with an average of 48,100 sequences per sample. Two subjects in the WG market basket treatment were excluded from the microbiota analysis because one each of their samples was not sequenced sufficiently to effectively represent the overall community structure.

Overall, *Firmicutes* was the most relatively abundant phylum detected in our subjects, as has previously been observed in studies examining urban adult human gut microbiota using stool samples [38,39]. The second most abundant phylum was *Actinobacteria* with *Bacteroidetes* coming in third. The high proportion of *Actinobacteria* in our samples was driven primarily by a high representation of the genus *Bifidobacterium*, which composed as much as 40% of one sample prior to whole grain market basket consumption and was present at a median 10% and 16% relative abundance at baseline prior to WG and RG market basket consumption, respectively. Change in abundance during market basket consumption was not significant and this might be explained by the high levels present prior to consumption (Figure 6).

Although there was no significant difference in the relative abundance of any particular taxa between experimental groups, six of eight individuals consuming a high proportion (50% or greater) of the WG market basket showed increased relative abundance of *Akkermansia* and *Lactobacillus*, while two of three individuals consuming a high proportion of the RG market basket showed decreased relative abundance of this organism. There was also a trend for increased abundance of order *Erysipelotrichales* ($p = 0.023$) with high (50% or greater) RG market basket consumption. In our dataset, order *Erysipelotrichales* included unidentified members of family *Erysipelotrichaceae* and the genera *Eubacterium* and *Catenibacterium* (Figure 7).

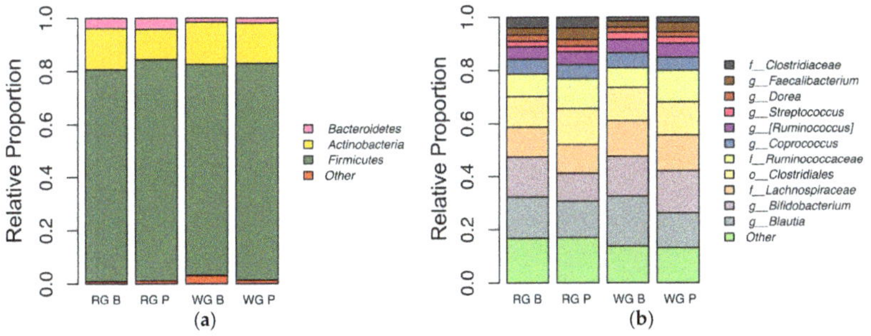

Figure 6. Relative proportion of taxa in each experimental group. The relative proportion of taxa at baseline (B) and post intervention (P) for the refined grain (RG) and whole (WG) treatments: (**a**) the relative proportion of bacteria at the phylum level; and (**b**) the relative abundance of bacteria at the most specific level of classification available. In both panels, taxa present at a median of 1% relative abundance in the data set are shown. Taxa present at lower than 1% median relative abundance are grouped into the "Other" category.

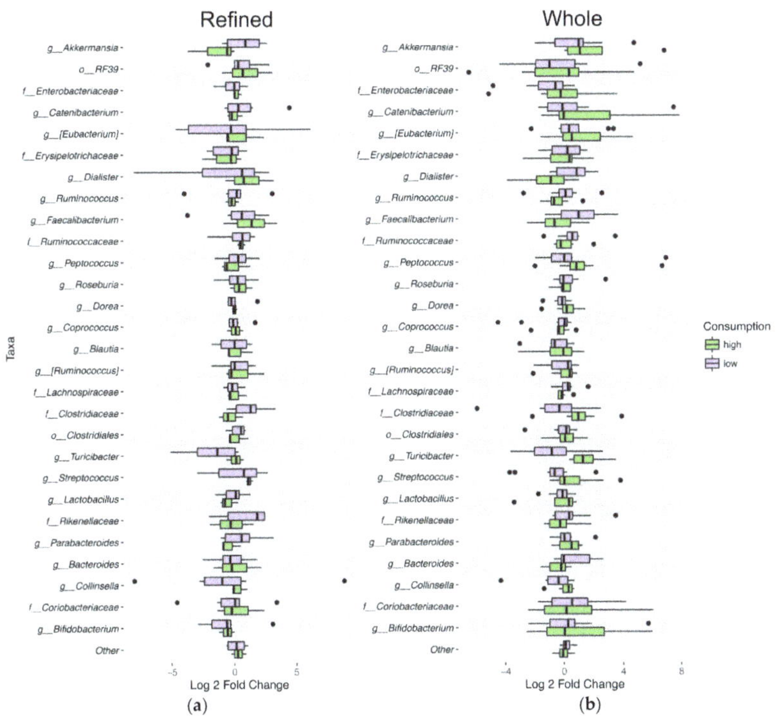

Figure 7. Variation in specific taxa during market basket consumption. Log2 fold change in abundance of bacteria at either high (50% or more) or low (49.99% or less) levels of consumption of the market baskets from baseline to post intervention for: refined grain (**a**); and whole grain (**b**). Taxa shown were present in at least 2% relative abundance in at least one sample. Dots seen in the graphs represent outliers. The findings of interest were an increase in the relative abundance of *Akkermansia* and *Lactobacillus* with high whole grain market basket consumption and a decrease with high refined grain consumption, as well as the increased abundance of the order *Erysipelotrichales* ($p = 0.023$) with high refined grain consumption.

4. Discussion

Consumption of the whole grain market basket products for six weeks was associated with a significant decrease in total, LDL, and non-HDL cholesterol compared to subjects consuming the refined grain market basket. Health parameters including fasting glucose, and bowel movement frequency were associated with a higher percentage of consumption of the whole grain market basket. No significant differences were seen when comparing the change from baseline to post intervention between treatment groups for the following parameters: BMI, fat mass, fat free mass, glucose, HDL, triglycerides, gas or bloating, abdominal pain, nausea, self-reported change in stool, feelings about changes in stool, bowel movement frequency, Bristol stool score, or abundance of microbiota.

4.1. Fiber Intake

Market baskets were designed to mimic the types of grain products typically consumed by Americans as closely as possible, which is why the baskets featured a majority of wheat products (~75%), some maize products (~15%), and rice (~10%), since those proportions are similar to the national availability of those grains as reported by USDA Economic Research Service [1]. The whole and the refined grain market baskets were matched as closely as possible in terms of types of foods provided, but the difference in the amount fiber between market baskets was substantial. At the 2000 kcal level, the whole grain market basket supplied 96 g of fiber, an average of 13.7 g per day, whereas the refined grain market basket supplied only 29.7 g of fiber, an average of 4.2 g per day, if all of the products were consumed. The average consumption of the market basket in this study, when rounded, was 47 percent. Thus, subjects in the refined grain group were consuming only about 2 g per day of fiber from the provided grain products whereas the whole grain subjects were consuming about 7 g per day of fiber from the grain products. Even though this is an average of a five-gram difference in fiber consumption between the grain treatments, whole grains at this percent consumption are not contributing a significant amount of fiber to the daily diet. Fibers such as beta glucan have been shown to reduce cholesterol and LDL with as small a dose as three grams per day [40]. However, the major sources of fiber in wheat are arabinoxylans, hemicellulose, and only very small amounts of beta glucan [41]; corn fibers are hemicellulose, arabinose, xylan, lignin, and resistant starch [42]; and rice contains cellulose, pectic fibers (arabinans, arabinogalactans, and galacturonans) and hemicellulose [21,43–46]. Not much is known about the dietary impacts of these individual fibers. Since background diet was not evaluated during the intervention it is possible that subjects in the whole and refined grain treatment groups were consuming vegetable and or fruit fiber at different levels from each other. Assuming we were successful at disqualifying habitual medium or high whole grain consumers, we were confident that the enrolled subjects were not consuming a large amount of cereal fiber outside of the intervention. Not having a reliable estimate of the subject's fiber intake outside of the intervention limits any conclusions we can draw about fiber intake during the study, and how the difference in fiber provided by the market baskets may have influenced the outcome of individual subjects.

4.2. Fasting Glucose

When comparisons were made taking into account what percentage of the market basket was consumed, a nearly significant trend was observed: as whole grain consumption increased fasting glucose levels decreased. A potential mechanism behind this theory is that due to the increased fiber of whole grains they remain as larger particles post mastication and so potentially are more challenging to mechanically and enzymatically degrade resulting in lower, longer releases of glucose into the blood stream and subsequently a more gradual secretion of insulin. However, this effect may not explain why a decrease in glucose might exist after something as long as a 12-h overnight fast [47–50]. Another potential mechanism that may explain the persistence of decreased glucose levels with increased consumption of whole grains, even after an overnight fast, is that the increase in fiber from whole grains may alter metabolism in the microbiota increasing the production of short chain fatty acids (SCFA) like propionate and acetate due to continued exposure to fiber from the whole grains. Propionate is known to stimulate enteroendocrine L cells to increase the release of glucagon-like peptide-1 (GLP-1) which increases the responsiveness of insulin to glucose as well as inhibiting gastric emptying [51–53]. In a human study, supplementation with propionate was shown to decrease glucose peaks and two-hour glucose area under the curve [54]. Acetate may be able to alter appetite and satiety signaling in the brain without use of gut hormone intermediaries, and has been shown to reduce fasting glucose levels in humans [55,56]. Reduced blood glucose has been seen postprandially in the literature with boiled barley, whole rye, whole wheat, and brown rice in comparison to refined grain interventions [46,57,58]. Fasting glucose has been shown to decrease with acute interventions of wheat bran in mice [50] and with acute interventions of whole wheat, whole oats, and whole barley in rats [59]. There is some literature suggesting that whole grains do not have an effect on glycemic control. For example Ampatzoglou and colleagues showed no significant impact of increasing whole grain consumption from 24 or more grams per day to at least 80 g per day for six weeks, on blood glucose [13]. Another study by Kristensen and colleagues compared acute whole grain wheat and refined grain wheat consumption and failed to show significant differences in blood glucose up to 180 min after feeding [60]. Since only a trend towards decreased glucose levels was observed in our study no strong conclusions can be drawn, but it is clear that future research will be needed to definitively understand if beginning or increasing whole grain consumption may effect glycemic control, and if so why.

4.3. Blood Lipids

Fasting total, LDL, and non-HDL cholesterol decreased with consumption of the whole grain market basket, whereas no significant changes were seen with these lipids in the refined grain group. Whole grain consumption has been shown to improve lipid profiles [12]. In rats diets high in maize have been shown to reduce LDL [61]. In humans diets rich in whole wheat have been shown to reduce total cholesterol when given at a dosage of 48 g per day [15,19]. Most of the research on the lipid lowering effects of whole grains has been performed with oats, which are rich in beta glucan, a fiber that has been clinically shown to lower cholesterol [40]. Oats were not featured in this study and while whole wheat contains very small amounts of beta glucan, maize and rice do not [21,41]. The current understanding of this lipid lowering property of whole grains is that it is due to their increased fiber content as compared to their refined grain counterparts [8,41].

Assuming whole grain intake replaces refined grain intake this diet alteration would be expected to increase fiber intake, thereby initiating the following signaling cascade. Fiber increases the viscosity of the foodstuffs in the stomach which may delay gastric emptying and affect satiety signaling. In the duodenum the increased viscosity may also alter nutrient release from the chyme and thus affect nutrient sensing, which could have far reaching consequences including lipid metabolism and processing [62]. The better established and accepted mechanism for increased fiber intake decreasing blood cholesterol levels is through sequestration of bile salts resulting in their loss in feces instead of their reabsorption back into the intestine, which results in the body needing to use cholesterol to manufacture more bile salts, thus decreasing blood cholesterol concentrations [58,63]. The existing literature suggests that in some cases increasing whole grains consumption does not affect lipid levels. This was seen in the previously discussed mixed increased whole grain consumption study by Ampatzoglou and colleagues [13]. Odes and colleagues also performed a study on humans using a mixed grain fiber supplement providing 12.5 g of fiber daily for two or four weeks and found that it had no effect on HDL or LDL cholesterol [64]. However, the findings of the current study indicate that inclusion of a combination of whole grain wheat, corn and rice in the diet for six weeks led to decreased fasting total, LDL, and non-HDL cholesterol levels compared to consuming the refined grain counterparts.

4.4. Fecal Frequency

While there was no difference in average bowel movement frequency across the six-week intervention, there was there a significant difference in frequency with relation to percent of the whole grain market basket consumed when looking at only the sixth week of intervention. Bowel movement frequency increased significantly with increased whole grain consumption in Week 6 while there was only a slight, non-significant increase in the refined grain intervention. Whole grains have been shown to decrease intestinal transit time, thereby increasing bowel movement frequency [8,41,65,66]. In a recent review of 65 intervention studies, it was found that intake of wheat fiber, such as is found in wheat bran, a component of whole grain wheat, was shown to decrease transit time by about 45 min per gram of wheat fiber consumed, if the initial transit time was more than 48 h [67]. In a meta-analysis of 65 intervention studies utilizing cereal fibers from wheat, rye, corn, oats, barley, sorghum, and rice, investigators reported that, if the initial transit time was more than 48 h, cereal fiber reduced transit time by 30 min per gram consumed [68]. The mechanism for this is generally thought to be fecal bulking due to the increased fiber from increasing whole grain intake causing water retention in the feces which improves transit time [8,69]. Consuming whole grain barley has been shown to increase average fecal weight compared to the stool weight of refined grain consumers [65] and consumption of a high fiber cereal made of wheat, corn, oats, and soybeans was shown to increase bowel movement frequency compared to a similar low fiber cereal in humans [70]. It must be noted that bowel movement frequency was self-reported in our study and was not measured pre-intervention at baseline. There was also a trend towards increased bowel movement frequency observed in the refined grain intervention, thus the validity of the increase should be interpreted with caution.

4.5. Microbiota

Increasing intake of whole grain wheat, maize, and barley have all been shown to alter the human gut microbiota, potentially through increasing the availability of fiber, but possibly due to other functional components in the whole grains such as polyphenols [14].

However, in this study no significant changes in microbial community composition were detected with consumption of the whole or refined grain market baskets. This is not necessarily surprising, given that in this pilot study subjects were free-living and the market basket comprised only about 16% of their expected calorie intake at the average level of consumption.

Although no significant differences were detected between the whole and refined grain treatments this does not empirically mean that there were not changes in the microbial community that were simply unable to reach statistical significance with our small sample size. Additionally, it is possible that changes occurred in the metabolic pathways or activity of the microbiota over the course of this investigation that could be detected with metatranscriptomic, metabolomics, or proteomic analysis [71]. For example, changes in the production of metabolic byproducts such as short chain fatty acids can occur without necessitating changes in bacterial composition [72–74]. Alterations in bacterial metabolism can occur due to changes in pH, oxygen tension, or substrate availability, to name a few [75].

Based on studies seen in the literature it was expected that the increase in dietary fiber from the consumption of 50% of more of the whole grain market basket would initiate an increase in the abundance in *Bifidobacterium* [19,76–78]. At baseline, high levels of *Actinobacteria* were seen, largely due to an enrichment of *Bifidobacterium*. Enrichment of *Actinobacteria* has previously been observed in expectant mothers in the third trimester of pregnancy [79], however since subjects were excluded if pregnant it is unclear to us why *Actinobacteria* was so abundant at baseline. It is possible that subjects were consuming a significant amount of dietary fiber from a non-whole grain source prior to the study, which could have selectively enriched *Bifidobacterium* [80]. If this were the case, background diet variability may have acted as a confounding factor obscuring the expected increase in the abundance of *Bifidobacterium*. The average fiber intake for American adults is 17.0 g per day with grain products as well as mixed dishes (containing grains) make up nearly half (46%) of the intake, whereas vegetables account for 16%, snacks and sweets for 13% and fruits 12% [81].

The trend towards increased relative abundance of *Akkermansia* and *Lactobacillus* with high whole grain consumption seen in this study has been previously observed with a whole grain barley feeding study in rats [82]. Increases in the abundance of *Lactobacillus* have also been seen in humans after a diet rich in whole grain barley [83] and whole grain wheat [19]. While this trend was not significant, we feel it is a noteworthy observation since increases in *Akkermansia* are associated with reduced endotoxemia, improved inflammatory tone, and potentially weight loss [84–87]. *Lactobacillus* are often taken as probiotics due to their ability to exclude pathogenic bacteria and prevent or shorten episodes of diarrhea [88].

An increase in the abundance of the order *Erysipelotrichales* was seen in this study in the three individuals that consumed 50% or more of the refined grain market basket. Increased abundance of *Erysipelotrichales* has also been reported in canines with a diet high in refined maize and low in fiber [89], in mice with high fat diets [90], in mouse models of acute inflammatory colitis [91], and in humans with Crohn's disease [92]. Within the order *Erysipelotrichales*, the genera *Eubacterium* and *Catenibacterium* as well as unidentified members of family *Erysipelotrichaceae* were observed, although no significant differences were detected at the family or genus levels. *Eubacterium* has been seen in lower abundance in individuals with metabolic syndrome [93] and advanced colorectal adenoma [94]. *Catenibacterium* has been observed to be enriched in individuals with end stage renal disease [95] and to be depleted in individuals with higher risk for cardiovascular disease [96]. *Erysipelotrichaceae* has been observed as being enriched with obesity, Western-type diets, and increased host cholesterol metabolites [97].

4.6. Limitations

A serious limitation of the study was the small sample size. The study enrolled 46 subjects but due to technical problems with instrumentation and only partial cooperation of some of our research volunteers, we have missing data for some variables reported here. Most notably fecal samples from only 28 subjects were available for microbiota analysis. Of those 28 subjects used for the microbiota analysis the ratio of sexes was not balanced. There was a 1:2 ratio of females to males in the refined grain treatment and about a 3:1 ratio of females to males in the whole grain treatment. When observing gut microbiota there is enormous variation between subjects, and within subjects, so it is difficult to detect the signal above the noise, as it were, especially with a small population of subjects. Only having one baseline and one post intervention blood draw and fecal collection was another limitation. Much of the data were collected through self-report which introduces its own complexities and errors, especially when it concerns dietary record keeping, however pre-weighing and re-weighing the market baskets was used to improve the accuracy of those data. Background diet was attempted to be assessed with phone interviews using the multi-pass 24 hour recall method, however subject cooperation was extremely poor so the data collected were not considered to be representative of the usual diet intake. Due to this limitation, we cannot say with certainty that subjects did maintain their habitual diet, creating another possible source of error. Estimated fiber intake from the market basket products was calculated, not determined directly by analysis, so it is possible that the quantity of grain fiber consumed was erroneous. However, since those values were then averaged across the week and by all subjects in the treatment group, this might improve the reliability of the estimations. Analysis was done for body composition, blood work, and GI symptoms using linear regression which can only be used to discover medium to large effects with a sample size as small as those utilized in this study; small changes many have occurred but would not have been detectable. This limits the ability to conclude with certainty that changes did not occur if no difference was detected in our analysis.

5. Conclusions

The results of this paper indicate that increasing the consumption of whole grains in habitual low-whole grain consumers may significantly lower fasting measures of total, LDL, and non-HDL cholesterol.

The trend towards decreased fasting glucose with increased whole grain consumption came tantalizingly close to significance, and was not seen when the same analysis was done with those receiving the refined grain intervention. Due to the tight regulation of blood glucose in healthy individuals, it is not surprising that changes to fasting levels would be subtle and challenging to detect without large groups of homogenous subjects. The fact that a strong trend was seen indicates that a true effect may be present and detectable with better study design.

The increase in bowel movement frequency seen with increased consumption of whole grains during the sixth week of the intervention is supported by existing literature and meta-analyses, however given that no baseline measurements were taken, the sample size was small ($n = 37$), the data rely solely on self-report, and that the same pattern was seen in the refined grain intervention this finding must be interpreted with some reservations.

Microbial analysis was conducted on 28 subjects, and we did not have the power needed to detect anything but very large changes in the microbial community. The only significant change seen was an increase in abundance of the order *Erysipelotrichales* in the three individuals that consumed 50% or more of the refined grain market basket. This finding cannot reasonably be interpreted to say that other changes to the microbiota were not occurring, since there was not enough power in the analysis to validate that inference. The microbial analysis performed in this study was exploratory and should not be interpreted without the many caveats discussed above.

6. Future Research

Given the small sample size and limited sample collection, future research would be necessary to definitively describe changes in health parameters seen with increased whole grain consumption. This study does indicate that whole grains may be an important food type for improving fasting cholesterol and glucose levels, as well as increasing bowel movement frequency. Due to the fact that some changes in health parameters only became apparent in subjects who consumed at least 50% of the whole grain market basket, another direction for future research would be to determine what level of whole grain consumption affords the most beneficial health effects. Due to differences in the composition and level of fibers, vitamins, minerals, and digestibility of different grains, it would also be important to consider exactly which whole grains are being studied and whether they are similar to the grains, and preparations of grains, seen in the population relevant to the study. Another possible direction for future research would be to compare the whole grains typically consumed in the US (wheat, corn, and rice) to other sources of whole grains such as oats, barley, and rye for which more definitive health effects have been documented. Then, recommendations could be further refined to include not only the total quantity of whole grains, but also more specifically for the types of grains consumed based on the potential health benefit.

It is likely that the improvements seen from increasing whole grain consumption come from the increases in fiber consumption, but future research is necessary to confirm this assertion and determine if other functional components of the whole grains contribute to health benefits. Regardless of how whole grains exert their effects, increasing whole grain consumption can reduce the gap between the recommended consumption of fiber and current fiber intake in the US.

Acknowledgments: Funding was contributed by USDA-ARS intramural funds from projects 5306-51530-019 and 2032-51530-022, as well as the University of California at Davis Henry A. Jastro Research Award (2012–2013).

Author Contributions: N.L.K., A.D.L., J.E.B. and B.R. conceived and designed the study; D.B. designed the sensory evaluation and market basket foods/recipes; A.D.L., B.R. and J.E.B. conducted the study visits; D.N.C., M.E.K. and W.H. performed sample analyses; A.D.L., M.E.K. and D.N.C. analyzed the data; N.L.K. and M.L.M. contributed reagents/materials/analysis tools; and D.N.C., M.E.K. and N.L.K. wrote the paper.

Conflicts of Interest: The authors declare no conflict of interest.

Appendix A

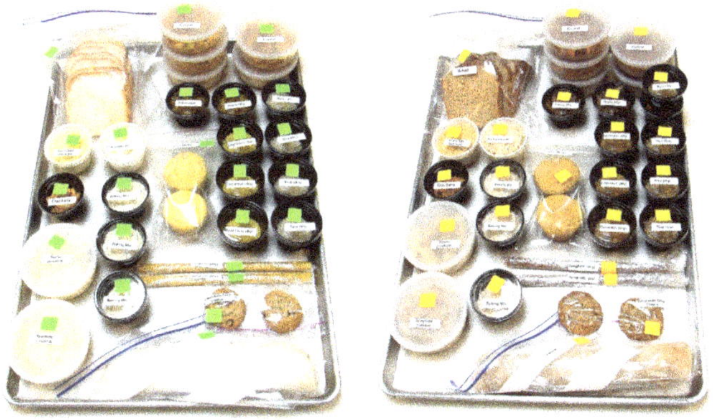

(a) (b)

Figure A1. Images of the 2000 kcal market baskets: (**a**) the refined grain basket; and (**b**) the whole grain basket.

References

1. Food Availability (Per Capita) Data System. Available online: http://ers.usda.gov/data-products/food-availability-per-capita-data-system.aspx (accessed on 20 April 2016).
2. Albertson, A.M.; Good, C.K.; Eldridge, A.L.; Holschuh, N.M. Whole grain consumption and food sources in the united states: Data from nhanes 1999–2000 and the usda's pyramid servings database for the usda survey food codes. *FASEB J.* **2005**, *19*, A87–A87.
3. McGill, C.; Fulgoni, V.L., III; Devareddy, L. Ten-year trends in fiber and whole grain intakes and food sources for the united states population: National health and nutrition examination survey 2001–2010. *Nutrients* **2015**, *7*, 1119–1130. [CrossRef] [PubMed]
4. Okarter, N.; Liu, R.H. Health benefits of whole grain phytochemicals. *Crit. Rev. Food Sci. Nutr.* **2010**, *50*, 193–208. [CrossRef] [PubMed]
5. Van der Kamp, J.W.; Poutanen, K.; Seal, C.J.; Richardson, D.P. The healthgrain definition of 'whole grain'. *Food Nutr. Res.* **2014**, *58*, 22100. [CrossRef] [PubMed]
6. International, AACC. Whole grain definition. *Cereal Foods World* **1999**, *45*, 79.
7. Bett-Garber, K.L.; Lea, J.M.; Champagne, E.T.; McClung, A.M. Whole-grain rice flavor associated with assorted bran colors. *J. Sens. Stud.* **2012**, *27*, 78–86. [CrossRef]
8. Slavin, J. Whole grains and digestive health. *Cereal Chem.* **2010**, *87*, 292–296. [CrossRef]
9. Slavin, J.L. Whole grains, refined grains and fortified refined grains: What's the difference? *Asia Pac. J. Clin. Nutr.* **2000**, *9*, S23–S27. [CrossRef] [PubMed]
10. Marquart, L.; Chan, H.W.; Orsted, M.; Schmitz, K.A.; Arndt, E.A.; Jacobs, D.R. Gradual incorporation of whole-grain flour into grain-based products. *Cereal Foods World* **2006**, *51*, 114–117. [CrossRef]
11. Montonen, J.; Knekt, P.; Jarvinen, R.; Aromaa, A.; Reunanen, A. Whole-grain and fiber intake and the incidence of type 2 diabetes. *Am. J. Clin. Nutr.* **2003**, *77*, 622–629. [PubMed]
12. Borneo, R.; Leon, A.E. Whole grain cereals: Functional components and health benefits. *Food Funct.* **2012**, *3*, 110–119. [CrossRef] [PubMed]
13. Ampatzoglou, A.; Atwal, K.K.; Maidens, C.M.; Williams, C.L.; Ross, A.B.; Thielecke, F.; Jonnalagadda, S.S.; Kennedy, O.B.; Yaqoob, P. Increased whole grain consumption does not affect blood biochemistry, body composition, or gut microbiology in healthy, low-habitual whole grain consumers. *J. Nutr.* **2015**, *145*, 215–221. [CrossRef] [PubMed]
14. Cooper, D.N.; Martin, R.J.; Keim, N.L. Does whole grain consumption alter gut microbiota and satiety? *Healthcare* **2015**, *3*, 364–392. [CrossRef] [PubMed]

15. Jackson, K.H.; West, S.G.; Vanden Heuvel, J.P.; Jonnalagadda, S.S.; Ross, A.B.; Hill, A.M.; Grieger, J.A.; Lemieux, S.K.; Kris-Etherton, P.M. Effects of whole and refined grains in a weight-loss diet on markers of metabolic syndrome in individuals with increased waist circumference: A randomized controlled-feeding trial. *Am. J. Clin. Nutr.* **2014**, *100*, 577–586. [CrossRef] [PubMed]
16. Modi, P. Benefits of low glycemic and high satiety index foods for obesity and diabetes control and management. In *Nutrients, Dietary Supplements, and Nutriceuticals*; Cost Analysis Versus Clinical Benefits; Springer: New York, NY, USA, 2011; pp. 403–424.
17. Zhou, A.L.; Hergert, N.; Rompato, G.; Lefevre, M. Whole grain oats improve insulin sensitivity and plasma cholesterol profile and modify gut microbiota composition in C57BL/6J mice. *J. Nutr.* **2015**, *145*, 222–230. [CrossRef] [PubMed]
18. Rebello, C.J.; Greenway, F.L.; Finley, J.W. Whole grains and pulses: A comparison of the nutritional and health benefits. *J. Agric. Food Chem.* **2014**, *62*, 7029–7049. [CrossRef] [PubMed]
19. Costabile, A.; Klinder, A.; Fava, F.; Napolitano, A.; Foglian, V.; Leonard, C.; Gibson, G.R.; Tuohy, K.M. Whole-grain wheat breakfast cereal has a prebiotic effect on the human gut microbiota: A double-blind, placebo-controlled, crossover study. *Br. J. Nutr.* **2008**, *99*, 110–120. [CrossRef] [PubMed]
20. Raninen, K.; Lappi, J.; Mykkanen, H.; Poutanen, K. Dietary fiber type reflects physiological functionality: Comparison of grain fiber, inulin, and polydextrose. *Nutr. Rev.* **2011**, *69*, 9–21. [CrossRef] [PubMed]
21. Nyman, M.; Siljestrom, M.; Pedersen, B.; Knudsen, K.E.B.; Asp, N.G.; Johansson, C.G.; Eggum, B.O. Dietary fiber content and composition in 6 cereals at different extraction rates. *Cereal Chem.* **1984**, *61*, 14–19.
22. Frankenfield, D.C.; Muth, E.R.; Rowe, W.A. The harris-benedict studies of human basal metabolism: History and limitations. *J. Am. Diet. Assoc.* **1998**, *98*, 439–445. [CrossRef]
23. Lewis, S.J.; Heaton, K.W. Stool form scale as a useful guide to intestinal transit time. *Scand. J. Gastroenterol.* **1997**, *32*, 920–924. [CrossRef] [PubMed]
24. Ferguson, L.W. A study of the likert technique of attitude scale construction. *J. Soc. Psychol.* **1941**, *13*, 51–57. [CrossRef]
25. Hsieh, Y.-H.; Peterson, C.M.; Raggio, A.; Keenan, M.J.; Martin, R.J.; Ravussin, E.; Marco, M.L. Impact of different fecal processing methods on assessments of bacterial diversity in the human intestine. *Front. Microbiol.* **2016**, *7*, 1–11. [CrossRef] [PubMed]
26. Salonen, A.; Nikkila, J.; Jalanka-Tuovinen, J.; Immonen, O.; Rajilic-Stojanovic, M.; Kekkonen, R.A.; Palva, A.; de Vos, W.M. Comparative analysis of fecal DNA extraction methods with phylogenetic microarray: Effective recovery of bacterial and archaeal DNA using mechanical cell lysis. *J. Microbiol. Methods* **2010**, *81*, 127–134. [CrossRef] [PubMed]
27. Wang, Q.; Garrity, G.M.; Tiedje, J.M.; Cole, J.R. Naive bayesian classifier for rapid assignment of rrna sequences into the new bacterial taxonomy. *Appl. Environ. Microbiol.* **2007**, *73*, 5261–5267. [CrossRef] [PubMed]
28. Caporaso, J.G.; Lauber, C.L.; Walters, W.A.; Berg-Lyons, D.; Lozupone, C.A.; Turnbaugh, P.J.; Fierer, N.; Knight, R. Global patterns of 16S rRNA diversity at a depth of millions of sequences per sample. *Proc. Natl. Acad. Sci. USA* **2011**, *108*, 4516–4522. [CrossRef] [PubMed]
29. Hamady, M.; Walker, J.J.; Harris, J.K.; Gold, N.J.; Knight, R. Error-correcting barcoded primers for pyrosequencing hundreds of samples in multiplex. *Nat. Methods* **2008**, *5*, 235–237. [CrossRef] [PubMed]
30. Caporaso, J.G.; Kuczynski, J.; Stombaugh, J.; Bittinger, K.; Bushman, F.D.; Costello, E.K.; Fierer, N.; Pena, A.G.; Goodrich, J.K.; Gordon, J.I.; et al. Qiime allows analysis of high-throughput community sequencing data. *Nat. Methods* **2010**, *7*, 335–336. [CrossRef] [PubMed]
31. Aronesty, E. Ea-utils: Command-Line Tools for Processing Biological Sequencing Data. Available online: https://github.com/ExpressionAnalysis/ea-utils (accessed on 17 April 2011).
32. Edgar, R.C.; Haas, B.J.; Clemente, J.C.; Quince, C.; Knight, R. Uchime improves sensitivity and speed of chimera detection. *Bioinformatics* **2011**, *27*, 2194–2200. [CrossRef] [PubMed]
33. Edgar, R.C. Search and clustering orders of magnitude faster than blast. *Bioinformatics* **2010**, *26*, 2460–2461. [CrossRef] [PubMed]
34. Bokulich, N.A.; Subramanian, S.; Faith, J.J.; Gevers, D.; Gordon, J.I.; Knight, R.; Mills, D.A.; Caporaso, J.G. Quality-filtering vastly improves diversity estimates from illumina amplicon sequencing. *Nat. Methods* **2013**, *10*, 57–59. [CrossRef] [PubMed]

35. Wu, G.D.; Lewis, J.D.; Hoffmann, C.; Chen, Y.Y.; Knight, R.; Bittinger, K.; Hwang, J.; Chen, J.; Berkowsky, R.; Nessel, L.; et al. Sampling and pyrosequencing methods for characterizing bacterial communities in the human gut using 16s sequence tags. *BMC Microbiol.* **2010**, *10*, 206. [CrossRef] [PubMed]
36. Segata, N.; Izard, J.; Waldron, L.; Gevers, D.; Miropolsky, L.; Garrett, W.S.; Huttenhower, C. Metagenomic biomarker discovery and explanation. *Genome Biol.* **2011**, *12*, R60. [CrossRef] [PubMed]
37. Kwong, K.S.; Holland, B.; Cheung, S.H. A modified benjamini-hochberg multiple comparisons procedure for controlling the false discovery rate. *J. Stat. Plan. Inference* **2002**, *104*, 351–362. [CrossRef]
38. De Filippo, C.; Cavalieri, D.; Di Paola, M.; Ramazzotti, M.; Poullet, J.B.; Massart, S.; Collini, S.; Pieraccini, G.; Lionetti, P. Impact of diet in shaping gut microbiota revealed by a comparative study in children from europe and rural africa. *Proc. Natl. Acad. Sci. USA* **2010**, *107*, 14691–14696. [CrossRef] [PubMed]
39. Mariat, D.; Firmesse, O.; Levenez, F.; Guimaraes, V.D.; Sokol, H.; Dore, J.; Corthier, G.; Furet, J.P. The firmicutes/bacteroidetes ratio of the human microbiota changes with age. *BMC Microbiol.* **2009**, *9*, 123. [CrossRef] [PubMed]
40. Lange, E. Oats products as functional food. *Zywnosc-Nauka Technol. Jakosc* **2010**, *17*, 7–24. [CrossRef]
41. Fardet, A. New hypotheses for the health-protective mechanisms of whole-grain cereals: What is beyond fibre? *Nutr. Res. Rev.* **2010**, *23*, 65–134. [CrossRef] [PubMed]
42. Bressani, R.; Breuner, M.; Ortiz, M.A. Acid-detergent and neutro-detergent fiber and mineral elements content of maize and tortilla. *Arch. Latinoam. Nutr.* **1989**, *39*, 382–391. [PubMed]
43. Sumczynski, D.; Bubelova, Z.; Fisera, M. Determination of chemical, insoluble dietary fibre, neutral-detergent fibre and in vitro digestibility in rice types commercialized in Czech markets. *J. Food Compos. Anal.* **2015**, *40*, 8–13. [CrossRef]
44. Lai, V.M.F.; Lu, S.; He, W.H.; Chen, H.H. Non-starch polysaccharide compositions of rice grains with respect to rice variety and degree of milling. *Food Chem.* **2007**, *101*, 1205–1210. [CrossRef]
45. Rose, D.J.; Patterson, J.A.; Hamaker, B.R. Structural differences among alkali-soluble arabinoxylans from maize (*Zea mays*), rice (*oryza sativa*), and wheat (*triticum aestivum*) brans influence human fecal fermentation profiles. *J. Agric. Food Chem.* **2010**, *58*, 493–499. [CrossRef] [PubMed]
46. Mohan, V.; Spiegelman, D.; Sudha, V.; Gayathri, R.; Hong, B.; Praseena, K.; Anjana, R.M.; Wedick, N.M.; Arumugam, K.; Malik, V.; et al. Effect of brown rice, white rice, and brown rice with legumes on blood glucose and insulin responses in overweight Asian Indians: A randomized controlled trial. *Diabetes Technol. Ther.* **2014**, *16*, 317–325. [CrossRef] [PubMed]
47. Tosh, S.M. Review of human studies investigating the post-prandial blood-glucose lowering ability of oat and barley food products. *Eur. J. Clin. Nutr.* **2013**, *67*, 310–317. [CrossRef] [PubMed]
48. Ranawana, V.; Clegg, M.E.; Shafat, A.; Henry, C.J. Postmastication digestion factors influence glycemic variability in humans. *Nutr. Res.* **2011**, *31*, 452–459. [CrossRef] [PubMed]
49. Bornhorst, G.M.; Stroebinger, N.; Rutherfurd, S.M.; Singh, R.P.; Moughan, P.J. Properties of gastric chyme from pigs fed cooked brown or white rice. *Food Biophys.* **2013**, *8*, 12–23. [CrossRef]
50. Oishi, K.; Yamamoto, S.; Itoh, N.; Nakao, R.; Yasumoto, Y.; Tanaka, K.; Kikuchi, Y.; Fukudome, S.; Okita, K.; Takano-Ishikawa, Y. Wheat alkylresorcinols suppress high-fat, high-sucrose diet-induced obesity and glucose intolerance by increasing insulin sensitivity and cholesterol excretion in male mice. *J. Nutr.* **2015**, *145*, 199–206. [CrossRef] [PubMed]
51. Arora, T.; Sharma, R.; Frost, G. Propionate. Anti-obesity and satiety enhancing factor? *Appetite* **2011**, *56*, 511–515. [CrossRef] [PubMed]
52. Everard, A.; Cani, P.D. Gut microbiota and GLP-1. *Rev. Endocr. Metab. Disord.* **2014**, *15*, 189–196. [CrossRef] [PubMed]
53. Chambers, E.S.; Viardot, A.; Psichas, A.; Morrison, D.J.; Murphy, K.G.; Sagen, E.K.; Varghese, Z.; MacDougall, K.; Preston, T. Effects of targeted delivery of propionate to the human colon on appetite regulation, body weight maintenance and adiposity in overweight adult. *BMJ* **2014**, 1–11. [CrossRef] [PubMed]
54. Todesco, T.; Rao, A.V.; Bosello, O.; Jenkins, D.J.A. Propionate lowers blood-glucose and alters lipid-metabolism in healthy-subjects. *Am. J. Clin. Nutr.* **1991**, *54*, 860–865. [PubMed]
55. Frost, G.; Sleeth, M.L.; Sahuri-Arisoylu, M.; Lizarbe, B.; Cerdan, S.; Brody, L.; Anastasovska, J.; Ghourab, S.; Hankir, M.; Zhang, S.; et al. The short-chain fatty acid acetate reduces appetite via a central homeostatic mechanism. *Nat. Commun.* **2014**, *5*, 3611. [CrossRef] [PubMed]

56. Venter, C.S.; Vorster, H.H.; Cummings, J.H. Effects of dietary propionate on carbohydrate and lipid-metabolism in healthy-volunteers. *Am. J. Gastroenterol.* **1990**, *85*, 549–553. [PubMed]
57. Johansson, E.V.; Nilsson, A.C.; Ostman, E.M.; Bjorck, I.M.E. Effects of indigestible carbohydrates in barley on glucose metabolism, appetite and voluntary food intake over 16 h in healthy adults. *Nutr. J.* **2013**, *12*, 46. [CrossRef] [PubMed]
58. McIntosh, G.H.; Noakes, M.; Royle, P.J.; Foster, P.R. Whole-grain rye and wheat foods and markers of bowel health in overweight middle-aged men. *Am. J. Clin. Nutr.* **2003**, *77*, 967–974. [PubMed]
59. Youn, M.; Csallany, A.S.; Gallaher, D.D. Whole grain consumption has a modest effect on the development of diabetes in the goto-kakisaki rat. *Br. J. Nutr.* **2012**, *107*, 192–201. [CrossRef] [PubMed]
60. Kristensen, M.; Jensen, M.G.; Riboldi, G.; Petronio, M.; Bugel, S.; Toubro, S.; Tetens, I.; Astrup, A. Wholegrain vs. Refined wheat bread and pasta. Effect on postprandial glycemia, appetite, and subsequent ad libitum energy intake in young healthy adults. *Appetite* **2010**, *54*, 163–169. [CrossRef] [PubMed]
61. Cano, J.M.M.; Aguilar, A.C.; Hernandez, J.C. Lipid-lowering effect of maize-based traditional mexican food on a metabolic syndrome model in rats. *Lipids Health Dis.* **2013**, *12*, 35. [CrossRef] [PubMed]
62. Mackie, A.; Bajka, B.; Rigby, N. Roles for dietary fibre in the upper gi tract: The importance of viscosity. *Food Res. Int.* **2016**, *88*, 234–238. [CrossRef]
63. Knudsen, K.E.B.; Laerke, H.N. Whole grain cereals and gut health. *Agro Food Ind. Hi-Tech* **2008**, *19*, 6–8.
64. Odes, H.S.; Lazovski, H.; Stern, I.; Madar, Z. Double-blind trial of a high dietary fiber, mixed grain cereal in patients with chronic constipation and hyperlipidemia. *Nutr. Res.* **1993**, *13*, 979–985. [CrossRef]
65. Bird, A.R.; Vuaran, M.S.; King, R.A.; Noakes, M.; Keogh, J.; Morell, M.K.; Topping, D.L. Wholegrain foods made from a novel high-amylose barley variety (himalaya 292) improve indices of bowel health in human subjects. *Br. J. Nutr.* **2008**, *99*, 1032–1040. [CrossRef] [PubMed]
66. Kim, J.Y.; Son, B.K.; Lee, S.S. Effects of adlay, buckwheat, and barley on transit time and the antioxidative system in obesity induced rats. *Nutr. Res. Pract.* **2012**, *6*, 208–212. [CrossRef] [PubMed]
67. De Vries, J.; Miller, P.E.; Verbeke, K. Effects of cereal fiber on bowel function: A systematic review of intervention trials. *World J. Gastroenterol.* **2015**, *21*, 8952–8963. [CrossRef] [PubMed]
68. De Vries, J.; Birkett, A.; Hulshof, T.; Verbeke, K.; Gibes, K. Effects of cereal, fruit and vegetable fibers on human fecal weight and transit time: A comprehensive review of intervention trials. *Nutrients* **2016**, *8*, 130. [CrossRef] [PubMed]
69. Slavin, J. Health aspects of dietary fibre. *Fibre-Rich Wholegrain Foods Improv. Qual.* **2013**, *237*, 61–75.
70. Belobrajdic, D.P.; Bird, A.R. The potential role of phytochemicals in wholegrain cereals for the prevention of type-2 diabetes. *Nutr. J.* **2013**, *12*, 62. [CrossRef] [PubMed]
71. Coughlin, S.S. Toward a road map for global -omics: A primer on -omic technologies. *Am. J. Epidemiol.* **2014**, *180*, 1188–1195. [CrossRef] [PubMed]
72. Scott, K.P.; Martin, J.C.; Duncan, S.H.; Flint, H.J. Prebiotic stimulation of human colonic butyrate-producing bacteria and bifidobacteria, in vitro. *Fems Microbiol. Ecol.* **2014**, *87*, 30–40. [CrossRef] [PubMed]
73. Mirande, C.; Kadlecikova, E.; Matulova, M.; Capek, P.; Bernalier-Donadille, A.; Forano, E.; Bera-Maillet, C. Dietary fibre degradation and fermentation by two xylanolytic bacteria bacteroides xylanisolvens xb1at and roseburia intestinalis xb6b4 from the human intestine. *J. Appl. Microbiol.* **2010**, *109*, 451–460. [PubMed]
74. Hamer, H.M.; De Preter, V.; Windey, K.; Verbeke, K. Functional analysis of colonic bacterial metabolism: Relevant to health? *Am. J. Physiol.-Gastrointest. Liver Physiol.* **2012**, *302*, G1–G9. [CrossRef] [PubMed]
75. Lozupone, C.A.; Stombaugh, J.I.; Gordon, J.I.; Jansson, J.K.; Knight, R. Diversity, stability and resilience of the human gut microbiota. *Nature* **2012**, *489*, 220–230. [CrossRef] [PubMed]
76. Bosscher, D.; Breynaert, A.; Pieters, L.; Hermans, N. Food-based strategies to modulate the composition of the intestinal microbiota and their associated health effects. *J. Physiol. Pharmacol.* **2009**, *60*, 5–11. [PubMed]
77. Cani, P.D.; Neyrinck, A.M.; Fava, F.; Knauf, C.; Burcelin, R.G.; Tuohy, K.M.; Gibson, G.R.; Delzenne, N.M. Selective increases of bifidobacteria in gut microflora improve high-fat-diet-induced diabetes in mice through a mechanism associated with endotoxaemia. *Diabetologia* **2007**, *50*, 2374–2383. [CrossRef] [PubMed]
78. Christensen, E.G.; Licht, T.R.; Kristensen, M.; Bahl, M.I. Bifidogenic effect of whole-grain wheat during a 12-week energy-restricted dietary intervention in postmenopausal women. *Eur. J. Clin. Nutr.* **2013**, *67*, 1316–1321. [CrossRef] [PubMed]

79. Koren, O.; Goodrich, J.K.; Cullender, T.C.; Spor, A.; Laitinen, K.; Backhed, H.K.; Gonzalez, A.; Werner, J.J.; Angenent, L.T.; Knight, R.; et al. Host remodeling of the gut microbiome and metabolic changes during pregnancy. *Cell* **2012**, *150*, 470–480. [CrossRef] [PubMed]
80. Gibson, G.R.; Probert, H.M.; Van Loo, J.; Rastall, R.A.; Roberfroid, M.B. Dietary modulation of the human colonic microbiota: Updating the concept of prebiotics. *Nutr. Res. Rev.* **2004**, *17*, 259–275. [CrossRef] [PubMed]
81. Mobley, A.R.; Jones, J.M.; Rodriguez, J.; Slavin, J.; Zelman, K.M. Identifying practical solutions to meet america's fiber needs: Proceedings from the food & fiber summit. *Nutrients* **2014**, *6*, 2540–2551. [PubMed]
82. Zhong, Y.; Nyman, M.; Fak, F. Modulation of gut microbiota in rats fed high-fat diets by processing whole-grain barley to barley malt. *Mol. Nutr. Food Res.* **2015**, *59*, 2066–2076. [CrossRef] [PubMed]
83. De Angelis, M.; Montemurno, E.; Vannini, L.; Cosola, C.; Cavallo, N.; Gozzi, G.; Maranzano, V.; Di Cagno, R.; Gobbetti, M.; Gesualdo, L. Effect of whole-grain barley on the human fecal microbiota and metabolome. *Appl. Environ. Microbiol.* **2015**, *81*, 7945–7956. [CrossRef] [PubMed]
84. Everard, A.; Belzer, C.; Geurts, L.; Ouwerkerk, J.P.; Druart, C.; Bindels, L.B.; Guiot, Y.; Derrien, M.; Muccioli, G.G.; Delzenne, N.M.; et al. Cross-talk between akkermansia muciniphila and intestinal epithelium controls diet-induced obesity. *Proc. Natl. Acad. Sci. USA* **2013**, *110*, 9066–9071. [CrossRef] [PubMed]
85. Joyce, S.A.; Gahan, C.G.M. The gut microbiota and the metabolic health of the host. *Curr. Opin. Gastroenterol.* **2014**, *30*, 120–127. [CrossRef] [PubMed]
86. Greer, R.L.; Dong, X.X.; Moraes, A.C.F.; Zielke, R.A.; Fernandes, G.R.; Peremyslova, E.; Vasquez-Perez, S.; Schoenborn, A.A.; Gomes, E.P.; Pereira, A.C.; et al. Akkermansia muciniphila mediates negative effects of ifn gamma on glucose metabolism. *Nat. Commun.* **2016**, *7*, 13329. [CrossRef] [PubMed]
87. Remely, M.; Tesar, I.; Hippe, B.; Gnauer, S.; Rust, P.; Haslberger, A.G. Gut microbiota composition correlates with changes in body fat content due to weight loss. *Benef. Microbes* **2015**, *6*, 431–439. [CrossRef] [PubMed]
88. Sarao, L.K.; Arora, M. Probiotics, prebiotics, and microencapsulation: A review. *Crit. Rev. Food Sci. Nutr.* **2017**, *57*, 344–371. [CrossRef] [PubMed]
89. Hang, I.; Rinttila, T.; Zentek, J.; Kettunen, A.; Alaja, S.; Apajalahti, J.; Harmoinen, J.; de Vos, W.M.; Spillmann, T. Effect of high contents of dietary animal-derived protein or carbohydrates on canine faecal microbiota. *BMC Vet. Res.* **2012**, *8*, 90. [CrossRef] [PubMed]
90. Magnusson, K.R.; Hauck, L.; Jeffrey, B.M.; Elias, V.; Humphrey, A.; Nath, R.; Perrone, A.; Bermudez, L.E. Relationships between diet-related changes in the gut microbiome and cognitive flexibility. *Neuroscience* **2015**, *300*, 128–140. [CrossRef] [PubMed]
91. Schwab, C.; Berry, D.; Rauch, I.; Rennisch, I.; Ramesmayer, J.; Hainzl, E.; Heider, S.; Decker, T.; Kenner, L.; Muller, M.; et al. Longitudinal study of murine microbiota activity and interactions with the host during acute inflammation and recovery. *ISME J.* **2014**, *8*, 1101–1114. [CrossRef] [PubMed]
92. Gevers, D.; Kugathasan, S.; Denson, L.A.; Vazquez-Baeza, Y.; Van Treuren, W.; Ren, B.Y.; Schwager, E.; Knights, D.; Song, S.J.; Yassour, M.; et al. The treatment-naive microbiome in new-onset crohn's disease. *Cell Host Microbe* **2014**, *15*, 382–392. [CrossRef] [PubMed]
93. Haro, C.; Garcia-Carpintero, S.; Alcala-Diaz, J.F.; Gomez-Delgado, F.; Delgado-Lista, J.; Perez-Martinez, P.; Zuniga, O.A.R.; Quintana-Navarro, G.M.; Landa, B.B.; Clemente, J.C.; et al. The gut microbial community in metabolic syndrome patients is modified by diet. *J. Nutr. Biochem.* **2016**, *27*, 27–31. [CrossRef] [PubMed]
94. Chen, W.G.; Liu, F.L.; Ling, Z.X.; Tong, X.J.; Xiang, C. Human intestinal lumen and mucosa-associated microbiota in patients with colorectal cancer. *PLoS ONE* **2012**, *7*, e39743. [CrossRef] [PubMed]
95. Vaziri, N.D.; Wong, J.; Pahl, M.; Piceno, Y.M.; Yuan, J.; DeSantis, T.Z.; Ni, Z.M.; Nguyen, T.H.; Andersen, G.L. Chronic kidney disease alters intestinal microbial flora. *Kidney Int.* **2013**, *83*, 308–315. [CrossRef] [PubMed]
96. Kelly, T.N.; Bazzano, L.A.; Ajami, N.J.; He, H.; Zhao, J.Y.; Petrosino, J.F.; Correa, A.; He, J. Gut microbiome associates with lifetime cardiovascular disease risk profile among bogalusa heart study participants. *Circ. Res.* **2016**, *119*, 956–964. [CrossRef] [PubMed]
97. Kaakoush, N.O. Insights into the role of erysipelotrichaceae in the human host. *Front. Cell. Infect. Microbiol.* **2015**, *5*, 84. [CrossRef] [PubMed]

nutrients

MDPI

Article

Intra Amniotic Administration of Raffinose and Stachyose Affects the Intestinal Brush Border Functionality and Alters Gut Microflora Populations

Sarina Pacifici [1], Jaehong Song [2], Cathy Zhang [3], Qiaoye Wang [4], Raymond P. Glahn [5], Nikolai Kolba [5] and Elad Tako [5,]*

1. Department of Animal Sciences, Cornell University, Ithaca, NY 14853, USA; sjp233@cornell.edu
2. Department of Biological Sciences, Cornell University, Ithaca, NY 14853, USA; js2833@cornell.edu
3. Division of Nutritional Sciences, Cornell University, Ithaca, NY 14853, USA; cz223@cornell.edu
4. Department of Food Science and Technology, Cornell University, Ithaca, NY 14853, USA; yw696@cornell.edu
5. USDA-ARS, Robert W. Holley Center for Agriculture and Health, Cornell University, Ithaca, NY 14853, USA; rpg3@cornell.edu (R.P.G.); nk598@cornell.edu (N.K.)

* Correspondence: et79@cornell.edu; Tel.: +1-607-255-5434

Received: 10 January 2017; Accepted: 17 March 2017; Published: 19 March 2017

Abstract: This study investigates the effectiveness of two types of prebiotics—stachyose and raffinose—which are present in staple food crops that are widely consumed in regions where dietary Fe deficiency is a health concern. The hypothesis is that these prebiotics will improve Fe status, intestinal functionality, and increase health-promoting bacterial populations in vivo (*Gallus gallus*). By using the intra-amniotic administration procedure, prebiotic treatment solutions were injected in ovo (day 17 of embryonic incubation) with varying concentrations of a 1.0 mL pure raffinose or stachyose in 18 MΩ H_2O. Four treatment groups (50, 100 mg·mL^{-1} raffinose or stachyose) and two controls (18 MΩ H_2O and non-injected) were utilized. At hatch the cecum, small intestine, liver, and blood were collected for assessment of the relative abundance of the gut microflora, relative expression of Fe-related genes and brush border membrane functional genes, hepatic ferritin levels, and hemoglobin levels, respectively. The prebiotic treatments increased the relative expression of brush border membrane functionality proteins ($p < 0.05$), decreased the relative expression of Fe-related proteins ($p < 0.05$), and increased villus surface area. Raffinose and stachyose increased the relative abundance of probiotics ($p < 0.05$), and decreased that of pathogenic bacteria. Raffinose and stachyose beneficially affected the gut microflora, Fe bioavailability, and brush border membrane functionality. Our investigations have led to a greater understanding of these prebiotics' effects on intestinal health and mineral metabolism.

Keywords: raffinose; stachyose; brush border membrane; iron; prebiotics

1. Introduction

Iron (Fe) deficiency is the most common nutrient deficiency worldwide, affecting between 30% and 40% of the world's population [1,2]. Those who suffer from this condition can experience fatigue, cognitive impairment, and death [3]. The prevalence of Fe deficiency in these geographical regions can be attributed to the populations' consumption of low-diversity plant-based diets including cereals and legumes, which contain low amounts of bioavailable Fe as well as compounds such as polyphenols that further inhibit Fe absorption [4,5]. Dietary Fe deficiency and other dietary mineral deficiencies stem from a lack of essential nutrients in staple food crops, and thus health sectors have turned to various agricultural interventions as potential solutions. A form of intervention that shows great promise is biofortification. Biofortification refers to the use of traditional breeding practices to bring about significant increases in bioavailable micronutrients in the edible portions of food crops [6,7]. Once biofortified, the seedlings of staple foods crops can be distributed to farmers who are already experienced in growing these particular crops. In fact, biofortified crops are found to have a multitude of agronomic benefits for farmers due to their high micronutrient stores, including disease resistance, improved seed viability, greater seedling vigor, lower seeding rate requirements, and faster root establishment—all of which lead to increased productivity relative to the original seedlings [7]. Another sustainable aspect of this solution is that once biofortified varieties are grown, they will not continue to require government attention or funding [7].

However, a major challenge associated with biofortification of staple food crops—namely cereal grains and legume seeds—in developing regions is that they contain factors such as polyphenols and phytic acid that inhibit the absorption of Fe [8]. When these crops are biofortified via conventional breeding, there is the potential for these inhibitory factors to increase along with Fe [9–11]. Despite containing inhibitory factors, cereal grains and legumes also carry other substances, referred to as promoters, which have the potential to counteract the effects of these inhibitory factors. Thus, one prospective solution to the aforementioned dilemma is to increase the content of these promoter substances to counteract the negative effects of the inhibitory factors such as polyphenols [9]. One of the most notable of these promoter substances is the prebiotic [9,12].

Prebiotics are polysaccharides that have been shown to enhance the growth and activities of probiotics, or beneficial gut microflora. These compounds are capable of surviving acidic and enzymatic digestion in the small intestine, and thus can be fermented by probiotics that reside in the colon/cecum [6]. The fermentation of prebiotics by probiotics leads to the production of short-chain fatty acids, which lower intestinal pH, inhibiting the growth of potentially pathogenic bacterial populations and improving the absorption of minerals such as Fe [7]. Raffinose and stachyose were chosen as the prebiotics for investigation in this study, since they are found in high concentrations in lentils and chickpeas [8], which are staple crops consumed by populations in which Fe deficiency is a health concern [5]. Previously, we demonstrated the effects of the wheat prebiotics arabinoxylans and fructans on intestinal probiotics [12] as a potential approach to improving Fe bioavailability in staple food crops and gut health.

In the current study, raffinose and stachyose effects were studied in vivo by utilizing the poultry model (*Gallus gallus*). The broiler chicken is a fast-growing animal with sensitivities to dietary deficiencies of trace minerals such as Fe [13], and is very receptive to dietary manipulations [9,12–14]. Additionally, there is >85% homology between gene sequences of human and chicken intestinal genes such as DMT1, DcytB, ZnT1, and Ferroportin [15]. Thus, one objective of this study is to assess the effects of intra-amniotic raffinose and stachyose administration on Fe status in vivo (*Gallus gallus*), an animal model that has been used to investigate the physiological effects of various nutritional solutions [16,17]. Specifically, the expression of Fe metabolism-related genes (DMT1, the major Fe intestinal transporter; DcytB, Fe reductase; and Ferroportin, the major intestinal enterocyte Fe exporter), in the duodenum (the major Fe absorption site). The second objective in using this model is to assess the effects of raffinose and stachyose on brush border membrane (BBM) development and functionality using biomarkers for BBM absorptive ability such as the relative expressions of aminopeptidase (AP), sucrase isomaltase (SI), and sodium glucose cotransporter-1 (SGLT1), as well as the surface areas of the intestinal villi. The third objective is to evaluate the effects of the intra-amniotic administration of these prebiotics on intestinal bacterial populations by measuring the relative abundances of probiotic health-promoting populations bacteria such as *Bifidobacterium* and *Lactobacillus* versus those of potentially pathogenic bacteria such as *E. coli* and *Clostridium*.

The goal in investigating these effects is to determine whether raffinose and stachyose may be candidates for biofortification in staple food crops. If they demonstrate the ability to improve Fe status, BBM functionality, and intestinal bacterial populations, breeding lentils and chickpeas for increased stachyose and raffinose content may potentially eliminate the need for exogenous Fe supplementation by increasing the bioavailability of Fe in these crops. The distribution of biofortified crop seedlings would serve as a sustainable means of combating malnutrition in developing regions where dietary Fe deficiency is common.

2. Materials and Methods

2.1. Animals and Design

Cornish cross-fertile broiler chicken eggs ($n = 120$) were obtained from a commercial hatchery (Moyer's chicks, Quakertown, PA, USA). The eggs were incubated under optimal conditions at the Cornell University Animal Science poultry farm incubator.

2.2. Intra-Amniotic Administration

All animal protocols were approved by Cornell University Institutional Animal Care and Use committee (ethic approval code: 2007-0129). Pure stachyose and raffinose in powder form were separately diluted in 18 MΩ H_2O to determine the concentrations necessary to maintain an osmolarity value of less than 320 Osm to ensure that the chicken embryos would not be dehydrated upon injection of the solution. This intra-amniotic administration procedure followed that of Tako et al. [12]. On day 17 of embryonic incubation, eggs containing viable embryos were weighed and divided into 6 groups ($n = 12$) with an approximately equal weight distribution. The intra-amniotic treatment solution (1 mL per egg) was injected with a 21-gauge needle into the amniotic fluid, which was identified by candling. After injection, the injection sites were sealed with cellophane tape. The six groups were assigned as follows: 1. 5% stachyose (in 18 MΩ H_2O); 2. 10% stachyose (in 18 MΩ H_2O); 3. 5% raffinose (in 18 MΩ H_2O); 4. 10% raffinose (in 18 MΩ H_2O); 5. 18 MΩ H_2O; 6. non-injected. Eggs were placed in hatching baskets such that each treatment was equally represented at each incubator location.

2.3. Tissue Collection

On the day of hatch (day 21), birds were euthanized by CO_2 exposure. The small intestines, ceca, blood, and livers were quickly removed from the carcasses and placed in separate tubes for storage. The samples were immediately frozen in liquid nitrogen and then stored in a −80 °C freezer until analysis.

2.4. Isolation of Total RNA

Total RNA was extracted from 30 mg of small intestine (duodenal) tissue using Qiagen RNeasy Mini Kit. RNA was quantified by absorbance at 260–280 nm. Integrity of the 28S and 18S rRNA was verified by 1.5% agarose gel electrophoresis followed by ethidium bromide staining.

2.5. Gene Expression Analysis

As was previously described [9,12,13], RT-PCR was carried out with primers chosen from the fragments of chicken duodenal tissues. After the completion of PCR, the results were run under gel electrophoresis on 2% agarose gel stained with ethidium bromide for separation of the target genes (DMT1, Ferroportin, DcytB, AP, SI, SGLT1). Quantity One 1D analysis software (Bio-Rad, Hercules, CA, USA) was utilized to quantify the resulting bands. Highly conserved tissue-specific 18S rRNA was used as internal standard to normalize the results.

2.6. Bacterial Analysis

As was previously described [18–20], the contents of the ceca were placed into a sterile 50 mL tube containing 9 mL of sterile phosphate-buffered saline (PBS) and homogenized by vortexing with glass beads. Debris was removed by centrifugation. For DNA purification, the pellet was treated with lysozyme. The bacterial genomic DNA was isolated using a Wizard Genomic DNA purification kit. Primers for *Lactobacillus*, *Bifidobacterium*, *Clostridium*, and *E. coli* were designed according to previously published data by Zhu et al. in 2002 [19]. The universal primers—which identify all known strains of bacteria in the intestine—were prepared with the invariant region in the 16S rRNA of bacteria, and were used as internal standard to normalize the results. The DNA samples underwent PCR, and the amplified results were loaded on 2% agarose gel stained with ethidium bromide and underwent electrophoresis for separation. Then, the bands were quantified using Quantity One 1-D analysis software (Bio-Rad, Hercules, CA, USA). Abundance of individual bacterial gene expression was measured relative to the universal primer product, where the total bacteria equaled 100%.

2.7. Assessment of Liver Ferritin

As was previously described [9,14], the collected liver samples were treated similarly to the procedures described in a previous study by Passaniti et al. in 1989 [21]. Approximately 0.25 g of liver sample was diluted into 0.5 mL of 50 mM Hepes buffer (pH 7.4) and homogenized on ice using an UltraTurrax homogenizer at maximum speed (5000× *g*) for 2 min. Each homogenate was subjected to heat treatment for 10 min at 75 °C to aid isolation of ferritin. The samples were immediately cooled on ice for 30 min after heat treatment, centrifuged at 13,000× *g* for 30 min until a clear supernatant was obtained, and the pellet containing insoluble denatured proteins was discarded. Native polyacrylamide gel electrophoresis was utilized for separation technique. Six percent separating gel and 5% stacking gel were prepared for the procedure. A constant 100 V voltage was administered throughout the process. The resulting gels were then treated with two specific stains: potassium ferricyanide ($K_3Fe(CN)_6$)—a stain specific for Fe—and Coomassie blue G-250 stain, specific for protein in general. The Fe-stained bands represented ferritin levels, and were compared to the corresponding bands in the Coomasie-stained gel to calculate relative abundance of ferritin (ferritin-to-total-protein ratio). Gels were scanned by using the Bio-Rad densitometer and measured using the Quantity-One 1-D analysis program (Bio-Rad, Hercules, CA, USA). Horse spleen ferritin was used as a standard to calibrate ferritin/Fe concentrations. Ferritin saturation levels were measured by calculating relative percentage of Fe present in the protein to the maximum number of Fe atoms that can be present per molecule of ferritin (approximately 4500 Fe atoms) [22].

2.8. Blood Analysis and Hb Measurements

Blood was collected using micro-hematocrit heparinized capillary tubes (Fisher Scientific, Waltham, MA, USA). Blood Hb concentrations were determined spectrophotometrically using the cyanmethemoglobin method (H7506-STD, Pointe Scientific Inc., Canton, MI, USA) following the kit manufacturer's instructions.

2.9. Morphological Examination of the Intestinal Villi

As was previously described [17], intestinal samples (duodenal region as the main intestinal Fe absorption site) at day of hatch from each treatment were fixed in fresh 4% (*vol/vol*) buffered formaldehyde, dehydrated, cleared, and embedded in paraffin. Serial sections were cut at 5 μm and placed on glass slides. Sections were deparaffinized in xylene, rehydrated in a graded alcohol series, stained with hematoxylin and eosin, and examined by light microscopy. Morphometric measurements of villus height and width were performed with an Olympus light microscope using EPIX XCAP software. Villus surface area was calculated from villus height and width at half height.

2.10. Goblet Cell Diameter

Morphometric measurements of goblet cell diameter were performed with an Olympus light microscope using EPIX XCAP software.

2.11. Statistical Analysis

Results were analyzed by one-way multiple analysis of variance (MANOVA) using the JMP software (SAS Institute Inc., Cary, NC, USA). Differences between treatments were compared by Tukey's test, and values were statistically different at $p < 0.05$ (values in the text are means ± SEM).

3. Results

3.1. Intestinal Content Bacterial Genera- and Species-Level Analysis

The relative abundance of both *Bifidobacterium* and *Lactobacillus*—which are known to be probiotics—significantly ($p < 0.05$) increased in the presence of both concentrations of stachyose and raffinose. The relative abundance of *E. coli* did not significantly ($p > 0.05$) increase or decrease in the presence of the prebiotic treatment solutions compared to the controls. *Clostridium*'s relative abundance significantly ($p < 0.05$) decreased in the presence of both concentrations of stachyose and raffinose compared to the controls (Figure 1). These results indicate that stachyose and raffinose improved gut health by promoting the survival of probiotics and limiting the existence of potentially pathogenic bacterial populations. The presence of these probiotics was expected to give rise to an increase in short-chain fatty acid production and an increase in Fe solubility, and in turn, Fe bioavailability.

3.2. BBM Functional Genes

The relative expressions of AP, SI, and SGLT1 were all significantly ($p < 0.05$) up-regulated in the presence of both concentrations of stachyose and raffinose (Figure 2). The up-regulation of the expression of BBM functional genes signifies increased absorptive ability of the BBM, which indicates improved functionality and gut health [23].

3.3. Fe Metabolism Genes

The relative expressions of DcytB, DMT1, and ferroportin were all significantly ($p < 0.05$) down-regulated in the presence of both concentrations of stachyose and raffinose (Figure 2). The down-regulation of these genes is in turn suggested to be an indicator of Fe-replete conditions. This is a potential biomarker for improved Fe status.

3.4. Cecum-to-Body-Weight Ratio

The cecum-to-bodyweight ratios were significantly ($p < 0.05$) higher in the prebiotic treatment groups compared to the controls. The ceca of subjects that received stachyose and raffinose increased, indicating an increase in their content of bacterial populations (Table 1).

3.5. Morphometric Data for Villi

The villus surface areas significantly ($p < 0.05$) increased in the presence of both concentrations of stachyose and raffinose (Table 2). This serves as a mechanical measurement of BBM absorptive ability and improvement in BBM functionality and gut health by indicating that the introduction of stachyose and raffinose enhanced proliferation of enterocytes.

3.6. Goblet Cell Diameters

The goblet cell diameters significantly ($p < 0.05$) increased in the presence of both concentrations of stachyose and raffinose (Table 2).

3.7. Liver Ferritin and Hb

There were no significant ($p > 0.05$) differences in ferritin or Hb values between treatment groups. The lack of a significant difference in these physiological measurements of Fe status between groups is posited to be because there was not enough Fe in the environment to create a significant change (Table 3).

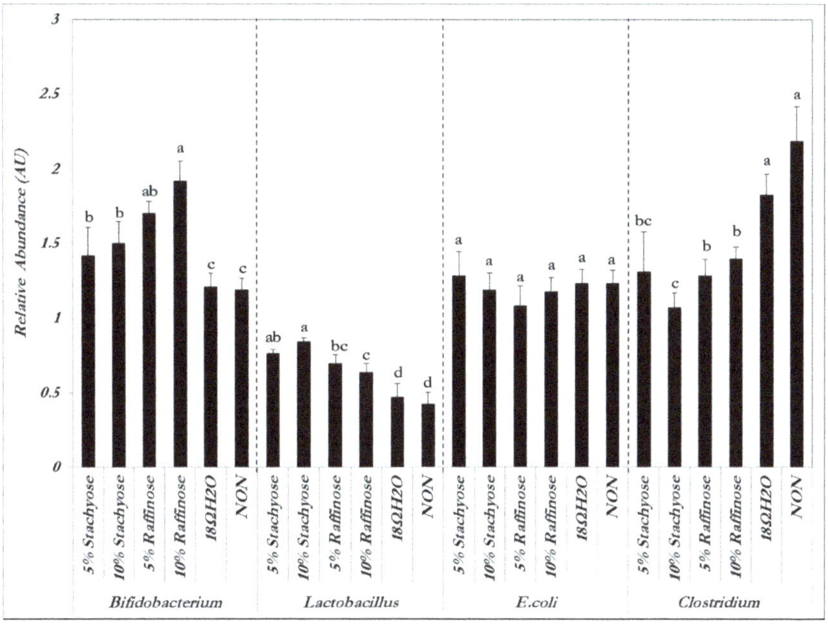

Figure 1. Genera and species-level bacterial populations (AU) from cecal contents measured on the day of hatch. Values are means ± SEM, n = 8. Per bacterial category, treatment groups not indicated by the same letter are significantly different ($p < 0.05$).

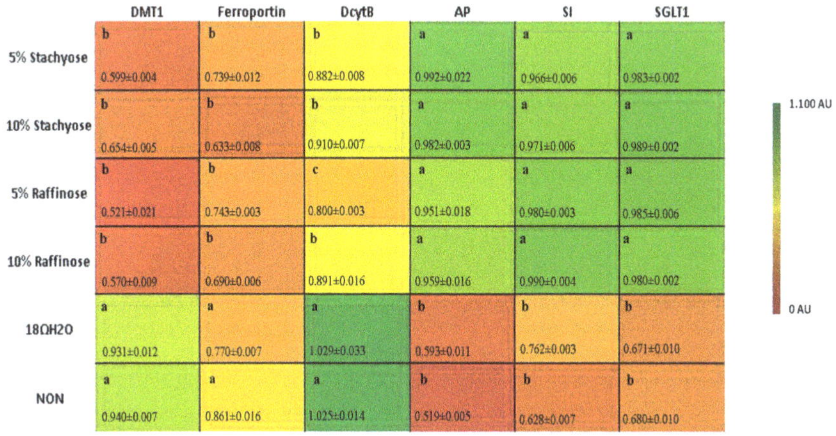
DMT1
Ferroportin
DcytB
AP
SI
SGLT1
5% Stachyose
0.599±0.004
0.739±0.012
0.882±0.008
0.992±0.022
0.966±0.006
0.983±0.002
10% Stachyose
0.654±0.005
0.633±0.008
0.910±0.007
0.982±0.003
0.971±0.006
0.989±0.002
5% Raffinose
0.521±0.021
0.743±0.003
0.800±0.003
0.951±0.018
0.980±0.003
0.985±0.006
10% Raffinose
0.570±0.009
0.690±0.006
0.891±0.016
0.959±0.016
0.990±0.004
0.980±0.002
18ΩH2O
0.931±0.012
0.770±0.007
1.029±0.033
0.593±0.011
0.762±0.003
0.671±0.010
NON
0.940±0.007
0.861±0.016
1.025±0.014
0.519±0.005
0.628±0.007
0.680±0.010
1.100 AU
0 AU

Figure 2. Duodenal mRNA expression (in AU) of measured brush border membrane (BBM) functional and Fe metabolism genes on the day of hatch. Values are means ± SEM, n = 8. Standard errors are represented by vertical bars. Per gene, treatments groups not indicated by the same letter are significantly different ($p < 0.05$). AP: aminopeptidase; SI: sucrase isomaltase; SGLT1: sodium glucose cotransporter-1.

Table 1. Cecum-to-body weight ratio (%). Values are means ± SEM, $n = 12$. [a,b] Treatment groups not indicated by the same letter are significantly different ($p < 0.05$).

Treatment Group	Cecum/Body Weight Ratio (%)
5% Stachyose	1.67 ± 0.21 [a]
10% Stachyose	1.63 ± 0.18 [a]
5% Raffinose	1.83 ± 0.20 [a]
10% Raffinose	1.55 ± 0.13 [a]
18ΩH_2O	1.35 ± 0.08 [b]
Non-injected	1.22 ± 0.07 [b]

Table 2. Effect of intra-amniotic administration of experimental solutions on the duodenal small intestinal villus surface area (mm^2) and goblet cells diameter (μm). Values are means ± SEM, $n = 6$. [a–e] Treatment groups not indicated by the same letter are significantly different ($p < 0.05$).

Treatment Group	Villus Surface Area (mm^2)	Goblet Cell Diameter (μm)
5% Stachyose	459.2 ± 32.09 [a,b]	18.2 ± 0.143 [c]
10% Stachyose	493.8 ± 10.31 [a]	19.1 ± 0.152 [b]
5% Raffinose	467.5 ± 35.55 [a,b]	22.5 ± 0.180 [a]
10% Raffinose	425.2 ± 24.04 [b,c]	19.5 ± 0.156 [b]
18ΩH_2O	384.4 ± 14.16 [c]	15.4 ± 0.123 [d]
Non-injected	353.1 ± 13.24 [c]	13.2 ± 0.105 [e]

Table 3. Liver Ferritin protein amounts (AU) and blood hemoglobin (Hb) concentrations (g/dL). Values are means ± SEM, $n = 10$. [a] Treatment groups not indicated by the same letter are significantly different ($p < 0.05$).

Treatment Group	Ferritin (AU)	Hb (g/dL)
5% Stachyose	0.48 ± 0.09 [a]	10.7 ± 0.54 [a]
10% Stachyose	0.48 ± 0.08 [a]	11.1 ± 0.55 [a]
5% Raffinose	0.47 ± 0.10 [a]	10.5 ± 0.68 [a]
10% Raffinose	0.48 ± 0.09 [a]	11.0 ± 0.56 [a]
18ΩH_2O	0.47 ± 0.09 [a]	10.4 ± 0.42 [a]
Non-injected	0.47 ± 0.07 [a]	10.3 ± 0.65 [a]

4. Discussion

This study utilized the *Gallus gallus* model, as it is a fast growing animal with relatively high mineral requirements, and hence can develop deficiency considerably quickly [13]. Previous studies have shown that intra-amniotic administration is useful for investigating the effects of specific nutrients at particular stages of intestinal development [16,17,24]. According to Ludwiczek et al., intracellular Fe concentrations play a role in regulating Fe absorption into the enterocytes and are beneficial to bacteria within the cecum [25].

There was an increased abundance of both *Lactobacillus* ($p < 0.05$) and *Bifidobacterium* ($p < 0.05$), and a decrease in *Clostridium* in the cecal contents of the birds that received the prebiotic treatments. However, there were no significant differences for *E. coli* between the groups ($p > 0.05$), and likewise a lack of significant differences within and between the raffinose and stachyose groups ($p > 0.05$) of same bacterial species (Figure 1). As previously mentioned, *Lactobacillus* and *Bifidobacterium* are known probiotics, whereas *Clostridium* is a potentially pathogenic genus and *E. coli* can be either pathogenic or beneficial, depending on the strain [20,26,27]. *Lactobacillus* and *Bifidobacterium* both produce short chain fatty acids (SCFA), potentially increasing Fe bioavailability and reducing the abundance of pathogenic bacteria that utilize dietary Fe in the colon [28,29]. Other prebiotic compounds such as inulin have been shown to enhance the proliferation of selected beneficial colonic microflora [26,30]. *Bifidobacterium* and *Lactobacillus* have an advantage over other intestinal microorganisms due to their β-1,2-glycosidase activity that allows them to break down prebiotics, resulting in their proliferation and possibly leading to greater SCFA production [18–20]. Therefore, it is reasonable to suspect that the intra-amniotic administration of stachyose and raffinose may improve Fe status by inducing a more efficient Fe uptake and intestinal transferring. In addition to the more efficient Fe uptake, the cecum-to-bodyweight ratios were higher in the prebiotic treatment groups versus the control groups ($p < 0.05$), indicating that the cecal content of chickens that received intra-amniotic prebiotic solutions was greater than those that did not. This observation is used as an indicator for a potential increase in cecal bacterial populations (Table 1) [12].

In addition, the expressions of duodenal (the major Fe absorption site) Fe metabolism-related proteins (DMT1, the major Fe intestinal transporter; DcytB, Fe reductase; and Ferroportin, the major intestinal enterocyte Fe exporter), was decreased in treatment groups receiving the raffinose and stachyose solutions versus controls ($p < 0.05$) (Figure 2). These results are comparable to those of a previous study conducted on late-term broiler embryos and hatchlings, in which treatment groups with improved Fe status expressed significantly less Fe-related proteins [31]. The results suggest that the increased Fe bioavailability led to Fe-sufficient conditions, meaning an increase in Fe metabolism-related transporters and enzymes were not required (as a compensatory mechanism). Furthermore, there was no significant differences ($p > 0.05$) between the two raffinose administered groups in DMT1 and ferroportin; whereas DcytB actually showed a significant decrease ($p < 0.05$) in the 10% versus 5% raffinose (Figure 2). One reasonable explanation is that SCFA produced from bacteria increases Fe^{3+} solubility, resulting in more bioavailable Fe that led to the decreased DcytB expression [16].

The significant increase in the expression of the BBM functionality genes (AP, SI, SGLT1, $p < 0.05$) is in agreement with the morphometric measurements, indicating that intra-amniotic administration of raffinose and stachyose improved BBM functionality and potentially enhanced the absorptive and digestive capacity of the villi (Table 2). As is evident in the current study, it was previously suggested that dietary prebiotics increase probiotics' butyrate production, which may lead to cellular (enterocyte) proliferation. It was also demonstrated that birds that received intra-amniotic administration of carbohydrates developed villi with greater surface areas compared to the untreated birds [32]. Scholz-Ahrens et al. (2007) and Preidis et al. (2012) support these results by concluding that some of their respective prebiotics increase cellular proliferation, which causes the increase in villi surface area [33,34]. Additionally, we also measured an increase in goblet cell diameter, which suggests an increased production of mucus that coats the intestinal lumen and effects bacterial composition and function [35,36].

Overall, the up-regulation of BBM functional proteins, down-regulation of Fe metabolism proteins, in addition to the increase in the relative abundance of beneficial probiotics, intestinal villi surface area, and goblet cell diameters, suggest that stachyose and raffinose are promising in their potential for improving Fe status and BBM functionality.

5. Conclusions

The current research validates the need for future studies that could incorporate these plant origin prebiotics in long-term feeding trials. The potential breeding of staple food crops such as lentils and chickpeas for increased stachyose and raffinose contents may serve as a sustainable means of combating malnutrition in developing regions, which is a strategy that has been proven effective in wheat [12]. This study served as a preliminary step to provide a greater understanding of the way that various prebiotics can alleviate dietary deficiencies.

Author Contributions: E.T. led the research conceived and designed the experiment, wrote and edited the manuscript, N.K., S.P. and Q.W. collected and analyzed the data and wrote the initial draft of the paper. J.S., C.Z. and R.G. analyzed the data. All authors critically reviewed the final draft.

Conflicts of Interest: The authors declare no conflict of interest.

Abbreviations

Fe	iron
Hb	hemoglobin
DMT1	divalent metal transporter 1
DcytB	duodenal cytochrome B
AP	amino peptidase
SI	sucrose isomaltase
SGLT-1	sodium glucose transporter 1
BBM	brush border membrane

References

1. World Health Organization. *Iron Deficiency Anemia: Assessment, Prevention and Control: A Guide for Programme Managers*; World Health Organization: Geneva, Switzerland, 2001; pp. 15–21.
2. World Health Organization. *The Global Prevalence of Anaemia in 2011*; World Health Organization: Geneva, Switzerland, 2015; pp. 3–6.
3. Pollitt, E.; Soemantri, A.G.; Yunis, F.; Scrimshaw, N.S. Cognitive effects of iron-deficiency Anaemia. *Lancet* **1985**, *325*, 158. [CrossRef]
4. Johnson, C.R.; Thavarajah, D.; Combs, G.F.; Thavarajah, P. Lentil (*Lens culinaris* L.): A prebiotic-rich whole food legume. *Food Res. Int.* **2013**, *51*, 107–113. [CrossRef]
5. Dwivedi, S.; Sahrawat, K.; Puppala, N.; Ortiz, R. Plant prebiotics and human health: Biotechnology to breed prebiotic-rich nutritious food crops. *Electron. J. Biotechnol.* **2014**, *17*, 238–245. [CrossRef]
6. Nestel, P.; Bouis, H.E.; Meenakshi, J.V.; Pfeiffer, W. Biofortification of staple food crops. *J. Nutr.* **2006**, *136*, 1064–1067. [PubMed]
7. Welch, R.M.; Graham, R.D. Breeding for micronutrients in staple food crops from a human nutrition perspective. *J. Exp. Bot.* **2004**, *55*, 353–364. [CrossRef] [PubMed]
8. Wiesinger, J.A.; Cichy, K.A.; Glahn, R.P.; Grusak, M.A.; Brick, M.A.; Thompson, H.J.; Tako, E. Demonstrating a Nutritional Advantage to the Fast-Cooking Dry Bean (*Phaseolus vulgaris* L.). *J. Agric. Food Chem.* **2016**, *64*, 8592–8603. [CrossRef] [PubMed]
9. Tako, E.; Beebe, S.E.; Reed, S.; Hart, J.J.; Glahn, R.P. Polyphenolic compounds appear to limit the nutritional benefit of biofortified higher iron black bean (*Phaseolus vulgaris* L.). *Nutr. J.* **2014**, *13*, 1. [CrossRef] [PubMed]
10. Petry, N.; Egli, I.; Zeder, C.; Walczyk, T.; Hurrell, R. Polyphenols and phytic acid contribute to the low iron bioavailability from common beans in young women. *J. Nutr.* **2010**, *140*, 1977–1982. [CrossRef] [PubMed]
11. Petry, N.; Egli, I.; Gahutu, J.B.; Tugirimana, P.L.; Boy, E.; Hurrell, R. Phytic acid concentration influences iron bioavailability from biofortified beans in Rwandese women with low iron status. *J. Nutr.* **2014**, *144*, 1681–1687. [CrossRef] [PubMed]
12. Tako, E.; Glahn, R.P.; Knez, M.; Stangoulis, J.C. The effect of wheat prebiotics on the gut bacterial population and iron status of iron deficient broiler chickens. *Nutr. J.* **2014**, *13*, 1. [CrossRef] [PubMed]
13. Tako, E.; Rutzke, M.A.; Glahn, R.P. Using the domestic chicken (*Gallus gallus*) as an in vivo model for iron bioavailability1. *Poult. Sci.* **2010**, *89*, 514–521. [CrossRef] [PubMed]
14. Tako, E.; Reed, S.M.; Budiman, J.; Hart, J.J.; Glahn, R.P. Higher iron pearl millet (*Pennisetum glaucum* L.) provides more absorbable iron that is limited by increased polyphenolic content. *Nutr. J.* **2015**, *14*, 1. [CrossRef] [PubMed]
15. Hillier, L.W.; Miller, W.; Birney, E.; Warren, W.; Hardison, R.C.; Ponting, C.P.; Bork, P.; Burt, D.W.; Groenen, M.A.M.; Delany, M.E.; et al. Sequence and comparative analysis of the chicken genome provide unique perspectives on vertebrate evolution. *Nature* **2004**, *432*, 695–716. [CrossRef] [PubMed]
16. Tako, E.; Glahn, R.P. Intra-amniotic administration and dietary inulin affect the iron status and intestinal functionality of iron-deficient broiler chickens. *Poult. Sci.* **2012**, *91*, 1361–1370. [CrossRef] [PubMed]
17. Tako, E.; Ferket, P.; Uni, Z. Changes in chicken intestinal zinc exporter mRNA expression and small intestinal functionality following intra-amniotic zinc-methionine administration. *J. Nutr. Biochem.* **2005**, *16*, 339–346. [CrossRef] [PubMed]

18. Hartono, K.; Reed, S.; Ankrah, N.A.; Glahn, R.P.; Tako, E. Alterations in gut microflora populations and brush border functionality following intra-amniotic daidzein administration. *RSC Adv.* **2015**, *5*, 6407–6412. [CrossRef]
19. Zhu, X.Y.; Zhong, T.; Pandya, Y.; Joerger, R.D. 16S rRNA-Based Analysis of Microbiota from the Cecum of Broiler Chickens. *Appl. Environ. Microbiol.* **2002**, *68*, 124–137. [CrossRef] [PubMed]
20. Tako, E.; Glahn, R.P.; Welch, R.M.; Lei, X.; Yasuda, K.; Miller, D.D. Dietary inulin affects the expression of intestinal enterocyte iron transporters, receptors and storage protein and alters the microbiota in the pig intestine. *Br. J. Nutr.* **2008**, *99*, 472–480. [CrossRef] [PubMed]
21. Passaniti, A.; Roth, T.F. Purification of chicken liver ferritin by two novel methods and structural comparison with horse spleen ferritin. *Biochem. J.* **1989**, *258*, 413–419. [CrossRef] [PubMed]
22. Mete, A.; van Zeeland, Y.R.A.; Vaandrager, A.B.; van Dijk, J.E.; Marx, J.J.M.; Dorrestein, G.M. Partial purification and characterization of ferritin from the liver and intestinal mucosa of chickens, turtledoves and mynahs. *Avian Pathol.* **2005**, *34*, 430–434. [CrossRef] [PubMed]
23. Reed, S.; Qin, X.; Ran-Ressler, R.; Brenna, J.; Glahn, R.; Tako, E. Dietary zinc deficiency affects blood linoleic acid: Dihomo-γ-linolenic acid (LA:DGLA) ratio; a sensitive physiological marker of zinc status in vivo (*Gallus gallus*). *Nutrients* **2014**, *6*, 1164–1180. [CrossRef] [PubMed]
24. Smirnov, A.; Tako, E.; Ferket, P.R.; Uni, Z. Mucin gene expression and mucin content in the chicken intestinal goblet cells are affected by in ovo feeding of carbohydrates. *Poult. Sci.* **2006**, *85*, 669–673. [CrossRef] [PubMed]
25. Ludwiczek, S.; Theurl, I.; Artner-Dworzak, E.; Chorney, M.; Weiss, G. Duodenal HFE expression and hepcidin levels determine body iron homeostasis: Modulation by genetic diversity and dietary iron availability. *J. Mol. Med.* **2004**, *82*, 373–382. [CrossRef] [PubMed]
26. Gibson, G.; Beatty, E.; Wang, X.; Cummings, J.H. Selective stimulation of Bifidobacteria in the Human Colon by Oligofructose and Inulin. *Gastroenterology* **1995**, *108*, 975–982. [CrossRef]
27. Roberfroid, M.; Van Loot, J.; Gibson, G. The bifidogenic nature of chicory inulin and its hydrolysis products. *J. Nutr.* **1998**, *128*, 11–19. [PubMed]
28. Patterson, J.K.; Lei, X.G.; Miller, D.D. The pig as an experimental model for elucidating the mechanisms governing dietary influence on mineral absorption. *Exp. Biol. Med.* **2008**, *233*, 651–664. [CrossRef] [PubMed]
29. Gibson, G.R.; Rastall, R.A. *Prebiotics: Development & Application*; John Wiley & Sons: Chichester, UK; Hoboken, NJ, USA, 2006.
30. Tzortzis, G.; Goulas, A.K.; Gibson, G.R. Synthesis of prebiotic galactooligosaccharides using whole cells of a novel strain, Bifidobacterium bifidum NCIMB 41171. *Appl. Microbiol. Biotechnol.* **2005**, *68*, 412–416. [CrossRef] [PubMed]
31. Tako, E.; Glahn, R.P. Iron status of the late term broiler (*Gallus gallus*) embryo and hatchling. *Int. J. Poul. Sci.* **2011**, *10*, 42–48. [CrossRef]
32. Tako, E.; Ferket, P.R.; Uni, Z. Effects of in ovo feeding of carbohydrates and beta-hydroxy-beta-methylbutyrate on the development of chicken intestine. *Poult. Sci.* **2004**, *83*, 2023–2028. [CrossRef] [PubMed]
33. Scholz-Ahrens, K.; Ade, P.; Marten, B.; Weber, P.; Timm, W.; Acil, Y.; Gluer, C.; Schrezenmeir, J. Prebiotics, probiotics, and synbiotics affect mineral absorption, bone mineral content, and bone structure. *J. Nutr.* **2007**, *137*, 838S–846S. [PubMed]
34. Preidis, G.A.; Saulnier, D.M.; Blutt, S.E.; Mistretta, T.-A.; Riehle, K.P.; Major, A.M.; Venable, S.F.; Finegold, M.J.; Petrosino, J.F.; Conner, M.E.; et al. Probiotics stimulate enterocyte migration and microbial diversity in the neonatal mouse intestine. *FASEB J.* **2012**, *26*, 1960–1969. [CrossRef] [PubMed]
35. Ouwehand, A.C.; Derrien, M.; de Vos, W.; Tiihonen, K.; Rautonen, N. Prebiotics and other microbial substrates for gut functionality. *Curr. Opin. Biotechnol.* **2005**, *16*, 212–217. [CrossRef] [PubMed]
36. Deplancke, B.; Gaskins, H.R. Microbial modulation of innate defense: Goblet cells and the intestinal mucus layer. *Am. J. Clin. Nutr.* **2001**, *73*, 1131S–1141S. [PubMed]

nutrients

Article

Effects of Commercial Apple Varieties on Human Gut Microbiota Composition and Metabolic Output Using an In Vitro Colonic Model

Athanasios Koutsos [1,2,*], Maria Lima [2], Lorenza Conterno [2], Mattia Gasperotti [3], Martina Bianchi [2], Francesca Fava [2], Urska Vrhovsek [3], Julie A. Lovegrove [1] and Kieran M. Tuohy [2]

1 Hugh Sinclair Unit of Human Nutrition and the Institute for Cardiovascular and Metabolic Research (ICMR), Department of Food and Nutritional Sciences, University of Reading, Whiteknights, P.O. Box 226, Reading RG6 6AP, UK; j.a.lovegrove@reading.ac.uk
2 Nutrition & Nutrigenomics Unit, Department of Food Quality and Nutrition, Research and Innovation Centre, Fondazione Edmund Mach (FEM), Via Mach 1, 38010 San Michele all'Adige, TN, Italy; Lima80in@yahoo.co.in (M.L.); lorenza.conterno@oliocru.it (L.C.); martina.bianchi.1@gmail.com (M.B.); francesca.fava@fmach.it (F.F.); kieran.tuohy@fmach.it (K.M.T.)
3 Metabolomics Unit, Department of Food Quality and Nutrition, Research and Innovation Centre, Fondazione Edmund Mach (FEM), Via Mach 1, 38010 San Michele all'Adige, TN, Italy; mattiagasperotti84@gmail.com (M.G.); urska.vrhovsek@fmach.it (U.V.)
* Correspondence: athanasios.koutsos@reading.ac.uk; Tel.: +44-118-378-7713

Received: 6 February 2017; Accepted: 15 May 2017; Published: 24 May 2017

Abstract: Apples are a rich source of polyphenols and fiber. A major proportion of apple polyphenols escape absorption in the small intestine and together with non-digestible polysaccharides reach the colon, where they can serve as substrates for bacterial fermentation. Animal studies suggest a synergistic interaction between apple polyphenols and the soluble fiber pectin; however, the effects of whole apples on human gut microbiota are less extensively studied. Three commercial apple varieties—Renetta Canada, Golden Delicious and Pink Lady—were digested and fermented in vitro using a batch culture colonic model (pH 5.5–6.0, 37 °C) inoculated with feces from three healthy donors. Inulin and cellulose were used as a readily and a poorly fermentable plant fiber, respectively. Fecal microbiota composition was measured by 16S rRNA gene Illumina MiSeq sequencing (V3-V4 region) and Fluorescence in Situ Hybridization. Short chain fatty acids (SCFAs) and polyphenol microbial metabolites were determined. The three apple varieties significantly changed bacterial diversity, increased Actinobacteria relative abundance, acetate, propionate and total SCFAs ($p < 0.05$). Renetta Canada and Golden Delicious significantly decreased Bacteroidetes abundance and increased Proteobacteria proportion and bifidobacteria population ($p < 0.05$). Renetta Canada also increased *Faecalibacterium prausnitzii*, butyrate levels and polyphenol microbial metabolites ($p < 0.05$). Together, these data suggest that apples, particularly Renetta Canada, can induce substantial changes in microbiota composition and metabolic activity in vitro, which could be associated with potential benefits to human health. Human intervention studies are necessary to confirm these data and potential beneficial effects.

Keywords: apples; polyphenols; proanthocyanidins; fiber; pectin; gut microbiota; in vitro batch culture fermentation; microbial metabolites; Illumina 16S rRNA gene sequencing; Fluorescence in situ hybridization (FISH)

1. Introduction

Evidence suggests that plant-derived dietary polyphenols and fiber possess health-promoting properties [1]. Apples are among the most popular and frequently consumed fruits in the world and a rich source of both polyphenols and fiber [2]. Epidemiological and dietary intervention studies suggest that frequent apple consumption is associated with a reduced risk of chronic pathologies such as cardiovascular disease, obesity and cancer [2,3]. However, up to 90–95% of dietary polyphenols are not absorbed in the small intestine [4] and together with non-digestible polysaccharides from apples reach the colon almost intact, where they can interact with the gut microbiota [2]. This interaction is reciprocal. Firstly, polyphenols and fiber undergo an extensive microbial bioconversion producing phenolic acids and short chain fatty acids (SCFAs), respectively, well-known to have positive health effects [5]. Secondly, polyphenols, fiber and/or their metabolic products modulate the gut microbiota composition by inhibiting pathogenic bacteria and stimulating beneficial bacteria, therefore acting as potential prebiotics [5].

Dietary fiber constituents in apples include insoluble fiber, mainly cellulose and hemicellulose and soluble fiber, mainly pectin. In vitro studies, using human fecal inoculum, have shown that pectin is fermented to SCFAs (acetate, propionate and butyrate) by several intestinal bacteria genera including *Bacteroides*, eubacteria, clostridia and bifidobacteria [6,7]. However, a recent study suggested a high selectivity at the species level [8]. Apples also contain a variety of polyphenols including dihydrochalcones, flavonols, hydroxycinnamates and flavanols (catechin and proanthocyanidins (PAs)) [9]. PAs, the major polyphenolic class in apples, also known as condensed tannins, are oligomers and polymers of flavanols and the most likely to reach the colon [2]. In an in vitro study, apple PAs have been shown to be converted to polyphenol microbial metabolites, mainly phenylpropionic, phenylacetic and benzoic acid derivatives. [10]. The study also reported reduced saccharolytic fermentation, suggesting potential antimicrobial properties of PAs. However, the specific bacteria composition was not explored [10].

In vivo, extraction juices from apple pomace, rich in polyphenols and fiber, have been shown to increase *Lactobacillus*, *Bifidobacterium*, *Bacteroidaceae* species, *Eubacterium rectale* cluster as well as SCFAs in rats [11,12]. Licht et al. (2010) [13] considered pectin, among apple components, responsible for a decrease in *Bacteroides* spp. and an increase in *Clostridium coccoides* and butyrate in rats [13]. Likewise, apple pectin restored the Firmicutes/Bacteroidetes ratio to normal in obesity-induced rats [14]. Decreased Firmicutes/Bacteroidetes ratio was similarly seen in mice with the administration of apple PAs, which also increased the proportion of *Akkermansia* [15]. However, a rat cecum fermentation showed that apple polyphenols and pectin are more effective in combination implying a synergistic effect [16]. Data available from human studies are still limited [2]. In a small scale trial of eight people, two apples per day for two weeks significantly increased bifidobacteria while reducing *Enterobacteriaceae* and lecithinace-positive clostridia, including *C. perfringens* [17]. In a more recent four-week study of 23 healthy subjects, whole apple and pomace intake lowered fecal pH but there were no changes in gut microbiota composition [18].

Thus, to date, the effects of apple components on gut microbiota have been explored mainly in animals and using extracted juices [11,12], PAs [15] or pectin [14] alone. There are no in vitro studies investigating the effects of whole apples using human fecal inoculum and only recently studies with apple components have focused on the entire gut community instead of targeted taxa [13,15]. The aim of the current work was to assess the effect of three commercial apple varieties—Renetta Canada, Golden Delicious and Pink Lady—on human gut microbiota composition and metabolic activity in vitro, compared to inulin (a prebiotic) and cellulose (poorly fermented). Illumina 16S rRNA sequencing was used to provide a broad picture of the microbial community architecture. Bacteria of specific interest (i.e., bifidobacteria and *Faecalibacterium prausnitzii*) were enumerated using the quantitative 16S rRNA probe based method, FISH. The production of SCFAs (acetate, propionate and butyrate) was also measured. Finally, disappearance of apple polyphenols and formation of microbial-derived metabolites were monitored throughout the fermentation using a targeted LC-MS based metabolomics approach.

2. Materials and Methods

2.1. Fecal Donors

Fecal donors, two males and one female, were in good health and aged between 30 and 50. They had not received antibiotic treatment for at least 3 months prior to stool collection, had not knowingly consumed pre- or probiotic supplements prior to experiment, and had no history of bowel disorders. The three healthy donors were informed of the study aims and procedures and provided their verbal consent for their fecal matter to be used for the experiments, in compliance with the ethics procedures required at the University of Reading and Fondazione Edmund Mach.

2.2. Materials

Enzymes for the apples digestion and chemicals for the batch culture basal nutrient medium were purchased from Sigma-Aldrich (St. Louis, MO, USA) and Applichem (Darmstadt, Germany), unless otherwise stated. For the chemical standards of polyphenols and microbial metabolites as well as the LC-MS reagents more information can be found in Vrhovsek et al. (2012) [19] and Gasperotti et al. (2014) [20].

2.3. Apples and Controls

The three commercial apple varieties, Renetta Canada, Golden Delicious and Pink Lady were purchased from a local shop in the Trentino region in north Italy. The apples' macronutrient composition was analyzed by Campden BRI laboratories, UK, whereas the detailed polyphenol content was measured in our laboratory in Fondazione Edmund Mach based on Vrhovsek et al. (2012) [19]. Inulin (from dahlia tubers) and cellulose were used as a readily and a poorly fermentable plant fiber, respectively.

2.4. Preparation of Phospholipid Vesicles

A protocol was followed according to Mandalari et al. (2008) [21], with some modifications, for the preparation of the phospholipid vesicles and the simulation of the in vitro gastric and duodenal digestion as described below. Egg L-α-phosphatidylcholine (PC, lecithin grade 1, 99% purity, Lipid Products, Surrey, UK), 6.5 mL of a stock solution (127 mmol/L in chloroform/methanol), was placed into a round-bottom flask, and dried under rotary evaporation to make a thin phospholipid film. The lipid film was further dried overnight under vacuum to remove any remaining solvent. Then, it was hydrated with the addition of 170 mL of warm saline (150 mmol/L NaCl, pH 2.5, at 37 °C). The flask was flushed with argon to prevent oxidation and was placed in an orbital shaker (170 rpm, 37 °C) for 30 min together with five 2 mm diameter glass beads. A PC nanoemulsion was then produced using a Branson Ultrasonics sonifier S-450 (Branson Ultrasonics, Danbury, CT, USA) equipped with a 13 mm titanium horn (30% of amplitude). The temperature of the liquid kept below 60 °C with ice.

2.5. In Vitro Gastric and Duodenal Digestion

A ratio of 4 g of apples for 12.4 mL gastric phase volume (acidic saline) considered appropriate after preliminary experiments and according to Mandalari et al. (2008) [21]. Initially, 96 g of each apple variety were grated with their skin and added to 146 mL of the sonicated and filtrated PC vesicle suspension. The pH was adjusted to 2.5 using HCl and acidic saline (150 mmol/L NaCl, pH 2.5) was added to a total volume of 298 mL. Then, the PC vesicle suspension together with gastric pepsin and lipase were added so that the final concentrations were 2.4 mmol/L, 146 units/mL and 60 units/mL, respectively. The digestion was performed in an orbital shaker (170 rpm, 37 °C) for 2 h. The in vitro gastric digestion was followed by duodenal digestion. The pH was raised to 6.5 using NaOH and the following were added: 4 mmol/L sodium taurocholate, 4 mmol/L sodium glycodeoxycholate,

11.7 mmol/L $CaCl_2$, 0.73 mmol/L Bis-Tris buffer (pH 6.5), 5.9 units/mL α-chymotrypsin, 104 units/mL trypsin, 3.2 μg/mL colipase, 54 units/mL pancreatic lipase and 25 units/mL alpha-amylase. The total volume of 340 mL was reached by the addition of saline (150 mmol/L NaCl, pH 6.5) and the final PC concentration was 2.1 mmol/L. The duodenal digestion was performed for 1 h in the shaking incubator (170 rpm, 37 °C). Then, samples were transferred to 1 kDa MWCO (molecular weight cut off) cellulose dialysis tubing (Spectra/Por® 6, Spectrum Europe, Breda, Netherlands) and dialyzed overnight against NaCl (10 mmol/L) at 4 °C to remove low molecular mass digestion products. The dialysis fluid was changed and dialysis continued for an additional 2 h. Finally, apples were frozen at −20 °C and then freeze-dried until use. Inulin and cellulose (19.2 g each, equivalent with the dry content of 96 g of apples) were also digested and dialyzed using the same protocol.

2.6. Fecal Batch-Culture Fermentation and Samples Collection

The fermentation profile of the three commercial apples, the prebiotic inulin and the poorly fermented cellulose was determined using anaerobic, stirred, pH and temperature controlled fecal batch cultures. Glass water-jacketed vessels (300 mL) were sterilized and filled aseptically with 180 mL of pre-sterilized basal nutrient medium according to Sanchez-Patan et al. 2012 [22]. The pH was adjusted to 5.5–6.0 and kept between this range throughout the experiment with the automatic addition of NaOH or HCI (0.5 M), to mimic the conditions located in the proximal region of the human large intestine. The medium was then gassed overnight with oxygen free nitrogen to maintain anaerobic conditions. The following day and before the inoculation, each of the 5 vessels was dosed with 2 g of the appropriate substrate/treatment (inulin, cellulose, Renetta Canada, Golden Delicious or Pink Lady) for a final concentration of 1% (*w*/*v*). Fresh human fecal samples were collected in an anaerobic jar and were processed within 1 h. Fecal slurry was prepared by homogenizing the feces in pre-reduced phosphate buffered saline (PBS). The temperature was set to 37 °C using a circulating water-bath and the vessels were inoculated with 20 mL fecal slurry (10% *w*/*v* of fresh human feces) to a final concentration of 1% (*w*/*v*). Batch cultures were run under these controlled conditions for a period of 24 h, during which samples were collected at 4 time points (0, 5, 10 and 24 h) for FISH, SCFA, precursors polyphenols and polyphenol microbial metabolites. Pellets were stored at −80 °C for DNA extraction. Fermentations were conducted in triplicate using three healthy fecal donors.

2.7. DNA Extraction, Amplification and Sequencing

DNA was extracted from each sample (available for 0, 10 and 24 h time points) using the FastDNA Spin Kit for Feces (MP Biomedicals, UK). Nucleic acid purity was tested on NanoDropTM 8000 Spectrophotometer (Thermo Fisher Scientific). Total genomic DNA was then subjected to PCR amplification by targeting a ~460-bp fragment of the 16S rRNA variable region V3-V4 using the specific bacterial primer set 341F (5′ CCTACGGGNGGCWGCAG 3′) and 806R (5′ GACTACNVGGGTWTCTAATCC 3′) with overhang Illumina adapters. PCR amplification of each sample was carried out using 25 μL reactions with 1 μM of each primer, following the Illumina Metagenomic Sequencing Library Preparation Protocol for 16S Ribosomal RNA Gene Amplicons. The PCR products were checked on 1.5% agarose gel and cleaned from free primers and primer dimer using the Agencourt AMPure XP system (Beckman Coulter, Brea, CA, USA) following the manufacturer's instructions. Subsequently dual indices and Illumina sequencing adapters Nextera XT Index Primer (Illumina) were attached by 7 cycles PCR (16S Metagenomic Sequencing Library Preparation, Illumina). The final libraries, after purification by the Agencourt AMPure XP system (Beckman), were analyzed on a Typestation 2200 platform (Agilent Technologies, Santa Clara, CA, USA) and quantified using the Quant-IT PicoGreen dsDNA assay kit (Thermo Fisher Scientific) by the Synergy2 microplate reader (Biotek). Finally, all the libraries were pooled in an equimolar way in a final amplicon library and analyzed on a Typestation 2200 platform (Agilent Technologies, Santa Clara, CA, USA). Barcoded library was sequenced on an Illumina® MiSeq (PE300) platform

(MiSeq Control Software 2.0.5 (Illumina, San Diego, CA, USA) and Real-Time Analysis software 1.16.18 (Illumina, San Diego, CA, USA)).

2.8. Sequence Data Analysis

Demultiplexed sequences were further processed using the Quantitative Insight Into Microbial Ecology (QIIME) open-source software package [23] using the following workflow: Forward and reverse Illumina reads (300 bp each) were joined using the fastq-join method [24], quality filtering was performed using 19 as the minimum Phred quality score and chimeric sequences were identified and removed using usearch 6.1. Then, sequences were assigned to operational taxonomic units (OTUs) using the QIIME implementation of UCLUST algorithm at 97% similarity threshold [25]. Representative sequences for each OTU were assigned to different bacterial taxonomic levels -phylum (p.), class (c.), order (o.), family (f.) and genus (g.)—by using Greengenes database release (May 2013).

The number of sequences collected that fulfilled quality control requirements (Phred quality score $\geq$20) yielded 1,647,935 (Sequence length mean $\pm$ SD, 450 $\pm$ 12). After removing chimeric sequences, a total of 1,621,799 reads remained, meaning that the used usearch61 algorithm reduced the dataset by approximately 1.6%. Using 97% as a homology cutoff value 4530 species-level OTUs were identified. For alpha and beta diversity tests all samples were subsampled to an equal number of reads (11,708 reads per sample which constitutes to 90% of the most indigent sample in the dataset). For further downstream analysis, the dataset was filtered to consider only those OTUs that were present in all samples at a relative abundance >0.005% (486 OTUs).

2.9. Enumeration of Bacterial Groups with Fluorescence In Situ Hybridization (FISH)

Changes in bacterial populations were determined using genus- and group-specific 16S rRNA gene-targeted oligonucleotide probes, labeled with Cy3 fluorescent dye, applying the FISH method [22]. The used oligonucleotide probes were: Bif164 specific for the *Bifidobacterium* spp. [26] and Fpra655 specific for the *Faecalibacterium prausnitzii* genus [27]. For total bacterial cell stain, the fixing of the samples onto the Teflon slides was performed as normal and the slides were incubated for 10 minutes in 50 mL of PBS with the addition of 50 µL of SYBR Green to a final concentration of 1:1000 [28].

2.10. Analysis of Short Chain Fatty Acids (SCFAs)

Analysis of SCFAs was performed using the method by Zhao et al. (2006) [29] with slight modifications. Briefly, 1 mL aliquots of 10% (w/v) fecal suspension in sterile 1 M PBS (pH 7.2) were dispensed into 1.5 mL tubes and centrifuged at 13,000$\times$ g for 5 min to pellet bacteria and other solids. Supernatants were then transferred into clean 1.5 mL tubes and frozen at 20 °C until required. On the day of the analysis samples were defrosted on ice and acidified to pH 2–3 by the addition of one volume of 6 M HCl to three volumes of sample. After 10 min incubation at room temperature, samples were centrifuged at 13,000$\times$ g for 5 min and filtered using a 0.2 µm polycarbonate syringe. One volume of 10 mM 2-ethylbutyirc acid was added to four volumes of sample as the internal standard. Calibration was done using standard solutions of acetic acid, propionic acid, i-butyric acid and n-butyric acid (Sigma-Aldrich, Schnelldorf, Germany) in acidified water (pH 2). SCFAs were determined by gas-liquid chromatography coupled with mass spectrometry on a Thermo Trace GC Ultra (Thermo Fisher Scientific, Austin, TX, USA) fitted with a FFAP column (Restek Stabilwax-DA; 30 m $\times$ 0.25 mm; 0.25 µm fth) and a flame-ionization detector. Peaks were integrated using Thermo Scientific Xcalibur data system (Thermo Fisher Scientific, Austin, TX, USA). All SCFAs showed a linear range between at least 0.5–20 mM with a coefficient of linearity $R^2 > 0.999$. LOD and LOQ were below 0.5 mM.

2.11. Analysis of Precursor Polyphenols and Polyphenol Microbial Metabolites

The determination of precursor polyphenols was performed according to Vrhovsek et al. (2012) [19] whereas the polyphenol microbial metabolites according to Gasperotti et al. (2014) [20].

Briefly, a previously developed targeted metabolomic method was performed with an ultra-performance liquid chromatographic system coupled to tandem mass spectrometry system with electrospray ionization (UHPLC-ESI-MS/MS). Before injection, batch culture supernatants were defrosted, centrifuged (13,000 rpm, 5 min), filtered (0.22 µm) and trans-cinnamic acid-d5 (5 µg/mL) was added as the first internal standard. Then, samples were dried under nitrogen and reconstituted in methanol:water (1:1, *v*/*v*) containing rosmarinic acid (1 µg/mL) as the second internal standard. Samples were finally shaken for 10 min in an orbital shaker, centrifuged for 5 min at 16,000 rpm and injected (2 µL) into the UHPLC–MS/MS system. Data processing was performed using Waters MassLynx 4.1 (Waters, Milford, CT, USA) and TargetLynx software (Waters, Milford, CT, USA). Details of the liquid chromatography and mass spectrometry are described in Vrhovsek et al. (2012) [19] and Gasperotti et al. (2014) [20].

2.12. Statistical Analysis

For the sequencing data analysis, the QIIME pipeline version 1.9.1 [23] was used. Within community diversity (alpha diversity) was calculated using observed OTUs, Chao1 and Shannon indexes with 10 sampling repetitions at each sampling depth. Analysis of similarity (ANOSIM) and the ADONIS test were used to determine statistical differences between samples (beta diversity) following the QIIME compare_categories.py script and using weighted and unweighted phylogenetic UniFrac distance matrices. Principal Coordinate Analysis (PCoA) plots were generated using the QIIME beta diversity plots workflow. The biplot function was used to visualize samples and taxa in the PCoA space. For the rest of the data analysis the SPSS IBM version 21 (SPSS Inc., Chicago, IL, USA) was used. One-way ANOVA was used to determine differences between fermentation treatments (inulin, cellulose, Renetta Canada, Golden Delicious and Pink Lady) at the same time point (0, 5, 10 or 24 h), followed by the least significant difference (LSD) *post hoc* test. A repeated measures ANOVA was used to explore the differences within the same treatment/vessel (inulin, cellulose, Renetta Canada, Golden Delicious or Pink Lady) with all the time points (0, 5, 10 and 24 h) as within factor and with LSD as the *post hoc* test. In addition to these analyses, the p values were corrected using false discovery rate (FDR) to account for multiple testing at the lower bacterial taxonomical level (67 taxa). $p \leq 0.05$ was considered statistically significant.

3. Results

3.1. Composition of Apples

The fiber and polyphenol content of the three fresh apples is shown in Table 1 (detailed nutrient composition analysis is presented in the Supplementary File, Table S1). Renetta Canada had the highest total polyphenol content (276 mg/100 g) followed by Golden Delicious (132 mg/100 g) and Pink Lady (94 mg/100 g). The total fiber content was similar among the apple varieties (Table 1).

Table 1. Composition analysis of Renetta Canada, Golden Delicious and Pink Lady *.

Components	Renetta Canada	Golden Delicious	Pink Lady
Total dietary fiber (AOAC) (g/100 g)	2.6	2.4	2.4
Soluble fiber (AOAC) (g/100 g)	1.6	1.3	0.9
Insoluble fiber (AOAC) (g/100 g)	1.0	1.1	1.5
Polyphenols (mg/100 g)			
Flavanols			
(+)—Catechin	1.07	0.16	0.17
(−)—Epicatechin	10.9	2.8	2.8
Procyanidin B1	6.6	0.95	0.78
Procyanidin B2 + B4 (as B2)	18.3	6.1	4.8
Proanthocyanidin (as cyanidin)	169.2	91.5	62.1

Table 1. *Cont.*

Components	Renetta Canada	Golden Delicious	Pink Lady
Hydroxycinnamates			
Chlorogenic acid	61	18.7	17.5
Neochlorogenic acid	0.04	0.04	0.01
Cryptochlorogenic acid	0.98	0.67	0.15
Flavonols			
Quercetin-3-glucoside	0.99	6.9	3.1
Quercetin-3-rhamnoside	0.65	2.7	1.7
Rutin	0.09	0.44	0.19
Kaempferol-3-rutinoside	0.002	0.011	0.002
Isorhamnetin-3-glucoside	0.001	0.002	0.001
Dihydrochalcones			
Phlorizin	5.9	1.5	0.8
Anthocyanins			
Cyanidin 3-galactoside	0.006	0.017	0.027
Benzoic Acid Derivatives			
Vanillin	0.008	0.006	0.003
Vanillic acid	0.001	0.003	0.002

* For each apple variety a mixture of three fresh whole apples was analyzed.

3.2. Changes in Fecal Bacterial Alpha and Beta Diversity

The diversity of gut microbiota within a community was measured with alpha diversity indices (within-sample richness), in particular the number of observed OTUs, the Chao1 estimator of species richness and the Shannon entropy and these are shown in Figure 1. At 0 h there were no differences between the treatments. At 10 h the observed OTUs, species richness (Chao1) as well as Shannon entropy were significantly lower with all the apple treatments compared to inulin or cellulose. At 24 h the same statistical differences as the 10 h time point were shown for the observed OTUs and species richness, with the exception of Shannon entropy, where Renetta Canada and inulin had lower values compared to the other apples or cellulose ($p < 0.05$). All alpha diversity indices decreased over time within every treatment throughout the fermentation ($p < 0.05$).

When the bacterial diversity between samples (for all the data set) was examined (beta diversity) a clustering was shown according to fecal donor (ANOSIM and ADONIS test, $p = 0.01$ and $p = 0.001$ ($R^2 = 34\%$), respectively) (Figure 2) and time point (ANOSIM and ADONIS test, $p = 0.01$ and $p = 0.001$ ($R^2 = 11\%$), respectively) (Figure S1), as demonstrated with principal coordinate analysis (PCoA) based on an unweighted (qualitative) phylogenetic UniFrac distance matrix. The clustering was less distinct but still significant according to donor (ANOSIM and ADONIS test, $p = 0.01$ and $p = 0.001$ ($R^2 = 29\%$), respectively) and time (ANOSIM and ADONIS test, $p = 0.01$ and $p = 0.001$ ($R^2 = 30\%$), respectively) when based on a weighted (quantitative) phylogenetic UniFrac distance matrix (Figure 2 and Figure S1, respectively). There was no significant effect of treatment on beta diversity for all the data set together (all time points and donors), ANOSIM test, $p = 0.81$ and $p = 0.59$ and ADONIS test, $p = 0.95$, $R^2 = 7\%$ and $p = 0.55$, $R^2 = 8.5\%$, according to an unweighted and a weighted UniFrac distance matrix, respectively (Figure S2). The 6 core genera which influenced overall variance the most in the samples were *Bacteroides, Bifidobacterium, Megamonas, Ruminococcaceae* unassigned genus, *Lachnospiraceae* unassigned *genus and Faecalibacterium* (Figure 2, Figures S1 and S2).

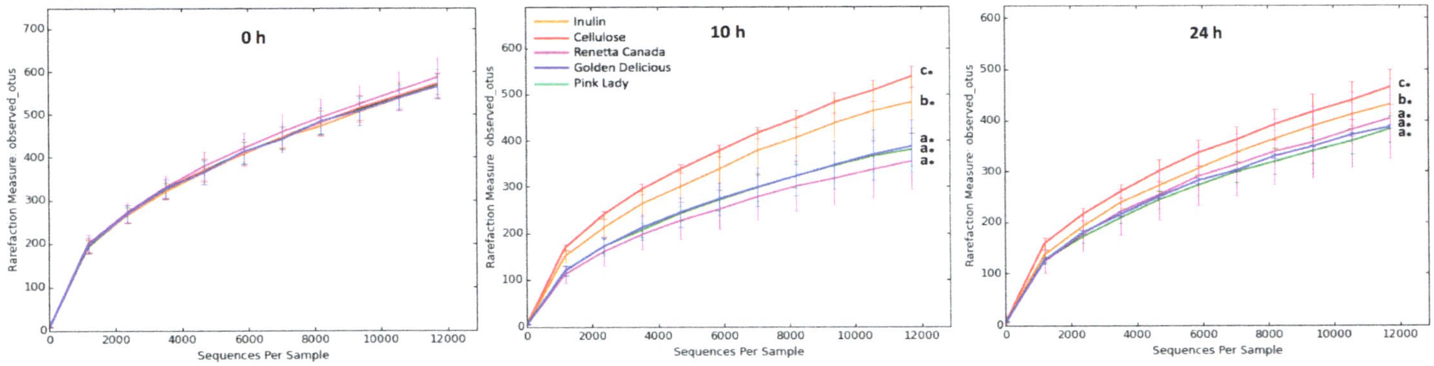

Treatment	Chao1 (0 h)	Shannon (0 h)	Chao1 (10 h)	Shannon (10 h)	Chao1 (24 h)	Shannon (24 h)
Inulin	1076 ± 43	6.36 ± 0.36	931 ± 91 ^{b,*}	5.32 ± 0.53 ^{b,*}	811 ± 37 ^{b,*}	4.88 ± 0.32 ^{a*}
Cellulose	1091 ± 26	6.39 ± 0.43	1030 ± 66 ^{c,*}	5.99 ± 0.27 ^{c,*}	849 ± 89 ^{c,*}	5.72 ± 0.29 ^{c,*}
Renetta Canada	1124 ± 84	6.49 ± 0.28	673 ± 113 ^{a,*}	4.28 ± 0.71 ^{a,*}	774 ± 135 ^{a,*}	4.78 ± 0.63 ^{a,*}
Golden Delicious	1064 ± 46	6.35 ± 0.41	724 ± 125 ^{a,*}	4.57 ± 0.64 ^{a,*}	737 ± 31 ^{a,*}	5.20 ± 0.07 ^{b,*}
Pink Lady	1115 ± 67	6.47 ± 0.27	748 ± 69 ^{a,*}	4.63 ± 0.66 ^{a,*}	769 ± 48 ^{a,*}	5.14 ± 0.47 ^{b,*}

Figure 1. Alpha diversity (within-sample richness) rarefaction curves based on the observed number of Operational Taxonomic Units, OTUs (image), average Chao1 and Shannon indexes (±SEM) in 24-h in vitro batch culture fermentations inoculated with human feces ($n = 3$ healthy donors) and administrated with inulin, cellulose, Renetta Canada, Golden Delicious and Pink Lady as the substrates (treatments). Samples were analyzed at 0, 10 and 24 h. Ten sampling repetitions were calculated at an even sampling depth of 11708 sequences. Significant differences ($p < 0.05$) between treatments at the same time point are indicated with different letters. * Significant differences ($p < 0.05$) from the 0 h time point within the same treatment.

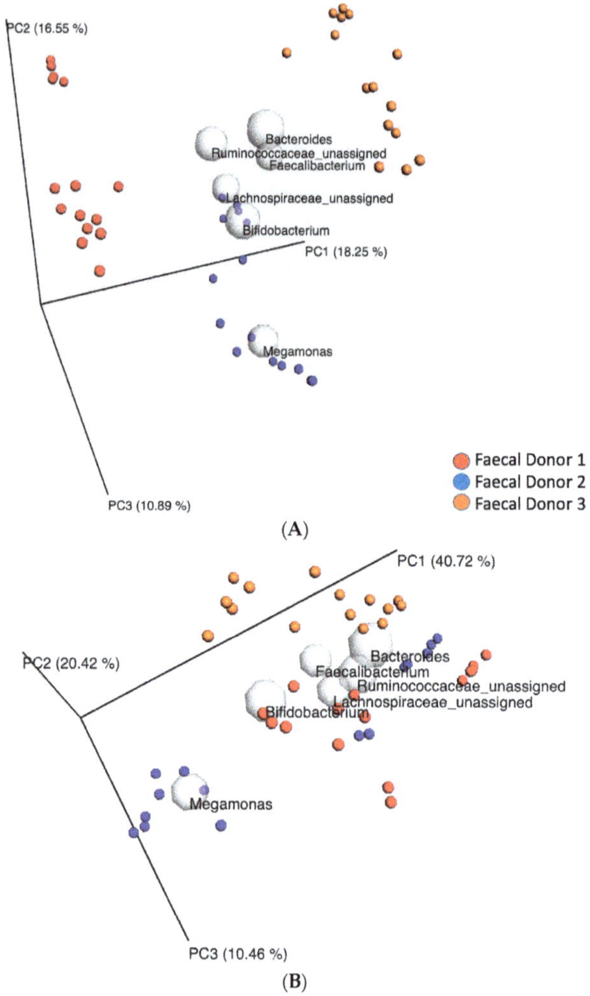

Figure 2. Principal coordinate analysis (PCoA) plots of 16S rRNA gene profiles based on (**A**) unweighted (qualitative) and (**B**) weighted (quantitative) phylogenetic UniFrac distance matrices calculated from a rarefied OTU table (11708 reads per sample) showing a clustering between donors (ANOSIM and ADONIS test, p = 0.01 and p = 0.001, respectively) for the whole data set (24-h in vitro batch culture fermentations inoculated with human feces (n = 3 healthy donors) and administrated with inulin, cellulose, Renetta Canada, Golden Delicious and Pink Lady as the substrates/treatments). Samples were analyzed at 0, 10 and 24 h. Each color represents a different donor. The gray spherical coordinates indicate taxonomic vectors of the 6 most prevalent taxa at the genus level. The size of each sphere is proportional to the mean relative abundance and approximates the causing variance throughout the plotted samples.

3.3. *Fecal Bacterial Relative Abundance at the Phylum Level*

The total sequence reads used in this study were classified into 7 phyla and one phylum was noted as unassigned. In particular, the bacterial communities, at time 0 h in all cultures, were dominated by bacteria belonging to Firmicutes (58–64%), Bacteroidetes (27–34%), Actinobacteria (5–7%) and Proteobacteria (1.5–2.0%) phylum, whereas a small percentage (0.1–0.3%) belonged to Cyanobacteria,

Lentisphaerae, Tenericutes and an unassigned phylum (Figure 3). Treatment did not have any significant effect on the relative abundance of phylum level at time 0 h and 10 h. However, at time 24 h Actinobacteria relative abundance differed significantly among all five treatments ($p = 0.017$), where supplementation with all the apple varieties led to a higher abundance compared to cellulose ($p < 0.05$). Focusing on changes over time for each treatment separately (Figure 3), Firmicutes abundance remained unaffected, whereas Bacteroidetes significantly decreased over time with inulin ($p = 0.012$), Renetta Canada ($p = 0.002$) and Golden Delicious ($p = 0.019$). Actinobacteria proportion was significantly increased over time with all the apple varieties (Renetta Canada, $p = 0.05$, Golden Delicious, $p = 0.011$ and Pink Lady, $p = 0.018$). Finally, Proteobacteria abundance was also significantly increased with cellulose ($p = 0.021$), Renetta Canada ($p = 0.012$) and Golden Delicious ($p = 0.02$) (Figure 3).

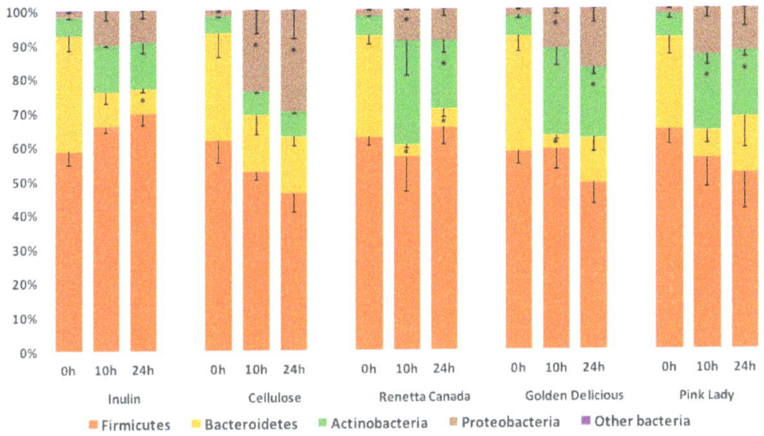

Figure 3. Changes in bacterial phyla (relative abundances (%)) throughout 24-h in vitro batch culture fermentations inoculated with human feces ($n = 3$ healthy donors) and administrated with inulin, cellulose, Renetta Canada, Golden Delicious and Pink Lady as the substrates (treatments). Samples were analyzed at 0, 10 and 24 h. Values are mean (%) with SEM (the negative error value is shown). Other bacteria represent Cyanobacteria, Lentisphaerae, Tenericutes and an unassigned phylum. * Significant differences from the 0 h time point within the same treatment ($p < 0.05$, FDR corrected).

3.4. Fecal Bacterial Relative Abundance at the Genus Level

At the lowest taxonomic level, 67 distinct bacterial taxa were detected. Of these, 46 were identified at the genus level, 15 at the family level, 5 at the order level and one was unassigned. At 0 h there were no differences between the treatments in bacterial taxa relative abundance. At 10 h, treatment had an effect on the abundance of g. *Oscillospira*, g. *Ruminococcus*, g. *Parabacteroides*, g. *Bilophila*, unassigned f. *Lachnospiraceae*, unassigned f. *Mogibacteriaceae* and unassigned and unclassified o. Clostridiales, which remained significant after the FDR correction for multiple testing for o. unassigned Clostridiales and f. *Mogibacteriaceae*, with cellulose administration showing higher proportions of these taxa compared to the other treatments (Table 2). Notably, *Bifidobacterium* g. abundance differed among all treatments at 10 h, with the highest proportion after Renetta Canada and Golden Delicious administration, however, this lost significance with FDR correction (Table 2). Significant differences, before correction, between treatments were also observed at 24 h on the relative abundance of g. *Faecalibacterium*, g. *Butyricimonas*, g. *Bifidobacterium* and unassigned o. Clostridiales. Additional details on the relative abundance of bacterial taxa at 10 and 24 h for the different treatments are shown in Table 2. Focusing on changes over time for each treatment separately, there were significant changes in the relative abundance of specific taxa however, these were not always significant after correction and presented as supplementary information (Table S2).

Table 2. Changes in bacterial taxa relative abundance (%) at 10 h and 24 h of in vitro batch culture fermentations inoculated with human feces ($n = 3$ healthy donors) and administrated with inulin, cellulose, Renetta Canada, Golden Delicious and Pink Lady as the substrates (treatments).

Phylum	Class	Order	Family	Genus	Time Point	Inulin (%)	Cellulose (%)	Renetta Canada (%)	Golden Delicious (%)	Pink Lady (%)	p *	p # (FDR-Corrected)
Firmicutes	Clostridia	Clostridiales	*Lachnospiraceae*	unassigned	10 h	4.3 ± 1.3^{a}	9 ± 0.9^{b}	2.6 ± 0.7^{a}	$5 \pm 2^{a,b}$	2.9 ± 1.2^{a}	0.040	0.336
Firmicutes	Clostridia	Clostridiales	[*Mogibacteriaceae*]	unassigned	10 h	0.15 ± 0.01^{b}	0.14 ± 0.01^{b}	0.08 ± 0.02^{a}	0.05 ± 0.01^{a}	0.06 ± 0.01^{a}	0.001	0.040
Firmicutes	Clostridia	Clostridiales	*Ruminococcaceae*	*Oscillospira*	10 h	0.66 ± 0.1^{b}	1 ± 0.1^{c}	0.32 ± 0.03^{a}	0.3 ± 0.1^{a}	0.23 ± 0.07^{a}	0.001	0.052
Firmicutes	Clostridia	Clostridiales	*Ruminococcaceae*	*Ruminococcus*	10 h	$1.4 \pm 0.3^{a,b}$	1.8 ± 0.5^{b}	0.63 ± 0.43^{a}	0.41 ± 0.18^{a}	0.45 ± 0.17^{a}	0.050	0.369
Firmicutes	Clostridia	Clostridiales	unassigned	unassigned	10 h	1.8 ± 0.1^{b}	2.8 ± 0.3^{c}	0.82 ± 0.24^{a}	0.76 ± 0.16^{a}	0.81 ± 0.12^{a}	0.000	0.009
Firmicutes	Clostridia	Clostridiales	unclassified	unclassified	10 h	0.68 ± 0.12^{b}	1.4 ± 0.23^{c}	$0.47 \pm 0.1^{a,b}$	$0.33 \pm 0.03^{a,b}$	$0.59 \pm 0.27^{a,b}$	0.013	0.215
Bacteroidetes	Bacteroidia	Bacteroidales	*Porphyromonadaceae*	*Parabacteroides*	10 h	0.72 ± 0.2^{b}	1.9 ± 0.6^{c}	$0.4 \pm 0.1^{a,b}$	$0.37 \pm 0.04^{a,b}$	$0.56 \pm 0.1^{a,b}$	0.022	0.264
Actinobacteria	Actinobacteria	Bifidobacteriales	*Bifidobacteriaceae*	*Bifidobacterium*	10 h	4.7 ± 2.4^{a}	2.8 ± 0.2^{a}	24.3 ± 8.7^{b}	19.4 ± 4.2^{b}	$16.2 \pm 2.1^{a,b}$	0.028	0.273
Proteobacteria	Deltaproteobacteria	Desulfovibrionales	*Desulfovibrionaceae*	*Bilophila*	10 h	0.33 ± 0.03^{a}	1.7 ± 0.6^{b}	0.17 ± 0.01^{a}	0.24 ± 0.08^{a}	0.26 ± 0.05^{a}	0.024	0.264
Firmicutes	Clostridia	Clostridiales	*Ruminococcaceae*	*Faecalibacterium*	24 h	17 ± 3.7^{c}	4.6 ± 2.2^{a}	$16 \pm 5.5^{b,c}$	$5.9 \pm 1.9^{a,b}$	5.4 ± 1.4^{a}	0.049	0.950
Firmicutes	Clostridia	Clostridiales	unassigned	unassigned	24 h	1.2 ± 0.3^{a}	2.5 ± 0.6^{b}	0.36 ± 0.05^{a}	0.75 ± 0.19^{a}	0.86 ± 0.19^{a}	0.007	0.482
Bacteroidetes	Bacteroidia	Bacteroidales	[*Odoribacteraceae*]	*Butyricimonas*	24 h	$0.04 \pm 0.01^{a,b}$	0.09 ± 0.03^{b}	0.03 ± 0.01^{a}	0.02 ± 0.01^{a}	0.02 ± 0.01^{a}	0.044	0.950
Actinobacteria	Actinobacteria	Bifidobacteriales	*Bifidobacteriaceae*	*Bifidobacterium*	24 h	$6.3 \pm 4.6^{a,b}$	2.6 ± 0.2^{a}	14.9 ± 2.5^{b}	15.2 ± 2.6^{b}	$10.4 \pm 3^{a,b}$	0.050	0.950

* ANOVA analysis to verify whether the relative abundance of a given taxa is different between the treatments within the same time point. # The p value after correction for multiple tests (67 taxa) with the false discovery rate (FDR) method. Different letters (a, b, c) indicate significant differences ($p < 0.05$) between treatments at the same time point. Brackets indicate suggested but not verified names. Values are mean ± SEM.

3.5. Changes in Selected Fecal Bacterial Populations Measured with FISH

Changes in *Bifidobacterium* spp., *Faecalibacterium prausnitzii* and total bacteria were also assessed by FISH (Figure 4). At 0 h there were no significant changes between the treatments. At 5 h bifidobacteria numbers increased significantly with Renetta Canada compared to cellulose ($p = 0.004$) and inulin ($p = 0.047$); bifidobacteria also increased with Golden Delicious as the treatment compared to cellulose ($p = 0.007$). At 10 h bifidobacteria and total bacteria increased significantly with all the apple varieties compared to cellulose ($p < 0.05$); with total bacteria also increasing with inulin compared to cellulose ($p = 0.009$). Bifidobacteria also increased at 10 h with Renetta Canada compared to inulin ($p = 0.036$). At 24 h *Faecalibacterium prausnitzii* increased significantly with Renetta Canada compared to the other apples ($p < 0.05$). All apple varieties and inulin increased *Faecalibacterium prausnitziii* compared to cellulose ($p < 0.05$). Inulin and Golden Delicious also had higher *Faecalibacterium prausnitziii* numbers at 24 h compared to Pink Lady ($p = 0.004$ and $p = 0.032$ respectively) (Figure 4). Finally, at 24 h total bacteria increased significantly with all the apple varieties and inulin compared to cellulose ($p < 0.05$).

Following changes over time for the same treatment, a significant increase in bifidobacteria population, from 0 h, was observed for Renetta Canada (compared to 5, 10 and 24 h ($p < 0.05$)) and Golden Delicious (compared to 10 and 24 h ($p < 0.05$)). Furthermore, inulin also increased *Bifidobacterium* spp. at 5 h ($p = 0.044$) compared to the 0 h value, but to a lesser extent compared to Renetta Canada and Golden Delicious. *Faecalibacterium prausnitzii* population was significantly higher after 24 h only for Renetta Canada compared to 0 h ($p = 0.049$), while it decreased significantly after the administration of cellulose (at 24 h compared to 0 h, $p = 0.02$). Apart from the cellulose treatment (significant decrease at 10 h, $p = 0.028$) there were no significant changes over time in total bacteria population with any of the other treatments (Figure 4).

A

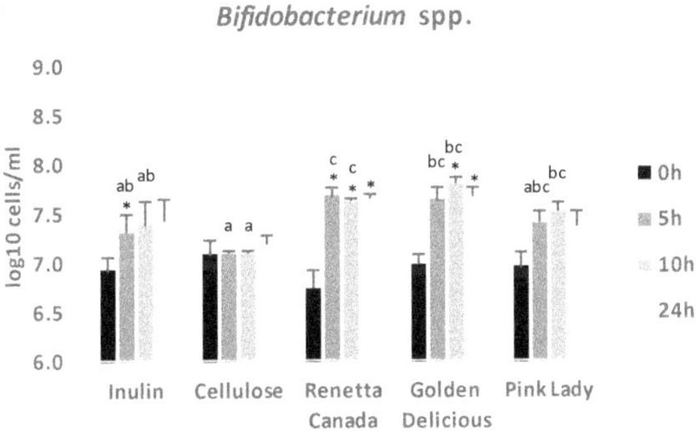

B

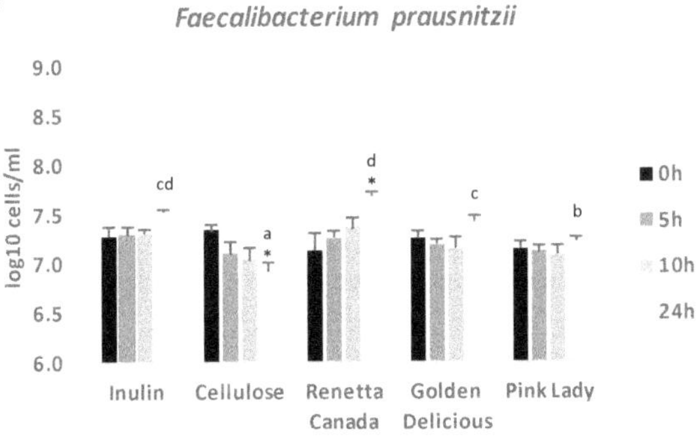

Figure 4. *Cont.*

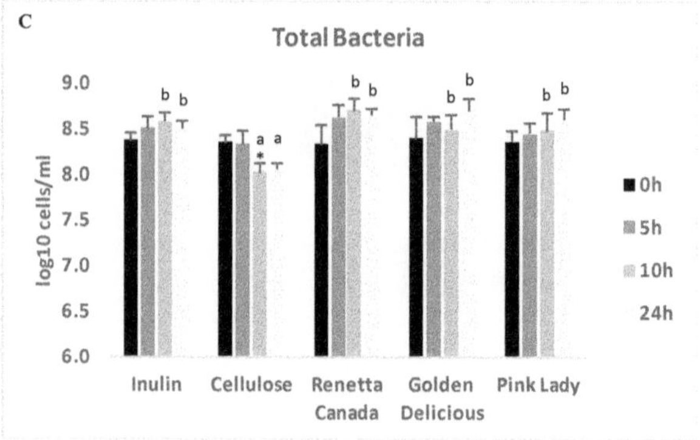

Figure 4. Changes in bacterial populations ((**A**) *Bifidobacterium* spp.; (**B**) *Faecalibacterium prausnitzii* and (**C**) Total Bacteria) throughout 24-h in vitro batch culture fermentations inoculated with human feces ($n = 3$ healthy donors) and administrated with inulin, cellulose, Renetta Canada, Golden Delicious and Pink Lady as the substrates (treatments). Samples were collected at 0, 5, 10 and 24 h. Results are expressed as $\log_{10}$ cells/mL of batch culture medium and values are mean ± SEM of the three fermentations. Significant differences ($p < 0.05$) between treatments at the same time point are indicated with different letters. * Significant differences ($p < 0.05$) from the 0 h time point within the same treatment.

3.6. SCFAs Production

Changes in SCFAs concentrations over time with the different treatments are shown in Table 3. All apples varieties significantly increased the concentration of acetic, propionic and total SCFAs ($p < 0.05$), but only Renetta Canada increased butyric acid among the apples ($p < 0.05$). Inulin significantly increased the concentrations of acetic, butyric and total SCFAs ($p < 0.05$) but these remained lower compared to the apple varieties. Cellulose increased butyric acid and total SCFAs but to a much lesser extent compared to inulin and the apple varieties ($p < 0.05$). There were no significant changes between the treatments at the same time point (0, 5, 10 or 24 h).

3.7. Changes in Precursor Polyphenols

A list of the precursor polyphenols and polyphenol microbial metabolites together with their multiple reaction monitoring (MRM) conditions are presented in Table S3. Changes in the concentration of precursor polyphenols, during the fecal fermentation, are shown in Table S4. Proanthocyanidin, kaempferol-3-rutinoside, rutin, isorhamentin-3-glucoside and cyanidin 3-galactoside were measured only in fresh apples whereas procyanidin A2, quercetin, kaempferol, isorhamnetin, laricitrin, phloretin, luteolin and ellagic acid were measured only in batch cultures.

Changes between the three apple varieties were observed at 0 h. In particular, Renetta Canada treatment resulted in significant higher concentrations of (+)-catechin, (−)-epicatechin, procyanidin A2, procyanidin B1, phloretin, phlorizin and vanillin compared to Golden Delicious and Pink Lady (Table S4). On the other hand, treatment with Golden Delicious resulted in higher ($p < 0.05$) levels of quercetin-3-glc compared to Pink Lady and Renetta Canada and higher quercetin-3-rha compared to Renetta Canada (Table S4). There were no significant changes in the concentration of precursor polyphenols at 5, 10 or 24 h.

Changes in the concentration of precursor polyphenols were observed over time throughout the fecal fermentation of the three apple varieties. In particular, significant reductions throughout the fermentation were detected for (+)-catechin (Renetta Canada), (−)-epicatechin (Renetta Canada and Golden Delicious), procyanidin A2 (Renetta Canada, Golden Delicious and Pink Lady), neochlorogenic acid (Golden Delicious), cryptochlorogenic acid (Golden Delicious), quercetin-3-glc (Renetta Canada,

Golden Delicious and Pink Lady), quercetin-3-rha (Renetta Canada, Golden Delicious and Pink Lady), kaempferol (Renetta Canada), isorhamnetin (Renetta Canada), phlorizin (Renetta Canada and Golden Delicious) and vanillin (Renetta Canada and Golden Delicious) (Table S4).

Table 3. SCFA concentrations (mmol/L) throughout 24-h in vitro batch culture fermentations inoculated with human feces (n = 3 healthy donors) and administrated with inulin, cellulose, Renetta Canada, Golden Delicious and Pink Lady as the substrates (treatments).

Substrate	Time (h)	Acetic Acid (mmol/L)	p [a]	Propionic Acid (mmol/L)	p [a]	Butyric Acid (mmol/L)	p [a]	Total SCFAs (mmol/L)	p [a]
Inulin	0	2.2 ± 0.1	0.050	0.8 ± 0.1	0.185	1 ± 0.3	0.013	4.1 ± 0.6	0.049
	5	9.5 ± 5.4		2.8 ± 1.4		4.4 ± 2.8		16.8 ± 9.6	
	10	11 ± 2.1		2.9 ± 0.8		5.5 ± 1 *		19.3 ± 3.3 *	
	24	17.3 ± 2.1 *		6.9 ± 2.6		11 ± 0.5 *		35.4 ± 4.6 *	
Cellulose	0	4.8 ± 2.9	0.062	1.4 ± 0.8	0.062	1.2 ± 0.6	0.041	7.5 ± 4.2	0.022
	5	5 ± 1.3		1.9 ± 0.5		2.3 ± 0.2 *		9.2 ± 2.3	
	10	13.5 ± 5.2		3.3 ± 1		2.8 ± 0.6		19.5 ± 5.6 *	
	24	13.1 ± 1.1		3.4 ± 0.1		3.5 ± 1		20 ± 1.5	
Renetta Canada	0	1 ± 0.1	0.034	0.5 ± 0.1	0.020	0.5 ± 0.1	0.025	3 ± 0.3	0.044
	5	11.5 ± 2.7		4.6 ± 2.6		2 ± 0.5		18.1 ± 3.9	
	10	19 ± 2.2 *		5.6 ± 2.1		3.7 ± 0.6 $^{*,\#}$		28.4 ± 1.8 *	
	24	28.1 ± 6 $^{*,\#}$		8.8 ± 2.6 $^{\#,\wedge}$		16.9 ± 6.1		53.7 ± 11.4 *	
Golden Delicious	0	2 ± 0.4	0.034	0.6 ± 0.1	0.016	0.5 ± 0.2	0.057	3.1 ± 0.7	0.008
	5	13.9 ± 5.8		4.2 ± 1.6		1.9 ± 0.7		20 ± 6.7	
	10	15.3 ± 3 *		4.7 ± 1.9		4.9 ± 1.6		25 ± 3.1 *	
	24	23.7 ± 2.8 *		7.8 ± 1.9 $^{\#,\wedge}$		13.3 ± 5.1		44.8 ± 7.2 $^{*,\#}$	
Pink Lady	0	1.8 ± 0.3	0.049	0.5 ± 0.1	0.020	0.4 ± 0.1	0.044	2.7 ± 0.5	0.040
	5	8.3 ± 2.3		3.2 ± 1.5		1.1 ± 0.2		12.6 ± 2.9	
	10	22.8 ± 8		6 ± 2.2		4 ± 1.2		32.8 ± 9.7	
	24	26.2 ± 3.8 $^{*,\#}$		8.8 ± 2 $^{\#,\wedge}$		13 ± 2.8		48 ± 7.9 $^{*,\#,\wedge}$	

Results are expressed as mmol/L of batch culture medium and values are mean ± SEM of the three fermentations. [a] Difference over time within the same treatment (ANOVA). * Significant different from 0 h time point $p < 0.05$, # Significant different from 5 h time point, $p < 0.05$, ^ Significant different from 10 h time point, $p < 0.05$.

3.8. Formation of Polyphenol Microbial Metabolites

The formation of polyphenol microbial metabolites throughout the fecal fermentation of the three apple varieties is shown in Figures 5 and 6. Significant increases were observed over time for 3-hydroxyphenylacetic acid (Renetta Canada and Pink Lady, p = 0.034 and p = 0.043, respectively), 3,4-dihydroxyphenylacetic acid (Renetta Canada, p = 0.05), 3-(4-hydroxyphenyl)propionic acid (Pink Lady, p = 0.009), hydroferulic acid (Renetta Canada, p = 0.046), 4-hydroxybenzoic acid (Pink Lady, p = 0.017) and pyrocatechol (Pink Lady, p = 0.049). In contrast, significant decreases throughout the fermentation were shown for caffeic acid (Renetta Canada and Golden Delicious, p = 0.000 and p = 0.001, respectively), p-coumaric acid (Renetta Canada and Golden Delicious, p = 0.001 and p = 0.001, respectively), trans-ferulic (Renetta Canada and Golden Delicious, p = 0.002 and p = 0.003, respectively) and trans-isoferulic (Renetta Canada, p = 0.001), as these metabolites can also appear as precursor polyphenols in apples (Figure S3). There were no significant changes in the concentration of the polyphenol microbial metabolites between the three apple varieties when each time point (0, 5, 10 or 24 h) was explored separately, with the exception of caffeic acid and p-coumaric acid (significantly higher concentration with Renetta Canada fermentation compared to Golden Delicious and Pink Lady at 0 h) and t-ferulic acid (significantly higher concentration with Renetta Canada compared to Pink Lady at 0 h).

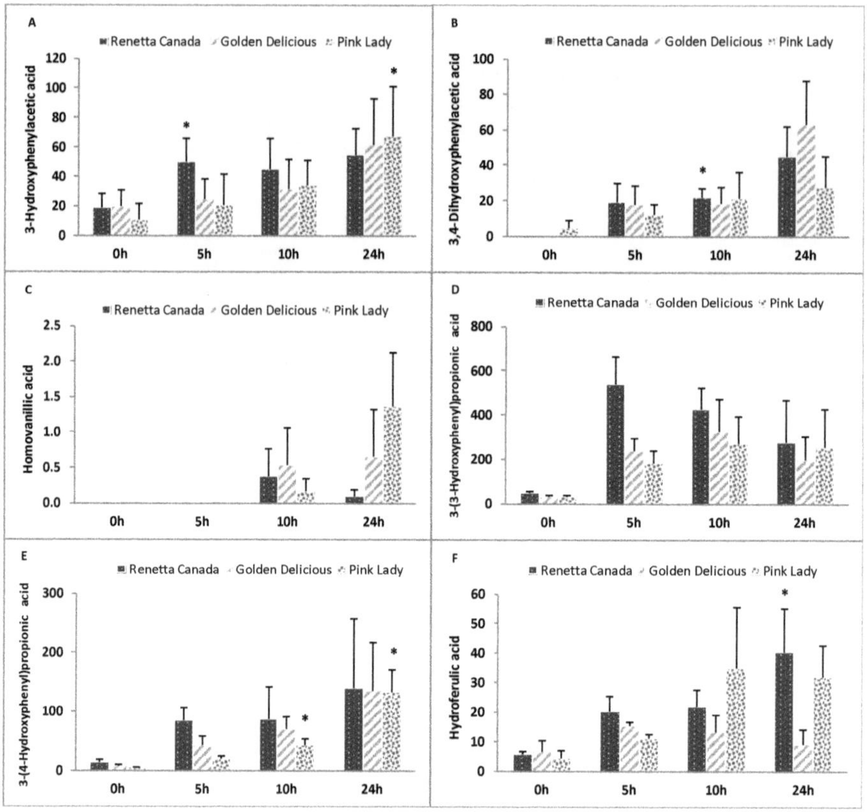

Figure 5. Changes in phenylacetic ((**A**) 3-Hydroxyphenylacetic acid; (**B**) 3,4-Dihydroxyphenylacetic acid and (**C**) Homovanillic acid) and phenylpropionic acid ((**D**) 3-(3-Hydroxyphenyl)propionic acid; (**E**) 3-(4-Hydroxyphenyl)propionic acid and (**F**) Hydroferulic acid) derivatives throughout 24-h in vitro batch culture fermentations inoculated with human feces (n = 3 healthy donors) and administrated with Renetta Canada, Golden Delicious and Pink Lady as the substrates (treatments). Samples were collected at 0, 5, 10 and 24 h. Results are expressed as ng/mL of batch culture medium and values are mean ± SEM of the three fermentations. * Significant differences ($p < 0.05$) from the 0 h time point within the same treatment.

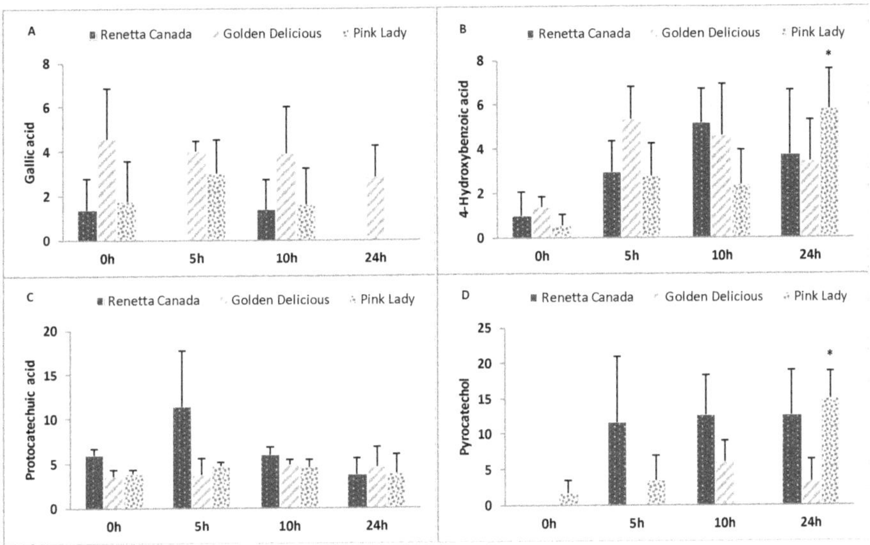

Figure 6. Changes in benzoic acid derivatives ((**A**) Gallic acid; (**B**) 4-Hydroxybenzoic acid; (**C**) Protocatechuic acid and (**D**) Pyrocatechol) throughout 24-h in vitro batch culture fermentations inoculated with human feces ($n = 3$ healthy donors) and administrated with Renetta Canada, Golden Delicious and Pink Lady as the substrates (treatments). Samples were collected at 0, 5, 10 and 24 h. Results are expressed as ng/mL of batch culture medium and values are mean ± SEM of the three fermentations. * Significant differences ($p < 0.05$) from the 0 h time point within the same treatment.

4. Discussion

The present in vitro study showed that whole apples can effectively modify both the human fecal microbiota composition and metabolic output. Effects on the bacterial community were observed at phylum and genus/species level. Actinobacteria relative abundance increased with all the tested apple varieties (Renetta Canada, Golden Delicious and Pink Lady). Increases in Actinobacteria have been observed in humans after intake of pectin [30], resistant starch [31] and pomegranate extract [32] and in rats fed with wild blueberries [33]. This increase can be explained by *Bifidobacterium* spp. growth, an important member of the Actinobacteria phylum. Although this did not remain significant with Illumina sequencing after multiple testing correction in the current study, the FISH results showed that *Bifidobacterium* spp. population increased significantly after the administration with Renetta Canada and Golden Delicious varieties. Notably, *Bifidobacterium* is considered a beneficial member of the gut microbiota by inhibiting the growth of pathogens, synthesizing certain vitamins (e.g., folate) and reducing serum cholesterol [2]. This observation is consistent with previous studies showing a bifidogenic effect with extraction juices from apple pomace in rats [12] and with the administration of two apples daily for two weeks in eight human subjects [17]. In contrast, Masumoto et al. (2016) [15], using a high throughput metagenomics technique, have reported decreased relative abundance of *Bifidobacterium* in diet-induced obese mice after the administration of apple PAs [15]. In our study, inulin, a known prebiotic, increased bifidobacteria to a lesser extent than apples. Inulin structure can affect its utilization by gut bacteria and many isolated bifidobacteria cannot utilize long-chain inulin [8] but they can grow on short-chain length structures (i.e., fructo-oligosaccharides) [34]. The inulin in the current study was a commercial isolate from dahlia tubers and details of its structure were not available.

Within the Firmicutes phylum, *Faecalibacterium prausnitzii* population (measured with the quantitative FISH) increased with Renetta Canada administration. *F. prausnitzii* is a key butyrate-producer, with anti-inflammatory properties, that may offer potential health benefits, especially in patients with inflammatory bowel disease (IBD) [35,36]. Renetta Canada increased butyrate, a major energy source for the colonocytes, which is particularly beneficial to the gut mucosa [37]. In support of our results *F. prausnitzii* strains have been shown to utilize apple pectin for growth [8,38] and increase butyrate concentration [13,39]. *F. prausnitzii* levels were unaffected by Golden Delicious and Pink Lady, and although the concentration of pectin was not determined, Renetta Canada had 19% and 44% higher soluble fiber content compared with Golden Delicious and Pink Lady, respectively. These data suggest that at least for *F. prausnitzii*, pectin may have played a major role.

Bacteroidetes relative abundance decreased with inulin, Renetta Canada and Golden Delicious. *Bacteroides* is considered a dominant bacterial group in the large intestine and the main Bacteroidetes member, along with the *Prevotella*. Licht et al. (2010) reported that both whole apples and isolated pectin decreased *Bacteroides* spp. in rats compared to a control diet [13]. Moreover, *Bacteroides* has been shown to decrease after the administration of other polyphenol sources, such as red wine [40] and cocoa [41] in rats, as well as with grape [42] and date extracts [43] in in vitro gut models inoculated with human feces. By contrast, *Bacteroides* species have been shown to increase with apple pomace juice extracts [11] and PAs from *Acacia angustissima* [44] in rats, as well as with red wine in humans [45].

The proportion of Proteobacteria increased after the administration of Renetta Canada and Golden Delicious but to a lesser extent compared to cellulose. However, an increase in *Enterobacteriaceae* family, a major member of Proteobacteria, was not observed. *Enterobacteriaceae*, includes numerous pathogenic bacteria genera, such as *Escherichia*, *Salmonella* and *Yersinia* and has been shown to increase in IBD patients. Increased Proteobacteria with inulin [8], resistant starch [46] and de-alcoholized wine [45] has also been reported elsewhere.

Interestingly, the alpha diversity of gut microbiota, at the OTU level, was lower with the apple treatments compared to inulin or cellulose. This may indicate the selective nature of the apple fermentations towards particular species. The beta diversify analysis showed a partitioning by donor and time, but not with treatment, which indicates that each individual possesses a specific starting population of gut bacteria, a finding consistent with the previously described inter-individual variation in the intestinal microbiota [47,48]. However, despite the variability between donors, there were still treatment-associated changes in gut microbiota composition at phylum and at genus/species level.

In the present study, the conditions of the proximal colon were simulated by creating an environment moderately acidic (pH 5.5–6.0) compared to a more neutral pH in the transverse and distal colon. The majority of the unabsorbed dietary carbohydrates are fermented in the proximal section producing SCFAs, leading to this reduced colonic pH, whereas in the distal section carbohydrate fermentation is generally assumed to be low. The pH affects bacterial growth and SCFA production, especially among bacteria that utilize the same polysaccharides [8,49]. For example, suppression in *Bacteroides* spp. growth was observed at pH values below six [8]. On the other hand, *F. prausnitzii* is more low-pH tolerant [8]. Moreover, a lower pH tends to favor butyrate production [49]. However, in our study, a significant increase in butyrate levels and *F. prausnitzii* population was only shown by Renetta Canada, indicating a treatment effect rather than a pH effect.

Pectin, the main soluble fiber found in apples, is extensively fermented by the gut microbiota to SCFAs, which are an important energy source for colonic health as well as for other tissues and organs [2]. Apart from the aforementioned butyrate increase by Renetta Canada, all apples significantly increased propionate and mainly acetate. Increased SCFAs have been shown with apple pomace juices [11,12]. Acetate serves as an energy source for the liver and peripheral tissues, but is also involved in the metabolic pathways of lipogenesis [50]. Pectin is known to produce relatively large amounts of acetate [51], which can also be utilized by butyrate producers such as *F. prausnitzii* as part of the cross feeding between bacteria [52]. A cross-feeding between *Bifidobacterium* strains and *F. prausnitzii* has been suggested, enhancing butyrate production [53]. Propionate on the other hand, may help to reduce hepatic cholesterol synthesis [54].

The effects of polyphenols on health depend on their bioavailability. Flavanol monomers (i.e., catechin and epicatechin) are readily absorbed in the small intestine, while high molecular weight polyphenols, such as the polymeric PAs, reach the colon almost intact, where they are transformed by the gut bacteria into a complex mixture of simple phenolic acids [55]. In the present study, the degradation of precursor apple polyphenols started as early as 5 h of fermentation and was complete throughout the 24 h for most of the polyphenolic compounds. Renetta Canada fermentation resulted in higher degradation of precursor polyphenols due to their initial high concentration.

The formation of polyphenol microbial products represent potential beneficial bioactive metabolites, not only locally in the gut but also systematically after their absorption in the colon and their appearance in the blood circulation. Renetta Canada was associated with the production of 3,4-dihydroxyphenylacetic acid and hydroferulic acid, which both have shown to possess anti-inflammatory properties [56]. It has been proposed that 3,4-dihydroxyphenylacetic acid can arise from the microbial catabolism of dimeric PAs [57]. Moreover, microbial metabolites of chlorogenic acids such as dihydroferulic acid showed a high antioxidant activity in vitro [58]. These results are in line with the higher concentration of PAs and chlorogenic acid in Renetta Canada apples. Pink Lady was associated with the formation of 3-(4-hydroxyphenyl)propionic acid and benzoic acid derivatives, in particular 4-hydroxybenzoic acid and pyrocatechol. Benzoic acids such as 4-hydroxybenzoic acid are considered to arise from beta oxidation of phenylpropionic acid derivatives and higher levels have been found after the in vitro fermentation of grape seed flavanols [59]. Pyrocatechol may arise from the dehydroxylation of gallic acid [60], which has been identified as a microbial metabolite and a native compound [61]. In our study, gallic acid concentration remained unaffected throughout the fermentation. Finally, both Renetta Canada and Pink Lady apples increased 3-hydroxyphenylacetic acid concentration. In vitro studies with human fecal inoculum are in line with the identified phenolic acids. In particular, PA catabolism has been associated with the production of 3-hydroxyphenylpropionic acid, 3-phenylpropionic acid, 4-hydroxyphenylpropionic acid and 4-hydroxyphenylacetic acid [62] as the main metabolites, whereas apples and apple components including isolated PAs formed 3-(3,4-dihydroxyphenyl)propionic acid, 3-(3-hydroxyphenyl)propionic acid, 3-phenylpropionic acid, benzoic acid, 2-(3,4-dihydroxyphenyl)acetic acid and 2-(3-hydroxyphenyl)acetic acid [10]. Furthermore, in human subjects, chocolate intake, a rich source of flavanols increased the urinary excretion of 3-hydroxyphenylpropionic acid, ferulic acid, 3,4-dihydroxyphenylacetic acid, 3-hydroxyphenylacetic acid, vanillic acid and 3-hydroxybenzoic acid [63].

In this study, we demonstrated that whole apples could modify the gut microbiota composition and affect the extent of degradation of soluble fiber and polyphenols through the production of SCFAs and phenolic acids, with Renetta Canada variety showing the most beneficial effects. In vitro batch culture models are a quick, simple and cost effective method of mimicking changes in gut microbiota numbers and metabolism [64], although they lack key metabolic functions, such as host immunological interactions, intestinal absorption and physiological components, such as epithelial mucosa, that exist in the human colon. The sample size ($n = 3$) is consistent with similar studies investigating polyphenols extracts [22,59], prebiotics [65,66] and fruits [43,67], with observed changes consistent with outcomes of human intervention studies [68]. Batch culture vessels contain a basal medium with limited carbohydrate and protein sources, therefore changes in microbiota composition and fermentation metabolites is known to be due to the added substrate, the apple varieties added to the vessels, even with different starting bacterial populations. Finally, although, donors were of similar age, with no gastrointestinal disorders, other characteristics that may affect gut microbiota composition such as diet, exercise and stress levels were not recorded and may have influenced the observed results, and it is recommended that these are provided in future studies.

5. Conclusions

In conclusion, whole apples beneficially modulate the gut microbiota composition and metabolic output in vitro. Renetta Canada variety in particular may have positive consequences for human health by increasing bifidobacteria, *Faecalibacterium prausnitzii* population and producing SCFAs and polyphenol microbial metabolites. It is recommended that the findings of this in vitro study should be confirmed in human intervention trials.

Supplementary Materials: The following are available online at www.mdpi.com/2072-6643/9/5/533/s1, Figure S1: Principal coordinate analysis (PCoA) plots of 16S rRNA gene profiles based on (A) unweighted (qualitative) and (B) weighted (quantitative) phylogenetic UniFrac distance matrices, colored by time, Figure S2: Principal coordinate analysis (PCoA) plots of 16SrRNA gene profiles based on (A) unweighted (qualitative) and (B) weighted (quantitative) phylogenetic UniFrac distance matrices, colored by treatment, Figure S3: Changes in cinnamic acid derivatives, Table S1: Composition analysis of Renetta Canada, Golden Delicious and Pink Lady, Table S2: Changes in bacterial taxa throughout 24-h in vitro batch culture fermentations inoculated with human feces (n = 3 healthy donors) and administrated with inulin, cellulose, Renetta Canada, Golden Delicious and Pink Lady as the substrates, Table S3: Multiple Reaction Monitoring (MRM) conditions of precursor polyphenols and polyphenol microbial metabolites, Table S4: Changes in precursor polyphenols throughout 24-h in vitro batch culture fermentations inoculated with human feces (n = 3 healthy donors) and administrated with inulin, cellulose, Renetta Canada, Golden Delicious and Pink Lady as the substrates.

Acknowledgments: This study was jointly funded by the University of Reading Research Endowment Trust Fund, Reading, United Kingdom and Fondazione Edmund Mach, San Michele all' Adige, Italy. We kindly thank Domenico Masuero and Evelyn Soini for measuring polyphenols in the three test apples and Silvia Carlin for helping with the SCFA analysis.

Author Contributions: K.M.T., J.A.L., A.K. and M.L. conceived the research and designed the study. A.K. wrote the manuscript. A.K. and M.L. performed the apple digestion and the in vitro batch cultures with the training of L.C. and F.F. A.K. performed the FISH analysis, the MiSeq Illumina sequencing data analysis and statistical analysis. A.K. performed the metabolites annotation, with the advice of L.C. and M.B. M.L. performed the SCFA analysis. M.G., M.L. and U.V. performed the metabolomics polyphenol analysis in fermentation samples. K.M.T. and J.A.L. coordinated the overall project and provided funding. J.A.L. and K.M.T. reviewed and edited the manuscript and all authors approved the final version.

Conflicts of Interest: The authors declare no conflict of interest.

References

1. Wang, X.; Ouyang, Y.Y.; Liu, J.; Zhu, M.M.; Zhao, G.; Bao, W.; Hu, F.B. Fruit and vegetable consumption and mortality from all causes, cardiovascular disease, and cancer: Systematic review and dose-response meta-analysis of prospective cohort studies. *BMJ* **2014**, *349*, 14. [CrossRef] [PubMed]
2. Koutsos, A.; Tuohy, K.M.; Lovegrove, J.A. Apples and cardiovascular health-is the gut microbiota a core consideration? *Nutrients* **2015**, *7*, 3959–3998. [CrossRef] [PubMed]
3. Gerhauser, C. Cancer chemopreventive potential of apples, apple juice, and apple components. *Planta Med.* **2008**, *74*, 1608–1624. [CrossRef] [PubMed]
4. Monagas, M.; Urpi-Sarda, M.; Sanchez-Patan, F.; Llorach, R.; Garrido, I.; Gomez-Cordoves, C.; Andres-Lacueva, C.; Bartolome, B. Insights into the metabolism and microbial biotransformation of dietary flavan-3-ols and the bioactivity of their metabolites. *Food Funct.* **2010**, *1*, 233–253. [CrossRef] [PubMed]
5. Ozdal, T.; Sela, D.A.; Xiao, J.B.; Boyacioglu, D.; Chen, F.; Capanoglu, E. The reciprocal interactions between polyphenols and gut microbiota and effects on bioaccessibility. *Nutrients* **2016**, *8*, 36. [CrossRef] [PubMed]
6. Olano-Martin, E.; Gibson, G.R.; Rastall, R.A. Comparison of the in vitro bifidogenic properties of pectins and pectic-oligosaccharides. *J. Appl. Microbiol.* **2002**, *93*, 505–511. [CrossRef] [PubMed]
7. Chen, J.; Liang, R.-H.; Liu, W.; Li, T.; Liu, C.-M.; Wu, S.-S.; Wang, Z.-J. Pectic-oligosaccharides prepared by dynamic high-pressure nnicrofluidization and their in vitro fermentation properties. *Carbohydr. Polym.* **2013**, *91*, 175–182. [CrossRef] [PubMed]
8. Chung, W.S.F.; Walker, A.W.; Louis, P.; Parkhill, J.; Vermeiren, J.; Bosscher, D.; Duncan, S.H.; Flint, H.J. Modulation of the human gut microbiota by dietary fibres occurs at the species level. *BMC Biol.* **2016**, *14*, 13. [CrossRef] [PubMed]
9. Vrhovsek, U.; Rigo, A.; Tonon, D.; Mattivi, F. Quantitation of polyphenols in different apple varieties. *J. Agric. Food Chem.* **2004**, *52*, 6532–6538. [CrossRef] [PubMed]
10. Bazzocco, S.; Mattila, I.; Guyot, S.; Renard, C.M.G.C.; Aura, A.-M. Factors affecting the conversion of apple polyphenols to phenolic acids and fruit matrix to short-chain fatty acids by human faecal microbiota in vitro. *Eur. J. Nutr.* **2008**, *47*, 442–452. [CrossRef] [PubMed]

11. Sembries, S.; Dongowski, G.; Jacobasch, G.; Mehrlander, K.; Will, F.; Dietrich, H. Effects of dietary fibre-rich juice colloids from apple pomace extraction juices on intestinal fermentation products and microbiota in rats. *Br. J. Nutr.* **2003**, *90*, 607–615. [CrossRef] [PubMed]
12. Sembries, S.; Dongowski, G.; Mehrlaender, K.; Will, F.; Dietrich, H. Physiological effects of extraction juices from apple, grape, and red beet pomaces in rats. *J. Agric. Food Chem.* **2006**, *54*, 10269–10280. [CrossRef] [PubMed]
13. Licht, T.R.; Hansen, M.; Bergstrom, A.; Poulsen, M.; Krath, B.N.; Markowski, J.; Dragsted, L.O.; Wilcks, A. Effects of apples and specific apple components on the cecal environment of conventional rats: Role of apple pectin. *BMC Microbiol.* **2010**, *10*. [CrossRef] [PubMed]
14. Jiang, T.; Gao, X.; Wu, C.; Tian, F.; Lei, Q.; Bi, J.; Xie, B.; Wang, H.Y.; Chen, S.; Wang, X. Apple-derived pectin modulates gut microbiota, improves gut barrier function, and attenuates metabolic endotoxemia in rats with diet-induced obesity. *Nutrients* **2016**, *8*, 126. [CrossRef] [PubMed]
15. Masumoto, S.; Terao, A.; Yamamoto, Y.; Mukai, T.; Miura, T.; Shoji, T. Non-absorbable apple procyanidins prevent obesity associated with gut microbial and metabolomic changes. *Sci. Rep.* **2016**, *6*, 31208. [CrossRef] [PubMed]
16. Aprikian, O.; Duclos, V.; Guyot, S.; Besson, C.; Manach, C.; Bernalier, A.; Morand, C.; Remesy, C.; Demigne, C. Apple pectin and a polyphenol-rich apple concentrate are more effective together than separately on cecal fermentations and plasma lipids in rats. *J. Nutr.* **2003**, *133*, 1860–1865. [PubMed]
17. Shinohara, K.; Ohashi, Y.; Kawasumi, K.; Terada, A.; Fujisawa, T. Effect of apple intake on fecal microbiota and metabolites in humans. *Anaerobe* **2010**, *16*, 510–515. [CrossRef] [PubMed]
18. Ravn-Haren, G.; Dragsted, L.O.; Buch-Andersen, T.; Jensen, E.N.; Jensen, R.I.; Nemeth-Balogh, M.; Paulovicsova, B.; Bergstrom, A.; Wilcks, A.; Licht, T.R.; et al. Intake of whole apples or clear apple juice has contrasting effects on plasma lipids in healthy volunteers. *Eur. J. Nutr.* **2012**. [CrossRef] [PubMed]
19. Vrhovsek, U.; Masuero, D.; Gasperotti, M.; Franceschi, P.; Caputi, L.; Viola, R.; Mattivi, F. A versatile targeted metabolomics method for the rapid quantification of multiple classes of phenolics in fruits and beverages. *J. Agric. Food Chem.* **2012**, *60*, 8831–8840. [CrossRef] [PubMed]
20. Gasperotti, M.; Masuero, D.; Guella, G.; Mattivi, F.; Vrhovsek, U. Development of a targeted method for twenty-three metabolites related to polyphenol gut microbial metabolism in biological samples, using spe and uhplc-esi-ms/ms. *Talanta* **2014**, *128*, 221–230. [CrossRef] [PubMed]
21. Mandalari, G.; Faulks, R.M.; Rich, G.T.; Lo Turco, V.; Picout, D.R.; Lo Curto, R.B.; Bisignano, G.; Dugo, P.; Dugo, G.; Waldron, K.W.; et al. Release of protein, lipid, and vitamin e from almond seeds during digestion. *J. Agric. Food Chem.* **2008**, *56*, 3409–3416. [CrossRef] [PubMed]
22. Sanchez-Patan, F.; Cueva, C.; Monagas, M.; Walton, G.E.; Gibson, G.R.; Quintanilla-Lopez, J.E.; Lebron-Aguilar, R.; Martin-Alvarez, P.J.; Moreno-Arribas, M.V.; Bartolome, B. In vitro fermentation of a red wine extract by human gut microbiota: Changes in microbial groups and formation of phenolic metabolites. *J. Agric. Food Chem.* **2012**, *60*, 2136–2147. [CrossRef] [PubMed]
23. Caporaso, J.G.; Kuczynski, J.; Stombaugh, J.; Bittinger, K.; Bushman, F.D.; Costello, E.K.; Fierer, N.; Pena, A.G.; Goodrich, J.K.; Gordon, J.I.; et al. Qiime allows analysis of high-throughput community sequencing data. *Nat. Methods* **2010**, *7*, 335–336. [CrossRef] [PubMed]
24. Aronesty, E. Comparison of sequencing utilitiy programs. *Open Bioinform. J.* **2013**, *7*, 1–8. [CrossRef]
25. Edgar, R.C. Search and clustering orders of magnitude faster than blast. *Bioinformatics* **2010**, *26*, 2460–2461. [CrossRef] [PubMed]
26. Langendijk, P.S.; Schut, F.; Jansen, G.J.; Raangs, G.C.; Kamphuis, G.R.; Wilkinson, M.H.F.; Welling, G.W. Quantitative fluorescence in-situ hybridization of *Bifidobacterium* spp. with genus-specific 16s ribosomal-rna-targeted probes and its application in fecal samples. *Appl. Environ. Microbiol.* **1995**, *61*, 3069–3075. [PubMed]
27. Hold, G.L.; Schwiertz, A.; Aminov, R.I.; Blaut, M.; Flint, H.J. Oligonucleotide probes that detect quantitatively significant groups of butyrate-producing bacteria in human feces. *Appl. Environ. Microbiol.* **2003**, *69*, 4320–4324. [CrossRef] [PubMed]
28. Daims, H.; Stoecker, K.; Wagner, M. Fluorescence In Situ Hybridization for the detection of prokaryotes. In *Molecular Microbial Ecology*; Osborn, A.M., Smith, C.J., Eds.; Taylor & Francis: New York, NY, USA, 2005.

29. Zhao, G.H.; Nyman, M.; Jonsson, J.A. Rapid determination of short-chain fatty acids in colonic contents and faeces of humans and rats by acidified water-extraction and direct-injection gas chromatography. *Biomed. Chromatogr.* **2006**, *20*, 674–682. [CrossRef] [PubMed]
30. Yang, J.; Martinez, I.; Walter, J.; Keshavarzian, A.; Rose, D.J. In vitro characterization of the impact of selected dietary fibers on fecal microbiota composition and short chain fatty acid production. *Anaerobe* **2013**, *23*, 74–81. [CrossRef] [PubMed]
31. Martinez, I.; Kim, J.; Duffy, P.R.; Schlegel, V.L.; Walter, J. Resistant starches types 2 and 4 have differential effects on the composition of the fecal microbiota in human subjects. *PLoS ONE* **2010**, *5*, 11. [CrossRef] [PubMed]
32. Li, Z.P.; Henning, S.M.; Lee, R.P.; Lu, Q.Y.; Summanen, P.H.; Thames, G.; Corbett, K.; Downes, J.; Tseng, C.H.; Finegold, S.M.; et al. Pomegranate extract induces ellagitannin metabolite formation and changes stool microbiota in healthy volunteers. *Food Funct.* **2015**, *6*, 2487–2495. [CrossRef] [PubMed]
33. Lacombe, A.; Li, R.W.; Klimis-Zacas, D.; Kristo, A.S.; Tadepalli, S.; Krauss, E.; Young, R.; Wu, V.C.H. Lowbush wild blueberries have the potential to modify gut microbiota and xenobiotic metabolism in the rat colon. *PLoS ONE* **2013**, *8*, 8. [CrossRef] [PubMed]
34. Rossi, M.; Corradini, C.; Amaretti, A.; Nicolini, M.; Pompei, A.; Zanoni, S.; Matteuzzi, D. Fermentation of fructooligosaccharides and inulin by bifidobacteria: A comparative study of pure and fecal cultures. *Appl. Environ. Microbiol.* **2005**, *71*, 6150–6158. [CrossRef] [PubMed]
35. Sokol, H.; Pigneur, B.; Watterlot, L.; Lakhdari, O.; Bermudez-Humaran, L.G.; Gratadoux, J.-J.; Blugeon, S.; Bridonneau, C.; Furet, J.-P.; Corthier, G.; et al. Faecalibacterium prausnitzii is an anti-inflammatory commensal bacterium identified by gut microbiota analysis of crohn disease patients. *Proc. Natl. Acad. Sci. USA* **2008**, *105*, 16731–16736. [CrossRef] [PubMed]
36. Machiels, K.; Joossens, M.; Sabino, J.; De Preter, V.; Arijs, I.; Eeckhaut, V.; Ballet, V.; Claes, K.; Van Immerseel, F.; Verbeke, K.; et al. A decrease of the butyrate-producing species roseburia hominis and faecalibacterium prausnitzii defines dysbiosis in patients with ulcerative colitis. *Gut* **2014**, *63*, 1275–1283. [CrossRef] [PubMed]
37. Pryde, S.E.; Duncan, S.H.; Hold, G.L.; Stewart, C.S.; Flint, H.J. The microbiology of butyrate formation in the human colon. *FEMS Microbiol. Lett.* **2002**, *217*, 133–139. [CrossRef] [PubMed]
38. Lopez-Siles, M.; Khan, T.M.; Duncan, S.H.; Harmsen, H.J.M.; Garcia-Gil, L.J.; Flint, H.J. Cultured representatives of two major phylogroups of human colonic faecalibacterium prausnitzii can utilize pectin, uronic acids, and host-derived substrates for growth. *Appl. Environ. Microbiol.* **2012**, *78*, 420–428. [CrossRef] [PubMed]
39. Waldecker, M.; Kautenburger, T.; Daumann, H.; Busch, C.; Schrenk, D. Inhibition of histone-deacetylase activity by short-chain fatty acids and some polyphenol metabolites formed in the colon. *J. Nutr. Biochem.* **2008**, *19*, 587–593. [CrossRef] [PubMed]
40. Dolara, P.; Luceri, C.; de Filippo, C.; Femia, A.P.; Giovannelli, L.; Caderni, G.; Cecchini, C.; Silvi, S.; Orpianesi, C.; Cresci, A. Red wine polyphenols influence carcinogenesis, intestinal microflora, oxidative damage and gene expression profiles of colonic mucosa in f344 rats. *Mutat. Res.-Fundam. Mol. Mech. Mutag.* **2005**, *591*, 237–246. [CrossRef] [PubMed]
41. Massot-Cladera, M.; Perez-Berezo, T.; Franch, A.; Castell, M.; Perez-Cano, F.J. Cocoa modulatory effect on rat faecal microbiota and colonic crosstalk. *Arch. Biochem. Biophys.* **2012**, *527*, 105–112. [CrossRef] [PubMed]
42. Kemperman, R.A.; Gross, G.; Mondot, S.; Possemiers, S.; Marzorati, M.; van de Wiele, T.; Dore, J.; Vaughan, E.E. Impact of polyphenols from black tea and red wine/grape juice on a gut model microbiome. *Food Res. Int.* **2013**, *53*, 659–669. [CrossRef]
43. Eid, N.; Enani, S.; Walton, G.; Corona, G.; Costabile, A.; Gibson, G.; Rowland, I.; Spencer, J.P. The impact of date palm fruits and their component polyphenols, on gut microbial ecology, bacterial metabolites and colon cancer cell proliferation. *J. Nutr. Sci.* **2014**, *3*, e46. [CrossRef] [PubMed]
44. Smith, A.H.; Mackie, R.I. Effect of condensed tannins on bacterial diversity and metabolic activity in the rat gastrointestinal tract. *Appl. Environ. Microbiol.* **2004**, *70*, 1104–1115. [CrossRef] [PubMed]

45. Isabel Queipo-Ortuno, M.; Boto-Ordonez, M.; Murri, M.; Miguel Gomez-Zumaquero, J.; Clemente-Postigo, M.; Estruch, R.; Cardona Diaz, F.; Andres-Lacueva, C.; Tinahones, F.J. Influence of red wine polyphenols and ethanol on the gut microbiota ecology and biochemical biomarkers. *Am. J. Clin. Nutr.* **2012**, *95*, 1323–1334. [CrossRef] [PubMed]
46. Lyte, M.; Chapel, A.; Lyte, J.M.; Ai, Y.F.; Proctor, A.; Jane, J.L.; Phillips, G.J. Resistant starch alters the microbiota-gut brain axis: Implications for dietary modulation of behavior. *PLoS ONE* **2016**, *11*, 22. [CrossRef] [PubMed]
47. Walker, A.W.; Ince, J.; Duncan, S.H.; Webster, L.M.; Holtrop, G.; Ze, X.L.; Brown, D.; Stares, M.D.; Scott, P.; Bergerat, A.; et al. Dominant and diet-responsive groups of bacteria within the human colonic microbiota. *ISME J.* **2011**, *5*, 220–230. [CrossRef] [PubMed]
48. Salonen, A.; Lahti, L.; Salojarvi, J.; Holtrop, G.; Korpela, K.; Duncan, S.H.; Date, P.; Farquharson, F.; Johnstone, A.M.; Lobley, G.E.; et al. Impact of diet and individual variation on intestinal microbiota composition and fermentation products in obese men. *ISME J.* **2014**, *8*, 2218–2230. [CrossRef] [PubMed]
49. Walker, A.W.; Duncan, S.H.; McWilliam Leitch, E.C.; Child, M.W.; Flint, H.J. Ph and peptide supply can radically alter bacterial populations and short-chain fatty acid ratios within microbial communities from the human colon. *Appl. Environ. Microbiol.* **2005**, *71*, 3692–3700. [CrossRef] [PubMed]
50. Zambell, K.L.; Fitch, M.D.; Fleming, S.E. Acetate and butyrate are the major substrates for de novo lipogenesis in rat colonic epithelial cells. *J. Nutr.* **2003**, *133*, 3509–3515. [PubMed]
51. Onumpai, C.; Kolida, S.; Bonnin, E.; Rastall, R.A. Microbial utilization and selectivity of pectin fractions with various structures. *Appl. Environ. Microbiol.* **2011**, *77*, 5747–5754. [CrossRef] [PubMed]
52. Duncan, S.H.; Barcenilla, A.; Stewart, C.S.; Pryde, S.E.; Flint, H.J. Acetate utilization and butyryl coenzyme a (coa): Acetate-coa transferase in butyrate-producing bacteria from the human large intestine. *Appl. Environ. Microbiol.* **2002**, *68*, 5186–5190. [CrossRef] [PubMed]
53. Rios-Covian, D.; Gueimonde, M.; Duncan, S.H.; Flint, H.J.; de los Reyes-Gavilan, C.G. Enhanced butyrate formation by cross-feeding between faecalibacterium prausnitzii and bifidobacterium adolescentis. *FEMS Microbiol. Lett.* **2015**, *362*. [CrossRef] [PubMed]
54. Cheng, H.H.; Lai, M.H. Fermentation of resistant rice starch produces propionate reducing serum and hepatic cholesterol in rats. *J. Nutr.* **2000**, *130*, 1991–1995. [PubMed]
55. Velderrain-Rodriguez, G.R.; Palafox-Carlos, H.; Wall-Medrano, A.; Ayala-Zavala, J.F.; Chen, C.Y.O.; Robles-Sanchez, M.; Astiazaran-Garcia, H.; Alvarez-Parrilla, E.; Gonzalez-Aguilar, G.A. Phenolic compounds: Their journey after intake. *Food Funct.* **2014**, *5*, 189–197. [CrossRef] [PubMed]
56. Larrosa, M.; Luceri, C.; Vivoli, E.; Pagliuca, C.; Lodovici, M.; Moneti, G.; Dolara, P. Polyphenol metabolites from colonic microbiota exert anti-inflammatory activity on different inflammation models. *Mol. Nutr. Food Res.* **2009**, *53*, 1044–1054. [CrossRef] [PubMed]
57. Appeldoorn, M.M.; Vincken, J.P.; Aura, A.M.; Hollman, P.C.H.; Gruppen, H. Procyanidin dimers are metabolized by human microbiota with 2-(3,4-dihydroxyphenyl)acetic acid and 5-(3,4-dihydroxyphenyl)-gamma-valerolactone as the major metabolites. *J. Agric. Food Chem.* **2009**, *57*, 1084–1092. [CrossRef] [PubMed]
58. Gomez-Ruiz, J.A.; Leake, D.S.; Ames, J.M. In vitro antioxidant activity of coffee compounds and their metabolites. *J. Agric. Food Chem.* **2007**, *55*, 6962–6969. [CrossRef] [PubMed]
59. Cueva, C.; Sanchez-Patan, F.; Monagas, M.; Walton, G.E.; Gibson, G.R.; Martin-Alvarez, P.J.; Bartolome, B.; Moreno-Arribas, M.V. In vitro fermentation of grape seed flavan-3-ol fractions by human faecal microbiota: Changes in microbial groups and phenolic metabolites. *FEMS Microbiol. Ecol.* **2013**, *83*, 792–805. [CrossRef] [PubMed]
60. Selma, M.V.; Espin, J.C.; Tomas-Barberan, F.A. Interaction between phenolics and gut microbiota: Role in human health. *J. Agric. Food Chem.* **2009**, *57*, 6485–6501. [CrossRef] [PubMed]
61. Dall'Asta, M.; Calani, L.; Tedeschi, M.; Jechiu, L.; Brighenti, F.; Del Rio, D. Identification of microbial metabolites derived from in vitro fecal fermentation of different polyphenolic food sources. *Nutrition* **2012**, *28*, 197–203. [CrossRef] [PubMed]
62. Deprez, S.; Brezillon, C.; Rabot, S.; Philippe, C.; Mila, I.; Lapierre, C.; Scalbert, A. Polymeric proanthocyanidins are catabolized by human colonic microflora into low-molecular-weight phenolic acids. *J. Nutr.* **2000**, *130*, 2733–2738. [PubMed]

63. Rios, L.Y.; Gonthier, M.P.; Remesy, C.; Mila, L.; Lapierre, C.; Lazarus, S.A.; Williamson, G.; Scalbert, A. Chocolate intake increases urinary excretion of polyphenol-derived phenolic acids in healthy human subjects. *Am. J. Clin. Nutr.* **2003**, *77*, 912–918. [PubMed]
64. Williams, C.F.; Walton, G.E.; Jiang, L.; Plummer, S.; Garaiova, I.; Gibson, G.R. Comparative analysis of intestinal tract models. In *Annual Review of Food Science and Technology*; Doyle, M.P., Klaenhammer, T.R., Eds.; Annual Reviews: Palo Alto, CA, USA, 2015; Volume 6, pp. 329–350.
65. Johnson, L.P.; Walton, G.E.; Psichas, A.; Frost, G.S.; Gibson, G.R.; Barraclough, T.G. Prebiotics modulate the effects of antibiotics on gut microbial diversity and functioning in vitro. *Nutrients* **2015**, *7*, 4480–4497. [CrossRef] [PubMed]
66. Rodrigues, D.; Walton, G.; Sousa, S.; Rocha-Santos, T.A.P.; Duarte, A.C.; Freitas, A.C.; Gomes, A.M.P. In vitro fermentation and prebiotic potential of selected extracts from seaweeds and mushrooms. *LWT -Food Sci. Technol.* **2016**, *73*, 131–139. [CrossRef]
67. Blatchford, P.; Stoklosinski, H.; Walton, G.; Swann, J.; Gibson, G.; Gearry, R.; Ansell, J. Kiwifruit fermentation drives positive gut microbial and metabolic changes irrespective of initial microbiota composition. *Bioact. Carbohydr. Diet. Fibre* **2015**, *6*, 37–45. [CrossRef]
68. Walton, G.E.; van den Heuvel, E.; Kosters, M.H.W.; Rastall, R.A.; Tuohy, K.M.; Gibson, G.R. A randomised crossover study investigating the effects of galacto-oligosaccharides on the faecal microbiota in men and women over 50 years of age. *Br. J. Nutr.* **2012**, *107*, 1466–1475. [CrossRef] [PubMed]

nutrients

MDPI

Review

Cell-Surface and Nuclear Receptors in the Colon as Targets for Bacterial Metabolites and Its Relevance to Colon Health

Sathish Sivaprakasam, Yangzom D. Bhutia, Sabarish Ramachandran and Vadivel Ganapathy *

Department of Cell Biology and Biochemistry, Texas Tech University Health Sciences Center, Lubbock, TX 79430, USA; sathish.sivaprakasam@ttuhsc.edu (S.S.); yangzom.d.bhutia@ttuhsc.edu (Y.D.B.); s.ramachandran@ttuhsc.edu (S.R.)

* Correspondence: vadivel.ganapathy@ttuhsc.edu; Tel.: +1-806-743-2518

Received: 27 June 2017; Accepted: 5 August 2017; Published: 10 August 2017

Abstract: The symbiotic co-habitation of bacteria in the host colon is mutually beneficial to both partners. While the host provides the place and food for the bacteria to colonize and live, the bacteria in turn help the host in energy and nutritional homeostasis, development and maturation of the mucosal immune system, and protection against inflammation and carcinogenesis. In this review, we highlight the molecular mediators of the effective communication between the bacteria and the host, focusing on selective metabolites from the bacteria that serve as messengers to the host by acting through selective receptors in the host colon. These bacterial metabolites include the short-chain fatty acids acetate, propionate, and butyrate, the tryptophan degradation products indole-3-aldehyde, indole-3-acetic, acid and indole-3-propionic acid, and derivatives of endogenous bile acids. The targets for these bacterial products in the host include the cell-surface G-protein-coupled receptors GPR41, GPR43, and GPR109A and the nuclear receptors aryl hydrocarbon receptor (AhR), pregnane X receptor (PXR), and farnesoid X receptor (FXR). The chemical communication between these bacterial metabolite messengers and the host targets collectively has the ability to impact metabolism, gene expression, and epigenetics in colonic epithelial cells as well as in mucosal immune cells. The end result, for the most part, is the maintenance of optimal colonic health.

Keywords: colonic bacteria; symbiotic relationship; bacterial metabolites; molecular targets; cell-surface receptors; nuclear receptors; immune tolerance; colitis; colon cancer

1. Introduction

Over millions of years, humans have co-evolved with microorganisms through co-habitation. Adult human harbors microflora that is equal or even greater than their human cells in number [1,2]. These microorganisms colonize different parts of the body that are exposed to external environment, which include skin, oral cavity, airway lumen, intestinal tract, and vagina. Among these, the colon is the site where the microorganisms are most abundant, with bacteria as the principal component. There are 800–1000 different species of colonic bacteria under normal physiological conditions, but the presence or absence of specific strains and the relative abundance of any given strain might vary from individual to individual, primarily influenced by the environmental factors such as the diet, air and water quality, medications, and mode of delivery (vaginal or Cesarean section) [3]. Because of the impact of multiple variables, the colonic bacteria might not remain the same even in a given individual over a long period of time. Despite these interpersonal variations, colonic bacteria are in general dominated by two phyla: Bacteroidetes and Firmicutes [4,5]. Normal microflora in the colon elicit significant influence on the host, in the colon and in other organs. Recent studies have implicated colonic bacteria in brain function (gut-brain axis), liver function (gut-liver axis), mucosal and systemic immune function, diabetes (type 1 and type 2) (gut-pancreas axis), nutrition and obesity, and cardiovascular diseases [6–10]. This broad spectrum of biological impact of colonic bacteria on the host is possible because of active communication between the two co-habitants. The impact of colonic bacteria on the host is not limited locally to the colon because of the changes the bacteria bring in terms of gene expression and biological function in colonic epithelial cells as well as mucosal immune cells. The colon releases a wide variety of biologically active molecules into circulation in response to changes in the density and phylogenic makeup of the bacterial population; these active molecules include hormones and cytokines that impact on the functions of distant organs including the liver, pancreas, and brain. Similarly, mucosal immune cells are also influenced in their behavior and function in response to colonic bacteria, which then travel to distant sites to modulate immune function and disease processes [11,12]. Furthermore, colonic bacteria themselves elaborate different classes of metabolites, which enter the portal and systemic circulations to regulate the biology of cells and tissues at distant sites through specific molecular targets that include enzymes and receptors [10,13,14].

Because of its close proximity to the bacteria, the colon is the most influenced organ as the result of this co-habitation. The presence of bacteria in the colon is absolutely necessary for optimal colonic health; normal bacteria in the colon offer protection against inflammation and cancer. As such, the beneficial effects of colonic bacteria are undeniable. Any imbalance in the normal density and phylogenetic composition in colonic bacteria, generally referred to as dysbiosis, is detrimental to colonic health [15–18]. Inflammatory bowel diseases (IBD) are chronic inflammatory disorders of the intestinal tract that develop as a result of deregulation of the immune response toward the intestinal/colonic bacteria. In particular, there is a marked decrease in the colonization of Firmicutes and Bacteroidetes in the gut microbiota in association with IBD. Crohn's disease and ulcerative colitis are the two major types of IBD, which are distinct diseases with different histological features and etiology that involve different immune cell types. Animal studies have shown that neither of these diseases develops under germ-free conditions, indicating that the presence of bacteria is obligatory for the disease process [19,20]. The findings that normal bacteria are essential for colonic health and that IBD does not develop in the absence of bacteria are not necessarily contradictory. The epithelial cells of the intestine/colon form an effective barrier between the bacteria and the host, and the communication between the two co-habitants occurs solely via chemical messengers to make sure that the mucosal immune system is not overly active in response to the bacterial antigens. However, if the barrier function is compromised for any reason, the ability of the mucosal immune system to tolerate the bacteria is at risk [21–23]. What causes the breakdown of the barrier in IBD is not completely understood, but changes in the normal bacterial phylogenetic composition are believed to be major determinants in the process. When the phylogenetic composition (i.e., dysbiosis) is altered in the colon, the chemical communication between the bacteria and the host also undergoes changes, thus initiating the inflammatory disease process. This phenomenon is also relevant to carcinogenesis in the colon because chronic inflammation as occurs in ulcerative colitis increases the risk of colorectal cancer [24].

2. Relationship between Microbiota and the Host: Parasitism, Commensalism, or Mutualism?

The relationship between the host and the microbiota could fall into three categories—parasitism, commensalism, and mutualism—depending on the specifics of the interaction. In parasitism, one of the co-habitants gets the benefits, while the other is harmed. In commensalism, one of the co-habitants reaps the benefits, while the co-habitation is neither beneficial nor harmful to the other partner. In mutualism, both partners get the benefits from the co-existence. The relationship between the host and the colonic bacteria falls under the third category, mutualism. The benefits to the bacteria as a result of this co-habitation include the availability of the colonic lumen for colonization and proliferation and provision of the nutrients by the host necessary for survival and growth. The host also benefits from the relationship [25–27]. Colonic bacteria synthesize a variety of vitamins (folic acid, biotin, vitamin K, etc.) that are made available to the host. The principal fermentation products of bacterial metabolism, called short-chain fatty acids, that are present in normal colonic lumen at concentrations as high as 100 mM serve as preferential metabolic fuel to colonic epithelial cells [28]. These short-chain fatty acids also function as signaling molecules eliciting a broad range of biological effects in colonic epithelium by targeting enzymes such histone deacetylases (HDACs), cell-surface receptors such as GPR109A and GPR43, and nuclear receptors such as AhR, PXR, FXR, and peroxisome proliferator-activated receptors (PPARs) [29]. The end result of this mutually beneficial co-habitation is a symbiotic relationship between the two partners. Notwithstanding this overwhelming evidence for mutualism between the host and colonic bacteria, too many investigators and published reports still continue to describe the relationship between the host and the bacteria as commensalism and the bacteria as commensals [30–32]. Surprisingly, the terms "commensalism" and "commensals" appear even in publications that provide data in support of the mutually beneficial relationship between the host and the colonic bacteria [25,30–32].

3. Bacterial Dysbiosis as a Cause of Colonic Diseases

Dysbiosis in the colon is a critical determinant in the pathogenesis of IBD. Research on colitis induction in germ-free mice with introduction of specific strains of bacteria has shown that microbial dysbiosis, rather than genetic factors, is the major factor for IBD pathogenesis. Many genetically-engineered mouse models that develop spontaneous colitis in the presence of bacteria in the colon are resistant to colitis when raised under germ-free conditions [33,34]. This suggests that the presence of bacteria in the intestinal tract is a critical requirement for IBD development. Most animal models of colitis show altered bacterial composition in the colon, providing evidence of dysbiosis [16,35]. However, the link between dysbiosis and IBD is only associative, and the cause-effect relationship has not yet been established beyond doubt. Nonetheless, administration of probiotics to patients with colonic inflammation has beneficial effects in terms of slowing or preventing progression of the disease process [36–38]. As these probiotics tend to favor colonization of normal bacterial flora and suppress the growth of pathogenic bacteria in the colon, the preventive effects of probiotics suggest effective reversal of the disease-associated dysbiosis and may actually point to a mechanistic model in which the dysbiosis is most likely the cause, rather than the result, of colonic inflammation [37,39,40].

4. Bacterial Metabolites with Impact on the Host: Relevance to Colitis and Colon Cancer

The communication between colonic bacteria and the host could be contact-dependent as well as contact-independent. The phylogenetic composition of the microflora in colonic lumen is not exactly the same as that of the microflora on the surface of the colonic epithelium. Which bacterial strains adhere to the colonic epithelial cells depends on multiple factors such as the presence or absence of cell-surface receptors for a given strain, ability of bacterial strains to traverse the thick mucin present on the luminal surface of the epithelial cell layer, as well as susceptibility of the bacterial strains to the bactericidal and bacteriostatic actions of the various molecules secreted by the epithelial cells and mucosal immune cells. The physical contact followed by insertion of specific bacterial proteins into the epithelial cell membrane could elicit signaling changes in the epithelium as a means of communication. Another mode of communication, probably more prevalent than the former, is through metabolites released into the lumen from live bacteria or from dead bacterial cells. The colon provides a favorable environment for anaerobic microbial growth, resulting in fermentation by resident bacteria of dietary constituents that reach the colon. The microbiota population in the colon is highly variable depending on the intestinal physiology, substrate availability, oxygen tension, and pH [28]. As a result, the microorganisms present in the colon are not the same all through the length of the large intestine. The phylogenetic composition of the bacteria is significantly different between the proximal colon and the distal colon [41]. As the metabolites elaborated by these bacteria depend on the repertoire of metabolic pathways in a given strain of the bacteria, different regions of the colon are exposed to different bacterial metabolites and hence respond differently. Furthermore, the phylogenetic composition of the colonic bacteria varies from individual to individual and also in the same individual in health and disease; this again impacts the biological response of the host colon to the presence of bacteria that could be significantly different on an individual basis and also depend on the health status of the individual.

Among these bacterial metabolites responsible for communication between the bacteria and the host, short-chain fatty acids (SCFAs) have received the most attention [42–45]. SCFAs are organic acids consisting of 2–4 carbon atoms. The principal components of SCFAs are acetate (C2), propionate (C3), and butyrate (C4). These fatty acids arise in the colon by bacterial fermentation of carbohydrates that reach the colon either in the form of dietary fiber or due to ineffective digestion and absorption in the small intestine. The relative ratio of acetate, propionate, and butyrate in colon is 6:3:1, and the total concentration of these three SCFAs in colonic lumen is in the range of 50–100 mM. SCFAs serve as an important energy source for colonocytes. These fatty acids enter the colonic epithelium across the lumen–facing apical membrane by diffusion, anion-exchange, $H^+/SCFA^-$ symport, and $Na^+/SCFA^-$ symport [46–49]. The relative contributions of each of these entry mechanisms might vary depending on the luminal concentrations of SCFAs because of the marked differences in the substrate affinities for the transport processes. Under physiological conditions with luminal concentrations of SCFAs in the range of 50–100 mM, diffusion is probably the major entry mechanism. When the concentrations decrease due to changes in the dietary intake of fibers or due to dysbiosis under disease conditions, the carrier-mediated entry mechanisms probably play the major role. Irrespective of the entry mechanism, most of the SCFAs generated by the bacteria are absorbed in the colon, with only a minimal amount excreted in feces. The biological effects of SCFAs in the colon are not restricted to their role as energy substrates for the epithelial cells. These bacterial metabolites promote water and electrolyte absorption in the colon, thus providing protection against potential diarrheagenic diseases [48]. They also modulate the mucosal immune system by helping the development of a tolerant environment to facilitate the co-habitation of the bacteria and the host [50–52]. They aid in the maintenance of the mucosal barrier, thus preventing the direct exposure of systemic organs to colonic bacteria. SCFAs also suppress colonic inflammation and carcinogenesis [43,46,53–56].

As the cell-surface receptors for SCFAs are located on the lumen-facing apical membrane of colonic epithelial cells (see below), the luminal concentrations of these agonists are physiologically relevant. SCFAs are low-affinity agonists for these receptors, and the normal luminal concentrations of these bacterial metabolites are in the millimolar levels, sufficient to activate these receptors from the luminal side. However, some of the molecular targets for these metabolites are either inside the cells (e.g., HDACs) or on the surface of the immune cells located in the lamina propria. Therefore, concentrations of these metabolites inside the colonic epithelial cells and in the lamina propria are relevant to impact these molecular targets. The intracellular target HDAC is inhibited by butyrate and propionate at low micromolar concentrations. There are effective transport systems for SCFAs in the apical membrane of colonic epithelial cells (e.g., proton-coupled and sodium-coupled monocarboxylate transporters) [47], thus making it very likely for these SCFAs to reach intracellular levels sufficient to inhibit HDACs. Even though the luminal concentrations of SCFAs are in the millimolar range, it is unlikely that they reach lamina propria at significant levels to activate the cell-surface receptors present on the mucosal immune cells. These metabolites are present only at micromolar levels in the portal blood [57], indicating that they undergo robust metabolism inside the colonic epithelial cells. This raises the question as to the physiological relevance of these bacterial metabolites to the activation of the cell-surface SCFA receptors in immune cells located in the lamina propria. With regard to this issue, it is important to note that colonic epithelial cells are highly ketogenic; they use acetate and butyrate to generate the ketone body β-hydroxybutyrate [58]. This ketone body is released from the cells into portal blood. As β-hydroxybutyrate is 3–4 times more potent than butyrate in activating its receptor GPR109A, it can be speculated that the colon-derived ketone body is most likely involved in the activation of the SCFA receptor in mucosal immune cells.

Lactate is another bacterial metabolite that is important to colonic health but has received much less attention than the SCFAs. Lactobacilli that generate lactate as a fermentation product form a significant constituent of normal bacterial flora in the colon. As such, in addition to the dietary sources of lactate from yogurt and other dairy products, bacterial metabolism constitutes an important source of lactate in the colonic lumen [36,59].

Bacterial metabolites arising from protein catabolism are receiving increasing attention in recent years, particularly the metabolites resulting from tryptophan degradation [60,61]. This includes indole, indole-3-aldehyde, indole-3-acetic acid, and indole-3-propionic acid. These metabolites also elicit beneficial effects on the host colon; they suppress inflammation and carcinogenesis [14,62]. Another important class of bacterial metabolites that impact on colonic health is the secondary bile acids [63]. Liver synthesizes two different bile acids, namely cholic acid and chenodeoxycholic acid, which are called primary bile acids. These bile acids are secreted into the bile and reach the small intestine to facilitate the digestion and absorption of dietary fat. Almost 95% of these bile acids are reabsorbed in the ileum to undergo entero-hepatic circulation. The remaining bile acids reach the colon where the resident bacteria metabolize them into secondary bile acids (deoxycholic acid and lithocholic acid). The bacteria-generated secondary bile acids get absorbed in the colon and enter the entero-hepatic circulation similar to the primary bile acids produced by the liver. Colonic bacteria also act on dietary lipids, generating metabolites such as conjugated linoleic and linolenic acids and trimethylamine [64–66]. All these molecules have marked biological effects on the host colon. In addition to these metabolites, the bacterial cell-wall components such as lipopolysaccharide, peptidoglycans, and polysaccharide A also serve signaling molecules in the colon.

5. Molecular Targets for Bacterial Metabolites in the Host

Even though the beneficial effects of colonic bacteria and their metabolites on the host have been recognized for a long time, it was not until recently that we began to understand the molecular mechanisms that underlie this important biological phenomenon. This was true even in the case of SCFAs for which there is a long history of investigations focusing on the role of these bacterial metabolites as the molecular link between colonic bacteria and the host. Inhibition of histone deacetylases (HDACs) by the SCFA butyrate is an exception; HDAC is probably the first molecular target discovered for bacterial metabolites in the colon to provide a mechanistic insight into the communication between colonic bacteria and the host [67]. HDACs are enzymes that modulate the epigenetics of the target cells, including the colonic epithelium. Butyrate is an inhibitor of HDAC1 and HDAC3, which belong to class I HDACs [68,69]. Propionate also possesses this inhibitory effect [68,69]. There is overwhelming evidence in the literature for overexpression of HDACs in cancer and for the therapeutic rationale and efficacy of HDAC inhibitors in cancer treatment [70,71]. As such, the biologic phenomenon of protection against colon carcinogenesis by SCFAs can be explained, at least in part, by the functions of butyrate and propionate as inhibitors of HDACs. This also provided a mechanistic explanation for the tumor-suppressive function of the Na^+-coupled SCFA transporter SMCT1 (SLC5A8) in the colon [46]. HDACs being intracellular enzymes, entry of SCFAs from the lumen into colonic epithelial cells is a prerequisite for these bacterial metabolites to reach their molecular targets inside the cells. As inhibition of HDACs causes tumor suppression, it is understandable why the transporter that facilitates this process functions as a tumor suppressor.

In the past decade, we have witnessed a burgeoning of literature describing identification of new and novel molecular targets in the colon for bacterial metabolites [29,50,51,60,61]. These new discoveries have expanded our current understanding and knowledge of the molecular mechanisms as the basis of effective communication between the colonic bacteria and the host. The newly identified molecular targets include the cell-surface G-protein-coupled receptors GPR109A, GPR43, GPR41, GPR 81, and GPR91, and the nuclear receptors AhR (aryl hydrocarbon receptor), PXR (pregnane X receptor), and FXR (farnesoid X receptor). Table 1 lists the bacterial metabolites and the corresponding endogenous metabolites that function as agonists for each of these molecular targets. There are additional molecular targets for bacterial metabolites such as the receptors for bacterial cell-wall components (TLR4 for lipopolysaccharide, NOD1/NOD2 for peptidoglycans, and TLR2 for polysaccharide A) and the receptors for lipid metabolites from bacteria (TAAR5 for trimethylamine and PPARs for conjugated linoleic and linolenic acids) [29]. The present review however will focus on the cell-surface G-protein-coupled receptors GPR109A, GPR43, GPR41, GPR81, and GPR91, and the nuclear receptors AhR, PXR, and FXR.

Table 1. Receptors involved in host-bacteria communication in the colon.

Receptor	Agonist	
	Bacterial Metabolite	**Endogenous Metabolite**
Cell-surface receptors		
GPR109A	Butyrate [72,73]	β-Hydroxybutyrate [74]
GPR43	Acetate, Propionate, Butyrate [75–77]	Acetate, Propionate [75–77]
GPR41	Acetate, Propionate, Butyrate [75]	Acetate, Propionate [75]
GPR81	Lactate [78]	Lactate [78]
GPR91	Succinate [79]	Succinate [79]
Nuclear receptors		
AhR	Tryptamine, Indole, Indole-3-aldehyde, Indole-3-acetic acid, Indole-3-propionic acid [60,61], Indole-3-acrylic acid [80]	Kynurenine [81]
PXR	Lithocholic acid, Indole-3-propionic acid [82]	Steroids [82]
FXR	Deoxycholic acid, Lithocholic acid [83–86]	Cholic acid, Chenodeoxycholic acid [83–86]

6. G-Protein-Coupled Receptors for Bacterial Metabolites

G-protein-coupled receptors are seven transmembrane domain–containing proteins involved in cellular signaling; most of them are expressed on the cell surface to interact with extracellular signals and transmit the signals into the cells via second messengers. The human genome encodes ~700 G-protein-coupled receptors. Even though physiological agonists have been identified for many of these receptors, a significant number of them still remain as orphan receptors with no information on the identity of their agonists. In the last decade, however, a distinct class of these "orphan" receptors has been found to be activated by normal physiological metabolites, which were never considered as signaling molecules; these include long-chain fatty acids, the ketone body β-hydroxybutyrate, the ubiquitous metabolite lactate, and the citric-acid-cycle intermediate succinate. Many of these metabolites are also found in the bacterial kingdom and hence are present in colonic lumen; consequently, if these receptors are expressed on the lumen-facing apical membrane of colonic epithelial cells, bacterial metabolites serve as the agonists for these receptors rather than the metabolites arising from the host metabolism. Examples of this category include GPR81, GPR91, GPR43, and GPR41 (Table 1). In some cases, the endogenous agonists for the receptors in non-colonic tissues are different from the bacterial metabolites, which activate the same receptors in the colon; in these cases, metabolites from bacteria that are structurally similar to endogenous agonists "hijack" the receptors for bacteria-host communication. Examples of this category include GPR109A, AhR, PXR, and FXR (Table 1).

7. GPR109A: Expression and Function in the Colon and the Mucosal Immune System

GPR109A was originally identified as a high-affinity receptor for the B-complex vitamin niacin (nicotinic acid) [87–89]. This provided a molecular mechanism for the niacin-induced correction of dyslipidemia because activation of the receptor in adipocytes inactivates the hormone-sensitive lipase and inhibits lipolysis. However, niacin is only a pharmacological agonist as the affinity of the receptor for niacin (~1 μM) is such that plasma concentrations of niacin under normal physiological conditions (~0.1 μM) are not sufficient to activate the receptor. Subsequently, β-hydroxybutyrate, the major ketone body in blood, was identified as the physiological agonist for the receptor [74]. GPR109A is expressed in a wide variety of tissues/cells including adipose tissue, skin, hepatocytes, retinal cells, and bones; it is also highly expressed in immune cells such as macrophages and dendritic cells [90,91]. Butyrate is the only known SCFA agonist for GPR109A, but it activates the receptor only with low affinity (EC_{50} value in low millimolar range) [72,73]. Acetate and propionate do not interact with the receptor. The receptor is expressed in the intestinal tract, most robustly in the colon where butyrate is present at concentrations high enough to activate the receptor [72,73]. The expression is restricted to the lumen-facing apical membrane of intestinal and colonic epithelial cells, thus having direct access to butyrate in the lumen. As such, the bacterial metabolite butyrate appears to be the principal agonist for GPR109A in the intestinal tract. Colonic bacteria regulate the expression of the receptor in the colon; the expression is markedly reduced in germ-free mice, but the expression comes back to normal when the colon gets re-colonized [73].

Upon ligand binding, GPR109A couples through the Gi pathway in most tissues, resulting in decreased levels of cAMP inside the cells [87,88]. The receptor functions as a suppressor of inflammation and carcinogenesis in the colon [72,92,93]. Deletion of the receptor in mice accelerates the progression of colonic inflammation and colon cancer in multiple experimental model systems [92,93]. The receptor is also expressed on mucosal immune cells, particularly in dendritic cells. Activation of the receptor in dendritic cells promotes the ability of these cells to convert naïve T cells into immunosuppressive Tregs and potentiates the production of the anti-inflammatory cytokine IL-10; Gpr109a-null mice have reduced number of Tregs in the colon, reduced levels of IL-10, and increased levels of the pro-inflammatory cytokine IL-17 [92,93]. Studies with NLRP6 knockout mice have shown that increased Prevotellaceae and decreased IL-18 levels are associated with colitis [94]. Gpr109a-null mice also show decreased IL-18 production and increased population of Prevotellaceae, both alterations leading to potentiation of experimentally induced colitis [92]. Recent studies show that NLRP3-mediated inflammasome plays an important role in IL-18 secretion and regulation of microbiota through GPR109A [93].

8. GPR43: Expression and Function in the Colon and the Mucosal Immune System

GPR43 was discovered in a cluster of four novel GPRs located in close proximity to CD22 on human chromosome 19 [95] and then cloned from mouse leukemia cells [96]. It has a widespread expression pattern, with most prominent expression in the adipose tissue, gastrointestinal tract, leukocytes and neutrophils [75]. The receptor is coupled to both Gq and Gi/o, leading to a decrease in cAMP levels and the activation of phospholipase-C [50,75]. Studies with reporter mice have shown that Gpr43 is highly expressed not only in colonic epithelial cells but also in immune cells present in the colon lamina propria [76]. The receptor is activated by all three major SCFAs, acetate, propionate, and butyrate [77], which is in contrast to GPR109A that is activated solely by butyrate.

The exact biological role of GPR43 under normal physiological conditions remains controversial with regard to whether the receptor suppresses or promotes inflammation and carcinogenesis in the colon. Several studies have demonstrated that the receptor plays a role in promoting inflammation and cancer [77,97–99]. GPR43 is expressed at higher levels in colorectal and gastric cancers and overexpression of the receptor in cancer cells potentiates their growth when xenografted in nude mice [97]. The receptor has also been shown to induce neutrophil chemotaxis and promote inflammation [77,98,99]. However, there are other reports that show the opposite; the receptor functions as a suppressor of colonic inflammation and carcinogenesis [55,100,101]. Tang et al. [100] have reported that GPR43 is silenced in colon cancer, both at the primary site and in metastatic spreads. Most colon cancer cells do not express the receptor, and when engineered to express the receptor ectopically, the cells undergo apoptosis upon exposure to the receptor agonists propionate or butyrate. These studies strongly demonstrate a tumor-suppressive function for the receptor. Maslowski et al. [55] and Masui et al. [101] have shown that Gpr43- null mice are more susceptible to experimental colitis, indicating an anti-inflammatory role for the receptor. Our own studies [102] also corroborated the function of the receptor as a suppressor of inflammation and carcinogenesis. The anti-inflammatory role is further supported by the findings that Gpr43 blocks inflammasomes [93] and deletion of the receptor in mice leads to dysbiosis in colonic microflora and increased susceptibility to colon cancer [102].

In contrast to GPR109A, which is expressed only in colonic epithelial cells, GPR43 is expressed in epithelial cells and in enteroendocrine cells, particularly L-cells [103–105]. This has significant biological implications. L-cells secrete two important gut hormones: glucagon-like peptide 1 and Peptide YY. Activation of GPR43 by SCFAs increases the secretion of both these gut hormones. As these hormones impact on the function of pancreas (insulin secretion) and brain (appetite control), SCFAs influence the biology of distant organs via GPR43 expressed in the intestinal tract.

9. GPR41: Expression and Function in the Colon

GPR41 is also a receptor for SCFAs: all three SCFAs activate the receptor [50]. However, similar to GPR43, GPR41 is expressed in enteroendocrine cells, but unlike GPR43, GPR41 is not expressed in colonic epithelial cells [104–106]. Furthermore, unlike GPR109A and GPR43, GPR41 is also in enteric neurons [107]. However, the intracellular signaling mechanism seems to be similar for all three SCFA receptors, which involve a decrease intracellular levels of cAMP in response to receptor activation. Activation of GPR41 by SCFAs present in the colonic lumen is capable of altering secretion of gut hormones to impact biology at distant organs. Studies have shown that activation of Gpr41 by SCFAs induces secretion of glucagon-like peptide 1 and Peptide YY to alter insulin secretion and appetite control [104,105].

10. GPR81 and GPR91: Expression and Function in the Colon

GPR81 is a cell-surface, G-protein-coupled receptor for the ubiquitous metabolite lactate [78] whereas GPR91, also present on cell-surface, is a G-protein-coupled receptor for the citric-acid cycle intermediate succinate [79]. Relatively less is known about the role of these receptors in the colon. Both these receptors are expressed in colonic epithelial cells and are likely to play a role in colonic biology because lactate is a major metabolite generated by normal colonic bacteria, particularly by Lactobacilli, and succinate is released by dead bacterial cells. The presence of these receptors in the colon and their ligands in the colonic lumen strongly suggest a potential connection between these receptors and colonic health. Further investigations are needed to understand the biological significance of these two receptors and their role in the communication between colonic bacteria and the host.

11. Nuclear Receptors AhR, PXR, and FXR and Their Modulation by Bacterial Metabolites

There are bacterial metabolites other than the SCFAs that are also important for the communication between the host and colonic bacteria and hence for optimal colonic health. These include tryptophan metabolites and bile acids (Table 1). While the SCFAs elicit their biological effects on the colon by serving as agonists for the cell-surface G-protein-coupled receptors GPR109A, GPR43, and GPR41, tryptophan metabolites and bile acids impact colonic health by serving as the ligands for the nuclear receptors AhR (aryl hydrocarbon receptor), PXR (pregnane X receptor), and FXR (farnesoid X receptor). Unlike the G-protein-coupled receptors, which regulate cellular function via changes in intracellular levels of the second messengers such as cAMP and calcium, the nuclear receptors modulate cellular function by altering gene transcription as they all function as transcription factors. However, the ability of these nuclear receptors to bind to their target genes is ligand-dependent; the receptors reside in the cytoplasm when not bound to their ligands, but in the presence of the ligands, the receptor-ligand complex translocates into the nucleus to act on the target genes.

AhR is expressed in colonic epithelial cells and functions as a suppressor of inflammation and carcinogenesis [62,108,109]. The bacterial metabolites that activate this receptor originate from tryptophan catabolism; these include tryptamine, indole, indole-3-aldehyde, indole-3-acetic acid, and indole-3-propionic acid (Table 1). Activation of AhR by these metabolites occurs at doses that are relevant to their concentrations found in the colonic lumen under normal physiological conditions [60,61]. AhR has received considerable attention for its activation by xenobiotics as a process related to xenobiotic biotransformation and their subsequent elimination from the body. However, recent studies have identified the endogenous tryptophan metabolite kynurenine as the physiological agonist for the receptor [81]. Kynurenine is a catabolic product of tryptophan in mammalian cells, generated by the intracellular enzyme indoleamine-2,3-dioxygenase-1 (IDO1); this enzyme is expressed at high levels in colonic epithelial cells. IDO1 is an immunosuppressive enzyme [110] and its robust expression in the colon contributes to the tolerance of the colonic bacteria by the host. Activation of AhR by kynurenine in the colon is obviously essential for the host-bacteria symbiotic relationship. The tryptophan metabolites produced by the colonic bacteria also contribute to this process via their ability to activate the same receptor. A more recent study has identified another tryptophan metabolite, indole-3-acrylic acid, in colonic lumen that is generated by a specific bacterial species, Peptostreptococcus [80]. This metabolite is an agonist for AhR and is also a potent activator of antioxidant machinery in cells [80]. Through these mechanisms, indole-3-acrylic acid promotes intestinal barrier function and attenuates inflammation.

PXR and FXR are also nuclear receptors and they are also activated by various xenobiotics. However, the endogenous agonists for these receptors are steroids and bile acids, respectively (Table 1). The bacterial metabolites that activate these receptors include the secondary bile acids deoxycholic acid and lithocholic acid and the tryptophan metabolite indole-3-propionic acid. The activation of both these receptors elicits protective effects in the colon against inflammation and cancer [82–86].

12. Relevance of Dietary Fiber to the Production of Tryptophan Metabolites in Colon

Colonic bacteria generate tryptophan metabolites via protein metabolism. In contrast, the short-chain fatty acids are generated via fermentation of carbohydrates that reach the colon mostly in the form of dietary fiber. However, the quantity and quality of dietary fiber can potentially impact the generation of tryptophan metabolites because fiber as the source of carbon and energy is a major determinant of the composition of bacterial species in the colon. It has been documented that restriction of sugar in the diet promotes expansion of Lactobacilli species that possess enzymatic machinery to generate selective tryptophan metabolites to activate AhR and stimulate IL22 production [14]. This cytokine alters mucosal immune response in such a manner that it facilitates colonization of selective bacterial species and at the same time prevents colonization of the fungus Candida albicans [14]. As such, alterations in dietary fiber intake have a major impact on the generation of tryptophan metabolites and possibly other metabolites as well.

13. Conclusions

The symbiotic relationship between colonic bacteria and the host is undeniable, and this mutually beneficial coexistence is made possible through effective communication between the two partners in this co-habitation. The primary mode of this communication is chemical, mediated by specific bacterial metabolites that elicit their biological effects on the host by activating selective molecular targets in the host colon. Some of these molecular targets (GPR41, GPR43, GPR109A, GPR81, and GPR91) are located on the lumen-facing apical membrane of colonic epithelial cells where they have direct access to bacterial metabolites generated in the lumen. Some are located intracellularly (e.g., HDACs, AhR, FXR, PXR, and PPARs), and there is evidence that the bacterial metabolites generated in the lumen enter the colonic epithelial cells, many of them via selective transporters expressed in the apical membrane of these cells. Mucosal immune cells present in the lamina propria also express the same molecular targets as in colonic epithelial cells for these bacterial metabolites, but it is questionable if all of these metabolites reach lamina propria at concentrations sufficient to act on these targets in immune cells. This question seems particularly appropriate for SCFAs because these metabolites are actively metabolized in colonic epithelial cells. This might not be an issue for tryptophan metabolites. Taken collectively, there is an overwhelming evidence for active dialogue between colonic bacteria and the host with selective bacterial metabolites functioning as messengers. The end result of this chemical communication is the tolerance of colonic bacteria by the host immune system, which is obligatory for the symbiosis. A beneficial byproduct of this co-habitation and symbiosis is the maintenance of optimal colonic health with a decreased risk of colonic inflammation and carcinogenesis.

Acknowledgments: This work was supported by the National Institutes of Health grant CA190710 and by the Welch Endowed Chair in Biochemistry, Grant No. BI-0028, at the Texas Tech University Health Sciences Center.

Author Contributions: Sathish Sivaprakasam prepared the first draft of the review; Yangzom D. Bhutia and Sabarish Ramachandran helped in the literature search and also worked on the first draft; Vadivel Ganapathy corrected, edited, and revised the first draft and prepared the final version.

Conflicts of Interest: The authors declare no conflict of interest.

References

1. Sender, R.; Fuchs, S.; Milo, R. Revised estimates for the number of human and bacterial cells in the body. *PLoS Biol.* **2016**, *14*, e1002533. [CrossRef] [PubMed]
2. Sender, R.; Fuchs, S.; Milo, R. Are we really vastly outnumbered? Revisiting the ratio of bacterial to host cells in humans. *Cell* **2016**, *164*, 337–340. [CrossRef] [PubMed]
3. Lozupone, C.A.; Stombaugh, J.I.; Gordon, J.I.; Jansson, J.K.; Knight, R. Diversity and resilience of the human gut microbiota. *Nature* **2012**, *489*, 220–230. [CrossRef] [PubMed]
4. Qin, J.; Li, R.; Raes, J.; Arumugam, M.; Burgdorf, K.S.; Manichanh, C.; Nielsen, T.; Pons, N.; Levenez, F.; Yamada, T.; et al. A human gut microbial gene catalogue established by metagenomic sequencing. *Nature* **2010**, *464*, 59–65. [CrossRef] [PubMed]
5. Arumugam, M.; Raes, J.; Pelletier, E.; Le Paslier, D.; Yamada, T.; Mende, D.R.; Fernandes, G.R.; Tap, J.; Bruls, T.; Batto, J.M.; et al. Enterotypes of the human gut microbiome. *Nature* **2011**, *473*, 174–180. [CrossRef] [PubMed]
6. Mu, C.; Yang, Y.; Zhu, W. Gut microbiota: The brain peacekeeper. *Front. Microbiol.* **2016**, *7*, 345. [CrossRef] [PubMed]
7. Haque, T.R.; Barritt, A.S. Intestinal microbiota in liver disease. *Best Pract. Res. Clin. Gastroenterol.* **2016**, *30*, 133–142. [CrossRef] [PubMed]
8. Leal-Lopes, C.; Velloso, F.J.; Campopiano, J.C.; Sogayar, M.C.; Correa, R.G. Roles of commensal microbiota in pancreas homeostasis and pancreatic pathologies. *J. Diabetes Res.* **2015**, *2015*, 284680. [CrossRef] [PubMed]
9. Khan, M.J.; Gerasimidis, K.; Edwards, C.A.; Shaikh, M.G. Role of gut microbiota in the aetiology of obesity: Proposed mechanisms and review of the literature. *J. Obes.* **2016**, *2016*, 7353642. [CrossRef] [PubMed]
10. Jonsson, A.L.; Backhed, F. Role of gut microbiota in atherosclerosis. *Nat. Rev. Cardiol.* **2017**, *14*, 79–87. [CrossRef] [PubMed]
11. Haghikia, A.; Jorg, S.; Duscha, A.; Berg, J.; Manzel, A.; Waschbisch, A.; Hammer, A.; Lee, D.H.; May, C.; Wilck, N.; et al. Dietary fatty acids directly impact central nervous system autoimmunity via the small intestine. *Immunity* **2015**, *43*, 817–829. [CrossRef] [PubMed]
12. Bhutia, Y.D.; Ganapathy, V. Short, but smart: SCFAs train T cells in the gut to fight autoimmunity in the brain. *Immunity* **2015**, *43*, 629–631. [CrossRef] [PubMed]
13. Rothhammer, V.; Mascanfroni, I.D.; Bunse, L.; Takenaka, M.C.; Kenison, J.E.; Mayo, L.; Chao, C.C.; Patel, B.; Yan, R.; Blain, M.; et al. Type I interferons and microbial metabolites of tryptophan modulate astrocyte activity and central nervous system inflammation via the aryl hydrocarbon receptor. *Nat. Med.* **2016**, *22*, 586–597. [CrossRef] [PubMed]
14. Zelante, T.; Iannitti, R.G.; Cunha, C.; De Luca, A.; Giovannini, G.; Pieraccini, G.; Zecchi, R.; D'Angelo, C.; Massi-Benedetti, C.; Fallarino, F.; et al. Tryptophan catabolites from microbiota engage aryl hydrocarbon receptor and balance mucosal reactivity via interleukin-22. *Immunity* **2013**, *39*, 372–385. [CrossRef] [PubMed]
15. Ohland, C.L.; Jobin, C. Microbial activities and intestinal homeostasis: A delicate balance between health and disease. *Cell. Mol. Gastroenterol. Hepatol.* **2015**, *1*, 28–40. [CrossRef] [PubMed]
16. Buttó, L.F.; Haller, D. Dysbiosis in intestinal inflammation: Cause or consequence. *Int. J. Med. Microbiol.* **2016**, *306*, 302–309. [CrossRef] [PubMed]
17. Gao, Z.; Guo, B.; Gao, R.; Zhu, Q.; Qin, H. Microbiota disbiosis is associated with colorectal cancer. *Front. Microbiol.* **2015**, *6*, 20. [CrossRef] [PubMed]

18. Arthur, J.C.; Jobin, C. The struggle within: Microbial influences on colorectal cancer. *Inflamm. Bowel Dis.* **2011**, *17*, 396–409. [CrossRef] [PubMed]
19. Sadlack, B.; Merz, H.; Schorle, H.; Schimpl, A.; Feller, A.C.; Horak, I. Ulcerative colitis-like disease with a disrupted interleukin-2 gene. *Cell* **1993**, *75*, 253–261. [CrossRef]
20. Madsen, K.L. Inflammatory bowel disease: Lessons from the IL-10 gene-deficient mouse. *Clin. Investig. Med.* **2001**, *24*, 250–257.
21. Cani, P.D.; Everard, A. Talking microbes: When gut bacteria interact with diet and host organs. *Mol. Nutr. Food Res.* **2016**, *60*, 58–66. [CrossRef] [PubMed]
22. Velcich, A.; Yang, W.; Heyer, J.; Fragale, A.; Nicholas, C.; Viani, S.; Kucherlapati, R.; Lipkin, M.; Yang, K.; Augenlicht, L. Colorectal cancer in mice genetically deficient in the mucin Muc2. *Science* **2002**, *295*, 1726–1729. [CrossRef] [PubMed]
23. Salim, S.Y.; Söderholm, J.D. Importance of disrupted intestinal barrier in inflammatory bowel diseases. *Inflamm. Bowel Dis.* **2011**, *17*, 362–381. [CrossRef] [PubMed]
24. Yashiro, M. Ulcerative colitis-associated colorectal cancer. *World J. Gastroenterol.* **2014**, *20*, 16389–16397. [CrossRef] [PubMed]
25. Mueller, C.; Macpherson, A.J. Layers of mutualism with commensal bacteria protect us from intestinal inflammation. *Gut* **2006**, *55*, 276–284. [CrossRef] [PubMed]
26. Shapira, M. Gut microbiotas and host evolution: Scaling up symbiosis. *Trends Ecol. Evol.* **2016**, *31*, 539–549. [CrossRef] [PubMed]
27. Cogen, A.L.; Nizet, V.; Gallo, R.L. Skin microbiota: A source of disease or defence? *Br. J. Dermatol.* **2008**, *158*, 442–455. [CrossRef] [PubMed]
28. Macfarlane, S.; Macfarlane, G.T. Regulation of short-chain fatty acid production. *Proc. Nutr. Soc.* **2003**, *62*, 67–72. [CrossRef] [PubMed]
29. Bhutia, Y.D.; Ogura, J.; Sivaprakasam, S.; Ganapathy, V. Gut microbiome and colon cancer: Role of bacterial metabolites and their molecular targets in the host. *Curr. Colorectal Cancer Rep.* **2017**, *13*, 111–118. [CrossRef]
30. Cario, E. Microbiota and innate immunity in intestinal inflammation and neoplasia. *Curr. Opin. Gastroenterol.* **2013**, *29*, 85–91. [CrossRef] [PubMed]
31. Shanahan, F. The colonic microbiota in health and disease. *Curr. Opin. Gastroenterol.* **2013**, *29*, 49–54. [CrossRef] [PubMed]
32. Wang, X.; Huycke, M.M. Colorectal cancer: Role of commensal bacteria and bystander effects. *Gut Microbes* **2015**, *6*, 370–376. [CrossRef] [PubMed]
33. Peloquin, J.M.; Nguyen, D.D. The microbiota and inflammatory bowel disease: Insights from animal models. *Anaerobe* **2013**, *24*, 102–106. [CrossRef] [PubMed]
34. Seksik, P.; Sokol, H.; Lepage, P.; Vasquez, N.; Manichanh, C.; Mangin, I.; Pochart, P.; Dore, J.; Marteau, P. Review article: The role of bacteria in onset and perpetuation of inflammatory bowel disease. *Aliment. Pharmacol. Ther.* **2006**, *24* (Suppl. 3), 11–18. [CrossRef] [PubMed]
35. Butto, L.F.; Schaubeck, M.; Haller, D. Mechanisms of microbe-host interaction in Crohn's disease: Dysbiosis vs. pathobiont selection. *Front. Immunol.* **2015**, *6*, 555. [CrossRef] [PubMed]
36. De Moreno de LeBlanc, A.; Del Carmen, S.; Chatel, J.M.; Miyoshi, A.; Azevedo, V.; Langella, P.; Bermudez-Humaran, L.G.; LeBlanc, J.G. Current review of genetically modified lactic acid bacteria for the prevention and treatment of colitis using murine models. *Gasteroenterol. Res. Pract.* **2015**, *2015*, 146972. [CrossRef] [PubMed]
37. Wasilewski, A.; Zielinska, M.; Storr, M.; Fichna, J. Beneficial effects of probiotics, prebiotics, synbiotics, and psychobiotics in inflammatory bowel disease. *Inflamm. Bowel Dis.* **2015**, *21*, 1674–1682. [CrossRef] [PubMed]
38. Bellaguarda, E.; Chang, E.B. IBD and the gut microbiota—From bench to personalized medicine. *Curr. Gastroenterol. Rep.* **2015**, *17*, 15. [CrossRef] [PubMed]
39. Patel, R.; DuPont, H.L. New approaches for bacteriotherapy: Prebiotics, new-generation probiotics, and synbiotics. *Clin. Infect. Dis.* **2015**, *60* (Suppl. 2), S108–S121. [CrossRef] [PubMed]
40. Grimm, V.; Riedel, C.U. Manipulation of the microbiota using probiotics. *Adv. Exp. Med. Biol.* **2016**, *902*, 109–117. [PubMed]

41. Stearns, J.C.; Lynch, M.D.; Senadheera, D.B.; Tenenbaum, H.C.; Goldberg, M.B.; Cvitkovitch, D.G.; Croitoru, K.; Moreno-Hagelsieb, G.; Neufeld, J.D. Bacterial biogeography of the human digestive tract. *Sci. Rep.* **2011**, *1*, 170. [CrossRef] [PubMed]
42. Vinolo, M.A.; Rodrigues, H.G.; Nachbar, R.T.; Curi, R. Regulation of inflammation by short-chain fatty acids. *Nutrients* **2011**, *3*, 858–876. [CrossRef] [PubMed]
43. Leonel, A.J.; Alvarez-Leite, J.I. Butyrate: Implications for intestinal function. *Curr. Opin. Clin. Nutr. Metab. Care* **2012**, *15*, 474–479. [CrossRef] [PubMed]
44. O'Keefe, S.J. Diet, microorganisms and their metabolites, and colon cancer. *Nat. Rev. Gastroenterol. Hepatol.* **2016**, *13*, 691–706. [CrossRef] [PubMed]
45. Rios-Covian, D.; Ruas-Madeido, P.; Margolles, A.; Gueimonde, M.; de Los Reyes-Gavilan, C.G.; Salazar, N. Intestinal short chain fatty acids and their link with diet and human health. *Front. Microbiol.* **2016**, *7*, 185. [CrossRef] [PubMed]
46. Gupta, N.; Martin, P.M.; Prasad, P.D.; Ganapathy, V. SLC5A8 (SMCT1)-mediated transport of butyrate forms the basis for the tumor-suppressive function of the transporter. *Life Sci.* **2006**, *78*, 2419–2425. [CrossRef] [PubMed]
47. Ganapathy, V.; Thangaraju, M.; Gopal, E.; Martin, P.M.; Itagaki, S.; Miyauchi, S.; Prasad, P.D. Sodium-coupled monocarboxylate transporters in normal tissues and in cancer. *AAPS J.* **2008**, *10*, 193–199. [CrossRef] [PubMed]
48. Binder, H.J. Role of colonic short-chain fatty acid transport in diarrhea. *Annu. Rev. Physiol.* **2010**, *72*, 297–313. [CrossRef] [PubMed]
49. Goncalves, P.; Martel, F. Butyrate and colorectal cancer: The role of butyrate transport. *Curr. Drug Metab.* **2013**, *14*, 994–1008. [CrossRef] [PubMed]
50. Tazoe, H.; Otomo, Y.; Kaji, I.; Tanaka, R.; Karaki, S.I.; Kuwahara, A. Roles of short-chain fatty acids receptors, GPR41 and GPR43 on colonic functions. *J. Physiol. Pharmacol.* **2008**, *59* (Suppl. 2), 252–262.
51. Ganapathy, V.; Thangaraju, M.; Prasad, P.D.; Martin, P.M.; Singh, N. Transporters and receptors for short-chain fatty acids as the molecular link between colonic bacteria and the host. *Curr. Opin. Pharmacol.* **2013**, *13*, 869–874. [CrossRef] [PubMed]
52. Tan, J.; McKenzie, C.; Potamitis, M.; Thorburn, A.N.; Mackay, C.R.; Macia, L. The role of short-chain fatty acids in health and disease. *Adv. Immunol.* **2014**, *121*, 91–119. [PubMed]
53. Arpaia, N.; Campbell, C.; Fan, X.; Dikiy, S.; van der Veeken, J.; deRoos, P.; Liu, H.; Cross, J.R.; Pfeffer, K.; Coffer, P.J.; et al. Metabolites produced by commensal bacteria promote peripheral regulatory T-cell generation. *Nature* **2013**, *504*, 451–455. [CrossRef] [PubMed]
54. Smith, P.M.; Howitt, M.R.; Panikov, N.; Michaud, M.; Gallini, C.A.; Bohlooly-Y, M.; Glickman, J.N.; Garrett, W.S. The microbial metabolites, short-chain fatty acids, regulate colonic Treg cell homeostasis. *Science* **2013**, *341*, 569–573. [CrossRef] [PubMed]
55. Maslowski, K.M.; Vieira, A.T.; Ng, A.; Kranich, J.; Sierro, F.; Yu, D.; Schilter, H.C.; Rolph, M.S.; Mackay, F.; Artis, D.; et al. Regulation of inflammatory responses by gut microbiota and chemoattractant receptor GPR43. *Nature* **2009**, *461*, 1282–1286. [CrossRef] [PubMed]
56. Sengupta, S.; Muir, J.G.; Gibson, P.R. Does butyrate protect from colorectal cancer? *J. Gastroenterol. Hepatol.* **2006**, *21*, 209–218. [CrossRef] [PubMed]
57. Cummings, J.H.; Pomare, E.W.; Branch, W.J.; Naylor, C.P.; Macfarlane, G.T. Short chain fatty acids in human large intestine, portal, hepatic and venous blood. *Gut* **1987**, *28*, 1221–1227. [CrossRef] [PubMed]
58. Helenius, T.O.; Misiorek, J.O.; Nystrom, J.H.; Fortelius, L.E.; Habtezion, A.; Liao, J.; Asghar, M.N.; Zhang, H.; Azhar, S.; Omary, M.B.; et al. Keratin 8 absence down-regulates colonocyte HMGCS2 and modulates colonic ketogenesis and energy metabolism. *Mol. Biol. Cell* **2015**, *26*, 2298–2310. [CrossRef] [PubMed]
59. Pace, F.; Pace, M.; Quartarone, G. Probiotics in digestive diseases: Focus on Lactobacillus GG. *Minerva Gastroenterol. Dietol.* **2015**, *61*, 273–292. [PubMed]
60. Hubbard, T.D.; Murray, I.A.; Perdew, G.H. Indole and tryptophan metabolism: Endogenous and dietary routes to Ah receptor activation. *Drug Metab. Dispos.* **2015**, *43*, 1522–1535. [CrossRef] [PubMed]
61. Jin, U.H.; Lee, S.O.; Sridharan, G.; Lee, K.; Davidson, L.A.; Jayaraman, A.; Chapkin, R.S.; Alaniz, R.; Safe, S. Microbiome-derived tryptophan metabolites and their aryl hydrocarbon receptor-dependent agonist and antagonist activities. *Mol. Pharmacol.* **2014**, *85*, 777–788. [CrossRef] [PubMed]

62. Díaz-Díaz, C.J.; Ronnekleiv-Kelly, S.M.; Nukaya, M.; Geiger, P.G.; Balbo, S.; Dator, R.; Megna, B.W.; Carney, P.R.; Bradfield, C.A.; Kennedy, G.D. The aryl hydrocarbon receptor is a repressor of inflammation-associated colorectal tumorigenesis in mouse. *Ann. Surg.* **2016**, *264*, 429–436. [CrossRef] [PubMed]
63. Ridlon, J.M.; Harris, S.C.; Bhowmik, S.; Kang, D.J.; Hylemon, P.B. Consequences of bile salt biotransformations by intestinal bacteria. *Gut Microbes* **2016**, *7*, 22–39. [CrossRef] [PubMed]
64. Brown, J.M.; Hazen, S.L. The gut microbial endocrine organ: Bacterially derived signals driving cardiometabolic diseases. *Annu. Rev. Med.* **2015**, *66*, 343–359. [CrossRef] [PubMed]
65. Wilson, A.; McLean, C.; Kim, R.B. Trimethylamine-N-oxide: A link between the gut microbiome, bile acid metabolism, and atherosclerosis. *Curr. Opin. Lipidol.* **2016**, *27*, 148–154. [CrossRef] [PubMed]
66. Gorissen, L.; Leroy, F.; De Vuyst, L.; De Smet, S.; Raes, K. Bacterial production of conjugated linoleic and linolenic acid in foods: A technological challenge. *Crit. Rev. Food Sci. Nutr.* **2015**, *55*, 1561–1574. [CrossRef] [PubMed]
67. Davie, J.R. Inhibition of histone deacetylase activity by butyrate. *J. Nutr.* **2003**, *133* (Suppl. 7), S2485–S2493.
68. Thangaraju, M.; Gopal, E.; Martin, P.M.; Ananth, S.; Smith, S.B.; Prasad, P.D.; Sterneck, E.; Ganapathy, V. SLC5A8 triggers tumor cell apoptosis through pyruvate-dependent inhibition of histone deacetylases. *Cancer Res.* **2006**, *66*, 11560–11564. [CrossRef] [PubMed]
69. Singh, N.; Thangaraju, M.; Prasad, P.D.; Martin, P.M.; Lambert, N.A.; Boettger, T.; Offermanns, S.; Ganapathy, V. Blockade of dendritic cell development by bacterial fermentation products butyrate and propionate through a transporter (Slc5a8)-dependent inhibition of histone deacetylases. *J. Biol. Chem.* **2010**, *285*, 27601–27608. [CrossRef] [PubMed]
70. Montezuma, D.; Henrique, R.M.; Jeronimo, C. Altered expression of histone deacetylases in cancer. *Crit. Rev. Oncog.* **2015**, *20*, 19–34. [CrossRef] [PubMed]
71. West, A.C.; Johnstone, R.W. New and emerging HDAC inhibitors for cancer treatment. *J. Clin. Investig.* **2014**, *124*, 30–39. [CrossRef] [PubMed]
72. Thangaraju, M.; Cresci, G.A.; Liu, K.; Ananth, S.; Gnanaprakasam, J.P.; Browning, D.D.; Mellinger, J.D.; Smith, S.B.; Digby, G.J.; Lambert, N.A.; et al. GPR109A is a G-protein-coupled receptor for the bacterial fermentation product butyrate and functions as a tumor suppressor in colon. *Cancer Res.* **2009**, *69*, 2826–2832. [CrossRef] [PubMed]
73. Cresci, G.A.; Thangaraju, M.; Mellinger, J.D.; Liu, K.; Ganapathy, V. Colonic gene expression in conventional and germ-free mice with a focus on the butyrate receptor GPR109A and the butyrate transporter SLC5A8. *J. Gastrointest. Surg.* **2010**, *14*, 449–461. [CrossRef] [PubMed]
74. Taggart, A.K.; Kero, J.; Gan, X.; Cai, T.Q.; Cheng, K.; Ippolito, M.; Ren, N.; Kaplan, R.; Wu, K.; Wu, T.J.; et al. (D)-β-hydroxybutyrate inhibits adipocyte lipolysis via the nicotinic acid receptor PUMA-G. *J. Biol. Chem.* **2005**, *280*, 26649–26652. [CrossRef] [PubMed]
75. Brown, A.J.; Goldsworthy, S.M.; Barnes, A.A.; Eilert, M.M.; Tcheang, L.; Daniels, D.; Muir, A.I.; Wigglesworth, M.J.; Kinghorn, I.; Fraser, N.J.; et al. The Orphan G protein-coupled receptors GPR41 and GPR43 are activated by propionate and other short chain carboxylic acids. *J. Biol. Chem.* **2003**, *278*, 11312–11319. [CrossRef] [PubMed]
76. Nøhr, M.K.; Pedersen, M.H.; Gille, A.; Egerod, K.L.; Engelstoft, M.S.; Husted, A.S.; Sichlau, R.M.; Grunddal, K.V.; Poulsen, S.S.; Han, S.; et al. GPR41/FFAR3 and GPR43/FFAR2 as cosensors for short-chain fatty acids in enteroendocrine cells vs. FFAR3 in enteric neurons and FFAR2 in enteric leukocytes. *Endocrinology* **2013**, *154*, 3552–3564. [CrossRef] [PubMed]
77. Le Poul, E.; Loison, C.; Struyf, S.; Springael, J.Y.; Lannoy, V.; Decobecq, M.E.; Brezillon, S.; Dupriez, V.; Vassart, G.; Van Damme, J.; et al. Functional characterization of human receptors for short chain fatty acids and their role in polymorphonuclear cell activation. *J. Biol. Chem.* **2003**, *278*, 25481–25489. [CrossRef] [PubMed]
78. Liu, C.; Wu, J.; Zhu, J.; Kuei, C.; Yu, J.; Shelton, J.; Sutton, S.W.; Li, X.; Yun, S.J.; Mirzadegan, T.; et al. Lactate inhibits lipolysis in fat cells through activation of an orphan G-protein-coupled receptor. *J. Biol. Chem.* **2009**, *284*, 2811–2822. [CrossRef] [PubMed]
79. He, W.; Miao, F.J.; Lin, D.C.; Schwandner, R.T.; Wang, Z.; Gao, J.; Chen, J.L.; Tian, H.; Ling, L. Citric acid cycle intermediates as ligands for orphan G-protein-coupled receptors. *Nature* **2004**, *429*, 188–193. [CrossRef] [PubMed]

80. Wlodarska, M.; Luo, C.; Kolde, R.; d'Hennezel, E.; Annand, J.W.; Heim, C.E.; Krastel, P.; Schmitt, E.K.; Omar, A.S.; Creasey, E.A.; et al. Indoleacrylic acid produced by commensal Peptostrreptococcus species suppresses inflammation. *Cell Host Microbe* **2017**, *22*, 25–37. [CrossRef] [PubMed]
81. Opitz, C.A.; Litzenburger, U.M.; Sahm, F.; Ott, M.; Tritschler, I.; Trump, S.; Schumacher, T.; Jestaedt, L.; Schrenk, D.; Weller, M.; et al. An endogenous tumour-promoting ligand of the human aryl hydrocarbon receptor. *Nature* **2011**, *478*, 197–203. [CrossRef] [PubMed]
82. Cheng, J.; Shah, Y.M.; Gonzalez, F.J. Pregnane X receptor as a target for treatment of inflammatory bowel disorders. *Trends Pharmacol. Sci.* **2012**, *33*, 323–330. [CrossRef] [PubMed]
83. Cheng, J.; Fang, Z.Z.; Nagaoka, K.; Okamoto, M.; Qu, A.; Tanaka, N.; Kimura, S.; Gonzalez, F.J. Activation of intestinal human pregnane X receptor protects against azoxymethane/dextran sulfate sodium-induced colitis. *J. Pharmacol. Exp. Ther.* **2014**, *351*, 559–567. [CrossRef] [PubMed]
84. Modica, S.; Murzilli, S.; Salvatore, L.; Schmidt, D.R.; Moschetta, A. Nuclear bile acid receptor FXR protects against intestinal tumorigenesis. *Cancer Res.* **2008**, *68*, 9589–9594. [CrossRef] [PubMed]
85. Maran, R.R.; Thomas, A.; Roth, M.; Sheng, Z.; Esterly, N.; Pinson, D.; Gao, X.; Zhang, Y.; Ganapathy, V.; Gonzalez, F.J.; et al. Farnesoid X receptor deficiency in mice leads to increased intestinal epithelial cell proliferation and tumor development. *J. Pharmacol. Exp. Ther.* **2009**, *328*, 469–477. [CrossRef] [PubMed]
86. Stojancevic, M.; Stankov, K.; Mikov, M. The impact of farnesoid X receptor activation on intestinal permeability in inflammatory bowel disease. *Can. J. Gastroenterol.* **2012**, *26*, 631–637. [CrossRef] [PubMed]
87. Tunaru, S.; Kero, J.; Schaub, A.; Wufka, C.; Blaukat, A.; Pfeffer, K.; Offermanns, S. PUMA-G and HM74 are receptors for nicotinic acid and mediate its anti-lipolytic effect. *Nat. Med.* **2003**, *9*, 352–355. [CrossRef] [PubMed]
88. Wise, A.; Foord, S.M.; Fraser, N.J.; Barnes, A.A.; Elshourbagy, N.; Eilert, M.; Ignar, D.M.; Murdock, P.R.; Steplewski, K.; Green, A.; et al. Molecular identification of high and low affinity receptors for nicotinic acid. *J. Biol. Chem.* **2003**, *278*, 9869–9874. [CrossRef] [PubMed]
89. Soga, T.; Kamohara, M.; Takasaki, J.; Matsumoto, S.; Saito, T.; Ohishi, T.; Hiyama, H.; Matsuo, A.; Matsushime, H.; Furuichi, K. Molecular identification of nicotinic acid receptor. *Biochem. Biophys. Res. Commun.* **2003**, *303*, 364–369. [CrossRef]
90. Gille, A.; Bodor, E.T.; Ahmed, K.; Offermanns, S. Nicotinic acid: Pharmacological effects and mechanisms of action. *Annu. Rev. Pharmacol. Toxicol.* **2008**, *48*, 79–106. [CrossRef] [PubMed]
91. Blad, C.C.; Ahmed, K.; IJzerman, A.P.; Offermanns, S. Biological and pharmacological roles of HCA receptors. *Adv. Pharmacol.* **2011**, *62*, 219–250. [PubMed]
92. Singh, N.; Gurav, A.; Sivaprakasam, S.; Brady, E.; Padia, R.; Shi, H.; Thangaraju, M.; Prasad, P.D.; Manicassamy, S.; Munn, D.H.; et al. Activation of Gpr109a, receptor for niacin and the commensal metabolite butyrate, suppresses colonic inflammation and carcinogenesis. *Immunity* **2014**, *40*, 128–139. [CrossRef] [PubMed]
93. Macia, L.; Tan, J.; Vieira, A.T.; Leach, K.; Stanley, D.; Luong, S.; Maruya, M.; Ian McKenzie, C.; Hijikata, A.; Wong, C.; et al. Metabolite-sensing receptors GPR43 and GPR109A facilitate dietary fibre-induced gut homeostasis through regulation of the inflammasome. *Nat. Commun.* **2015**, *6*, 6734. [CrossRef] [PubMed]
94. Elinav, E.; Strowig, T.; Kau, A.L.; Henao-Mejia, J.; Thaiss, C.A.; Booth, C.J.; Peaper, D.R.; Bertin, J.; Eisenbarth, S.C.; Gordon, J.I.; et al. NLRP6 inflammasome regulates colonic microbial ecology and risk for colitis. *Cell* **2011**, *145*, 745–757. [CrossRef] [PubMed]
95. Sawzdargo, M.; George, S.R.; Nguyen, T.; Xu, S.; Kolakowski, L.F.; O'Dowd, B.F. A cluster of four novel human G protein-coupled receptor genes occurring in close proximity to CD22 gene on chromosome 19q13.1. *Biochem. Biophys. Res. Commun.* **1997**, *239*, 543–547. [CrossRef] [PubMed]
96. Senga, T.; Iwamoto, S.; Yoshida, T.; Yokota, T.; Adachi, K.; Azuma, E.; Hamaguchi, M.; Iwamoto, T. LSSIG is a novel murine leukocyte-specific GPCR that is induced by the activation of STAT3. *Blood* **2003**, *101*, 1185–1187. [CrossRef] [PubMed]
97. Hatanaka, H.; Tsukui, M.; Takada, S.; Kurashina, K.; Choi, Y.L.; Soda, M.; Yamashita, Y.; Haruta, H.; Hamada, T.; Ueno, T.; et al. Identification of transforming activity of free fatty acid receptor 2 by retroviral expression screening. *Cancer Sci.* **2010**, *101*, 54–59. [CrossRef] [PubMed]
98. Vinolo, M.A.; Ferguson, G.J.; Kulkarni, S.; Damoulakis, G.; Anderson, K.; Bohlooly, Y.M.; Stephens, L.; Hawkins, P.T.; Curi, R. SCFAs induce mouse neutrophil chemotaxis through the GPR43 receptor. *PLoS ONE* **2011**, *6*, e21205. [CrossRef] [PubMed]

99. Sina, C.; Gavrilova, O.; Förster, M.; Till, A.; Derer, S.; Hildebrand, F.; Raabe, B.; Chalaris, A.; Scheller, J.; Rehmann, A.; et al. G protein-coupled receptor 43 is essential for neutrophil recruitment during intestinal inflammation. *J. Immunol.* **2009**, *183*, 7514–7522. [CrossRef] [PubMed]
100. Tang, Y.; Chen, Y.; Jiang, H.; Robbins, G.T.; Nie, D. G-protein-coupled receptor for short-chain fatty acids suppresses colon cancer. *Int. J. Cancer* **2011**, *128*, 847–856. [CrossRef] [PubMed]
101. Masui, R.; Sasaki, M.; Funaki, Y.; Ogasawara, N.; Mizuno, M.; Iida, A.; Izawa, S.; Kondo, Y.; Ito, Y.; Tamura, Y.; et al. G protein-coupled receptor 43 moderates gut inflammation through cytokine regulation from mononuclear cells. *Inflamm. Bowel Dis.* **2013**, *19*, 2848–2856. [CrossRef] [PubMed]
102. Sivaprakasam, S.; Gurav, A.; Paschall, A.V.; Coe, G.L.; Chaudhary, K.; Cai, Y.; Kolhe, R.; Martin, P.; Browning, D.; Huang, L.; et al. An essential role of Ffar2 (Gpr43) in dietary fibre-mediated promotion of healthy composition of gut microbiota and suppression of intestinal carcinogenesis. *Oncogenesis* **2016**, *5*, e238. [CrossRef] [PubMed]
103. Psichas, A.; Sleeth, M.L.; Murphy, K.G.; Brooks, L.; Bewick, G.A.; Hanyaloglu, A.C.; Ghatei, M.A.; Bloom, S.R.; Frost, G. The short chain fatty acid propionate stimulates GLP-1 and PYY secretion via free fatty acid receptor 2 in rodents. *Int. J. Obes.* **2015**, *39*, 424–429. [CrossRef] [PubMed]
104. Tolhurst, G.; Heffron, H.; Lam, Y.S.; Parker, H.E.; Habib, A.M.; Diakogiannaki, E.; Cameron, J.; Grosse, J.; Reimann, F.; Gribble, F.M. Short-chain fatty acids stimulate glucagon-like peptide-1 secretion via the G-protein-coupled receptor FFAR2. *Diabetes* **2012**, *61*, 364–371. [CrossRef] [PubMed]
105. Kaji, I.; Karaki, S.; Kuwahara, A. Short-chain fatty acid receptor and its contribution to glucagon-like peptide-1 release. *Digestion* **2014**, *89*, 31–36. [CrossRef] [PubMed]
106. Tazoe, H.; Otomo, Y.; Karaki, S.; Kato, I.; Fukami, Y.; Terasaki, M.; Kuwahara, A. Expression of short-chain fatty acid receptor GPR41 in the human colon. *Biomed. Res.* **2009**, *30*, 149–156. [CrossRef] [PubMed]
107. Kimura, I.; Inoue, D.; Maeda, T.; Hara, T.; Ichimura, A.; Miyauchi, S.; Kobayashi, M.; Hirasawa, A.; Tsujimoto, G. Short-chain fatty acids and ketones directly regulate sympathetic nervous system via G protein-coupled receptor 41 (GPR41). *Proc. Natl. Acad. Sci. USA* **2011**, *108*, 8030–8035. [CrossRef] [PubMed]
108. Stockinger, B.; Di Meglio, P.; Gialitakis, M.; Duarte, J.H. The aryl hydrocarbon receptor: Multitasking in the immune system. *Annu. Rev. Immunol.* **2014**, *32*, 403–432. [CrossRef] [PubMed]
109. Xie, G.; Raufman, J.P. Role of the aryl hydrocarbon receptor in colon neoplasia. *Cancers* **2015**, *7*, 1436–1446. [CrossRef] [PubMed]
110. Munn, D.H.; Mellor, A.L. IDO in the tumor microenvironment: Inflammation, counter-regulation, and tolerance. *Trends Immunol.* **2016**, *37*, 193–207. [CrossRef] [PubMed]

Section 2:
Cancer Prevention and Treatment

nutrients

Article

Novel Combination of Prebiotics Galacto-Oligosaccharides and Inulin-Inhibited Aberrant Crypt Foci Formation and Biomarkers of Colon Cancer in Wistar Rats

Tahir Rasool Qamar [1], Fatima Syed [1], Muhammad Nasir [1], Habib Rehman [2], Muhammad Nauman Zahid [3], Rui Hai Liu [4] and Sanaullah Iqbal [1,*]

1 Department of Food Science and Human Nutrition, University of Veterinary & Animal Sciences, Lahore 54000, Punjab, Pakistan; tahirnutritionist@gmail.com (T.R.Q.); syed199146@gmail.com (F.S.); nasir@uvas.edu.pk (M.N.)
2 Department of Physiology, University of Veterinary & Animal Sciences, Lahore 54000, Punjab, Pakistan; habibrehman@uvas.edu.pk
3 Department of Population Medicine and Diagnostic Sciences, Cornell University, Ithaca, NY 14850, USA; mnz9@cornell.edu
4 Department of Food Science, Cornell University, Ithaca, NY 14850, USA; rl23@cornell.edu
* Correspondence: sanaullah.iqbal@uvas.edu.pk; Tel.: +92-42-9921-1449 (ext. 283); Fax: +92-42-9921-1449

Received: 23 May 2016; Accepted: 20 July 2016; Published: 1 August 2016

Abstract: The selectivity and beneficial effects of prebiotics are mainly dependent on composition and glycosidic linkage among monosaccharide units. This is the first study to use prebiotic galacto-oligosaccharides (GOS) that contains β-1,6 and β-1,3 glycosidic linkages and the novel combination of GOS and inulin in cancer prevention. The objective of the present study is to explore the role of novel GOS and inulin against various biomarkers of colorectal cancer (CRC) and the incidence of aberrant crypt foci (ACF) in a 1,2-dimethyl hydrazine dihydrochloride (DMH)-induced rodent model. Prebiotic treatments of combined GOS and inulin (57 mg each), as well as individual doses (GOS: 76–151 mg; inulin 114 mg), were given to DMH-treated animals for 16 weeks. Our data reveal the significant preventive effect of the GOS and inulin combination against the development of CRC. It was observed that inhibition of ACF formation (55.8%) was significantly ($p \leqslant 0.05$) higher using the GOS and inulin combination than GOS (41.4%) and inulin (51.2%) treatments alone. This combination also rendered better results on short-chain fatty acids (SCFA) and bacterial enzymatic activities. Dose-dependent effects of prebiotic treatments were also observed on cecum and fecal bacterial enzymes and on SCFA. Thus, this study demonstrated that novel combination of GOS and inulin exhibited stronger preventive activity than their individual treatments alone, and can be a promising strategy for CRC chemoprevention.

Keywords: prebiotics; galacto-oligosaccharides; inulin; biomarkers; colon cancer

1. Introduction

Colorectal cancer (CRC) is one of the major causes of mortality in both genders among cancer-related deaths worldwide. Being quite a complex process, many factors contribute to the onset of colon cancer and the major risk factors include family history, age, pre-carcinogens present in the food chain and environment [1,2], inflammatory bowel diseases, low intake of vegetables, fruits and fibers, high consumption of red meat and processed meat [3,4], as well as hereditary genetic factors [5]. Epidemiological studies suggest that high intake of fruits and vegetables in human diets has been linked to a lower risk of colon cancer. Excessive scientific and public concerns have been shown in earlier studies to identify naturally-occurring substances in food for CRC chemoprevention [6,7]. In chemoprevention, those natural or synthetic bioactive compounds are used to prevent, delay, or reverse the formation of adenomas, as well as their progression into carcinomas through signal transduction pathways in tumor cells. Recently, prebiotics have gained much attention as natural dietary ingredients which have the potential to maintain a healthy environment in gastrointestinal tract to improve intestinal functions and to prevent colon cancer [8].

Prebiotics are emerging as bioactive ingredients in foods and can positively influence the gastrointestinal microbiota and metabolism [9]. The beneficial bacteria residing in the colon causes fermentation of prebiotics to produce short chain fatty acids (SCFA), including acetate, propionate, and butyrate, which are further involved in prevention of CRC [10,11]. Prebiotic galacto-oligosaccharides (GOS) are produced through transgalactosylation of lactose catalyzed by β-galactosidase (EC 3.2.1.23). During this process various products may be produced having β-1,3, β-1,4, or β-1,6 glycosidic linkages depending upon the source of the enzyme [12]. Previous studies have demonstrated that GOS having different glycosidic linkages have different health effects on the host [13], so glycosidic linkages used between monosaccharide residues is of high importance in imparting health benefits.

The current study was performed to assess, for the first time, the combined effects of prebiotics GOS and inulin, as well as their individual effect on the various biomarkers of the initiation process of rat colon carcinogenesis. Several previously-performed experimental studies have shown that administration of prebiotics, probiotics [14], and synbiotics [15] provide protective and preventive effects against early biomarkers and tumor development in the colon of carcinogen-induced rats [16–18]. Research on GOS' role in colon cancer prevention is very limited to date. GOS used in previous studies had β-1,4 as the primary glycosidic linkage [19,20] and no product with β-1,3 or β-1,6 linkages have yet been used against any cancer treatment. To the best of our knowledge, this is the first time to use prebiotic GOS that contains β-1,6 and β-1,3 glycosidic linkages in a cancer prevention study.

Inulin-type prebiotics have been extensively studied for their potential benefits, and a large number of experimental studies have shown anti-carcinogenic effects of inulin this is the reason we added inulin as the positive control in our experiment to compare GOS anti-carcinogenic effects with inulin, as very limited data is available for the efficacy of GOS against CRC. No study is available on the combined effect of GOS and inulin against CRC prevention. The objectives of the present study were to investigate the preventive effects of inulin and GOS supplementation separately and in combination against the incidence of aberrant crypt foci (ACF) in a 1,2-dimethyl hydrazine dihydrochloride (DMH)-induced rodent model and to evaluate their effects on various biomarkers of colon cancer. Our study suggests that GOS had a dose-dependent preventive effect on biomarkers of colon cancer and the combined effect of GOS and inulin exhibited stronger preventive activity than their individual treatments alone.

2. Materials and Methods

2.1. Chemicals

All chemicals and reagents were analytical grade and were purchased form Merck Chemicals (Darmstadt, Germany) unless otherwise stated. The DMH, m-nitrobenzoic acid, phenolphthalein-β-D-glucuronide, nitrophenyl-β-D-glucoside, and *ortho*-nitrophenyl-β-D-galactopyranoside (*o*NPG) were purchased from Sigma-Aldrich (St. Louis, MO, USA). The prebiotic inulin extracted from chicory roots was purchased from Cargill® (Minneapolis, MN, USA).

2.2. Animals

Six-week old male Wister rats were purchased from the University of Agriculture, Faisalabad-Pakistan and were housed in temperature and humidity control room (22 ± 2 °C and 55% ± 10%) under 12 h light and dark cycle. All rats received basal diet for one week acclimatization period before beginning the actual experiment. The experimental protocols used herein were approved by the University Ethics Committee for Animal Research.

2.3. Experimental Design

Rats were randomly divided into seven groups (12 per group); G1 was control group fed on AIN-93G/M as basal diet [21]. G2 (DMH alone) was DMH control group fed on basal diet, and Groups G3–G7 were treatment groups. Treatments with prebiotic GOS were given to Groups G3–G5. Group G6 was given inulin and Group G7 received combination of GOS and inulin along with basal diet. Dose was calculated using the human equivalent dose (HED) equation: HED = animal dose in mg/kg × (animal weight in kg/human weight in kg)$^{0.33}$ [22]. Groups G3, G4, and G5 received 76 mg (HED = 4 g), 114 mg (HED = 6 g), and 151 mg (HED = 8 g) GOS, respectively. Group G6 received 114 mg (HED = 6 g) of inulin and group G7 was given combination of GOS and inulin (GOS 57 mg + inulin 57 mg) 114 mg (HED = 6 g). The doses of prebiotics were given orally through tube feeding for a period of 16 weeks according to each group's mean body weight at beginning of experiment and were adjusted at the end of each week according to body weight changes. In order to make experimental conditions similar, groups G1 and G2 were administered the same amount of water orally. After 16 weeks, all animals were sacrificed by injection of 45 mg/kg body weight of sodium pentobarbital anesthesia.

2.4. Carcinogenic Injection

After acclimatization period of one week, respective groups were given prebiotics daily and after completion of four weeks of prebiotics doses, groups G2–G7 received four subcutaneous injections of DMH, 40 mg/kg body weight, twice a week for 2 weeks [23,24]. While G1, control group received similar subcutaneous injections of Ethylenediaminetetraacetic acid (EDTA) solution of pH 6.0 (DMH vehicle). All prebiotic doses were continued during DMH administration.

2.5. Preparation of Prebiotic GOS

The *Escherichia coli* BL21 (DE3) containing β-galactosidase (β-gal) gene from *Lactobacillus reuteri* L103 was courtesy of Dietmar Haltrich, Food Biotechnology Laboratory, University of Natural Resources and Life Sciences, Vienna Austria and was used for β-gal production. The enzyme, β-gal was produced by following the procedure explained by Iqbal et al. [25] and enzyme activity was measured for *o*NPG and lactose. The crude cell extract of β-gal was used for the production of prebiotic GOS through transgalactosylation of lactose (250 g/L) prepared in 50 mM sodium phosphate buffer, pH 6.5 at 37 °C. The reaction was carried out for 5 h and immediately stopped by heating at 95 °C for 5 min and stored at −20 °C for further analysis. The Megazyme assay kits (Wicklow, Ireland) were used to analyze glucose (GOPOD assay kit, K-GLUC), galactose and lactose (Lactose/Galactose assay kit, K-LACGAR) in the transgalactosylated mixture by following standard protocol given in the manual and GOS were calculated by subtraction method. The maximum GOS were produced at 75% lactose conversion after 5 h of reaction and the final mixture contained 30% GOS, 30% D-glucose, 15% D-galactose and 25% untransgalactosylated lactose. Furthermore, the mixture of GOS was composed of mainly disaccharide (allolactose) and tri-saccharides followed by tetra-saccharides. It was also observed that maximum GOS were produced at 5 h of lactose conversion and as the reaction continued, all GOS were converted to monosaccharides, glucose, and galactose.

2.6. Measurement of Body Weight Changes

The body weight changes of rats were recorded weekly on weighing scale (Model No. SCL66110 Olympia Plus Kent Scientific Corporation, Torrington, CT, USA).

2.7. pH and Ammonia

The pH of cecal and fecal digesta were measured using a microelectrode and a pH/ION meter (Model No. HI 111, Hanna Instruments, Ann Arbor, MI, USA). The ammonia concentration was determined by the method described by Lin and Visek [26].

2.8. Aberrant Crypt Foci (ACF) Analysis

After animals were sacrificed, the colon was carefully removed, opened longitudinally, and gently rinsed with saline to remove residual bowel contents followed by fixing flat in 10% buffered formalin for 24 h at room temperature. The colon was divided into proximal (near the cecum), middle, and distal colon (near the rectum). Methylene blue (0.2%) was used to stain all these three sections and ACF counting was performed under light microscope. The total number of ACF per rat were calculated as the sum of small, medium, and large ACF in colon [27].

2.9. Samples Collection and Enzyme Analysis

To ensure fresh fecal samples, before sacrificing animals fecal samples were collected by gently squeezing the rectal region of rats and cecum samples were collected after sacrificing each animal, which were processed immediately after collection. Azoreductase activity was determined according to the method described by Goldin and Gorbach [28] and for nitroreductase, β-glucuronidase, β-glucosidase, and azoreductase activities minor modifications were made in methods described by Goldin and Gorbach [28].

2.9.1. Nitroreductase Assay

Cold pre-reduced (0.2 M; pH 7.8) Tris-HCl buffer was used to suspend fresh cecum and fecal samples. Specimens were disrupted using spatula and were agitated by adding glass beads of 0.2-mm diameter in a tightly stoppered tube for several minutes on a vortex mixer. The supernatant was collected anaerobically by centrifuging the suspension at 500× g for 10 min. This supernatant was further processed for enzyme assay. The reaction was carried out anaerobically for 1 h at 30 °C (pH 7.8). The total volume of reaction mixture was 500 μL containing 0.08 M Tris-HCl buffer, 0.35 mM m-nitrobenzoic acid, 0.5 mM NADPH, 1 mM NADH and 200 μL fecal and cecum extracts. At the end of reaction 750 μL HCl of 1.2 N concentration was added in reaction mixture to stop chemical process. To measure the amount of m-aminobenzoic acid produced, readings were taken at 550 nm. A standard curve was prepared by using the Bratton-Marshall reaction on known concentrations of m-aminobenzoic acid.

2.9.2. β-Glucuronidase Assay

Fresh cecal and fecal samples were thawed in cold potassium phosphate buffer (0.1 M) having pH 7.0. The cecal and fecal suspensions were homogenized in a pre-chilled homogenizer. The filtrate was sonicated for 30 s (six times) bursts at 4 °C and then supernatant was collected by centrifuging at 500× g for 15 min. The enzyme reaction was carried out using supernatant at 37 °C (pH 6.8), 500 μL was the total volume of reaction mixture containing 0.02 M potassium phosphate buffer, 0.1 mM EDTA, 1 mM phenolphthalein-β-D-glucuronide, and 50 μL cecal and fecal extracts. At the end of reaction 2.5 mL glycine buffer (0.2 M) having pH 10.4 containing NaCl (0.2 M) was added to stop the reaction. A standard curve of phenolphthalein was prepared for comparison to determine the amount of phenolphthalein released, all readings were taken at 540 nm.

2.9.3. β-Glucosidase Assay

The samples for β-glucosidase assay were prepared as described for the β-glucuronidase assay. Reaction was carried out at 37 °C (pH 7.0), 500 μL was the total volume of reaction mixture containing 0.1 M potassium phosphate buffer, 1 mM nitrophenyl-β-D-glucoside and 100 μL cecal and fecal extracts.

At the end of reaction 2.5 mL sodium hydroxide of 0.01 M concentration was added in reaction mixture to stop chemical process. A standard curve of nitrophenol was prepared for comparison to determine the amount of nitrophenol released, all readings were taken at 420 nm.

2.10. Short Chain Fatty Acids

After collection, cecal and fecal contents were stored at −80 °C until analysis of SCFAs using gas chromatography (Agilent 6890 Plus gas chromatograph, Santa Clara, CA, USA) and expressed as μmol/g of cecal/fecal material [29]. One gram of cecal/fecal sample was thawed and suspended in 5 mL of distilled water followed by homogenization (UltraTurrax T 25, Staufen, Germany) for 3 min, resulting in a 20% (*w*/*v*) cecal/fecal suspension. The HCl (5 M) was used to adjust the pH of suspension to 2–3 and was placed on shaker for 10 min at room temperature followed by centrifugation (5000 rpm) for 20 min and the clear supernatant was separated. 2-ethylbutyric acid solution was added in supernatant as internal standard having final concentration of 1 mM and this prepared supernatant was used for the quantification of acetic, propionic, and butyric acids using standards of these fatty acids.

2.11. Statistical Analysis

All of the results were expressed as mean ± standard error (SE). The inter group variation was assessed by one way analysis of variance (ANOVA) using SPSS software (ver. 18). In all significant results, post hoc comparison was performed using the Duncan Multiple Range test (DMRt). Differences were considered significant at $p < 0.05$.

3. Results

3.1. Body Weight and Food Intake

All groups were provided with a basal diet, along with DMH and different treatments of prebiotics, GOS, and inulin, except group G1 (fed only on basal diet) and G2 (basal diet and DMH without prebiotics). There were no significant differences in food intake among all groups (Table 1).

Table 1. Average food intake in different groups of animals throughout the experiment.

Groups	Food Intake (g/Rat/Day)
G1 (Basal Diet Control Group)	20.0 ± 0.5 [a]
G2 (DMH Control Group)	20.6 ± 0.6 [a]
G3 (DMH + GOS 76 mg)	21.0 ± 0.6 [a]
G4 (DMH + GOS 114 mg)	20.3 ± 0.5 [a]
G5 (DMH + GOS 151 mg)	20.1 ± 0.5 [a]
G6 (DMH + Inulin 114 mg)	21.0 ± 0.6 [a]
G7 (DMH + GOS 57 mg + Inulin 57 mg)	20.7 ± 0.6 [a]

Note: Values are expressed as mean ± SE. Means with the same letters are not significantly different ($p \leqslant 0.05$).

Group G1 gained significant body weight ($p \leqslant 0.05$) as compared to all other groups. DMH administration significantly reduced the body weight compared to group G1 as shown in Figure 1 (Body weight gain = final body wt. − initial body wt.). Group G2 gained the lowest body weight as compared to all other groups. Groups G3–G5, given GOS treatments, showed resistance to DMH-induced body weight loss and manifested dose-dependent alleviation of their body weights ($p \leqslant 0.05$) as compared to Group G2. Moreover, inulin, at a dose of 114 mg, exerted a better effect on body weight recovery than GOS treatment at the same dose. Interestingly, the combination of GOS and inulin achieved the best results in preventing DMH-induced body weight loss (Figure 1).

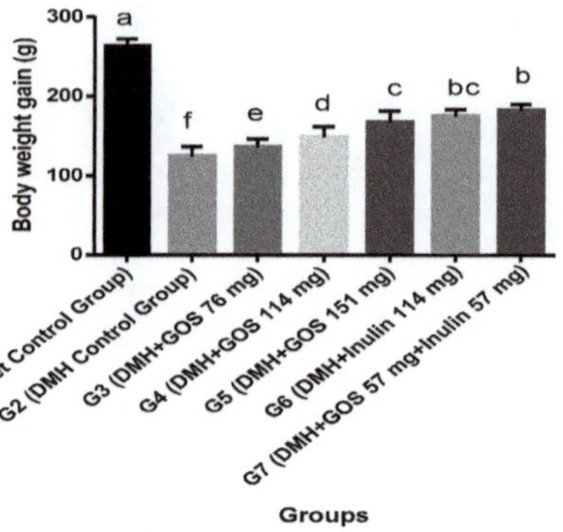

Figure 1. Change in body weights in DMH-initiated and non-initiated animals. Among DMH-treated animals, group G7 attained highest body weight. Body weight loss was maximum in the DMH control group. Values are expressed as mean ± SE. Bars with no letters in common are significantly different ($p \leqslant 0.05$).

3.2. *Individual Effect of GOS and Inulin on Aberrant Crypt Foci (ACF)*

ACF analysis was carried out at the end of 16 weeks and results are shown in Table 2 and Figure 2. The effect of prebiotics on the occurrence and distribution of ACF among different parts of the colon is shown in Table 2. There was no ACF detected in basal diet control group (G1). With DMH treatment, total numbers of ACF in the colon in Group G2 were 170.4 ± 7.34. A prominent reduction in the numbers of ACF was observed in DMH + prebiotic treated animals as compared to Group G2. Groups G4 and G5, given GOS, showed significant ($p \leqslant 0.05$) reductions in total ACF as compared to G2. Group G5 saw a significant ($p \leqslant 0.05$) reduction of total ACF as compared to other GOS groups (G3 and G4). Group G6 also showed a significant ($p \leqslant 0.05$) reduction of total ACF as compared to G2, G3, and G4, however, it was statistically similar to G5. The maximum percentage of total ACF inhibition was achieved in G6 (51.2%) in case of individual effects of prebiotics, followed by G5 (41.4%) and G4 (22.8%).

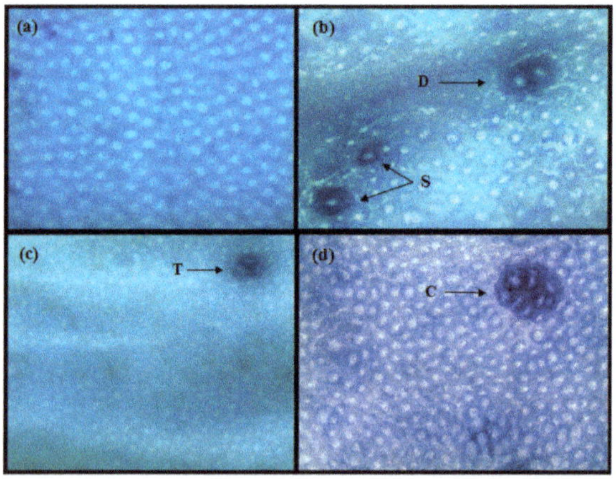

Figure 2. Histological examination of colon for ACF. (**a**) Normal crypts of control group animals; (**b–d**) DMH-treated animals showing aberrant crypt foci. Arrows indicate ACF: singlet (S); doublet (D); triplet (T); and cluster (C).

Table 2. Effect of prebiotic treatments on aberrant crypt foci (ACF) in proximal, middle, and distal colon in DMH-initiated and non-initiated animals ($n = 12$).

ACF	G1 (Basal Diet Control Group)	G2 (DMH Control Group)	G3 (DMH + GOS 76 mg)	G4 (DMH + GOS 114 mg)	G5 (DMH + GOS 151 mg)	G6 (DMH + Inulin 114 mg)	G7 (DMH + GOS 57 mg + Inulin 57 mg)
ACF/proximal colon	ND	24.6 ± 2.73^{a}	23.8 ± 2.87^{a}	12.6 ± 2.13^{b}	$8.7 \pm 1.47^{b,c}$	$7.5 \pm 1.05^{b,c}$	5.3 ± 0.63^{c}
ACF/middle colon	ND	39.6 ± 4.03^{a}	33.3 ± 3.09^{a}	23.8 ± 2.82^{b}	15.2 ± 1.86^{c}	$16.2 \pm 1.92^{b,c}$	$18.8 \pm 2.72^{b,c}$
ACF/distal colon	ND	106.3 ± 6.77^{a}	92.3 ± 5.50^{a}	95.2 ± 5.63^{a}	76.0 ± 5.32^{b}	59.6 ± 4.98^{c}	51.2 ± 4.14^{c}
Total ACF/colon	ND	170.4 ± 7.34^{a}	153.1 ± 9.23^{a}	131.6 ± 9.77^{b}	99.8 ± 8.93^{c}	$83.3 \pm 5.52^{c,d}$	75.3 ± 6.95^{d}
% of total ACF inhibition	-	-	10.2	22.8	41.4	51.2	55.8

Note: Values are expressed as m ± SE. Means in the same row with different superscript letters are significantly different ($p \leqslant 0.05$); DMH = 1,2 dimethylhydrazine dihydrochloride (4 × 40 mg/kg body weight, subcutaneous); ND = Not detected.

3.3. *Combined Effect of Inulin and GOS on ACF*

The combined effects of GOS and inulin showed much better results in ACF inhibition than their individual treatments. Group G7 showed a significant ($p \leqslant 0.05$) reduction of ACF in all parts of colon (proximal, middle and distal). The combination of GOS and inulin treatment showed 55.8% inhibition of ACF formation in animals, which is significantly ($p \leqslant 0.05$) higher than the GOS treatment alone.

3.4. *SCFA, pH, and Ammonia*

Groups G3–G5, which were receiving GOS, showed significant ($p \leqslant 0.05$) increases in cecum acetate levels as compared to Group G2, while groups G4 and G5 were higher ($p \leqslant 0.05$) in cecum butyrate, fecal acetate, and propionate levels, only G5 among GOS groups showed significant ($p \leqslant 0.05$) higher concentrations of fecal butyrate compared to the DMH control (G2) group, as shown in Table 3. Inulin (G6) treatment showed significantly higher levels ($p \leqslant 0.05$) of cecum and fecal acetate, propionate, and butyrate concentrations when compared with the DMH control group (G2). Interestingly, the combination of GOS and inulin treatment (G7) exhibited the highest cecum and fecal levels of acetate, propionate, and butyrate among all of the treatment groups. In addition to SCFA, pH and ammonia levels are also indicators of fermentation status. The fecal and cecal pH was not significantly altered among all groups (Table 3). Nevertheless, prebiotic treatments significantly reduced ($p \leqslant 0.05$) the ammonia levels in cecum and fecal overall. The combination of GOS and inulin significantly ($p \leqslant 0.05$) reduced the levels of cecal and fecal ammonia than GOS groups alone at doses of 114 mg and 76 mg, respectively.

3.5. *Bacterial Enzymes*

Overall, Group G2 showed higher levels of enzyme activities in cecum and fecal contents. Among those groups which were given GOS as treatments, G5 showed significantly ($p \leqslant 0.05$) lower concentrations of β-glucoronidase, and both G4 and G5 showed significantly ($p \leqslant 0.05$) lower concentrations of nitroreductase and azoreductase in cecum contents compared to G2. Regarding fecal content, G4 and G5 were able to significantly ($p \leqslant 0.05$) reduce the concentrations of β-glucoronidase, nitroreductase, and azoreductase, while only G5 was able to reduce ($p \leqslant 0.05$) the concentration of β-glucosidase compared to G2. Group G6, which was given inulin, also showed significantly ($p \leqslant 0.05$) lower concentrations of all enzymes in cecum and fecal contents as compared to DMH control group (G2). We observed that combination treatment of GOS and inulin (G7) resulted in the lowest concentrations of all enzymes in cecal and fecal samples, as shown in Table 4. Specifically, addition of a GOS and inulin mixture in both cecum and feces reduced the activity of all enzymes more efficiently, compared to individual treatments of GOS and inulin.

Table 3. Effect of prebiotic treatments on SCFA, pH, and ammonia concentrations of cecal and fecal contents in DMH-initiated and non-initiated animals (n = 12).

Parameters		G1 (Basal Diet Control Group)	G2 (DMH Control Group)	G3 (DMH + GOS 76 mg)	G4 (DMH + GOS 114 mg)	G5 (DMH + GOS 151 mg)	G6 (DMH + Inulin 114 mg)	G7 (DMH + GOS 57 mg + Inulin 57 mg)
CECUM	Acetate	$82.6 \pm 2.73^{c,d}$	80.5 ± 3.30^{e}	$86.8 \pm 3.66^{c,d}$	$91.4 \pm 3.08^{b,c}$	$97.1 \pm 2.89^{a,b}$	$99.3 \pm 3.55^{a,b}$	104.0 ± 3.95^{a}
	Propionate	23.3 ± 1.89^{c}	22.7 ± 1.96^{c}	$24.7 \pm 2.21^{b,c}$	$27.8 \pm 1.41^{b,c}$	$28.2 \pm 1.54^{b,c}$	$29.3 \pm 1.58^{a,b}$	33.6 ± 1.79^{a}
	Butyrate	$15.7 \pm 0.79^{c,d}$	15.4 ± 1.08^{d}	$16.3 \pm 1.13^{c,d}$	$18.8 \pm 1.08^{b,c}$	$19.7 \pm 1.19^{a,b}$	$20.2 \pm 0.99^{a,b}$	22.7 ± 1.44^{a}
	pH	6.6 ± 0.15	6.7 ± 0.14	6.5 ± 0.12	6.5 ± 0.07	6.4 ± 0.11	6.4 ± 0.13	6.3 ± 0.18
	Ammonia	15.3 ± 1.48^{a}	15.6 ± 1.69^{a}	14.9 ± 2.05^{a}	$12.8 \pm 1.62^{a,b}$	$11.1 \pm 1.06^{a,b,c}$	$10.3 \pm 1.15^{b,c}$	7.7 ± 0.64^{c}
FECAL	Acetate	55.4 ± 2.60^{c}	53.8 ± 2.84^{c}	$57.5 \pm 3.08^{b,c}$	$63.7 \pm 2.38^{a,b}$	67.1 ± 3.16^{a}	69.6 ± 2.58^{a}	70.4 ± 2.64^{a}
	Propionate	$15.4 \pm 0.83^{b,c}$	15.3 ± 0.78^{c}	$16.8 \pm 0.98^{b,c}$	18.4 ± 1.05^{b}	21.3 ± 1.04^{a}	22.3 ± 1.07^{a}	24.3 ± 1.27^{a}
	Butyrate	5.5 ± 0.51^{c}	5.3 ± 0.53^{c}	6.2 ± 0.67^{c}	$7.3 \pm 0.66^{b,c}$	$8.4 \pm 0.73^{a,b}$	$8.8 \pm 0.73^{a,b}$	9.8 ± 0.94^{a}
	pH	6.6 ± 0.16	6.6 ± 0.14	6.5 ± 0.10	6.4 ± 0.08	6.4 ± 0.11	6.4 ± 0.13	6.3 ± 0.11
	Ammonia	10.1 ± 1.13^{a}	10.6 ± 1.34^{a}	$8.8 \pm 0.84^{a,b}$	$6.8 \pm 0.87^{b,c}$	$5.9 \pm 0.95^{b,c}$	5.5 ± 0.92^{c}	4.2 ± 0.37^{c}

Note: Values are expressed as mean ± SE. Means in the same row with different letters are significantly different ($p \leqslant 0.05$); DMH = 1,2 dimethylhydrazine dihydrochloride (4 × 40 mg/kg body weight, subcutaneous); SCFAs = μmol/g; ammonia = mM.

Table 4. Effect of prebiotic treatments on cecal and fecal enzyme activities in DMH-initiated and non-initiated animals (n = 12).

Enzymes		G1 (Basal Diet Control Group)	G2 (DMH Control Group)	G3 (DMH + GOS 76 mg)	G4 (DMH + GOS 114 mg)	G5 (DMH + GOS 151 mg)	G6 (DMH + Inulin 114 mg)	G7 (DMH + GOS 57 mg + Inulin 57 mg)
CECUM	β-Glucosidase	$0.97 \pm 0.12^{a,b}$	1.13 ± 0.21^{a}	1.09 ± 0.11^{a}	$0.83 \pm 0.11^{a,b,c}$	$0.77 \pm 0.11^{a,b,c}$	$0.64 \pm 0.12^{b,c}$	0.52 ± 0.13^{c}
	β-Glucoronidase	3.15 ± 0.19^{a}	3.19 ± 0.19^{a}	2.94 ± 0.18^{a}	$2.57 \pm 0.18^{a,b}$	2.19 ± 0.27^{b}	2.27 ± 0.25^{b}	1.94 ± 0.19^{b}
	Nitroreductase	4.17 ± 0.65^{a}	4.33 ± 0.53^{a}	4.16 ± 0.82^{a}	2.58 ± 0.54^{b}	2.17 ± 0.27^{b}	2.02 ± 0.21^{b}	1.68 ± 0.19^{b}
	Azoreductase	10.75 ± 1.14^{a}	10.58 ± 1.06^{a}	$8.42 \pm 0.97^{a,b}$	7.25 ± 0.93^{b}	$5.67 \pm 0.69^{b,c}$	$6.08 \pm 0.86^{b,c}$	4.33 ± 0.58^{c}
FECAL	β-Glucosidase	$0.80 \pm 0.12^{a,b}$	1.12 ± 0.13^{a}	$0.73 \pm 0.08^{b,c}$	$0.81 \pm 0.10^{a,b}$	$0.57 \pm 0.10^{b,c}$	$0.47 \pm 0.10^{b,c}$	0.43 ± 0.11^{c}
	β-Glucoronidase	2.56 ± 0.33^{a}	2.64 ± 0.35^{a}	$2.14 \pm 0.26^{a,b}$	$1.71 \pm 0.19^{b,c}$	$1.50 \pm 0.25^{b,c}$	1.37 ± 0.12^{c}	1.17 ± 0.11^{c}
	Nitroreductase	$2.67 \pm 0.36^{a,b}$	2.92 ± 0.45^{a}	$2.66 \pm 0.62^{a,b}$	$1.75 \pm 0.18^{b,c}$	1.27 ± 0.16^{c}	1.14 ± 0.17^{c}	0.97 ± 0.16^{c}
	Azoreductase	6.58 ± 0.85^{a}	6.83 ± 0.81^{a}	$5.75 \pm 0.79^{a,b}$	$4.33 \pm 0.54^{b,c}$	$3.67 \pm 0.33^{c,d}$	$3.42 \pm 0.23^{c,d}$	2.17 ± 0.28^{d}

Note: Values are expressed as mean ± SE. Means in the same row with different letters are significantly different ($p \leqslant 0.05$); DMH = 1,2 dimethylhydrazine dihydrochloride (4 × 40 mg/kg body weight, subcutaneous); β-Glucosidase = μg/min/mg cecal or fecal protein; β-Glucoronidase = μg/min/mg cecal or fecal protein; Nitroreductase = μg/h/mg cecal or fecal protein; Azoreductase = μg/h/mg cecal or fecal protein.

4. Discussion

CRC is one of the most common cancers and is the leading cause for morbidity and mortality, even in developed countries. Scientists have focused on various bioactive components in foods to evaluate their role in prevention of CRC. Our data demonstrate that the combination of GOS and inulin provided a significant preventive effect against the development of CRC. Furthermore, the inhibition of ACF formation was significantly higher using this novel combination than inulin and GOS treatments alone. The results of current study also suggest that, in comparison to GOS or inulin individually in different doses, the combination of GOS and inulin rendered better resistance against DMH-induced body weight loss and showed higher levels of cecal and fecal SCFA (acetate, propionate, and butyrate).

ACF are pre-adenomatous morphological putative lesions within the colonic mucosa that may lead to progression to colon cancer. In the present study colon samples were collected after 16 weeks for ACF analysis and, as reported in previous literature, this time period is sufficient for the development of ACF and to observe the effects of treatments. Our results indicated that various doses of prebiotics significantly ($p > 0.05$) inhibited DMH-induced colonic ACF formation in rats. We also showed that GOS inhibited ACF formation in rats in a dose-dependent manner; among all GOS groups, G5 had the maximum effect on ACF inhibition (55.8%), followed by G4 (41.4%) and G3 (22.8%) when compared to the G2 group. Only one previous study [20] reported a high dose of commercial GOS (β-1,4 linkage), at 20% concentration in the diet, inhibited ACF formation. Interestingly, our results showed that the combination of prebiotics with both GOS and inulin (G7) had not only reduced the number of ACF in the proximal, middle, and distal colon, but also altered the distribution of ACF in the entire colon (Table 2). This suggests that administration of prebiotics in combination is able to exert a pronounced chemopreventive effect on preneoplastic ACF formation. Previous experimental studies also support our findings and suggest that prebiotics are effective enough to inhibit total ACF counts chemically-induced in the colon [8,20,30–32]. As it is observed that inulin was better than GOS in reducing ACF counts, it might be due to inulin being slowly degraded and passing further along the colon before being completely degraded in the upper parts of intestine [33]. Another reason might be the monosaccharides in GOS which promote the growth of microbes without discriminating beneficial and harmful microbes. A previous study reported that inulin was able to inhibit 78.8% ACF formation in rats [30]. The reduced ACF counts in prebiotic-treated animals may be due to the modulation of microbiota and increased concentrations of SCFAs, as these are important for normal development of colonic epithelial cells [16,31].

Those groups which were receiving prebiotics, particularly G5–G7, showed higher levels of SCFA production and reductions in ammonia in cecal and fecal contents of rats (Table 3). The SCFA, especially acetate, propionate, and butyrate, are the major products of prebiotic anaerobic fermentation, which results in the lowering of colon pH and increasing the growth of beneficial bacteria, and ultimately attribute to the health benefits of prebiotics [34]. Among these SCFA, butyrate has received much attention in colon cancer prevention with multiple roles, including intestinal barrier function, minerals absorption, cell growth and differentiation [35], as well as its immuno-modulatory activity through its histone deacetylase (HDAC) inhibitory activity on nuclear factor κB (NF-κB) and its expression in colon carcinoma cells [36]. The butyrigenic effect of prebiotic GOS and inulin is very much desirable and has been suggested to be a major contributor to prevent/inhibit colon carcinogenesis [37]. Higher dietary protein can raise ammonia levels in the colon [38] and increase CRC risk through enhancing colonocyte proliferation [26]. Prebiotic supplementation or increased levels of butyrate in the colon may reduce ammonia-mediated toxicity [39,40]. In the present study, significant ($p > 0.05$) reduction in ammonia and increase in SCFA's production in cecum and fecal samples (Table 3) during prebiotic treatments indicated a degree of shift from proteolytic activity to saccharolytic fermentation. This is particularly important in the distal colon where proteolytic fermentation predominates, leading to the accumulation of toxic metabolites. A previous study using prebiotic fructans was consistent with our results with lower levels of ammonia in the prebiotic-treated groups [8,40]. In our findings, high concentrations of dietary GOS (G5 151 mg,

HED 8 g), inulin (G6 114 mg, HED 6 g), and GOS + inulin (G7, 57 mg each, HED 6 g) significantly ($p > 0.05$) enhanced the production of SCFA with reduction of ammonia and, interestingly, without a change in pH. Similar findings have been observed in earlier studies using prebiotics and probiotics in combination and ITF against CRC [8,16,32].

The gastrointestinal tract (GIT), particularly the colon, is considered a complex natural ecosystem occupied by large number of micro-organisms. This microbiota is known to play a key role in the well-being and health of the host [41]. The substances produced by colonic microflora have different effects on the host, such as carcinogenic, genotoxic, tumor-promoting, and anti-carcinogenic activities [15]. Enzymes, particularly β-glucuronidase, β-glucosidase, azoreductase, nitroreductase, 7-β-dehydrogenase, and 7-β-dehydrolase, are involved in conversions of endogenous toxins and genotoxic compounds [34]. It is proven that changes in concentrations of these bacterial enzymes is an indication of change in GIT microbiota [42] In our findings, the levels of enzymes (β-glucuronidase, β-glucosidase, azoreductase and nitroreductase) in cecal and fecal contents were lower in treatment groups. It is well documented that the higher levels of β-glucuronidase and β-glucosidase are considered as biomarkers of colon cancer playing a significant role in colon carcinogenesis and are involved in the carcinogenesis of neoplasms [28], as β-glucuronidase is involved in restoration of the toxic properties of some xenobiotics in colon, its reduced level is taken as a positive effect for colon cancer prevention [43]. Higher levels of bacterial nitroreductase are considered harmful as it is involved in the synthesis of nitrosamines in the colon produced by the interaction of amines with the product of nitrate/nitrite reduction [43]. The decreased activity of β-glucosidase and β-glucuronidase in the present study with prebiotic treatment may be due to the improved intestinal microbiota and many other in vivo factors like pH, ammonia production and substrate availability. Moreover, earlier in vivo studies have also documented that inulin and oligofructose supplementation in fecal bacterial cultures led to enhanced growth of bifidobacterium, having low β-glucuronidase and β-glucosidase activity, and reduced growth of *Escherichia coli* and *Clostridium* sp. that are known to have higher β-glucuronidase activity [30]. The previous study [30] using inulin and lactulose prebiotics also found significantly ($p \leqslant 0.05$) decreased activity of β-glucuronidase and β-glucosidase in animals belonging to the inulin + DMH group compared with the lactulose + DMH-treated group strengthens our findings.

5. Conclusions

In conclusion, this study reveals that GOS prebiotic treatment has a dose-dependent chemo-preventive effect against DMH-induced ACF formation and CRC-related bio-markers. A GOS dose of 8 g (HED) per day is more effective at producing these outcomes than lower doses of 4 and 6 g per day. Novelty of the present study is utilization of GOS containing β-1,6 and β-1,3 glycosidic linkages, which have never been used before in any cancer prevention study. A novel combination of GOS and inulin exhibited stronger preventive activity than their individual treatments alone. As epidemiological data indicates increasing prevalence of CRC throughout the world, and dietary patterns are considered one of major risk factors, it time to focus on dietary strategies for chemoprevention of CRC. Results of the present study encourage inclusion of prebiotic combinations in routine diet and can be a promising strategy for CRC chemoprevention. Further studies are needed to understand the mechanisms of action of different prebiotics containing a variety of linkages in CRC prevention.

Acknowledgments: We are really thankful to Dietmar Haltrich, Food Biotechnology Laboratory, University of Natural Resources and Life Sciences, Vienna-Austria for providing us *E. coli* BL21 (DE3) containing β-galactosidase (β-gal) gene from *Lactobacillus reuteri* L103. Authors are very much thankful to Higher Education Commission, Islamabad—Pakistan for funding this study under project (112-25974-2AV1-346).

Author Contributions: Tahir Rasool Qamar conceptualized, designed, and conducted all analyses. Fatima Syed helped in performing efficacy study. Muhammad Nasir assisted in data collecting management. Habib-ur-Rehman contributed to analysis design. Muhammad Nauman Zahid contributed to the study concept and design and interpretation of the data. Rui Hai Liu helped in statistical analysis, and manuscript writing and Sanaullah Iqbal supervised the study and helped in manuscript writing.

Conflicts of Interest: The author declares no conflict of interest.

References

1. Benson, A.L. Epidemiology, disease progression, and economic burden of colorectal cancer. *J. Manag. Care Pharm.* **2007**, *13*, S5–S18. [CrossRef] [PubMed]
2. Watson, A.J.; Collins, P.D. Colon cancer: A civilization disorder. *Dig. Dis.* **2011**, *29*, 222–228. [CrossRef] [PubMed]
3. Bastide, N.M.; Pierre, F.H.; Corpet, D.E. Heme iron from meat and risk of colorectal cancer: A meta-analysis and a review of the mechanisms involved. *Cancer Prev. Res.* **2011**, *4*, 177–184. [CrossRef] [PubMed]
4. Khan, N.; Afaq, F.; Mukhtar, H. Lifestyle as risk factor for cancer: Evidence from human studies. *Cancer Lett.* **2010**, *293*, 133–143. [CrossRef] [PubMed]
5. Van Engeland, M.; Derks, S.; Smits, K.M.; Meijer, G.A.; Herman, J.G. Colorectal cancer epigenetics: Complex simplicity. *J. Clin. Oncol.* **2011**, *29*, 1382–1391. [CrossRef] [PubMed]
6. Poulsen, M.; Mortensen, A.; Binderup, M.L.; Langkilde, S.; Markowski, J.; Dragsted, L.O. The effect of apple feeding on markers of colon carcinogenesis. *Nutr. Cancer* **2011**, *63*, 402–409. [CrossRef] [PubMed]
7. Tarapore, R.S.; Siddiqui, I.A.; Mukhtar, H. Modulation of wnt/beta-catenin signaling pathway by bioactive food components. *Carcinogenesis* **2012**, *33*, 483–491. [CrossRef] [PubMed]
8. Fotiadis, C.I.; Stoidis, C.N.; Spyropoulos, B.G.; Zografos, E.D. Role of probiotics, prebiotics and synbiotics in chemoprevention for colorectal cancer. *World J. Gastroenterol.* **2008**, *14*, 6453–6457. [CrossRef] [PubMed]
9. Macfarlane, G.T.; Macfarlane, S. Fermentation in the human large intestine: Its physiologic consequences and the potential contribution of prebiotics. *J. Clin. Gastroenterol.* **2011**, *45*, S120–S127. [CrossRef] [PubMed]
10. Campbell, J.M.; Fahey, G.C., Jr.; Wolf, B.W. Selected indigestible oligosaccharides affect large bowel mass, cecal and fecal short-chain fatty acids, pH and microflora in rats. *J. Nutr.* **1997**, *127*, 130–136. [PubMed]
11. Ebert, M.N.; Beyer-Sehlmeyer, G.; Liegibel, U.M.; Kautenburger, T.; Becker, T.W.; Pool-Zobel, B.L. Butyrate induces glutathione s-transferase in human colon cells and protects from genetic damage by 4-hydroxy-2-nonenal. *Nutr. Cancer* **2001**, *41*, 156–164. [CrossRef] [PubMed]
12. Torres, D.P.M.; Gonçalves, M.d.P.F.; Teixeira, J.A.; Rodrigues, L.R. Galacto-oligosaccharides: Production, properties, applications, and significance as prebiotics. *Compr. Rev. Food Sci. Food Saf.* **2010**, *9*, 438–454. [CrossRef]
13. Laparra, J.M.; Diez-Municio, M.; Herrero, M.; Moreno, F.J. Structural differences of prebiotic oligosaccharides influence their capability to enhance iron absorption in deficient rats. *Food Funct.* **2014**, *5*, 2430–2437. [CrossRef] [PubMed]
14. Sivieri, K.; Spinardi-Barbisan, A.L.T.; Barbisan, L.F.; Bedani, R.; Pauly, N.D.; Carlos, I.Z.; Benzatti, F.; Vendramini, R.C.; Rossi, E.A. Probiotic *Enterococcus faecium* CRL 183 inhibit chemically induced colon cancer in male Wistar rats. *Eur. Food Res. Technol.* **2008**, *228*, 231–237. [CrossRef]
15. Gallaher, D.D.; Khil, J. The effect of synbiotics on colon carcinogenesis in rats. *J. Nutr.* **1999**, *129*, 1483S–1487S. [PubMed]
16. Femia, A.P.; Luceri, C.; Dolara, P.; Giannini, A.; Biggeri, A.; Salvadori, M.; Clune, Y.; Collins, K.J.; Paglierani, M.; Caderni, G. Antitumorigenic activity of the prebiotic inulin enriched with oligofructose in combination with the probiotics lactobacillus rhamnosus and bifidobacterium lactis on azoxymethane-induced colon carcinogenesis in rats. *Carcinogenesis* **2002**, *23*, 1953–1960. [CrossRef] [PubMed]
17. Pool-Zobel, B.; van Loo, J.; Rowland, I.; Roberfroid, M.B. Experimental evidences on the potential of prebiotic fructans to reduce the risk of colon cancer. *Br. J. Nutr.* **2002**, *87* (Suppl. S2), S273–S281. [CrossRef] [PubMed]
18. Reddy, B.S. Prevention of colon cancer by pre- and probiotics: Evidence from laboratory studies. *Br. J. Nutr.* **1998**, *80*, S219–S223. [PubMed]

19. Wijnands, M.V.; Appel, M.J.; Hollanders, V.M.; Woutersen, R.A. A comparison of the effects of dietary cellulose and fermentable galacto-oligosaccharide, in a rat model of colorectal carcinogenesis: Fermentable fibre confers greater protection than non-fermentable fibre in both high and low fat backgrounds. *Carcinogenesis* **1999**, *20*, 651–656. [CrossRef] [PubMed]
20. Wijnands, M.V.; Schoterman, H.C.; Bruijntjes, J.B.; Hollanders, V.M.; Woutersen, R.A. Effect of dietary galacto-oligosaccharides on azoxymethane-induced aberrant crypt foci and colorectal cancer in fischer 344 rats. *Carcinogenesis* **2001**, *22*, 127–132. [CrossRef] [PubMed]
21. Reeves, P.G.; Rossow, K.L.; Lindlauf, J. Development and testing of the ain-93 purified diets for rodents: Results on growth, kidney calcification and bone mineralization in rats and mice. *J. Nutr.* **1993**, *123*, 1923–1931. [PubMed]
22. Reagan-Shaw, S.; Nihal, M.; Ahmad, N. Dose translation from animal to human studies revisited. *FASEB J.* **2008**, *22*, 659–661. [CrossRef] [PubMed]
23. Dias, M.C.; Spinardi-Barbisan, A.L.; Rodrigues, M.A.; de Camargo, J.L.; Teran, E.; Barbisan, L.F. Lack of chemopreventive effects of ginger on colon carcinogenesis induced by 1,2-dimethylhydrazine in rats. *Food Chem. Toxicol.* **2006**, *44*, 877–884. [CrossRef] [PubMed]
24. Dias, M.C.; Vieiralves, N.F.; Gomes, M.I.; Salvadori, D.M.; Rodrigues, M.A.; Barbisan, L.F. Effects of lycopene, synbiotic and their association on early biomarkers of rat colon carcinogenesis. *Food Chem. Toxicol.* **2010**, *48*, 772–780. [CrossRef] [PubMed]
25. Iqbal, S.; Nguyen, T.H.; Nguyen, T.T.; Maischberger, T.; Haltrich, D. Beta-galactosidase from *Lactobacillus plantarum* WCFS1: Biochemical characterization and formation of prebiotic galacto-oligosaccharides. *Carbohydr. Res.* **2010**, *345*, 1408–1416. [CrossRef] [PubMed]
26. Lin, H.C.; Visek, W.J. Large intestinal ph and ammonia in rats: Dietary fat and protein interactions. *J. Nutr.* **1991**, *121*, 832–843. [PubMed]
27. Bird, R.P. Role of aberrant crypt foci in understanding the pathogenesis of colon cancer. *Cancer Lett.* **1995**, *93*, 55–71. [CrossRef]
28. Goldin, B.R.; Gorbach, S.L. The relationship between diet and rat fecal bacterial enzymes implicated in colon cancer. *J. Natl. Cancer Inst.* **1976**, *57*, 371–375. [PubMed]
29. Zhao, G.; Nyman, M.; Åke Jönsson, J. Rapid determination of short-chain fatty acids in colonic contents and faeces of humans and rats by acidified water-extraction and direct-injection gas chromatography. *Biomed. Chromatogr.* **2006**, *20*, 674–682. [CrossRef] [PubMed]
30. Verma, A.; Shukla, G. Administration of prebiotic inulin suppresses 1,2 dimethylhydrazine dihydrochloride induced procarcinogenic biomarkers fecal enzymes and preneoplastic lesions in early colon carcinogenesis in sprague dawley rats. *J. Funct. Foods* **2013**, *5*, 991–996. [CrossRef]
31. Aachary, A.A.; Gobinath, D.; Srinivasan, K.; Prapulla, S.G. Protective effect of xylooligosaccharides from corncob on 1,2-dimethylhydrazine induced colon cancer in rats. *Bioact. Carbohydr. Diet. Fibre* **2015**, *5*, 146–152. [CrossRef]
32. Pool-Zobel, B.L.; Sauer, J. Overview of experimental data on reduction of colorectal cancer risk by inulin-type fructans. *J. Nutr.* **2007**, *137*, 2580S–2584S. [PubMed]
33. Van de Wiele, T.; Boon, N.; Possemiers, S.; Jacobs, H.; Verstraete, W. Inulin-type fructans of longer degree of polymerization exert more pronounced in vitro prebiotic effects. *J. Appl. Microbiol.* **2007**, *102*, 452–460. [CrossRef] [PubMed]
34. Macfarlane, G.T.; Macfarlane, S. Bacteria, colonic fermentation, and gastrointestinal health. *J. AOAC Int.* **2012**, *95*, 50–60. [CrossRef] [PubMed]
35. Daly, K.; Cuff, M.A.; Fung, F.; Shirazi-Beechey, S.P. The importance of colonic butyrate transport to the regulation of genes associated with colonic tissue homoeostasis. *Biochem. Soc. Trans.* **2005**, *33*, 733–735. [CrossRef] [PubMed]
36. Vinolo, M.A.; Rodrigues, H.G.; Nachbar, R.T.; Curi, R. Regulation of inflammation by short chain fatty acids. *Nutrients* **2011**, *3*, 858–876. [CrossRef] [PubMed]
37. Fung, K.Y.; Cosgrove, L.; Lockett, T.; Head, R.; Topping, D.L. A review of the potential mechanisms for the lowering of colorectal oncogenesis by butyrate. *Br. J. Nutr.* **2012**, *108*, 820–831. [CrossRef] [PubMed]
38. Lupton, J.R.; Marchant, L.J. Independent effects of fiber and protein on colonic luminal ammonia concentration. *J. Nutr.* **1989**, *119*, 235–241. [PubMed]

39. De Preter, V.; Vanhoutte, T.; Huys, G.; Swings, J.; de Vuyst, L.; Rutgeerts, P.; Verbeke, K. Effects of *Lactobacillus casei* shirota, *Bifidobacterium breve*, and oligofructose-enriched inulin on colonic nitrogen-protein metabolism in healthy humans. *Am. J. Physiol. Gastrointest. Liver Physiol.* **2007**, *292*, G358–G368. [CrossRef] [PubMed]
40. Geboes, K.P.; de Hertogh, G.; de Preter, V.; Luypaerts, A.; Bammens, B.; Evenepoel, P.; Ghoos, Y.; Geboes, K.; Rutgeerts, P.; Verbeke, K. The influence of inulin on the absorption of nitrogen and the production of metabolites of protein fermentation in the colon. *Br. J. Nutr.* **2006**, *96*, 1078–1086. [CrossRef] [PubMed]
41. Tappenden, K.A.; Deutsch, A.S. The physiological relevance of the intestinal microbiota—Contributions to human health. *J. Am. Coll. Nutr.* **2007**, *26*, 679S–683S. [CrossRef] [PubMed]
42. Klewicka, E.; Zduńczyk, Z.; Juśkiewicz, J. Effect of lactobacillus fermented beetroot juice on composition and activity of cecal microflora of rats. *Eur. Food Res. Technol.* **2009**, *229*, 153–157. [CrossRef]
43. Ayesh, R.; Weststrate, J.A.; Drewitt, P.N.; Hepburn, P.A. Safety evaluation of phytosterol esters. Part 5. Faecal short-chain fatty acid and microflora content, faecal bacterial enzyme activity and serum female sex hormones in healthy normolipidaemic volunteers consuming a controlled diet either with or without a phytosterol ester-enriched margarine. *Food Chem. Toxicol.* **1999**, *37*, 1127–1138. [PubMed]

nutrients

MDPI

Article

The Effects of Early Post-Operative Soluble Dietary Fiber Enteral Nutrition for Colon Cancer

Rui Xu, Zhi Ding, Ping Zhao, Lingchao Tang, Xiaoli Tang and Shuomeng Xiao *

Department of Gastrointestinal Surgery, Sichuan Cancer Hospital, Chengdu 610041, China; xrscu2012@163.com (R.X.); dzscch@sina.com (Z.D.); zpscch@sina.com (P.Z.); scch2015@163.com (L.T.); txlscch@sina.com (X.T.)

* Correspondence: ambition123@foxmail.com; Tel.: +86-28-8542-0845

Received: 12 August 2016; Accepted: 13 September 2016; Published: 21 September 2016

Abstract: We examined colon cancer patients who received soluble dietary fiber enteral nutrition (SDFEN) to evaluate the feasibility and potential benefit of early SDFEN compared to EN. Sixty patients who were confirmed as having colon cancer with histologically and accepted radical resection of colon cancer were randomized into an SDFEN group and an EN group. The postoperative complications, length of hospital stay (LOH), days for first fecal passage, and the difference in nutritional status, immune function and inflammatory reaction between pre-operation and post-operation were all recorded. The statistical analyses were performed using the *t*-test and the chi square test. Statistical significance was defined as $p < 0.05$. After the nutrition support, differences in the levels of albumin, prealbumin and transferrin in each group were not statistically significant ($p > 0.05$); the levels of CD4+, IgA and IgM in the SDFEN group were higher than that of the EN group at seven days ($p < 0.05$); the levels of TNF-α and IL-6 in the SDFEN group were lower than that of the EN group at seven days ($p < 0.05$); and patients in the SDFEN group had a significantly shorter first flatus time than the EN group ($p < 0.05$). Early post-operative SDFEN used in colon cancer patients was feasible and beneficial in immune function and reducing inflammatory reaction, gastrointestinal function and speeding up the recovery.

Keywords: colon cancer; dietary fiber; early enteral nutrition

1. Introduction

In the 21st century, cancer incidence and mortality has not reduced; moreover, it has even increased year by year. The total number of patients with colorectal cancer increased to 1.23 million globally in 2008; it is ranked third in cancer incidence and fourth in mortality [1]. However, the incidence and mortality of colorectal cancer were ranked third and fifth, respectively [2] in China. Many studies showed that the incidence of malnutrition in patients with a malignant tumor was as high as 31%–97% [3,4], especially for gastrointestinal cancer, so choosing a proper nutrition therapy for colorectal cancer patients with malnutrition is necessary. Early enteral nutrition support is promoted after gastrointestinal surgery, and there are many kinds of nutrient elements, such as probiotics, ω-3PUFA, Gln and fiber. We know that dietary fiber is a kind of nutrient, which is divided into soluble dietary fiber and insoluble dietary fiber and can protect the intestinal barrier, modulate immune function, induce inflammatory response and postoperative complications [5,6]. SCFA is the main source of energy for intestinal epithelial cells and plays a key role in maintaining colonic health and moderating cell growth and differentiation. This depends on the fermentation of dietary fiber. Soluble dietary fiber is fermented, but insoluble dietary fiber is difficult to ferment. The relationship between dietary fiber and colon cancer prevention was studied widely, but there is little study about the early postoperative application of soluble dietary fiber in colon cancer [7–9]. Thus, we decide to add soluble dietary fiber to verify the feasibility and potential benefit of SDFEN for colon cancer for the postoperative course.

2. Patients and Methods

2.1. Patient Selection

We recruited 60 subjects from the department of gastrointestinal surgery of the Sichuan cancer Hospital between June 2014 and June 2015. All patients who confirmed colon cancer with histologically and accepted radical resection of colon cancer were randomized into an SDFEN group (30 cases) and EN group (30 cases). Informed consents were obtained according to the Declaration of Helsinki. Patients suffering from diabetes or underlying cardiopulmonary diseases were excluded. Moreover, the patients whose tumor staging was Stage IV (the cancer had spread to other parts of the body) were also excluded.

2.2. Methods

No patients had a decompression tube before the operation, and all were given sequential nutrition support for 7 days consecutively after the operation. The total daily calories for all the patients should reach 125.52 kJ (30 kcal)/kg. All enteral nutrition was ingested through mouth, and if energy was insufficient, we would obtain residual energy by infusing the Fat Emulsion, Amino Acids (17) and Glucose (1%) Injection (1440 mL/bag) made by Sino-Swed Pharmaceutical Corp. (Wuxi, China). Intervention in detail is in the following Table 1.

Table 1. Intervention of the cases and control.

Time	Nutrients	SDFEN	EN
Day 1	5% GNS dietary fiber Probiotics	500 mL 25 g 4g	500 mL - 4 g
Day 2–3	Enteral Nutrition dietary fiber Probiotics	500 mL 25 g 4 g	500 mL - 4 g
Day 4–7	Enteral Nutrition dietary fiber Probiotics	1000 mL 25 g 4 g	1000 mL - 4 g
Total energy	125.52 kJ (30 kcal)/kg		
Insufficient energy	Amino Acids (17) and Glucose (1%) Injection (1440 mL/bag)		

SDFEN: soluble dietary fiber enteral nutrition. EN: enteral nutrition. Dietary fiber: Soluble dietary fiber from fruit and vegetables made by Beijing yikang Biotechnology Corp. (Beijing, China); Enteral Nutrition: Enteral Nutritional Emulsion (TP-HE) (500 mL/bag, 750 kcal) made by Sino-Swed Pharmaceutical Corp; Probiotics: Live Combined Bifidobacterium and Lactobacillus Tablets made by Inner Mongolia shuangqi Pharmaceutical Corp. (Huhhot, China).

2.3. Clinical Assessment

Clinical factors included age, gender, smoking, drinking habits, and tumor stage according to the tumor-node-metastasis classification of the International Union against Cancer (7th edition) [10]. Peripheral blood was collected on the pre-operative day, and post-operative second and seventh day. Nutritional status was expressed by the levels of albumin, prealbumin and transferring; and immune function was shown by the levels of CD3+, CD4+, CD8+, CD4+/CD8+, IgA, IgM and IgG; The levels of TNF-α, IL-6 and PCT reflected the immune function. Length of hospital stay (LOH), and bowel movement recovery were expressed as days and the first fecal passage was recorded. Postoperative complications including pneumonia, anastomotic fistula and severe abdominal distension were also recorded.

2.4. Statistical Analysis

All analyses were carried out with the SPSS 19.0 software package (IBM, New York, NY, USA), and measurement data were indicated with the mean ± standard deviation. The *t*-test was used to examine measurement data, the chi-square test was used to categorize data. p value < 0.05 was considered significant for statistical analysis.

3. Results

3.1. Demography

Among 30 colon cancer cases, there were 16 males and 14 females, and the mean age was 52.20 ± 14.20 years; among the 30 control cases, there were 19 males and 11 females, and the mean age was 53.20 ± 13.10 years. The characteristics of the cases and controls are summarized in Table 2. There was no significant difference between the distributions of the age, gender, smoking, drinking habits and TNM stage of the two groups.

Table 2. Characteristics of the cases and control.

Variable	SDFEN (n = 30)	EN (n = 30)	p
Gender (%)			
Male	16 (53.3)	19 (63.3)	0.735
Female	14 (46.7)	11 (36.7)	0.690
Age mean (SD) year	52.2 ± 14.2	53.2 ± 13.1	0.750
Smoking status (%)			
Smokers	12 (40)	9 (30)	0.664
Nonsmokers	18 (60)	21 (70)	0.749
Drinking (%)			
Drinkers	10 (33)	13 (43.3)	0.678
Nondrinkers	20 (67)	17 (56.7)	0.868
TNM stage (%)			
I, II	13 (43.3)	11 (36.7)	0.839
III	17 (56.7)	19 (63.3)	0.868

SDFEN: soluble dietary fiber enteral nutrition; EN: enteral nutrition; SD: standard deviation.

3.2. Pre-Operative and Post-Operative Nutritional Index

After the nutrition support, differences of the levels of albumin, prealbumin and transferrin in each group were not statistically significant (p > 0.05) (Table 3).

Table 3. Comparison of the two groups' nutrition index.

	Pre Op	POD 2	POD 7
ALB (g/L)			
SDFEN	40.15 ± 2.45	32.64 ± 2.32	35.45 ± 2.21
EN	39.39 ± 2.87	31.81 ± 1.72	34.30 ± 1.86
p	0.22	0.09	0.05
PAB (mg/L)			
SDFEN	194.78 ± 31.74	177.32 ± 22.82	192.67 ± 21.30
EN	191.47 ± 30.61	178.09 ± 28.24	189.97 ± 25.32
p	0.62	0.88	0.58
TRF (g/L)			
SDFEN	2.58 ± 0.50	2.05 ± 0.39	2.29 ± 0.33
EN	2.55 ± 0.39	2.09 ± 0.20	2.23 ± 0.28
p	0.75	0.57	0.30

Pre Op: pre-operation; POD: postoperative day; SDFEN: soluble dietary fiber enteral nutrition; EN: enteral nutrition; ALB; albumin; PAB; prealbumin; TRF; transferring.

3.3. *Pre-Operative and Post-Operative Immune Index*

Differences of CD3+, CD8+, CD4+/CD8+ and IgG in each group were not statistically significant at two and seven days. The levels of CD4+, IgA and IgM in SDFEN group were higher than the EN group at seven days ($p < 0.05$) (Table 4).

Table 4. Comparison of the two groups' immune index.

	Pre Op	POD 2	POD 7
CD3+ (%)			
SDFEN	62.77 ± 6.46	54.32 ± 6.95	61.34 ± 4.32
EN	60.99 ± 7.00	53.59 ± 6.42	59.80 ± 6.23
p	0.321	0.669	0.285
CD4+ (%)			
SDFEN	34.28 ± 4.83	28.40 ± 3.32	35.90 ± 2.24
EN	33.70 ± 5.31	29.76 ± 3.32	34.41 ± 2.64
p	0.61	0.155	0.024
CD8+ (%)			
SDFEN	23.20 ± 4.83	21.58 ± 3.91	21.30 ± 3.03
EN	22.03 ± 3.83	21.11 ± 2.72	21.35 ± 1.94
p	0.377	0.659	0.949
CD4+/CD8+			
SDFEN	1.55 ±0.43	1.36 ± 0.31	1.72 ± 0.29
EN	1.58 ±0.41	1.44 ± 0.27	1.62 ± 0.20
p	0.766	0.387	0.190
IgA (g/L)			
SDFEN	2.13 ± 0.95	1.81 ± 0.94	2.25 ± 0.79
EN	2.03 ± 0.56	1.69 ± 0.59	1.88 ± 0.54
p	0.622	0.567	0.045
IgM (g/L)			
SDFEN	1.26 ± 0.64	0.94 ± 0.20	1.30 ± 0.33
EN	1.12 ± 0.19	0.96 ± 0.13	1.11 ± 0.15
p	0.241	0.693	0.002
IgG (g/L)			
SDFEN	11.22 ± 1.54	9.57 ± 1.59	11.55 ± 1.44
EN	11.12 ± 1.73	9.74 ± 0.87	11.41 ± 1.32
p	0.799	0.618	0.590

Pre Op: pre-operation; POD: postoperative day; SDFEN: soluble dietary fiber enteral nutrition; EN: enteral nutrition.

3.4. *Pre-Operative and Post-Operative Inflammatory Index*

The levels of TNF-α and IL-6 in the SDFEN group were lower than the EN group at seven days ($p < 0.05$) (Table 5).

Table 5. Comparison of the two groups' immune index.

	Pre Op	POD 2	POD 7
TNF-α (pg/mL)			
SDFEN	12.88 ± 5.62	20.32 ± 6.35	13.02 ± 2.85
EN	13.91 ± 6.47	22.14 ± 6.81	14.73 ± 4.07
p	0.524	0.333	0.045
IL-6(pg/mL)			
SDFEN	47.54 ± 34.30	110.72 ± 46.86	58.75 ± 24.82
EN	45.83 ± 42.14	115.57 ± 56.93	70.83 ± 35.65
p	0.850	0.682	0.044
PCT (ng/mL)			
SDFEN	0.11 ± 0.11	0.26 ± 0.18	0.15 ± 0.07
EN	0.15 ± 0.15	0.28 ± 0.18	0.16 ± 0.08
p	0.086	0.489	0.539

Pre Op: pre-operation; POD: postoperative day; SDFEN: soluble dietary fiber enteral nutrition; EN: enteral nutrition.

3.5. Post-Operative Recovery

Patients in the SDFEN group had a significantly shorter first flatus time than the EN group ($p < 0.05$). However, abdominal distension, pneumonia, Anastomotic fistula and total postoperative hospitalization time were similar between the two groups (Table 6).

Table 6. Post-operative recovery.

	SDFEN	EN	p
First flatus time (h)	58.93 ± 6.5	63.03 ± 4.8	0.015
Abdominal distension	1	2	-
Pneumonia	1	2	-
Anastomotic fistula	0	1	-
Length of hospital stay (day)	7.4 ± 0.72	7.63 ± 0.61	0.257

SDFEN: soluble dietary fiber enteral nutrition; EN: enteral nutrition.

4. Discussion

Colon cancer is a common gastrointestinal malignancy, the incidence of which has increased year by year. Seventy percent of patients with GI cancer may be suffering from malnutrition and 39.3% of patients with colon cancer had different degrees of malnutrition [11,12]. Surgery is still the first choice for treatment, but surgical trauma and anesthesia can cause body metabolic disorder and aggravated malnutrition. Widespread attention has been given on how to further improve the postoperative nutritional status and the prognosis.

Early enteral nutrition began at 24 h after surgery in our study. ASPEN [13] suggested that ideal enteral nutrition should begin within 24 to 48 h after surgery. Actually, intestine had recovered its absorption function and EMG activity within 4 to 8 h after surgery [14]. The gastrointestinal tract can not only absorb nutrients, but also plays an important role in immunity because it is a central organ after surgical stress [15] and it is also the motor of the MODS. Intestine mucosal atrophy and abnormal intestinal permeability can occur after not eating for several days. Early enteral nutrition is more close to the human physiological needs. The application of enteral nutrition can reverse the loss of gut mucosal integrity resulting from surgical trauma [16], and early enteral nutrition support is associated with a decreased infection risk, a reduced hospital stay, and a clear trend of a reduction in anastomotic breakdown [17,18]. Therefore, it could be the first choice for patients who have had an operation.

Some studies proposed that early application of soluble dietary fiber enteral nutrition could increase nutritional indicators, make patients' weight decline slowly and reduce the incidence of digestive tract complications [19,20]. However, there was no obvious difference in post-operative nutrition status and complication between the SDFEN group and EN group in our study. Fortunately, there was a trend of an increased post-operative nutrition status and declined incidence of complications. Dietary fiber are not a static collection of indigestible plant materials that pass through the human GI tract without any function; instead, they bind potential nutrients, result in new metabolites, and modulate nutrient absorption/metabolism, and they can promote the growth of the small intestinal villus to increase the absorption of nutrients to improve nutrition status. Dietary fiber is divided into soluble dietary fiber and insoluble dietary fiber. In general, soluble dietary fiber is fermented, but insoluble dietary fiber is difficult to ferment. Studies found that dietary fiber could be fermented into SCFAs in colon and unoxidized SCFA through the portal system into the liver. They can thus be converted to glutamine, and then glutamine enters into the circulation of blood to nourish the small intestine [21]. Therefore, statistical differences in post-operative nutrition status and complication will exist between the SDFEN group and EN group, if observation time is enough.

A large amount of research has reported that soluble dietary fiber had health benefits with immunomodulatory and anti-inflammatory effects [8,22]. In our study, there were significant differences in the indicators of immune conditions including deviations in CD4+, IgA and IgG at seven days between the SDFEN group and EN group (35.90% ± 2.24% vs. 34.41% ± 2.64%, 2.25% ± 0.79 g/L vs. 1.88 ± 0.54 g/L, and 11.55 ± 1.44 g/L vs. 11.41 ± 1.32 g/L, respectively, $p < 0.05$), and the levels of TNF-α and IL-6 in the SDFEN group was lower than those in the EN group (13.02 ± 2.85 pg/mL vs. 14.73 ± 4.07 pg/mL, and 58.75 ± 24.82 pg/mL vs. 70.83 ± 35.65 pg/mL, respectively, $p < 0.05$). These health benefits can be attributed to the fermentation of soluble dietary fiber into SCFAs in the colon. The three major colonic SCFAs are acetate, propionate and butyrate, which is the main source of energy for intestinal epithelial cells and plays a key role in maintaining colonic health and moderating cell growth and differentiation [23]. Acetate plays a role in the host immune system through interacting with the G protein-coupled receptor (GPCR43, 41) in immune cells [24]. Butyrate exhibits strong anti-inflammatory properties, and this effect is likely mediated by inhibition of TNF-α production, NF-κB activation, and IL-8, IL-10, and IL-12 expression in immune and colonic epithelial cells [25,26]. Leukocytes are recruited and migrate from the bloodstream to the inflamed tissue through a multistep process that involves expression and activation of several proteins such as adhesion molecules and chemokines, and SCFAs modify this leukocyte recruitment [27,28] by modulating the amount or type of adhesion molecules and chemokines. SCFAs may alter the recruitment of leukocytes to reduce the chronic GI tract inflammatory response. Therefore, intakes of dietary fiber can reduce inflammatory reaction and improve the postoperative immune function.

Under the stimulation of mixed dietary fiber food, the gastrointestinal hormone is increased, such as gastrin and cholecystokinin, which can promote recovery of intestinal movement. Furthermore, SCFAs also have the same function; Kamath et al. [29] found that the movement of the free small bowel was increased after being stimulated with SCFAs. In our study, patients in the SDFEN group had a significantly shorter first flatus time than the EN group (58.93 ± 6.5 h vs. 63.03 ± 4.8 h, $p < 0.05$), so that SDFEN can promote recovery of intestinal movement.

5. Conclusions

Early post-operative soluble dietary fiber enteral nutrition used in colon cancer patients was feasible and has advantages in improving immune function, reducing inflammatory response and promoting early recovery of intestinal movement.

Acknowledgments: Thanks to the support of gastrointestinal surgery centre, department of pathology and nutrition in Sichuan cancer hospital.

Author Contributions: R.X. and S.X. designed the study; R.X. and S.X. collected the data; X.T. and S.X. entered the data; R.X. and S.X. drafted the manuscript; and Z.D., L.T. and P.Z. undertook the statistical analysis. All authors read and approved the final manuscript.

Conflicts of Interest: The authors declare no conflicts of interest.

References

1. Ferlay, J.; Shin, H.R.; Bray, F.; Forman, D.; Mathers, C.; Parkin, D.M. Estimates of worldwide burden of cancer in 2008: GLOBOCAN 2008. *Int. J. Cancer* **2010**, *127*, 2893–2917. [CrossRef] [PubMed]
2. Chen, W.Q.; Zhang, S.W.; Zheng, R.S.; Zhao, P.; Li, G.; Wu, L.; He, J. Report of cancer incidence and mortality in China, 2009. *Chin. J. Cancer Res.* **2013**, *22*, 1–12.
3. Huhmann, M.B.; Cunningham, R.S. Importance of nutritional screening in treatment of cancer related weight loss. *Lancet Oncol.* **2005**, *6*, 334–343. [CrossRef]
4. Segura, A.; Pardo, J.; Jara, C.; Zugazabeitia, L.; Carulla, J.; de Las Peñas, R.; García-Cabrera, E.; Luz Azuara, M.; Casadó, J.; Gómez-Candela, C. An epidemiological evaluation of the prevalence of malnutrition in Spanish patients with locally advanced or metastatic cancer. *Clin. Nutr.* **2005**, *24*, 801–814. [CrossRef] [PubMed]
5. Zeng, H.W.; Lazarova, D.L.; Bordonaro, M. Mechanisms linking dietary fiber, gut microbiota and colon cancer prevention. *World J. Gastrointest. Oncol.* **2014**, *6*, 41–51. [CrossRef] [PubMed]
6. Vieira, A.T.; Galvão, I.; Macia, L.M.; Sernaglia, E.M.; Vinolo, M.A.; Garcia, C.C.; Tavares, L.P.; Amaral, F.A.; Sousa, L.P.; Martins, F.S.; et al. Dietary fiber and the short-chain fatty acid acetate promote resolution of neutrophilic inflammation in a model of gout in mice. *J. Leukoc. Biol.* **2016**. [CrossRef] [PubMed]

7. Kaczmarczyk, M.M.; Miller, M.J.; Freund, G.G. The health benefis of dietary fiber: Beyond the usual suspects of type 2 diabetes mellitus, cardiovascular disease and colon cancer. *Metabolism* **2012**, *61*, 1058–1066. [CrossRef] [PubMed]
8. Peters, U.; Sinha, R.; Chatterjee, N.; Subar, A.F.; Ziegler, R.G.; Kulldorff, M.; Bresalier, R.; Weissfeld, J.L.; Flood, A.; Schatzkin, A.; Hayes, R.B.; et al. Dietary fire and colorectal adenoma in a colorectal cancer early detection programme. *Lancet* **2003**, *361*, 1491–1495. [CrossRef]
9. Nomura, A.M.; Hankin, J.H.; Henderson, B.E.; Wilkens, L.R.; Murphy, S.P.; Pike, M.C.; Le Marchand, L.; Stram, D.O.; Monroe, K.R.; Kolonel, L.N. Dietary fier and colorectal cancer risk: The multiethnic cohort study. *Cancer Causes Control* **2007**, *18*, 753–764. [CrossRef] [PubMed]
10. Sobin, L.H.; Gospodarowicz, M.K.; Wittekind, C. *TNM Classification of Malignant Tumors*, 7th ed.; Wiley: New York, NY, USA, 2010.
11. Yang, Z.H.; Li, G.N. Clinical analysis of perioperative enteral nutrition in patients with gastrointestinal tumor. *Appl. J. Gen. Prac.* **2008**, *6*, 483–484.
12. Schwegler, I.; von Holzen, A.; Gutzwiller, J.P.; Schlumpf, R.; Mühlebach, S.; Stanga, Z. Nutritional risk is a clinical predictor of postoperative mortality and morbidity in surgery for colorectal cancer. *Br. J. Surg.* **2010**, *97*, 92–97. [CrossRef] [PubMed]
13. McClave, S.A.; Martindale, R.G.; Vanek, V.W.; McCarthy, M.; Roberts, P.; Taylor, B.; Ochoa, J.B.; Napolitano, L.; Cresci, G. Guidelines for the provision and assessment of nutritionsupport therapyintheadult critically ill patient: Society of Critical Caremedicine (SCCM) and American Society for Parenteral and Enteral Nutrition (ASPEN). *J. Parenter. Enter. Nutr.* **2009**, *33*, 277–316. [CrossRef] [PubMed]
14. Sakurai, Y.; Kanaya, S.; Komori, Y.; Uyama, I. Is postoperative early enteral nutrition with regular or disease-specific enteral formula really beneficial in patients undergoing esophagectomy? *Esophagus* **2009**, *3*, 149–154. [CrossRef]
15. Wilmore, D.W.; Smith, R.J.; O'Dwyer, S.T.; Jacobs, D.O.; Ziegler, T.R.; Wang, X.D. The gut: A central organ after surgical stress. *Surgery* **1988**, *104*, 917–923. [PubMed]
16. Jiang, X.H.; Li, N.; Li, J.S. Intestinal permeability in patients after surgical trauma and effect of enteral nutrition versus parenteral nutrition. *World J. Gastroenterol.* **2003**, *9*, 1878–1880. [CrossRef] [PubMed]
17. Ochoa, J.B.; Caba, D. Advances in surgical nutrition. *Surg. Clin. N. Am.* **2006**, *86*, 1483–1493. [CrossRef] [PubMed]
18. Fearon, K.C.; Ljungqvist, O.; Von Meyenfeldt, M.; Revhaug, A.; Dejong, C.H.; Lassen, K.; Nygren, J.; Hausel, J.; Soop, M.; Andersen, J.; et al. Enhanced recovery after surgery: A consensus review of clinical care for patients undergoing colonic resection. *Clin. Nutr.* **2005**, *24*, 466–477. [CrossRef] [PubMed]
19. Yan, M.; Li, S.F.; Li, C.; Zhang, J.; Ji, F.; Xu, H.; Cao, W.H. Clinical studies on early post-operative enteral nutrition with dietary fibers for GI tumor. *Parenter. Enter. Nutr.* **2001**, *8*, 15–18.
20. Lu, J.; Zhao, Z.M.; Wang, F.; Ding, Y.P.; Ma, D.N.; Ye, X.L.; Song, X.L. High dietary fiber enteral nutrition improves the nutritional status and tolerance in critically ill patients. *Chin. J. Crit. Care Med.* **2011**, *5*, 300–305.
21. Dosmoulin, F.; Caninoni, P.; Cozzone, P.J. Glutamate-glutamine metabolism in the perfused rat liver. ^{13}C NMR study using ^{13}C-enriched acetate. *FEBS Lett.* **1985**, *185*, 29–32. [CrossRef]
22. Macfarlane, G.T.; Steed, H.; Macfarlane, S. Bacterial metabolism and health-related effects of galacto-oligosaccharides and other prebiotics. *Appl. Microbiol.* **2008**, *104*, 305–344. [CrossRef] [PubMed]
23. Macfarlane, G.T.; Macfarlane, S. Fermentation in the human large intestine: Its physiologic consequences and the potential contribution of prebiotics. *Clin. Gastroenterol.* **2011**, *45*, S120–S127. [CrossRef] [PubMed]
24. Brown, A.J.; Goldsworthy, S.M.; Barnes, A.A.; Eilert, M.M.; Tcheang, L.; Daniels, D.; Muir, A.I.; Wigglesworth, M.J.; Kinghorn, I.; Fraser, N.J.; et al. The orphan G protein-coupled receptors GPR41 and GPR4 are activated by propionate and other short chain carboxylic acids. *J. Biol. Chem.* **2003**, *278*, 11312–11319. [CrossRef] [PubMed]
25. Bailón, E.; Cueto-Sola, M.; Utrilla, P.; Rodríguez-Cabezas, M.E.; Garrido-Mesa, N.; Zarzuelo, A.; Xaus, J.; Gálvez, J.; Comalada, M. Butyrate in vitro immune-modulatory effects might be mediated through a proliferation-related induction of apoptosis. *Immunobiology* **2010**, *215*, 863–873. [CrossRef] [PubMed]
26. Lührs, H.; Gerke, T.; Müller, J.G.; Melcher, R.; Schauber, J.; Box-berge, F.; Scheppach, W.; Menzel, T. Butyrate inhibits NF-kappaB activation in lamina propria macrophages of patients with ulcerative colitis. *Scand. J. Gastroenterol.* **2002**, *37*, 458–466. [CrossRef] [PubMed]

27. Maslowski, K.M.; Vieira, A.T.; Ng, A.; Kranich, J.; Sierro, F.; Yu, D.; Schilter, H.C.; Rolph, M.S.; Mackay, F.; Artis, D.; et al. Regulation of inflmmatory responses by gut microbiota and chemoattractant receptor GPR4. *Nature* **2009**, *461*, 1282–1286. [CrossRef] [PubMed]
28. Vinolo, M.A.; Rodrigues, H.G.; Hatanaka, E.; Hebeda, C.B.; Farsky, S.H.; Curi, R. Short-chain fatty acids stimulate the migration of neutrophils to inflmmatory sites. *Clin. Sci.* **2009**, *117*, 331–338. [CrossRef] [PubMed]
29. Kamath, P.S.; Hoepfner, M.T.; Phillips, S.F. Short-chain fatty acids stimulate ileal motility in humans. *Gastroenterology* **1988**, *95*, 1496–1502. [CrossRef]

nutrients

MDPI

Article

The Interaction between Dietary Fiber and Fat and Risk of Colorectal Cancer in the Women's Health Initiative

Sandi L. Navarro [1,*], Marian L. Neuhouser [1,2], Ting-Yuan David Cheng [3], Lesley F. Tinker [1], James M. Shikany [4], Linda Snetselaar [5], Jessica A. Martinez [6], Ikuko Kato [7], Shirley A. A. Beresford [1,2], Robert S. Chapkin [8] and Johanna W. Lampe [1,2]

1 Division of Public Health Sciences, Fred Hutchinson Cancer Research Center, Seattle, WA 98109, USA; mneuhous@fredhutch.org (M.L.N.); ltinker@whi.org (L.F.T.); beresfrd@uw.edu (S.A.A.B.); jlampe@fredhutch.org (J.W.L.)
2 Department of Epidemiology, School of Public Health, University of Washington, Seattle, WA 98105, USA
3 Division of Cancer Prevention and Population Sciences, Roswell Park Cancer Institute, Buffalo, NY 14263, USA; david.cheng@roswellpark.org
4 Division of Preventive Medicine, University of Alabama at Birmingham, Birmingham, AL 35294, USA; jshikany@uabmc.edu
5 Department of Epidemiology, University of Iowa, Iowa City, IA 52242, USA; linda-snetselaar@uiowa.edu
6 Department of Nutritional Sciences, University of Arizona Cancer Center, Tucson, AZ 85724, USA; jam1@email.arizona.edu
7 Department of Oncology and Pathology, Wayne State University, Detroit, MI 48201, USA; katoi@karmanos.org
8 Program in Integrative Nutrition and Complex Diseases, Texas A&M University, College Station, TX 77843, USA; r-chapkin@tamu.edu
* Correspondence: snavarro@fredhutch.org; Tel.: +1-206-667-6583

Received: 1 November 2016; Accepted: 25 November 2016; Published: 30 November 2016

Abstract: Combined intakes of specific dietary fiber and fat subtypes protect against colon cancer in animal models. We evaluated associations between self-reported individual and combinations of fiber (insoluble, soluble, and pectins, specifically) and fat (omega-6, omega-3, and docosahexaenoic acid (DHA) and eicosapentaenoic acid (EPA), specifically) and colorectal cancer (CRC) risk in the Women's Health Initiative prospective cohort (n = 134,017). During a mean 11.7 years (1993–2010), 1952 incident CRC cases were identified. Cox regression models computed multivariate adjusted hazard ratios to estimate the association between dietary factors and CRC risk. Assessing fiber and fat individually, there was a modest trend for lower CRC risk with increasing intakes of total and insoluble fiber (*p-trend* 0.09 and 0.08). An interaction (p = 0.01) was observed between soluble fiber and DHA + EPA, with protective effects of DHA + EPA with lower intakes of soluble fiber and an attenuation at higher intakes, however this association was no longer significant after correction for multiple testing. These results suggest a modest protective effect of higher fiber intake on CRC risk, but not in combination with dietary fat subtypes. Given the robust results in preclinical models and mixed results in observational studies, controlled dietary interventions with standardized intakes are needed to better understand the interaction of specific fat and fiber subtypes on colon biology and ultimately CRC susceptibility in humans.

Keywords: butyrate; colorectal cancer; DHA; EPA; fat; fiber; omega-3; pectin

1. Introduction

Colorectal cancer (CRC) is the third most common type of cancer in the U.S., accounting for roughly 8% of new cancer cases and 8% of all cancer deaths in 2015 [1]. Lifestyle factors such as diet, physical activity, and body weight contribute substantially to CRC, and it is generally held that risk could be greatly reduced through dietary modification [2]. Dietary fiber and fat are two of the most well-studied dietary components in this regard [3]. Although many case-control studies have found inverse associations between fiber and fat intakes and CRC [4], data from epidemiologic studies are mixed [4–25], possibly due to differences in intake assessment, the type of fiber or fat analyzed, and residual confounding by other lifestyle and dietary factors. More recent studies have attempted to control for dietary confounders such as folate, alcohol, and red meat consumption, yet the contradictions in outcomes persist [7,15,26,27]. Finally, within the Women's Health Initiative (WHI) Dietary Modification Trial, a low fat dietary pattern intervention which included a focus on increasing servings of whole grains, vegetables, and fruits, was found to have no significant benefit on CRC incidence over an average of 8.1 years [28].

There is a growing recognition that dietary exposures are complex with synergistic and antagonistic effects between different dietary components contributing to chronic disease risk. Interactions between dietary constituents and microbial metabolites may also partially explain differences in population-level study outcomes [29,30]. In contrast to the equivocal data from observational studies in humans—in which each dietary component is evaluated separately—strong evidence for a combined effect of the subtypes of fat and fiber in relation to reduced colon tumorigenesis has been demonstrated in preclinical animal models [31–35]. Gut bacteria ferment dietary fiber (e.g., pectins, a type of fermentable soluble fiber) to butyrate [36–49], a potent histone deacetylase (HDAC) inhibitor [29,30] associated with reduced CRC risk [50–52]. Omega 6 (*n*-6) polyunsaturated fatty acids (PUFA), commonly found in refined vegetables oils, processed and fast foods, and red meat, typical in Western diets [53], and omega 3 (*n*-3) PUFA in fish oils [54] are structural precursors of eicosanoids; those derived from n-6 are mainly pro-inflammatory, whereas those produced from *n*-3 tend to have opposing effects [55,56]. Given the strong correlation between inflammation and CRC [56], higher intakes of long-chain *n*-3 PUFA provide biologic validity for a chemoprotective effect [57].

Preclinical research suggests that the combined effects of *n*-3 PUFA in fish oils (e.g., docosahexaenoic acid (DHA) and eicosapentaenoic acid (EPA)) and butyrate from fermentable fiber (e.g., pectin) may work in concert to enhance the chemopreventive potential of either dietary component alone, primarily by increasing apoptosis [31,33,34,58–62]. While other factors, such as low dietary intakes of fiber and certain fatty acid subtypes, may contribute to the mixed results in humans, the lack of evaluation of the interaction between subtypes of dietary fat and fiber, i.e., pectins in soluble fiber and marine-derived *n*-3 PUFA, may also explain why the chemoprotective effects of fiber and fat have not been consistently detected in prospective cohort studies. Therefore, our objectives for this study were to determine the associations between the individual and combinations of subtypes of fiber (soluble, and pectins specifically, which leads to the production of butyrate, vs. insoluble) and fat (*n*-3, and DHA + EPA, specifically, vs. *n*-6), and risk of CRC in the WHI.

2. Materials and Methods

2.1. Study Population

The WHI is a large prospective study focused on understanding preventive strategies for major chronic diseases in postmenopausal women [63]. WHI includes both a multi-component randomized Clinical Trial (CT) and an Observational Study (OS). The CT (n = 68,132) was actually three overlapping randomized controlled trials evaluating combined hormone therapy or estrogen alone versus placebo (HRT), a low-fat dietary pattern versus comparison (Dietary Modification), and calcium and vitamin D supplementation versus placebo (CaD), on the risk of breast and colorectal cancers, coronary heart disease, and osteoporotic fractures. The OS (n = 93,676) examines a broader range of lifestyle, health, and risk factors and risk of common chronic diseases in postmenopausal women initially interested in but ineligible for one or more of the clinical trials. Postmenopausal women aged 50–79 years were recruited from the general population at 40 different Clinical Centers between

1993 and 1998, with trial follow-up information and outcome data available through 2005, and post-trial follow-up information and outcome data for these analyses available through September, 2010, the end of the first WHI Extension Study. All participants in the CT and OS were included in the present analysis except women who were randomized to the intervention arm of the Dietary Modification trial (n = 19,541). Further details on recruitment, study design, and baseline measures have been published elsewhere [63–66]. Institutional review board approval was obtained from all clinical sites, and women provided written informed consent prior to participation and for follow-up in the Extension period. The WHI ClinicalTrials.gov identifier is NCT00000611.

2.2. Data Collection and Dietary Assessment

Detailed information on demographic characteristics, medical, reproductive and familial CRC history, and lifestyle factors were collected at baseline. Weight and height were assessed with a standardized protocol using a calibrated balance beam scale and stadiometer, respectively, and body mass index (BMI) was computed as weight in kg/height in m^2. Physical activity was assessed by computing average weekly metabolic equivalents of moderate and vigorous leisure-time physical activity.

Dietary intake over the past three months was measured from the WHI food frequency questionnaire (FFQ) [67] using a standardized protocol at baseline for all women, and at year one for Dietary Modification CT participants. Follow-up FFQs were completed in years two through nine for a rotating proportion (33%) of Dietary Modification CT participants. The baseline FFQ data were used for the current study. The FFQs contained 122 food and food group items, and 19 adjustment questions, the majority of which ask about food practices pertaining to types and amounts of added fats (e.g., fat added at the table and in cooking), and three summary questions on food purchasing and preparation methods [67]. The WHI nutrient database was derived from Nutrition Data Systems for Research (NDS-R, version 2005, Nutrition Coordinating Center, University of Minnesota, Minneapolis, MN, USA). The database has over 140 nutrient values including total fat, total PUFA, n-6 and n-3 PUFA, total DHA and EPA from food sources; and total, insoluble and soluble fiber, and pectins.

2.3. Colorectal Cancer Case Ascertainment

Clinical outcomes, including cancer diagnoses, were updated annually in the OS and semi-annually in the CT until 2005 when the outcomes were thereafter reported annually using mail or telephone questionnaires. Self-reports of CRC were verified by trained physician adjudicators at the Clinical Centers who reviewed medical records and pathology reports [68]. All CRC diagnoses were then confirmed by blinded review at the WHI Clinical Coordinating Center at the Fred Hutchinson Cancer Research Center.

2.4. Statistical Analysis

Exclusions were made for women who reported history of colon or rectal cancers prior to baseline enrollment or who were missing these data (n = 946). Further exclusions were made for women with FFQs containing incomplete information, or data that suggested biologically implausible daily energy intakes of <2512 or >20,930 kJ (n = 4649), or extreme BMIs (<15 or >50 kg/m^2; n = 2069). Finally, women who were missing data for smoking, physical activity, and education variables combined (n = 9), or were lost to follow up (n = 577), were excluded, leaving a sample of 134,017 for analysis.

Cox proportional hazards models were used to estimate hazard ratios (HR) and 95% confidence intervals (95% CI) for the association of fiber (total, insoluble, soluble, and pectins) and fat (total, n-6, n-3, and DHA + EPA) intakes and CRC risk. Dietary variables were evaluated as separate main effects, as quintiles of intake, using the lowest quintile as the reference group. Quintile assignments of dietary variables from the baseline FFQ were calculated based on the distribution in non-cases. Tests for trend were performed in a separate Cox model treating quintiles 1–5 as linear. Fat variables were analyzed both as g intake/day with energy adjusted in the models, and as % energy. As the results for both were similar (data not shown) we present only fat as g intake/day. Interactions (a total of seven determined a priori: total fat × total fiber; insoluble fiber × *n*-6 PUFA; soluble fiber × *n*-3 PUFA; insoluble fiber × *n*-3 PUFA; soluble fiber × DHA + EPA; pectins × *n*-3 PUFA; pectins × DHA + EPA) were assessed by adding the multiplicative interaction term between linear quintiles of dietary fat and fiber variables to the final multivariate model. For the significant interaction of soluble fiber and DHA + EPA, post-hoc HRs and 95% CIs were computed for each quintile comparison for each of the 25 fat × fiber groups.

All models were adjusted for established or suggestive risk factors for CRC: (age (years, continuous); family history of CRC (yes/no); red and processed meat consumption (g/day, continuous); BMI (kg/m^2, continuous); leisure physical activity (total metabolic equivalent-h/week, continuous); smoking (current or past/never); alcohol use (g/day, continuous); current use of non-steroidal anti-inflammatory drugs (NSAIDs; yes/no); folate (food plus supplements; μg dietary folate equivalents/day, continuous); calcium (food plus supplements; mg/day; continuous)) [69,70], and confounders that altered point estimates for dietary outcome measures by more than 10%: total energy intake (kcal/day, continuous); history of screening colonoscopy (yes/no); education level (high school; technical school or some college; college grad or post); ever use of menopausal hormones (yes/no); and study component (OS, CT) and CT randomization assignment (HRT, Dietary Modification or CaD). We created a "missing" category for covariates with data missing for <0.5% of the participant population (NSAIDs, $n = 91$, smoking, $n = 1737$, education level, $n = 1005$, and colonoscopy screening, $n = 4736$), and imputed the median values for physical activity ($n = 5230$) to reduce the number of participants who would be dropped from the analysis. All tests for individual dietary factors were two sided and statistical significance was set at $p < 0.05$. Tests for interaction were adjusted for multiple testing using Bonferroni correction (0.05/7 tests conducted = $p < 0.007$). All analyses were conducted using Stata (v14.1; StataCorp, College Station, TX, USA).

3. Results

The distribution of baseline participant characteristics and dietary intake for CRC cases and non-cases are given in Table 1. During a mean follow up of 11.7 years (±3.5; range: 0.02–17.5 years), a total of 1952 CRC cases were reported. Women with CRC appeared less likely to have ever used hormone therapy and consumed less calcium. Intakes of all other dietary variables were very similar in cases and non-cases.

Table 1. Baseline characteristics, colorectal cancer risk factors, and dietary constituents for participants in the Women's Health Initiative 1993–2010 [1].

Characteristic	Cases (n = 1952)	Non-Cases (n = 132,065)
Age, (years)	66 (6.9)	63 (7.3)
Height (cm)	162 (6.3)	162 (6.4)
Body mass index (kg/m^2)	28 (5.7)	28 (5.5)
Race (%)		
White	85	84
Black	9	8
Other/Unknown [2]	6	8
Education (% college graduate)	38	40
Screening colonoscopy (%)	49	51
Family history of CRC (%)	19	15
NSAID (% current use)	17	19
Alcohol use at baseline (g/day)	5 (11.3)	5 (10.8)
Never smokers (%)	49	50
Physical activity (MET-h/week) [3]	12 (12.6)	13 (13.7)
Ever used post-menopausal Hormone therapy (%)	48	56
Dietary intake		
Total energy (kJ/day)	6766 (2671)	6787 (2642)
Total fiber (g/day)	16 (6.9)	16 (6.9)
Soluble fiber (g/day)	4.3 (1.8)	4.3 (1.8)
Pectins (g/day)	2.5 (1.2)	2.5 (1.2)
Insoluble fiber (g/day)	11.5 (5.1)	11.8 (5.1)

Table 1. *Cont.*

Characteristic	Cases (n = 1952)	Non-Cases (n = 132,065)
Total fat (g/day)	60 (32.7)	59 (32.0)
n-3 (g/day)	1.41 (0.8)	1.41 (0.8)
DHA + EPA (g/day)	0.12 (0.12)	0.13 (0.12)
n-6 (g/day)	10.8 (6.2)	10.7 (6.2)
Linoleic acid (g/day)	10.8 (6.2)	10.7 (6.1)
Linolenic acid (g/day)	1.3 (0.7)	1.3 (0.7)
Calcium (mg/day)	803 (439)	827 (453)
Folate (DFE, μg/day)	478 (206)	488 (207)
Red meat (g/day)	0.69 (0.57)	0.67 (0.55)

[1] Means (Standard Deviation) unless otherwise specified; [2] Includes Hispanic, American Indian, Asian/Pacific Islander, Mixed races, and Refused; [3] Total metabolic equivalent-hours/week. CRC, colorectal cancer; DFE, dietary folate equivalents; DHA, docosahexaenoic acid; EPA, eicosapentaenoic acid; NSAIDs, non-steroidal anti-inflammatory drugs.

Table 2 provides data on associations of total, insoluble, and soluble fiber, and pectins, with CRC risk. When assessing fiber as a main effect, higher versus lower total soluble and insoluble fibers were associated with modest, but non-significant lower risk of CRC. There was a suggestion of inverse linear trends for total and insoluble fiber, (*p-trend* = 0.09 for total fiber; *p-trend* = 0.08 for insoluble fiber).

Table 2. Multivariate-adjusted hazard ratios and 95% CIs for the association of fiber with colorectal cancer in the Women's Health Initiative (n = 134,017) 1993–2010.

Quintiles of Dietary Intake	No. Cases	Person-Years	Multivariate Adjusted HR (95% CI) [1]
		Total fiber (g/day)	
<10.3	420	302,828	1.00 (Reference)
10.3–13.6	426	312,546	1.00 (0.87, 1.15)
13.6–17.0	354	316,244	0.83 (0.71, 0.97)
17.0–21.5	372	318,893	0.87 (0.74, 1.03)
>21.5	380	318,844	0.90 (0.73, 1.10)
p-trend			0.09
		Soluble fiber (g/day)	
<2.8	408	304,051	1.00 (Reference)
2.8–3.7	409	312,599	0.97 (0.84, 1.12)
3.7–4.6	361	316,928	0.85 (0.73, 1.00)
4.6–5.8	410	318,628	0.96 (0.81, 1.13)
>5.8	364	317,148	0.84 (0.69, 1.03)
p-trend			0.14
		Insoluble fiber (g/day)	
<7.4	433	302,242	1.00 (Reference)
7.4–9.8	413	312,804	0.93 (0.81, 1.07)
9.8–12.3	357	316,721	0.81 (0.69, 0.94)
12.3–15.7	370	318,704	0.84 (0.72, 1.00)
>15.7	379	318,884	0.87 (0.72, 1.06)
p-trend			0.08
		Pectin (g/day)	
<1.4	399	303,832	1.00 (Reference)
1.4–2.0	397	313,746	0.97 (0.84, 1.12)
2.0–2.6	379	316,302	0.92 (0.79, 1.06)
2.6–3.5	396	318,847	0.97 (0.83, 1.13)
>3.5	381	316,626	0.94 (0.80, 1.11)
p-trend			0.56

[1] The following variables were included in both the multivariate and continuous models: total energy intake (continuous), age (continuous), body mass index (continuous), education (high school, technical school or some college, college graduate or post-graduate), family history of colorectal cancer (yes/no), history of colonoscopy (yes/no), current NSAID use (yes/no), alcohol intake (continuous), smoking history (never, former, current), physical activity (total metabolic equivalent-hours, continuous), ever use of hormone therapy (never, current/former), folate (DFE; μg/day, continuous), calcium (mg/day, continuous), and red meat intake (g/day, continuous), and study component (OS, CT) and CT randomization assignment and treatment arm. OS, observational study; CT, clinical trial; DFE, dietary folate equivalents; NSAIDs, non-steroidal anti-inflammatory drugs.

The associations of total fat, *n*-6 PUFA, *n*-3 PUFA, and EPA + DHA with CRC risk were null with most HRs near the null value of 1.0 (Table 3).

Table 3. Multivariate-adjusted hazard ratios and 95% CIs for the association of fat with colorectal cancer in the Women's Health Initiative (*n* = 134,017) 1993–2010.

Quintiles of Dietary Intake	No. Cases	Person-Years	Multivariate Adjusted HR (95% CI) [1]
		Total fat (g/day)	
<33.1	345	309,005	1.00 (Reference)
33.1–45.6	432	318,884	1.20 (1.04, 1.39)
45.6–59.7	394	316,808	1.05 (0.90, 1.24)
59.7–80.6	381	316,629	0.98 (0.82, 1.18)
>80.6	400	313,067	0.98 (0.76, 1.27)
p-trend			0.44
		n-6 PUFA (g/day)	
<5.9	375	309,046	1.00 (Reference)
5.9–8.1	405	314,292	1.02 (0.88, 1.18)
8.1–10.7	390	316,554	0.95 (0.81, 1.11)
10.7–14.6	394	317,021	0.92 (0.78, 1.09)
>14.6	388	312,441	0.84 (0.68, 1.05)
p-trend			0.10
		n-3 PUFA (g/day)	
<0.80	401	308,532	1.00 (Reference)
0.80–1.09	389	314,521	0.94 (0.82, 1.08)
1.09–1.41	383	316,931	0.90 (0.78, 1.05)
1.41–1.90	377	316,759	0.87 (0.75, 1.03)
>1.90	402	312,611	0.90 (0.74, 1.09)
p-trend			0.16
		DHA + EPA (g/day)	
<0.04	402	307,408	1.00 (Reference)
0.04–0.07	389	312,402	0.97 (0.84, 1.12)
0.07–0.11	393	315,998	0.98 (0.85, 1.13)
0.11–0.18	389	318,148	0.99 (0.85, 1.14)
>0.18	379	315,397	0.98 (0.84, 1.13)
p-trend			0.87

[1] The following variables were included in both the multivariate and continuous models: total energy intake (continuous), age (continuous), body mass index (continuous), education (high school, technical school or some college, college graduate or post-graduate), family history of colorectal cancer (yes/no), history of colonoscopy (yes/no), current NSAID use (yes/no), alcohol intake (continuous), smoking history (never, former, current), physical activity (total metabolic equivalent-hours, continuous), ever use of hormone therapy (never, current/former), folate (DFE μg/day, continuous), calcium (mg/day, continuous), and red meat intake (g/day, continuous), and study component (OS, CT) and CT randomization assignment and treatment arm. OS, observational study; CT, clinical trial; DFE, dietary folate equivalents; DHA, docosahexaenoic acid; EPA, eicosapentaenoic acid; NSAIDs, non-steroidal anti-inflammatory drugs. PUFA, polyunsaturated fatty acids.

We next examined the interaction of fat and fiber subtypes in relation to CRC risk. The interaction between DHA + EPA and soluble fiber was statistically significant (*p-interaction* = 0.01), with a significant decreased risk of CRC with increasing DHA + EPA intake among those in the lowest quintile of soluble fiber intake (*p-trend* = 0.02; Table 4) and a borderline increased risk of CRC with increasing DHA + EPA among those in the highest quintile of soluble fiber (*p-trend* = 0.07; Table 4). There was a marginal statistically significant association between pectins and DHA + EPA (p = 0.05), with a similar pattern of attenuation, whereby the protective effects of higher intakes of pectins were no longer apparent with higher intakes of DHA + EPA (data not shown). However, these interactions were no longer significant when adjusted for multiple comparisons. There were no other significant interactions between the various dietary fiber and fat combinations.

Table 4. Soluble fiber and DHA + EPA stratified by quintile of intake, and association with colorectal cancer in the Women's Health Initiative (n = 134,017) 1993–2010.

		DHA + EPA (g/Day)					HR (95% CI) [1]	p-Trend [2]
		Q1	Q2	Q3	Q4	Q5		
Soluble fiber (g/day)	Q1	1.00 (Ref) [3]	0.88 (0.68, 1.13)	0.78 (0.59, 1.04)	0.88 (0.65, 1.20)	0.59 (0.40, 0.88)	0.91 (0.84, 0.98)	0.02
	Q2	0.81 (0.62, 1.06)	0.82 (0.63, 1.07)	0.91 (0.70, 1.18)	0.80 (0.60, 1.06)	0.91 (0.69, 1.23)	1.03 (0.96, 1.11)	0.44
	Q3	0.71 (0.53, 0.96)	0.84 (0.63, 1.11)	0.73 (0.55, 0.97)	0.65 (0.48, 0.87)	0.79 (0.59, 1.06)	0.99 (0.91, 1.06)	0.70
	Q4	0.76 (0.56, 1.05)	0.86 (0.65, 1.15)	0.87 (0.66, 1.15)	0.90 (0.68, 1.18)	0.77 (0.57, 1.02)	1.00 (0.93, 1.07)	0.96
	Q5	0.70 (0.49, 1.01)	0.53 (0.37, 0.78)	0.73 (0.53, 1.00)	0.81 (0.60, 1.08)	0.80 (0.60, 1.08)	1.08 (1.00, 1.17)	0.07
HR (95% CI) [1]		0.97 (0.89, 1.08)	0.90 (0.81, 1.00)	1.02 (0.92, 1.13)	0.99 (0.89, 1.09)	1.00 (0.89, 1.11)		
p-trend [2]		0.62	0.05	0.72	0.80	0.95		

[1] HR and 95% CI across quintiles of soluble fiber and DHA + EPA; [2] p-trend values from linear interactions across each row and column. The following variables were included in the model: total energy intake (continuous), age (continuous), body mass index (continuous), education (high school, technical school or some college, college graduate or post-graduate), family history of colorectal cancer (yes/no), history of colonoscopy (yes/no), current NSAID use (yes/no), alcohol intake (continuous), smoking history (never, former, current), physical activity (total metabolic equivalent-hours, continuous), ever use of hormone therapy (never, current/former), folate (μg/day, continuous), calcium (mg/day, continuous), and red meat intake (g/day, continuous), and study component (OS, CT) and CT randomization assignment and treatment arm; [3] the combination of the first quintiles for soluble fiber and DHA + EPA is the reference group for all comparisons within quintiles. OS, observational study; CT, clinical trial; DFE, dietary folate equivalents; DHA, docosahexaenoic acid; EPA, eicosapentaenoic acid; NSAIDs, non-steroidal anti-inflammatory drugs. PUFA, polyunsaturated fatty acids.

4. Discussion

The results of the present analysis in a large, prospective cohort of postmenopausal women do not support the results obtained in preclinical studies demonstrating that combinations of higher fiber and fat subtypes are associated with reduced risk of CRC. While there was a modest additional protective effect of either dietary component when intake of the other was low, this protective effect was attenuated with greater consumption in our study population. Intakes and ranges were very low such that only women in the highest quintile of fiber were consuming adequate intakes for this age group (21 g/day for women ages 51–70 years), with a very small percentage consuming high intakes [71]. Further, intakes of n-3 PUFA, and DHA and EPA, specifically, were substantially lower than the levels used in experimental diets. These factors may have prevented detection of an association.

It is generally thought that CRC risk could be reduced through dietary modification, including increased dietary fiber intake and reduced fat intake [3]. Dietary fiber mainly includes remnants of plant foods resistant to digestion by human enzymes and therefore arrives in the colon relatively intact, where it undergoes metabolism by gut microbiota. In the 2011 Colorectal Cancer Report, part of the Continuous Update Project, the World Cancer Research Fund/American Institute for Cancer Research Expert Panel classified evidence supporting consumption of fiber-containing foods and CRC protection as 'convincing' [72], noting that for every 10 g/day increase in fiber, there was a 10% decrease in CRC risk. Mechanisms hypothesized to explain how dietary fiber may reduce CRC include increased stool bulk and reduced intestinal transit time, resulting in reduced exposure to potential carcinogens; decreased secondary bile acids and subsequent generation of reactive oxygen species; and fiber fermentation by gut microbiota to short-chain fatty acids, particularly butyrate [73–75]. It is now well-documented that butyrate induces apoptosis in tumor cells through inhibition of HDAC and subsequent activation of the Fas receptor-mediated extrinsic death pathway [31,76–79]. Given the potential importance of fiber fermentation on CRC risk, consideration of fiber subtypes may be important; however, few studies have examined fiber subtype (i.e., soluble and insoluble, or more and less fermentable), and associations are similar, with both null [9,10] and inverse associations [80–83] reported.

When evaluating total fiber and subtypes in the present study, CRC risk was reduced for all quintiles of increased consumption and a marginal linear trend was observed; however, most quintiles did not reach statistical significance. Inconsistencies across epidemiologic studies may be attributed in part to lower overall fiber intakes and narrow ranges of fiber intakes in Western populations which reduce statistical power [13]. Mean fiber intake in the U.S. is ~15 g/day [4]. Intakes at or above current recommended intakes (25 g/day for women and 38 g/day for men) [71] show robust protection against CRC with relative risks ranging from 0.72 to 0.90 [4,6,26]. Only 10% of our study population reported intakes of dietary fiber >25 g/day, thus our ability to detect a protective effect was compromised.

Overlaying the conflicting data observed with dietary fiber and CRC is a similar body of inconsistent literature on the association between subtypes of fat, particularly *n*-3 PUFA, and CRC risk. In addition to the anti-inflammatory effects promulgated by changes in the eicosanoid milieu, other putative actions of *n*-3 PUFA have been proposed. These include alterations in membrane fluidity and lipid raft composition, which may affect receptor signaling involved in proliferation and apoptosis [84], and modulation of oxidative stress [57,85]. As with dietary fiber, laboratory data consistently show reduced CRC risk with marine *n*-3 PUFA [58], while epidemiologic data are less convincing. Whereas two meta-analyses reported reduced CRC risk with *n*-3 PUFA from fish intake [86,87], two systematic reviews concluded that there is insufficient [15] or limited [7] evidence to suggest an association between long-chain *n*-3 PUFA intake and CRC risk. A more recent publication reported no overall association between *n*-3 PUFA and CRC risk among 123,529 individuals; however, among women in the same cohort, *n*-3 PUFA intake after CRC diagnosis had a protective effect on survival [88].

In the WHI population, we did not observe an association between any dietary fat subtypes and CRC risk. As with fiber, intakes of *n*-3 PUFA were very low; mean intakes were 1.4 g/day (range 0.1–10.4) for *n*-3, and 0.04 and 0.08 g/day (range 0–1.4 and 0–3.1, respectively) for EPA and DHA. While specific recommendations for *n*-3 PUFA intake have not been determined, the Food and Nutrition Board of the Institute of Medicine established adequate intake levels for alpha-linolenic acid (ALA), the precursor of long-chain *n*-3 PUFA, of 1.1 g/day for women over the age of 19 [71]. Only about half of our study population had intakes at that level. Furthermore, the Academy of Nutrition and Dietetics recommends a minimum intake of 0.5 g/day of combined EPA and DHA [89]. Less than 2% of the women in our study cohort reached an intake level above 0.5 g/day.

Despite the inconsistent epidemiologic data for dietary fiber and fat, studies in preclinical animal models have shown that combinations of fiber and fat work synergistically to protect against colon cancer [58–62]. In a series of experiments, the effects of different types of fat (fish oil or corn oil; 15 g/100 g) and fiber (pectin or cellulose; 6 g/100 g) diets were tested on tumorigenesis and various other aspects of colonocyte physiology [58,90]. Both fish oil and pectin alone, relative to corn oil and cellulose feeding, resulted in a significantly lower proportion of animals with adenocarcinomas; however, the combination of fish oil and pectin led to an even greater reduction [58]. Additional work showed changes to the re-dox environment within rat colonocytes with a concomitant reduction in DNA damage [35,59,91]. Serving as the primary energy source for colonic epithelial cells, butyrate induces cellular reactive oxygen species (ROS) generation, creating a pro-oxidant environment [31]. At the same time, long chain *n*-3 PUFA from fish oil (e.g., DHA) incorporated into cell membranes, are susceptible to oxidation due to their high degree of unsaturation [33]. These physiological attributes of butyrate and DHA are relevant as lipid peroxidation can directly trigger the release of pro-apoptotic factors from mitochondria into the cytosol, through a p53-independent, calcium-mediated cell death pathway [33]. Given that butyrate independently induces apoptosis through an extrinsic, HDAC inhibition-mediated pathway, the combination of dietary constituents, and subsequent effects on intrinsic apoptotic pathways, would be expected to exponentially increase apoptosis.

Dietary fiber and fatty acids, in combination, and risk of CRC in humans has only recently begun to be evaluated. In a large cohort study (n = 96,354) of Seventh Day Adventists, risk of CRC was reduced by 22% among all vegetarians combined compared to non-vegetarians, but protection was greatest among pescovegetarians who consume high amounts of both fiber and n-3 PUFA-containing fish (HR: 0.57; 95% CI: 0.40, 0.82) [92]. Furthermore, striking reciprocal changes in gut mucosal cancer risk biomarkers, the microbiome, and the metabolome were reported after African Americans were given a high-fiber (primarily in the form of resistant starch, including pectin), low-fat diet and rural Africans were given a high-fat, low-fiber Western-style diet [93]. Significantly increased butyrate production and suppressed secondary bile acid synthesis were also noted after the diet exchange to high-fiber, low-fat intake in African Americans [93].

An analysis in the Rotterdam prospective cohort (n = 4967) lends support to the hypothesis that higher intakes of fat and fiber are an important factor mediating the relationship between these dietary variables. An increased risk of CRC was observed with n-3 PUFA intake and dietary fiber intakes below the median, but not when fiber intakes were above [22]. It is noteworthy that the levels of fiber intakes were markedly lower (mean 26 g/day) relative to the intakes among pescovegetarians in the Seventh Day Adventist population (mean 40 g/day) and the African American intervention participants (mean 55 g/day), but higher than the intakes in our population (mean 16 g/day). Adding to the complexity of the relationship, when evaluated by food sources of n-3 PUFA in the Rotterdam study, increased CRC risk was restricted to intake from non-marine sources which contain ALA; there was no association when n-3 PUFA from marine-derived (e.g., EPA and DHA) sources were evaluated [22]. Contrary to these results, evaluation by n-3 PUFA source in a case-control study did not show any difference between non-marine and marine sources and interaction with dietary fiber. In this instance, greater protection of n-3 PUFA was found among individuals with lower dietary fiber intakes although overall intake was low (median 18.6 g/day) [94], consistent with our observation of the significant reduced risk of CRC among women with the lowest soluble fiber and highest DHA + EPA intakes. The authors speculated that high fiber intake may interfere with lipid absorption, offsetting potential beneficial effects of certain fatty acids [94].

While intakes in animal models do not directly translate to human intakes, the amount of fiber and fat used in preclinical experiments is comparable, as a proportion of intake, to what is currently recommended for humans. For example, the amount of fiber in the rat diets was 6% by weight, which is approximately equivalent to 30 g/day for humans [58]. This level of intake was only approached in the highest quintile of total fiber intake (>21.5 g/day). Similarly, all rat diets contained fat at 15% by weight and 30% of energy, with fish oil comprising approximately 1%–5% [58]. Women in WHI consumed 33% of their calories from fat on average, but less than 1% from n-3 PUFA and even less from combined DHA and EPA from fish oil (highest quintile >0.18 g/day). In the VITamins And Lifestyle (VITAL) cohort (n = 68,109), individuals using fish oil supplements on 4+ days/week for 3+ years experienced 49% lower CRC risk than non-users (HR = 0.51, 95% CI = 0.26–1.00; *p-trend* = 0.06) [17]. An average serving of oily fish (e.g., salmon or mackerel) provides 1.5–3 g of marine fish oil [95]. Thus, it may be difficult to achieve the levels of n-3 PUFA needed for a chemoprotective effect through diet alone.

Strengths of this study include the large, well-characterized prospective cohort. As CRC was one of the primary outcomes of WHI, incident cases were expertly adjudicated and confirmed. Additionally, detailed information was collected on a wide range of exposures, including diet, with reliability subsequently assessed [65]. Finally, this is the largest prospective cohort to evaluate the interactions of subtypes of fiber and fat on CRC to date.

As with all observational studies, there are limitations. First, we relied on self-report via FFQ to capture usual dietary intake, therefore we cannot rule out measurement error. FFQs are subject to lack of precision and inaccurate recall of dietary intake [96]. As dietary intakes were only assessed at baseline, it is possible that diets changed over time. However, we performed a sensitivity analysis using FFQ from women in the Dietary Modification comparison arm (the only group for which FFQ data from multiple time-points were collected) between years 0, 1, 3, 6, and 9, and found that correlations were 0.62 for fiber intake and 0.44 for total fat intake, suggesting that intake remained relatively stable during the follow-up. The WHI FFQ has been shown to yield nutrient estimates that are similar to those obtained from short-term dietary recall and recording methods, and test-retest reliability for most nutrients was high (e.g., FFQ estimates for total, saturated, and polyunsaturated fat variables were all within 10% of those from food records and 24-h recalls, although dietary fiber was slightly higher ~17%, and information on fat and fiber subtypes was not evaluated) [67]. Our fiber exposure also did not include the integration of dietary fiber supplement use, which is known to be higher with age and among women [97]. Lastly, measurement of the level of EPA/DHA incorporation in plasma or the tissue level was not conducted. It is widely known that the biological activities of these compounds depend on their bioavailability [98] and FFQ estimates only provide a surrogate for exposure.

Finally, while we adjusted for several potential confounders, we did not directly evaluate antioxidant content of the diet. Because the combination of butyrate and n-3 PUFA drive apoptosis via an oxidative-dependent mechanism, higher antioxidant intakes might antagonize this protective effect. In addition, there is some evidence that high antioxidants promote CRC in both preclinical [59,91] and epidemiologic [99–101] studies. Although mean intakes for several individual nutrients with antioxidant capacity (e.g., vitamins C, E, and beta-carotene) were very similar between cases and controls at baseline (<1% difference), total antioxidant capacity of dietary intakes was not considered.

5. Conclusions

In summary, at the levels of dietary intake consumed by women in WHI, we did not find evidence of a protective association between increased subtypes of fiber and fat intakes in combination, and reduced risk of CRC. Our results for fat and fiber separately are in agreement with what has been reported previously, namely modest inverse associations with fiber, but no consistent trends across intakes. Given the biologic plausibility of a protective effect for fiber and n-3 PUFA, the robust results from preclinical models, and the mixed results in observational studies, controlled feeding trials with standardized intakes and consideration of the potential impact of the gut microbiome are urgently needed.

Acknowledgments: We acknowledge the WHI Investigator Group, short list: Program Office: (National Heart, Lung, and Blood Institute, Bethesda, Maryland); Jacques Rossouw, Shari Ludlam, Dale Burwen, Joan McGowan, Leslie Ford, and Nancy Geller; Clinical Coordinating Center: (Fred Hutchinson Cancer Research Center, Seattle, WA, USA) Garnet Anderson, Ross Prentice, Andrea LaCroix, and Charles Kooperberg; Investigators and Academic Centers: (Brigham and Women's Hospital, Harvard Medical School, Boston, MA, USA) JoAnn E. Manson; (MedStar Health Research Institute/Howard University, Washington, DC, USA) Barbara V. Howard; (Stanford Prevention Research Center, Stanford, CA, USA) Marcia L. Stefanick; (The Ohio State University, Columbus, OH, USA) Rebecca Jackson; (University of Arizona, Tucson/Phoenix, AZ, USA) Cynthia A. Thomson; (University at Buffalo, Buffalo, NY, USA) Jean Wactawski-Wende; (University of Florida, Gainesville/Jacksonville, FL, USA) Marian Limacher; (University of Iowa, Iowa City/Davenport, IA, USA) Robert Wallace; (University of Pittsburgh, Pittsburgh, PA, USA) Lewis Kuller; (Wake Forest University School of Medicine, Winston-Salem, NC, USA) Sally Shumaker. Women's Health Initiative Memory Study: (Wake Forest University School of Medicine, Winston-Salem, NC, USA) Sally Shumaker; WHI is supported by National Heart, Lung, and Blood Institute, National Institutes of Health, U.S. Department of Health and Human Services through contracts, HHSN268201100046C (Fred Hutch), HHSN268201100001C (SUNY Buffalo), HHSN268201100002C (The Ohio State University), HHSN268201100003C (Stanford), HHSN268201100004C (Wake Forest), and HHSN271201100004C (WHI Memory Study), and grants P30 CA015704, R35 CA197707, and T32 CA09168.

Author Contributions: Author contributions: S.L.N., J.W.L., M.L.N., S.A.A.B., T.-Y.D.C., L.F.T. and R.S.C. conceived the study; S.L.N., T.-Y.D.C. and M.L.N. conducted the data analysis; S.L.N., M.L.N., T.-Y.D.C., R.S.C. and J.W.L. interpreted the results; S.L.N. wrote the manuscript; M.L.N., J.W.L., R.S.C., T.-Y.D.C., L.F.T., J.M.S., L.S., J.A.M., I.K. and S.A.A.B. critically revised the manuscript.

Conflicts of Interest: The authors declare no conflict of interest.

References

1. American Cancer Society. *Cancer Facts & Figures 2016*; American Cancer Society: Atlanta, GA, USA, 2016.
2. World Cancer Research Fund. *Food, Nutrition, Physical Activity, and the Prevention of Cancer: A Global Perspective*; American Institute for Cancer Research: Washington, DC, USA, 2007.

3. Perez-Cueto, F.J.; Verbeke, W. Consumer implications of the WCRF's permanent update on colorectal cancer. *Meat. Sci.* **2012**, *90*, 977–978. [CrossRef] [PubMed]
4. Ben, Q.; Sun, Y.; Chai, R.; Qian, A.; Xu, B.; Yuan, Y. Dietary fiber intake reduces risk for colorectal adenoma: A meta-analysis. *Gastroenterology* **2014**, *146*, 689–699. [CrossRef] [PubMed]
5. Michels, K.B.; Fuchs, C.S.; Giovannucci, E.; Colditz, G.A.; Hunter, D.J.; Stampfer, M.J.; Willett, W.C. Fiber intake and incidence of colorectal cancer among 76,947 women and 47,279 men. *Cancer Epidemiol. Biomark. Prev.* **2005**, *14*, 842–849. [CrossRef] [PubMed]
6. Murphy, N.; Norat, T.; Ferrari, P.; Jenab, M.; Bueno-de-Mesquita, B.; Skeie, G.; Dahm, C.C.; Overvad, K.; Olsen, A.; Tjonneland, A.; et al. Dietary fibre intake and risks of cancers of the colon and rectum in the european prospective investigation into cancer and nutrition (epic). *PLoS ONE* **2012**, *7*, e39361. [CrossRef] [PubMed]
7. Gerber, M. Omega-3 fatty acids and cancers: A systematic update review of epidemiological studies. *Br. J. Nutr.* **2012**, *107*, S228–S239. [CrossRef] [PubMed]
8. Kunzmann, A.T.; Coleman, H.G.; Huang, W.Y.; Kitahara, C.M.; Cantwell, M.M.; Berndt, S.I. Dietary fiber intake and risk of colorectal cancer and incident and recurrent adenoma in the prostate, lung, colorectal, and ovarian cancer screening trial. *Am. J. Clin. Nutr.* **2015**, *102*, 881–890. [CrossRef] [PubMed]
9. Wakai, K.; Date, C.; Fukui, M.; Tamakoshi, K.; Watanabe, Y.; Hayakawa, N.; Kojima, M.; Kawado, M.; Suzuki, K.; Hashimoto, S.; et al. Dietary fiber and risk of colorectal cancer in the japan collaborative cohort study. *Cancer Epidemiol. Biomark. Prev.* **2007**, *16*, 668–675. [CrossRef] [PubMed]
10. Uchida, K.; Kono, S.; Yin, G.; Toyomura, K.; Nagano, J.; Mizoue, T.; Mibu, R.; Tanaka, M.; Kakeji, Y.; Maehara, Y.; et al. Dietary fiber, source foods and colorectal cancer risk: The fukuoka colorectal cancer study. *Scand. J. Gastroenterol.* **2010**, *45*, 1223–1231. [CrossRef] [PubMed]
11. Park, Y.; Hunter, D.J.; Spiegelman, D.; Bergkvist, L.; Berrino, F.; van den Brandt, P.A.; Buring, J.E.; Colditz, G.A.; Freudenheim, J.L.; Fuchs, C.S.; et al. Dietary fiber intake and risk of colorectal cancer: A pooled analysis of prospective cohort studies. *JAMA* **2005**, *294*, 2849–2857. [CrossRef] [PubMed]
12. Willett, W.C.; Stampfer, M.J.; Colditz, G.A.; Rosner, B.A.; Speizer, F.E. Relation of meat, fat, and fiber intake to the risk of colon cancer in a prospective-study among women. *N. Engl. J. Med.* **1990**, *323*, 1664–1672. [CrossRef] [PubMed]
13. Schatzkin, A.; Mouw, T.; Park, Y.; Subar, A.F.; Kipnis, V.; Hollenbeck, A.; Leitzmann, M.F.; Thompson, F.E. Dietary fiber and whole-grain consumption in relation to colorectal cancer in the nih-aarp diet and health study. *Am. J. Clin. Nutr.* **2007**, *85*, 1353–1360. [PubMed]
14. Fuchs, C.S.; Giovannucci, E.L.; Colditz, G.A.; Hunter, D.J.; Stampfer, M.J.; Rosner, B.; Speizer, F.E.; Willett, W.C. Dietary fiber and the risk of colorectal cancer and adenoma in women. *N. Engl. J. Med.* **1999**, *340*, 169–176. [CrossRef] [PubMed]
15. MacLean, C.H.; Newberry, S.J.; Mojica, W.A.; Khanna, P.; Issa, A.M.; Suttorp, M.J.; Lim, Y.W.; Traina, S.B.; Hilton, L.; Garland, R.; et al. Effects of omega-3 fatty acids on cancer risk: A systematic review. *JAMA* **2006**, *295*, 403–415. [CrossRef] [PubMed]
16. Daniel, C.R.; McCullough, M.L.; Patel, R.C.; Jacobs, E.J.; Flanders, W.D.; Thun, M.J.; Calle, E.E. Dietary intake of omega-6 and omega-3 fatty acids and risk of colorectal cancer in a prospective cohort of US men and women. *Cancer Epidemiol. Biomark. Prev.* **2009**, *18*, 516–525. [CrossRef] [PubMed]
17. Kantor, E.D.; Lampe, J.W.; Peters, U.; Vaughan, T.L.; White, E. Long-chain omega-3 polyunsaturated fatty acid intake and risk of colorectal cancer. *Nutr. Cancer* **2014**, *66*, 716–727. [CrossRef] [PubMed]
18. Ward, H.A.; Norat, T.; Overvad, K.; Dahm, C.C.; Bueno-de-Mesquita, H.B.; Jenab, M.; Fedirko, V.; van Duijnhoven, F.J.; Skeie, G.; Romaguera-Bosch, D.; et al. Pre-diagnostic meat and fibre intakes in relation to colorectal cancer survival in the european prospective investigation into cancer and nutrition. *Br. J. Nutr.* **2016**, *116*, 316–325. [CrossRef] [PubMed]
19. Liu, L.; Wang, S.; Liu, J. Fiber consumption and all-cause, cardiovascular, and cancer mortalities: A systematic review and meta-analysis of cohort studies. *Mol. Nutr. Food Res.* **2015**, *59*, 139–146. [CrossRef] [PubMed]
20. Hajishafiee, M.; Saneei, P.; Benisi-Kohansal, S.; Esmaillzadeh, A. Cereal fibre intake and risk of mortality from all causes, cvd, cancer and inflammatory diseases: A systematic review and meta-analysis of prospective cohort studies. *Br. J. Nutr.* **2016**, *116*, 343–352. [CrossRef] [PubMed]

21. Song, M.; Chan, A.T.; Fuchs, C.S.; Ogino, S.; Hu, F.B.; Mozaffarian, D.; Ma, J.; Willett, W.C.; Giovannucci, E.L.; Wu, K. Dietary intake of fish, omega-3 and omega-6 fatty acids and risk of colorectal cancer: A prospective study in U.S. Men and women. *Int. J. Cancer* **2014**, *135*, 2413–2423. [CrossRef] [PubMed]
22. Kraja, B.; Muka, T.; Ruiter, R.; de Keyser, C.E.; Hofman, A.; Franco, O.H.; Stricker, B.H.; Kiefte-de Jong, J.C. Dietary fiber intake modifies the positive association between *n*-3 pufa intake and colorectal cancer risk in a Caucasian population. *J. Nutr.* **2015**, *145*, 1709–1716. [CrossRef] [PubMed]
23. Trock, B.; Lanza, E.; Greenwald, P. Dietary fiber, vegetables, and colon cancer: Critical review and meta-analyses of the epidemiologic evidence. *J. Natl. Cancer Inst.* **1990**, *82*, 650–661. [CrossRef] [PubMed]
24. Vargas, A.J.; Neuhouser, M.L.; George, S.M.; Thomson, C.A.; Ho, G.Y.; Rohan, T.E.; Kato, I.; Nassir, R.; Hou, L.; Manson, J.E. Diet quality and colorectal cancer risk in the women's health initiative observational study. *Am. J. Epidemiol.* **2016**, *184*, 23–32. [CrossRef] [PubMed]
25. Makarem, N.; Nicholson, J.M.; Bandera, E.V.; McKeown, N.M.; Parekh, N. Consumption of whole grains and cereal fiber in relation to cancer risk: A systematic review of longitudinal studies. *Nutr. Rev.* **2016**, *74*, 353–373. [CrossRef] [PubMed]
26. Aune, D.; Chan, D.S.; Lau, R.; Vieira, R.; Greenwood, D.C.; Kampman, E.; Norat, T. Dietary fibre, whole grains, and risk of colorectal cancer: Systematic review and dose-response meta-analysis of prospective studies. *BMJ* **2011**, *343*, d6617. [CrossRef] [PubMed]
27. Aune, D.; Lau, R.; Chan, D.S.; Vieira, R.; Greenwood, D.C.; Kampman, E.; Norat, T. Nonlinear reduction in risk for colorectal cancer by fruit and vegetable intake based on meta-analysis of prospective studies. *Gastroenterology* **2011**, *141*, 106–118. [CrossRef] [PubMed]
28. Beresford, S.A.; Johnson, K.C.; Ritenbaugh, C.; Lasser, N.L.; Snetselaar, L.G.; Black, H.R.; Anderson, G.L.; Assaf, A.R.; Bassford, T.; Bowen, D.; et al. Low-fat dietary pattern and risk of colorectal cancer: The women's health initiative randomized controlled dietary modification trial. *JAMA* **2006**, *295*, 643–654. [CrossRef] [PubMed]
29. Donohoe, D.R.; Bultman, S.J. Metaboloepigenetics: Interrelationships between energy metabolism and epigenetic control of gene expression. *J. Cell. Physiol.* **2012**, *227*, 3169–3177. [CrossRef] [PubMed]
30. Donohoe, D.R.; Garge, N.; Zhang, X.X.; Sun, W.; O'Connell, T.M.; Bunger, M.K.; Bultman, S.J. The microbiome and butyrate regulate energy metabolism and autophagy in the mammalian colon. *Cell Metab.* **2011**, *13*, 517–526. [CrossRef] [PubMed]
31. Kolar, S.; Barhoumi, R.; Jones, C.K.; Wesley, J.; Lupton, J.R.; Fan, Y.Y.; Chapkin, R.S. Interactive effects of fatty acid and butyrate-induced mitochondrial Ca(2)(+) loading and apoptosis in colonocytes. *Cancer* **2011**, *117*, 5294–5303. [CrossRef] [PubMed]
32. Kansal, S.; Negi, A.K.; Bhatnagar, A.; Agnihotri, N. Ras signaling pathway in the chemopreventive action of different ratios of fish oil and corn oil in experimentally induced colon carcinogenesis. *Nutr. Cancer* **2012**, *64*, 559–568. [CrossRef] [PubMed]
33. Kolar, S.S.; Barhoumi, R.; Callaway, E.S.; Fan, Y.Y.; Wang, N.; Lupton, J.R.; Chapkin, R.S. Synergy between docosahexaenoic acid and butyrate elicits p53-independent apoptosis via mitochondrial Ca(2+) accumulation in colonocytes. *Am. J. Physiol. Gastrointest. Liver Physiol.* **2007**, *293*, G935–G943. [CrossRef] [PubMed]
34. Kolar, S.S.; Barhoumi, R.; Lupton, J.R.; Chapkin, R.S. Docosahexaenoic acid and butyrate synergistically induce colonocyte apoptosis by enhancing mitochondrial Ca2+ accumulation. *Cancer Res.* **2007**, *67*, 5561–5568. [CrossRef] [PubMed]
35. Ng, Y.; Barhoumi, R.; Tjalkens, R.B.; Fan, Y.Y.; Kolar, S.; Wang, N.; Lupton, J.R.; Chapkin, R.S. The role of docosahexaenoic acid in mediating mitochondrial membrane lipid oxidation and apoptosis in colonocytes. *Carcinogenesis* **2005**, *26*, 1914–1921. [CrossRef] [PubMed]
36. Hooda, S.; Boler, B.M.; Serao, M.C.; Brulc, J.M.; Staeger, M.A.; Boileau, T.W.; Dowd, S.E.; Fahey, G.C., Jr.; Swanson, K.S. 454 pyrosequencing reveals a shift in fecal microbiota of healthy adult men consuming polydextrose or soluble corn fiber. *J. Nutr.* **2012**, *142*, 1259–1265. [CrossRef] [PubMed]
37. Ross, A.B.; Bruce, S.J.; Blondel-Lubrano, A.; Oguey-Araymon, S.; Beaumont, M.; Bourgeois, A.; Nielsen-Moennoz, C.; Vigo, M.; Fay, L.B.; Kochhar, S.; et al. A whole-grain cereal-rich diet increases plasma betaine, and tends to decrease total and ldl-cholesterol compared with a refined-grain diet in healthy subjects. *Br. J. Nutr.* **2011**, *105*, 1492–1502. [CrossRef] [PubMed]

38. Costabile, A.; Klinder, A.; Fava, F.; Napolitano, A.; Fogliano, V.; Leonard, C.; Gibson, G.R.; Tuohy, K.M. Whole-grain wheat breakfast cereal has a prebiotic effect on the human gut microbiota: A double-blind, placebo-controlled, crossover study. *Br. J. Nutr.* **2008**, *99*, 110–120. [CrossRef] [PubMed]
39. Finley, J.W.; Burrell, J.B.; Reeves, P.G. Pinto bean consumption changes scfa profiles in fecal fermentations, bacterial populations of the lower bowel, and lipid profiles in blood of humans. *J. Nutr.* **2007**, *137*, 2391–2398. [PubMed]
40. Smith, S.C.; Choy, R.; Johnson, S.K.; Hall, R.S.; Wildeboer-Veloo, A.C.; Welling, G.W. Lupin kernel fiber consumption modifies fecal microbiota in healthy men as determined by rrna gene fluorescent in situ hybridization. *Eur. J. Nutr.* **2006**, *45*, 335–341. [CrossRef] [PubMed]
41. Johnson, S.K.; Chua, V.; Hall, R.S.; Baxter, A.L. Lupin kernel fibre foods improve bowel function and beneficially modify some putative faecal risk factors for colon cancer in men. *Br. J. Nutr.* **2006**, *95*, 372–378. [CrossRef] [PubMed]
42. Tuohy, K.M.; Kolida, S.; Lustenberger, A.M.; Gibson, G.R. The prebiotic effects of biscuits containing partially hydrolysed guar gum and fructo-oligosaccharides—A human volunteer study. *Br. J. Nutr.* **2001**, *86*, 341–348. [CrossRef] [PubMed]
43. Hylla, S.; Gostner, A.; Dusel, G.; Anger, H.; Bartram, H.P.; Christl, S.U.; Kasper, H.; Scheppach, W. Effects of resistant starch on the colon in healthy volunteers: Possible implications for cancer prevention. *Am. J. Clin. Nutr.* **1998**, *67*, 136–142. [PubMed]
44. Arumugam, M.; Raes, J.; Pelletier, E.; Le Paslier, D.; Yamada, T.; Mende, D.R.; Fernandes, G.R.; Tap, J.; Bruls, T.; Batto, J.M.; et al. Enterotypes of the human gut microbiome. *Nature* **2011**, *473*, 174–180. [CrossRef] [PubMed]
45. Faust, K.; Raes, J. Microbial interactions: From networks to models. *Nat. Rev. Microbiol.* **2012**, *10*, 538–550. [CrossRef] [PubMed]
46. Faust, K.; Sathirapongsasuti, J.F.; Izard, J.; Segata, N.; Gevers, D.; Raes, J.; Huttenhower, C. Microbial co-occurrence relationships in the human microbiome. *PLoS Comput. Biol.* **2012**, *8*, e1002606. [CrossRef] [PubMed]
47. Lozupone, C.; Faust, K.; Raes, J.; Faith, J.J.; Frank, D.N.; Zaneveld, J.; Gordon, J.I.; Knight, R. Identifying genomic and metabolic features that can underline early successional and opportunistic lifestyles of human gut symbionts. *Genome Res.* **2012**, *22*, 1974–1984. [CrossRef] [PubMed]
48. Bolca, S.; van de Wiele, T.; Possemiers, S. Gut metabotypes govern health effects of dietary polyphenols. *Curr. Opin. Biotechnol.* **2013**, *24*, 220–225. [CrossRef] [PubMed]
49. Heinzmann, S.S.; Merrifield, C.A.; Rezzi, S.; Kochhar, S.; Lindon, J.C.; Holmes, E.; Nicholson, J.K. Stability and robustness of human metabolic phenotypes in response to sequential food challenges. *J. Proteome Res.* **2012**, *11*, 643–655. [CrossRef] [PubMed]
50. Wang, T.; Cai, G.; Qiu, Y.; Fei, N.; Zhang, M.; Pang, X.; Jia, W.; Cai, S.; Zhao, L. Structural segregation of gut microbiota between colorectal cancer patients and healthy volunteers. *ISME J.* **2012**, *6*, 320–329. [CrossRef] [PubMed]
51. Weir, T.L.; Manter, D.K.; Sheflin, A.M.; Barnett, B.A.; Heuberger, A.L.; Ryan, E.P. Stool microbiome and metabolome differences between colorectal cancer patients and healthy adults. *PLoS ONE* **2013**, *8*, e70803. [CrossRef] [PubMed]
52. Wu, N.; Yang, X.; Zhang, R.; Li, J.; Xiao, X.; Hu, Y.; Chen, Y.; Yang, F.; Lu, N.; Wang, Z.; et al. Dysbiosis signature of fecal microbiota in colorectal cancer patients. *Microb. Ecol.* **2013**, *66*, 462–470. [CrossRef] [PubMed]
53. Simopoulos, A.P. Importance of the omega-6/omega-3 balance in health and disease: Evolutionary aspects of diet. *World Rev. Nutr. Diet.* **2011**, *102*, 10–21. [PubMed]
54. Strobel, C.; Jahreis, G.; Kuhnt, K. Survey of *n*-3 and *n*-6 polyunsaturated fatty acids in fish and fish products. *Lipids Health Dis.* **2012**, *11*, 144. [CrossRef] [PubMed]
55. Skender, B.; Hyrslova Vaculova, A.; Hofmanova, J. Docosahexaenoic fatty acid (dha) in the regulation of colon cell growth and cell death: A review. *Biomed. Pap. Med. Fac. Univ. Palacky Olomouc Czech. Repub.* **2012**, *156*, 186–199. [CrossRef] [PubMed]
56. Azer, S.A. Overview of molecular pathways in inflammatory bowel disease associated with colorectal cancer development. *Eur. J. Gastroenterol. Hepatol.* **2012**, *25*, 271–281. [CrossRef] [PubMed]

57. Cockbain, A.J.; Toogood, G.J.; Hull, M.A. Omega-3 polyunsaturated fatty acids for the treatment and prevention of colorectal cancer. *Gut* **2012**, *61*, 135–149. [CrossRef] [PubMed]
58. Chang, W.C.; Chapkin, R.S.; Lupton, J.R. Predictive value of proliferation, differentiation and apoptosis as intermediate markers for colon tumorigenesis. *Carcinogenesis* **1997**, *18*, 721–730. [CrossRef] [PubMed]
59. Sanders, L.M.; Henderson, C.E.; Hong, M.Y.; Barhoumi, R.; Burghardt, R.C.; Wang, N.; Spinka, C.M.; Carroll, R.J.; Turner, N.D.; Chapkin, R.S.; et al. An increase in reactive oxygen species by dietary fish oil coupled with the attenuation of antioxidant defenses by dietary pectin enhances rat colonocyte apoptosis. *J. Nutr.* **2004**, *134*, 3233–3238. [PubMed]
60. Vanamala, J.; Glagolenko, A.; Yang, P.; Carroll, R.J.; Murphy, M.E.; Newman, R.A.; Ford, J.R.; Braby, L.A.; Chapkin, R.S.; Turner, N.D.; et al. Dietary fish oil and pectin enhance colonocyte apoptosis in part through suppression of ppardelta/pge2 and elevation of pge3. *Carcinogenesis* **2008**, *29*, 790–796. [CrossRef] [PubMed]
61. Crim, K.C.; Sanders, L.M.; Hong, M.Y.; Taddeo, S.S.; Turner, N.D.; Chapkin, R.S.; Lupton, J.R. Upregulation of p21waf1/cip1 expression in vivo by butyrate administration can be chemoprotective or chemopromotive depending on the lipid component of the diet. *Carcinogenesis* **2008**, *29*, 1415–1420. [CrossRef] [PubMed]
62. Cho, Y.; Kim, H.; Turner, N.D.; Mann, J.C.; Wei, J.; Taddeo, S.S.; Davidson, L.A.; Wang, N.; Vannucci, M.; Carroll, R.J.; et al. A chemoprotective fish oil- and pectin-containing diet temporally alters gene expression profiles in exfoliated rat colonocytes throughout oncogenesis. *J. Nutr.* **2011**, *141*, 1029–1035. [CrossRef] [PubMed]
63. The Women's Health Initiative Study Group. Design of the women's health initiative clinical trial and observational study. *Control. Clin. Trials* **1998**, *19*, 61–109.
64. Anderson, G.L.; Manson, J.; Wallace, R.; Lund, B.; Hall, D.; Davis, S.; Shumaker, S.; Wang, C.Y.; Stein, E.; Prentice, R.L. Implementation of the women's health initiative study design. *Ann. Epidemiol.* **2003**, *13*, S5–S17. [CrossRef]
65. Langer, R.D.; White, E.; Lewis, C.E.; Kotchen, J.M.; Hendrix, S.L.; Trevisan, M. The women's health initiative observational study: Baseline characteristics of participants and reliability of baseline measures. *Ann. Epidemiol.* **2003**, *13*, S107–S121. [CrossRef]
66. Hays, J.; Hunt, J.R.; Hubbell, F.A.; Anderson, G.L.; Limacher, M.; Allen, C.; Rossouw, J.E. The women's health initiative recruitment methods and results. *Ann. Epidemiol.* **2003**, *13*, S18–S77. [CrossRef]
67. Patterson, R.E.; Kristal, A.R.; Tinker, L.F.; Carter, R.A.; Bolton, M.P.; Agurs-Collins, T. Measurement characteristics of the women's health initiative food frequency questionnaire. *Ann. Epidemiol.* **1999**, *9*, 178–187. [CrossRef]
68. Curb, J.D.; McTiernan, A.; Heckbert, S.R.; Kooperberg, C.; Stanford, J.; Nevitt, M.; Johnson, K.C.; Proulx-Burns, L.; Pastore, L.; Criqui, M.; et al. Outcomes ascertainment and adjudication methods in the women's health initiative. *Ann. Epidemiol.* **2003**, *13*, S122–S128. [CrossRef]
69. Haggar, F.A.; Boushey, R.P. Colorectal cancer epidemiology: Incidence, mortality, survival, and risk factors. *Clin. Colon Rectal Surg.* **2009**, *22*, 191–197. [CrossRef] [PubMed]
70. Edwards, B.K.; Ward, E.; Kohler, B.A.; Eheman, C.; Zauber, A.G.; Anderson, R.N.; Jemal, A.; Schymura, M.J.; Lansdorp-Vogelaar, I.; Seeff, L.C.; et al. Annual report to the nation on the status of cancer, 1975–2006, featuring colorectal cancer trends and impact of interventions (risk factors, screening, and treatment) to reduce future rates. *Cancer* **2010**, *116*, 544–573. [CrossRef] [PubMed]
71. National Academy of Sciences-Institute of Medicine. Food and Nutrition Board. *Dietary Reference Intakes for Energy, Carbohydrate, Fiber, Fat, Fatty Acids, Cholesterol, Protein, and Amino Acids*; National Academy Press: Washington, DC, USA, 2005.
72. American Institute For Cancer Research. Available online: http://www.Aicr.Org/continuous-update-project/colorectal-cancer.Html (accessed on 4 November 2016).
73. Bingham, S.A. Diet and large bowel cancer. *J. R. Soc. Med.* **1990**, *83*, 420–422. [PubMed]
74. Young, G.P.; Hu, Y.; Le Leu, R.K.; Nyskohus, L. Dietary fibre and colorectal cancer: A model for environment–gene interactions. *Mol. Nutr. Food Res.* **2005**, *49*, 571–584. [CrossRef] [PubMed]
75. Slavin, J.L. Dietary fiber and body weight. *Nutrition* **2005**, *21*, 411–418. [CrossRef] [PubMed]
76. Donohoe, D.R.; Collins, L.B.; Wali, A.; Bigler, R.; Sun, W.; Bultman, S.J. The warburg effect dictates the mechanism of butyrate-mediated histone acetylation and cell proliferation. *Mol. Cell* **2012**, *48*, 612–626. [CrossRef] [PubMed]

77. Bultman, S.J. Molecular pathways: Gene-environment interactions regulating dietary fiber induction of proliferation and apoptosis via butyrate for cancer prevention. *Clin. Cancer Res.* **2014**, *20*, 799–803. [CrossRef] [PubMed]
78. Triff, K.; Kim, E.; Chapkin, R.S. Chemoprotective epigenetic mechanisms in a colorectal cancer model: Modulation by *n*-3 pufa in combination with fermentable fiber. *Curr. Pharmacol. Rep.* **2015**, *1*, 11–20. [CrossRef] [PubMed]
79. Chapkin, R.S.; Seo, J.; McMurray, D.N.; Lupton, J.R. Mechanisms by which docosahexaenoic acid and related fatty acids reduce colon cancer risk and inflammatory disorders of the intestine. *Chem. Phys. Lipids* **2008**, *153*, 14–23. [CrossRef] [PubMed]
80. Levi, F.; Pasche, C.; Lucchini, F.; la Vecchia, C. Dietary fibre and the risk of colorectal cancer. *Eur. J. Cancer* **2001**, *37*, 2091–2096. [CrossRef]
81. Freudenheim, J.L.; Graham, S.; Horvath, P.J.; Marshall, J.R.; Haughey, B.P.; Wilkinson, G. Risks associated with source of fiber and fiber components in cancer of the colon and rectum. *Cancer Res.* **1990**, *50*, 3295–3300. [PubMed]
82. Le Marchand, L.; Hankin, J.H.; Wilkens, L.R.; Kolonel, L.N.; Englyst, H.N.; Lyu, L.C. Dietary fiber and colorectal cancer risk. *Epidemiology* **1997**, *8*, 658–665. [CrossRef] [PubMed]
83. Negri, E.; Franceschi, S.; Parpinel, M.; La Vecchia, C. Fiber intake and risk of colorectal cancer. *Cancer Epidemiol. Biomark. Prev.* **1998**, *7*, 667–671.
84. Turk, H.F.; Monk, J.M.; Fan, Y.Y.; Callaway, E.S.; Weeks, B.; Chapkin, R.S. Inhibitory effects of omega-3 fatty acids on injury-induced epidermal growth factor receptor transactivation contribute to delayed wound healing. *Am. J. Physiol. Cell Physiol.* **2013**, *304*, C905–C917. [CrossRef] [PubMed]
85. Larsson, S.C.; Kumlin, M.; Ingelman-Sundberg, M.; Wolk, A. Dietary long-chain *n*-3 fatty acids for the prevention of cancer: A review of potential mechanisms. *Am. J. Clin. Nutr.* **2004**, *79*, 935–945. [PubMed]
86. Wu, S.; Feng, B.; Li, K.; Zhu, X.; Liang, S.; Liu, X.; Han, S.; Wang, B.; Wu, K.; Miao, D.; et al. Fish consumption and colorectal cancer risk in humans: A systematic review and meta-analysis. *Am. J. Med.* **2012**, *125*, 551–559. [CrossRef] [PubMed]
87. Geelen, A.; Schouten, J.M.; Kamphuis, C.; Stam, B.E.; Burema, J.; Renkema, J.M.; Bakker, E.J.; van't Veer, P.; Kampman, E. Fish consumption, *n*-3 fatty acids, and colorectal cancer: A meta-analysis of prospective cohort studies. *Am. J. Epidemiol.* **2007**, *166*, 1116–1125. [CrossRef] [PubMed]
88. Song, M.; Zhang, X.; Meyerhardt, J.A.; Giovannucci, E.L.; Ogino, S.; Fuchs, C.S.; Chan, A.T. Marine omega-3 polyunsaturated fatty acid intake and survival after colorectal cancer diagnosis. *Gut* **2016**. [CrossRef] [PubMed]
89. Vannice, G.; Rasmussen, H. Position of the academy of nutrition and dietetics: Dietary fatty acids for healthy adults. *J. Acad. Nutr. Diet.* **2014**, *114*, 136–153. [CrossRef] [PubMed]
90. Jiang, Y.H.; Lupton, J.R.; Chapkin, R.S. Dietary fat and fiber modulate the effect of carcinogen on colonic protein kinase c lambda expression in rats. *J. Nutr.* **1997**, *127*, 1938–1943. [PubMed]
91. Fan, Y.Y.; Ran, Q.; Toyokuni, S.; Okazaki, Y.; Callaway, E.S.; Lupton, J.R.; Chapkin, R.S. Dietary fish oil promotes colonic apoptosis and mitochondrial proton leak in oxidatively stressed mice. *Cancer Prev. Res.* **2011**, *4*, 1267–1274. [CrossRef] [PubMed]
92. Orlich, M.J.; Singh, P.N.; Sabate, J.; Fan, J.; Sveen, L.; Bennett, H.; Knutsen, S.F.; Beeson, W.L.; Jaceldo-Siegl, K.; Butler, T.L.; et al. Vegetarian dietary patterns and the risk of colorectal cancers. *JAMA Intern. Med.* **2015**, *175*, 767–776. [CrossRef] [PubMed]
93. O'Keefe, S.J.; Li, J.V.; Lahti, L.; Ou, J.; Carbonero, F.; Mohammed, K.; Posma, J.M.; Kinross, J.; Wahl, E.; Ruder, E.; et al. Fat, fibre and cancer risk in African americans and rural Africans. *Nat. Commun.* **2015**, *6*, 6342. [CrossRef] [PubMed]
94. Kato, I.; Majumdar, A.P.; Land, S.J.; Barnholtz-Sloan, J.S.; Severson, R.K. Dietary fatty acids, luminal modifiers, and risk of colorectal cancer. *Int. J. Cancer* **2010**, *127*, 942–951. [CrossRef] [PubMed]
95. US Department of Agriculture, Agriculture Research Services. Nutrient Intakes from Food: Mean Amounts Consumed per Individual, by Gender and Age. Available online: http://www.ars.usda.gov/ba/bhnrc/fsrg (accessed on 4 November 2016).
96. Kristal, A.R.; Shattuck, A.L.; Williams, A.E. Food Frequency Questionnaires for Diet Intervention Research. In Proceedings of the 17th National Nutrient Databank Conference, Baltimore, MD, USA, 7–10 June 1992.

97. Satia-Abouta, J.; Kristal, A.R.; Patterson, R.E.; Littman, A.J.; Stratton, K.L.; White, E. Dietary supplement use and medical conditions: The vital study. *Am. J. Prev. Med.* **2003**, *24*, 43–51. [CrossRef]
98. Fasano, E.; Serini, S.; Cittadini, A.; Calviello, G. Long-chain *n*-3 pufa against breast and prostate cancer: Which are the appropriate doses for intervention studies in animals and humans? *Crit. Rev. Food Sci. Nutr.* **2015**. [CrossRef] [PubMed]
99. Vece, M.M.; Agnoli, C.; Grioni, S.; Sieri, S.; Pala, V.; Pellegrini, N.; Frasca, G.; Tumino, R.; Mattiello, A.; Panico, S.; et al. Dietary total antioxidant capacity and colorectal cancer in the italian epic cohort. *PLoS ONE* **2015**, *10*, e0142995. [CrossRef] [PubMed]
100. La Vecchia, C.; Decarli, A.; Serafini, M.; Parpinel, M.; Bellocco, R.; Galeone, C.; Bosetti, C.; Zucchetto, A.; Polesel, J.; Lagiou, P.; et al. Dietary total antioxidant capacity and colorectal cancer: A large case-control study in italy. *Int. J. Cancer* **2013**, *133*, 1447–1451. [CrossRef] [PubMed]
101. Bjelakovic, G.; Nikolova, D.; Simonetti, R.G.; Gluud, C. Antioxidant supplements for prevention of gastrointestinal cancers: A systematic review and meta-analysis. *Lancet* **2004**, *364*, 1219–1228. [CrossRef]

nutrients

MDPI

Article

Butyrate Inhibits Cancerous HCT116 Colon Cell Proliferation but to a Lesser Extent in Noncancerous NCM460 Colon Cells

Huawei Zeng [1,*], David P. Taussig [1], Wen-Hsing Cheng [2], LuAnn K. Johnson [1] and Reza Hakkak [3,4]

1 United States Department of Agriculture, Agricultural Research Service, Grand Forks Human Nutrition Research Center, Grand Forks, ND 58203, USA; dtaussig@gmail.com (D.P.T.); luann.johnson@ars.usda.gov (L.K.J.)
2 Department of Food Science, Nutrition and Health Promotion, Mississippi State University, Starkville, MS 39762, USA; wcheng@fsnhp.msstate.edu
3 Departments of Dietetics and Nutrition, University of Arkansas for Medical Sciences, Little Rock, AR 72205, USA; RHakkak@uams.edu
4 Arkansas Children Research Institute, Little Rock, AR 72202, USA
* Correspondence: huawei.zeng@ars.usda.gov; Tel.: +1-701-795-8465

Received: 20 October 2016; Accepted: 23 December 2016; Published: 1 January 2017

Abstract: Butyrate, an intestinal microbiota metabolite of dietary fiber, exhibits chemoprevention effects on colon cancer development. However, the mechanistic action of butyrate remains to be determined. We hypothesize that butyrate inhibits cancerous cell proliferation but to a lesser extent in noncancerous cells through regulating apoptosis and cellular-signaling pathways. We tested this hypothesis by exposing cancerous HCT116 or non-cancerous NCM460 colon cells to physiologically relevant doses of butyrate. Cellular responses to butyrate were characterized by Western analysis, fluorescent microscopy, acetylation, and DNA fragmentation analyses. Butyrate inhibited cell proliferation, and led to an induction of apoptosis, genomic DNA fragmentation in HCT116 cells, but to a lesser extent in NCM460 cells. Although butyrate increased H3 histone deacetylation and p21 tumor suppressor expression in both cell types, p21 protein level was greater with intense expression around the nuclei in HCT116 cells when compared with that in NCM460 cells. Furthermore, butyrate treatment increased the phosphorylation of extracellular-regulated kinase 1/2 (p-ERK1/2), a survival signal, in NCM460 cells while it decreased p-ERK1/2 in HCT116 cells. Taken together, the activation of survival signaling in NCM460 cells and apoptotic potential in HCT116 cells may confer the increased sensitivity of cancerous colon cells to butyrate in comparison with noncancerous colon cells.

Keywords: apoptosis; butyrate; colon cancer; cell proliferation; microbiota

1. Introduction

Colon cancer is the third most frequently occurring cancer in men and women in the United States. In 2016 about 134,490 people are predicted to be diagnosed with colorectal cancer in the US, and it is likely that half the Western population will develop at least one colorectal tumor by the age of 70 years [1,2]. It has been reported that high intake of dietary fiber and resistant starches reduces the risk of colon cancer in human populations and animal models [3,4]. This effect may be related to butyrate, a short chain fatty acid (SCFA), which is produced in the colonic lumen by the bacterial fermentation of dietary fiber [3–6]. Colonic luminal SCFA concentration can reach 10 mmol/L when humans consume diets containing moderate levels of fiber [7,8]. Conceivably, there is continuous butyrate exposure in the colonic epithelium, and butyrate may exert several anticarcinogenic effects through the modulation of colon cell proliferation and apoptosis [9–12].

A successful chemoprevention agent should have a minimal effect on normal cells but a strong inhibitory effect on cell proliferation and carcinogenic pathways in cancer cells. While much has been studied on the effect of butyrate on colon cancer cells, little is known about its effect on noncancerous cells, which is essential for understanding butyrate's anticancer properties. Several studies have shown that histone deacetylase (HDAC) activity represses transcriptional activity by condensing the chromatin package leading to an epigenetically mediated silencing of tumor suppressor genes like p21 [13,14]. Butyrate is an HDAC inhibitor (HDACi) and a potential anti-tumor agent. HDACi strongly activates the expression of the cyclin-dependent kinase inhibitor p21, a tumor suppressor [13,15]. In addition, previous data have shown that the extracellular-regulated kinase 1/2 (ERK1/2) and myelocytomatosis (c-Myc) signaling pathways are both required to drive cell cycle progression during cell proliferation [16–18]; c-Myc may also modulate p21 expression [19,20]. To study the effects of butyrate on these signaling pathways related to colon cancer proliferation, two human colon cell lines were employed in this study. The NCM460 colon cell line is an epithelial cell line which is noncancerous and derived from normal colon mucosa [21]. This cell line has not been infected or transfected with any genetic information, and is widely used because there are few other noncancerous colon cell lines [21]. Although there are several cancerous colon cell lines (e.g., HCT116, HT29, and Caco-2) available, most of these cell lines are derived from adenocarcinoma, and only the HCT116 cell line is derived from carcinoma [22,23]. It is known that adenocarcinoma develops in glands whereas carcinoma originates in the epithelial tissue, and there are differences between colorectal carcinoma and advanced adenomas [24]. Given the fact that NCM460 and HCT116 cells were both originally derived from (male adult) colon epithelial tissues and are the same cell subtypes, we believe that NCM460 and HCT116 cells are the best cell-line pair to use in our present study.

In view of the critical role of butyrate in colon cancer prevention [3–6], we hypothesize that butyrate inhibits cancerous cell proliferation but to a lesser extent in noncancerous colon cells through signaling pathways regulating apoptosis and cellular survival [21,22]. Colon crypt cells divide rapidly and travel to the top of the epithelium where they differentiate, proliferate, and undergo cell cycle progression and apoptosis within 48 h. Thus, we focused on the effects of butyrate on colon cell growth and apoptosis for up to 48 h in the present study whereas signaling molecules were examined at early time points (e.g., 1.5 h) to limit the bystander effect.

2. Materials and Methods

2.1. Cell Cultures

HCT116 colorectal carcinoma cells were obtained from American Type Culture Collection and maintained in Dulbecco's Modified Eagle Medium (DMEM) (Invitrogen, Carlsbad, CA, USA) with 10% fetal bovine serum (FBS; Sigma Chemical Co., St. Louis, MO, USA). The nontransformed, noncancerous colon NCM460 cells derived from human normal colon mucosa [21,25] were maintained in M3 Base medium (INCELL Corp., San Antonio, TX, USA) with 10% FBS. Sodium butyrate (purity > 98.5%) was purchased from Sigma Chemical Corporation (St. Louis, MO, USA). Stock cells were passaged twice weekly at ~<80% confluency in Ca-Mg-free Hanks' balanced salt solution (Sigma Chemical Co., St. Louis, MO, USA) containing 0.25% trypsin (Invitrogen) and 1 mmol/L ethylenediamine tetra-acetic acid (EDTA). Cell viability was determined by trypan blue exclusion based on hemocytometer counts and cells were incubated in a humidified chamber at 36.5 °C with 5% CO_2. Cultures were tested and found to be mycoplasma free [26]. HCT116 cells at passages 22–40 and NCM460 cells at passages 34–50 were used. Importantly, both HCT116 and NCM460 cell lines were grown in DMEM medium with 10% FBS in all subsequent assays.

2.2. Cell Count/Growth Assay

HCT116 and NCM460 cell lines were both cultured in DMEM medium with 10% FBS, harvested with 0.25% trypsin (Invitrogen) and 1 mmol/L EDTA, and resuspended in 1 mL medium. Cells were then diluted 1:2 (or 1:4) in 0.2% trypan blue and counted in duplicate using a hemocytometer. At least 200 cells per sample were counted.

2.3. Apoptosis Analysis

Apoptosis was analyzed using a Guava Nexin™ Kit (Guava Technologies, Inc. Hayward, CA, USA). HCT116 and NCM460 cell lines were tryspinized, and then suspended in growth media (DMEM with 10% FBS). Annexin V is a calcium-dependent phospholipid binding protein with high affinity to phosphatidylserine (PS), which has translocated from the internal to external side of the cell membrane upon induction of apoptosis. The cell impermeant dye 7-amino-actinomycin D (7-AAD) is included in the assay kit as an indicator of membrane structural integrity [27]. Therefore, [Annexin V (+), 7-AAD (−)] cells are in the early stages of apoptosis, and [Annexin V (+) and 7-AAD (+)] cells are in the late stages of apoptosis. At least 2000 single cell events per sample were analyzed by the Guava PCA System (Hayward, CA, USA).

2.4. DNA Fragmentation Assay

Each DNA sample was extracted from about 1,000,000 cells by overnight incubation at 50–55 °C in a lysis buffer (50 mmol/L Tris-HCl, pH 8.0, 10 mmol/L EDTA, 150 mmol/L NaCl, 100 μg/mL proteinase K). These DNA samples were recovered by isopropanol precipitation, resuspended in Tris-EDTA-RNase (6 units/mL), analyzed using 1.9% agarose gels, and visualized by ethidium bromide staining. The intensity signals of genomic DNA fragmentation were analyzed by the UVP Bioimaging Systems (Upland, CA, USA).

2.5. Western Blotting Analysis

After butyrate treatment for 1.5 or 15 h, adherent cells were scraped, pooled with the detached cells in 5 mL media, and then these cells were collected by centrifugation at 350× *g* for 10 min at 4 °C. At least four independent experimental cell sample sets were collected. The cell pellet (about 1,000,000 cells) was washed once in ice-cold PBS and lysed in a cell lysis buffer (20 mmol/L Tris-HCT, pH 7.5, 150 mmol/L NaCl, 1 mmol/L Na2EDTA, 1 mmol/L EGTA, 1% Triton, 2.5 mmol/L sodium pyrophosphate, 1 mmol/L Na_3VO_4, 1 μg/mL leupeptin, 1 mmol/L phenylmethylsulfonyl fluoride) (Cell Signaling Technology, Inc., Danvers, MA, USA). After 15 s sonication, the cell lysate was centrifuged at 14,000× *g* for 30 min at 4 °C. The supernatant was designated as whole cell protein extract and kept at −80 °C. The protein concentration was quantified by the Bradford dye-binding assay (Bio-Rad laboratories, Richmond, CA, USA). Protein extracts with equal amount (~40 μg) were resolved over 4%–20% Tris-glycine gradient gels under denaturing and reducing conditions and electroblotted onto polyvinylidene difluoride (PVDF) membranes (Invitrogen, Carlsbad, CA, USA). Membrane blots were blocked in phosphate-buffered saline (PBS)—0.05% Tween (*v*/*v*) supplemented with 1% (*wt*/*v*) nonfat dry milk (BioRad, Hercules, CA, USA) overnight at 4 °C. Membranes were probed with antibodies against c-Myc (Epitomics, Inc., Burlingame, CA, USA), phosphorylated ERK1/2 (p-ERK1/2), ERK1/2, acetyl-Histone H3 (Lys9), and p21 antibodies (Cell Signaling Technology, Inc., Danvers, MA, USA), and then incubated with an anti-mouse/rabbit (1:3000 dilution) horseradish peroxidase (HRP)-conjugated secondary antibody (Cell Signaling Technology, Inc., Danvers, MA, USA) in blocking solution for 1 h at room temperature. Blots were washed as above and proteins were incubated with an ECL plus kit (Amersham Pharmacia Biotech, Piscataway, NJ, USA) and imaged by the Molecular Dynamics Image-Quant system (Sunnyvale, CA, USA).

2.6. Immunfluorescent Staining

HCT116 and NCM460 colon cells were seeded on microscope slides (about 200,000 cells per cell culture chamber slide) in DMEM media supplemented with 10% FBS under an atmosphere of 5% CO_2 at 37 °C overnight. For the observation of p21 and its nuclear localization, the cells were pretreated with butyrate for 15 h. After the treatment, cells were fixed using 4% paraformaldehyde for 15 min, they were permeabilized with ice-cold 100% methanol for 10 min at −20 °C with PBS rinse for 5 min. Cells were then blocked with 10% goat serum (Sigma Chemical Corporation, St. Louis, MO, USA) for 1 h, and then incubated with an anti-p21 antibody (Cell Signaling Technology, Inc., Danvers, MA, USA) overnight at 4 °C. Cells, after washing with PBS, were incubated with anti-rabbit Immunoglobulin G (IgG, H and L), F(ab')$_2$ Fragment (Alexa Fluor® 488 Conjugate) (green fluorescence) (Cell Signaling Technology, Inc., Danvers, MA, USA) for 1 h at room temperature with propidium iodide (PI) (25 μg/mL). Finally, fluoroshield with PI (Sigma Chemical Corporation, St. Louis, MO, USA), an aqueous mounting medium, was used for preserving fluorescence and producing a red fluorescence as counter stain for overall cell morphology. The fluorescence images and intensity quantification of at least more 2000 cells (per sample) were analyzed by Nikon E400 microscope and Image Pro Plus version 9.1 (North Central Instruments, Plymouth, MN, USA).

2.7. Statistical Analysis

Results are given as means ± SDs. The concentration of butyrate needed to inhibit cell growth by 50% (IC_{50}) was estimated by fitting a three-parameter logistic model to percent inhibition using concentration as the independent variable. The resulting model was used to predict the concentration at which 50% inhibition was expected to occur. Proc NLIN in SAS was used to fit the model. The HCT116 and NCM460 data for 24 h and 48 h were analyzed by two-way analysis of variance with cell type (HCT116 or NCM460), treatment concentration, and their interaction as fixed effects and experiment as a blocking factor. Data were log-transformed prior to analysis in order to test whether changes were proportional across treatment concentrations. Dunnett's multiple comparison procedure was used to compare individual HCT116 or NCM460 group means with their respective control group (untreated cells). The Proc Mixed procedure in SAS v. 9.4 (SAS Institute, Inc., Cary, NC, USA) was used for all analyses. Differences with a p value < 0.05 were considered statistically significant.

3. Results

3.1. Differential Effects of Butyrate (NaB) on Cell Growth

The cell growth rate was inhibited in a dose-dependent manner with a maximum of 58% at 24 h, and 84% at 48 h, respectively, in HCT116 cells treated with 0.5, 1, 1.5, or 2 mmol/L NaB when compared with that of untreated cells (Figure 1). In contrast, the cell growth rate was inhibited to a lesser extent in a dose-dependent manner with a maximum of 38% at 24 h, and 47% at 48 h, respectively, in NCM460 cells treated with 0.5, 1, 1.5, or 2 mmol/L NaB when compared with that of untreated cells (Figure 1). At 48 h, the IC50 of butyrate to inhibit HCT116 cell growth was 0.91 mmol/L, and the 95% confidence interval around this estimate was (0.81, 1.02). In contrast, the IC50 of butyrate to inhibit NCM460 cell growth was greater than 2 mmol/L; we could not precisely determine the value because 2 mmol/L was the highest concentration of NaB used in this study (Figure 1B).

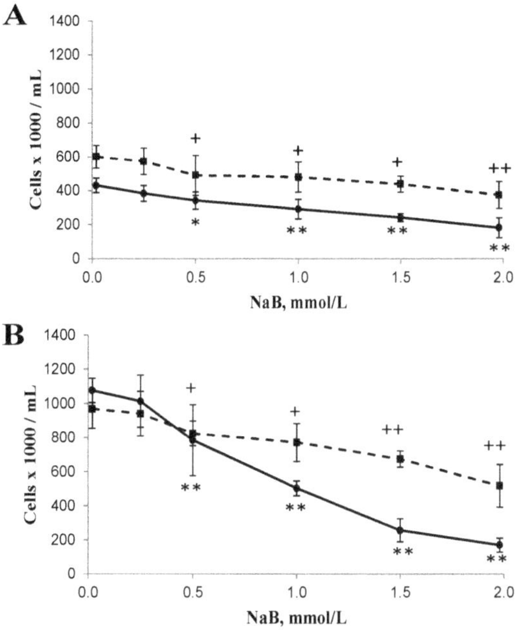

Figure 1. Effect of sodium butyrate (NaB) treatment for (**A**) 24 h and (**B**) 48 h on the growth of cancerous HCT116 (solid lines) and non-cancerous NCM460 (dashed lines) colon cells. Values are means ± SD, $n = 5$ to 6. There was a significant interaction between cell type and concentration at 24 h ($p = 0.01$) and at 48 h ($p < 0.0001$) by two-way ANOVA. * Different from HCT116 control (0 mmol/L NaB); * $p < 0.05$, ** $p < 0.0001$. + Different from NCM460 control (0 mmol/L NaB); $^{+}$ $p < 0.05$, $^{++}$ $p < 0.0001$.

3.2. *Differential Effects of Butyrate (NaB) on Apoptosis*

Apoptotic cells (including both early and late apoptosis) were increased in a dose-dependent manner with a maximum 1.7 fold increase at 24 h, and 5.4 fold increase at 48 h, respectively, in HCT116 cells treated with 1, 1.5, or 2 mmol/L NaB when compared with that of untreated cells (Figure 2). In contrast, apoptotic cells were increased in a dose-dependent manner with a maximum 0.2 fold increase at 24 h, and 0.4 fold increase at 48 h, respectively, in NCM460 cells treated with 1, 1.5, or 2 mmol/L NaB when compared with that of untreated cells (Figure 2). Furthermore, the early and late apoptotic cells were also increased in a dose-dependent manner, respectively. The percentage of early apoptotic cells was greater ($p < 0.05$) in HCT116 cells treated with 1, 1.5, or 2 mmol/L NaB when compared with that of untreated cells (9.05 ± 5.07, 16.05 ± 5.76, 21.63 ± 6.84 vs. 2.36 ± 0.75, respectively) at 48 h. The percentage of early apoptotic cells was greater ($p < 0.05$) in NCM460 cells treated with 0.5, 1, 1.5, or 2 mmol/L NaB when compared to untreated cells (5.23 ± 1.45, 6.21 ± 1.86, 6.37 ± 2.04, 6.59 ± 1.83 vs. 3.91 ± 1.27) at 48 h. Similarly, the percentage of late apoptotic cells was greater ($p < 0.05$) in HCT116 cells treated with 1, 1.5, or 2 mmol/L NaB when compared with that of untreated cells (8.89 ± 2.76, 13.48 ± 2.78, 17.09 ± 3.09 vs. 3.70 ± 1.36, respectively) at 48 h. In contrast, in NCM460 cells, the percentage of late apoptotic cells was greater ($p < 0.05$) only in cells treated with the highest concentration of NaB (2 mmol/L) when compared to untreated cells (7.93 ± 1.02 vs. 6.49 ± 1.20) at 48 h.

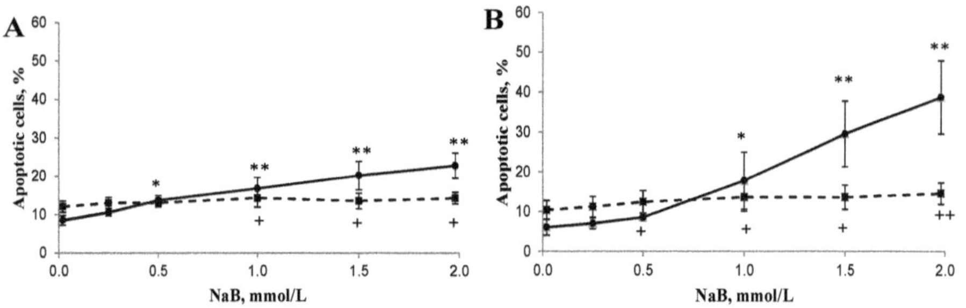

Figure 2. Effect of sodium butyrate (NaB) treatment for (**A**) 24 h and (**B**) 48 h on the apoptosis (including both early and late apoptosis) of cancerous HCT116 (solid lines) and non-cancerous NCM460 (dashed lines) colon cells. Values are means ± SD, n = 5 to 6. There was a significant interaction between cell type and concentration at 24 h ($p < 0.0001$) and at 48 h ($p < 0.0001$) by two-way ANOVA. * Different from HCT116 control (0 mmol/L NaB); * $p < 0.05$, ** $p < 0.0001$. + Different from NCM460 control (0 mmol/L NaB); $^{+}$ $p < 0.05$, $^{++}$ $p < 0.0001$.

3.3. *Differential Effects of Butyrate (NaB) on DNA Fragmentation*

The intensity of genomic DNA fragmentation was increased by 1.3 and 2.1 fold in HCT116 cells treated with 1.5 or 2 mmol/L NaB, respectively, for 15 h (Figure 3B) but not 1.5 h (Figure 3A) when compared with that of untreated cells (Figure 3). There was no NaB-induced genomic DNA fragmentation at 1.5 or 15 h in NCM460 cells.

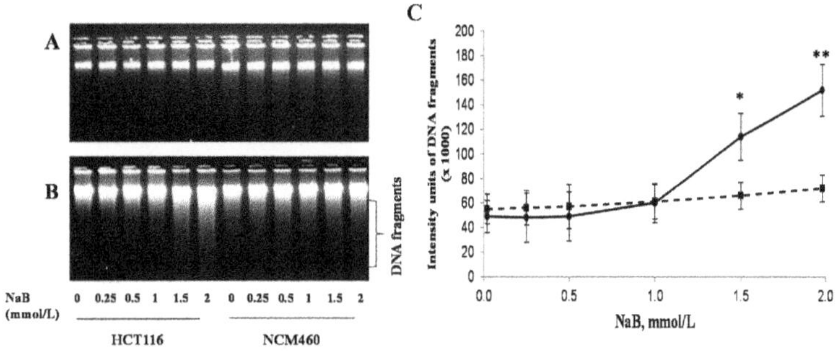

Figure 3. Effect of sodium butyrate (NaB) on the genomic DNA fragmentation of cancerous HCT116 and non-cancerous NCM460 colon cells. A representative DNA image showing DNA fragmentation at (**A**) 1.5 h; (**B**) 15 h; (**C**) the intensity signals of genomic DNA fragmentation (at 15 h) of cancerous HCT116 (solid lines) and non-cancerous NCM460 (dashed lines) colon cells were analyzed by the UVP Bioimaging Systems (there was no DNA fragmentation at 1.5 h). Values are means ± SD, n = 4. There was a significant interaction between cell type and concentration ($p < 0.0001$) by two-way ANOVA. * Different from HCT116 control (0 mmol/L NaB); * $p < 0.05$, ** $p < 0.0001$.

3.4. *Differential Effects of Butyrate (NaB) on Signaling Molecules*

While the p-ERK1/2 level was decreased dose-dependently at 15 h after treatment with NaB in HCT116 cells, the opposite trend was observed in NCM460 cells (Figure 4). Except for the p21 level at 1.5 h in HCT116 cells, there were NaB dose-dependent increases in levels of p21 and acetyl-H3 at Lys 9 at 1.5 and 15 h in both HCT116 and NCM460 cells (Figure 4). Except for the level of acetyl-H3 at Lys 9 in HCT116 cells, the extent of p21 and acetyl-H3 at Lys 9 induction was greater at 15 h than 1.5 h in both types of cells. In contrast, there were NaB dose-dependent decreases in c-Myc protein level at 1.5 and 15 h in HCT116 cells and 15 h in NCM460 cells (Figure 4). The β-actin and total ERK1/2 protein levels did not differ at 1.5 and 15 h in HCT116 and NCM460 cells because of NaB treatment (Figure 4).

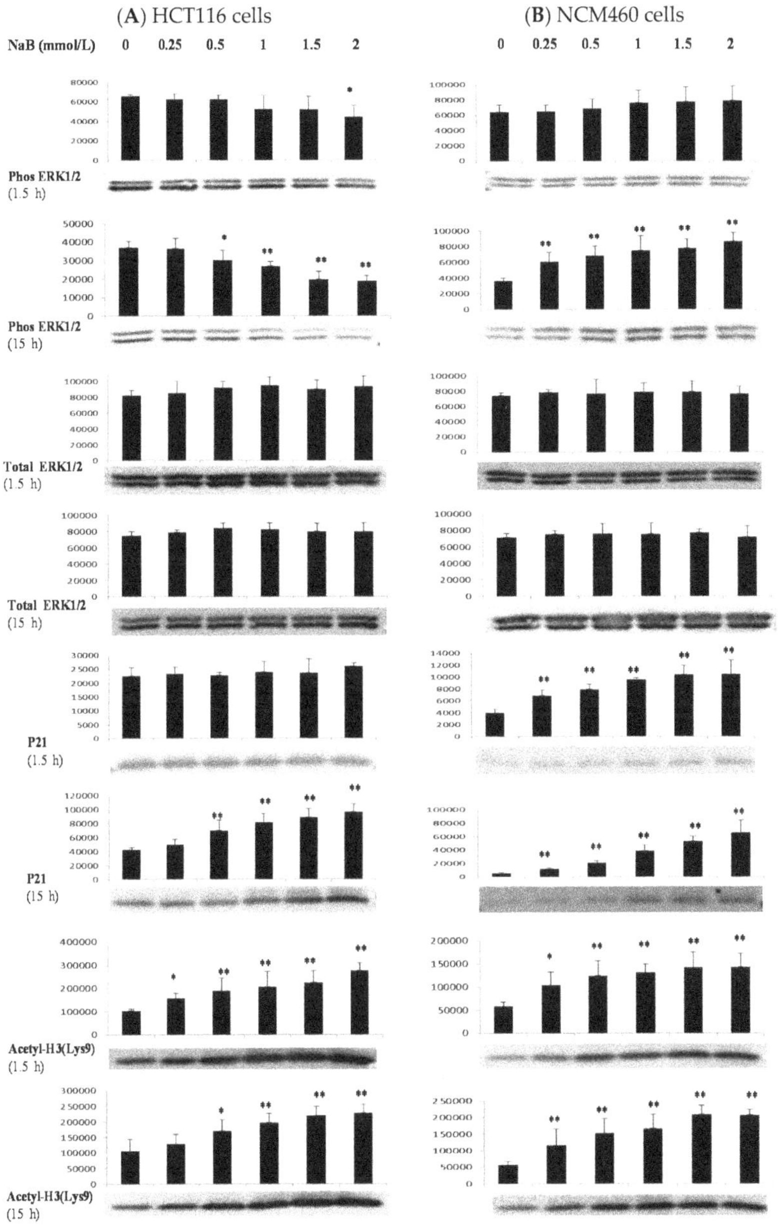

Figure 4. *Cont.*

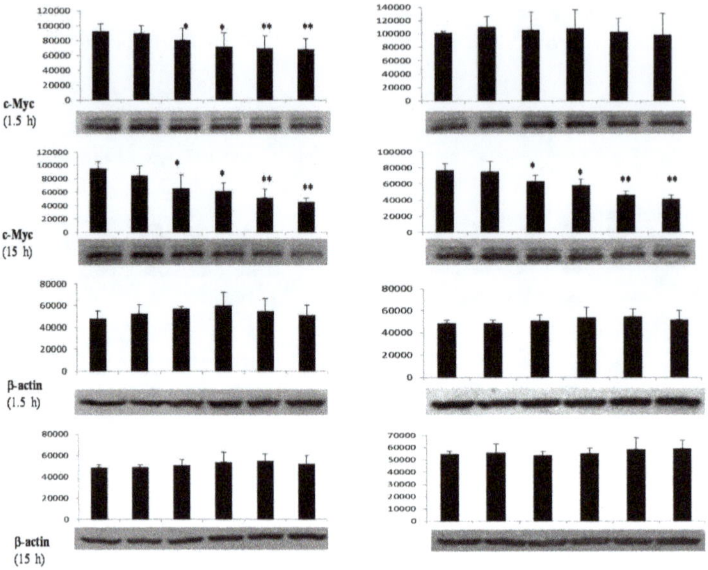

Figure 4. Effect of butyrate on the cell-proliferation proteins. Western blot analyses of the effects of sodium butyrate (NaB) treatment for 1.5 h or 15h on intracellular signaling proteins (densitometric units) in (**A**) HCT116 colon cells and (**B**) NCM460 colon cells. Values are means ± SD, n = 4, * Different from control (0 mmol/L NaB); * $p < 0.05$, ** $p < 0.0001$. A representative Western blotting image was from four independent experiments for a given antibody assay.

3.5. *Differential Effects of Butyrate (NaB) on p21 Protein Level and Cellular Localization*

The ratio percentage (composite image) of p21 protein level (green signals) vs. overall cell background (red signals) at 15 h was 69%, 81%, and 93%, respectively, in HCT116 cells treated with 1, 1.5, or 2 mmol/L NaB when compared with that of untreated cells. To a lesser extent, the ratio percentage (composite image) of p21 protein level (green signals) vs. overall cell background (red signals) at 15 h was 42%, 56%, and 62%, respectively, in NCM460 cells treated with 1, 1.5, or 2 mmol/L NaB when compared with that of untreated cells (Figure 5A,B). In addition, the overall p21 protein level (green signals) was greater with intense expression around the nuclei in HCT116 cells when compared with that in NCM460 cells (Figure 5C,D).

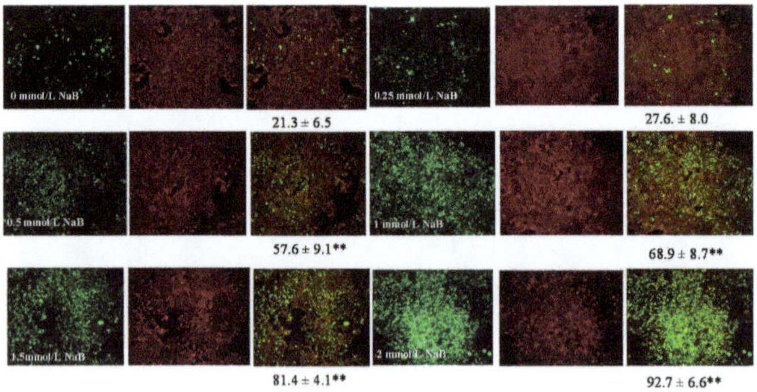

(**A**)

Figure 5. *Cont.*

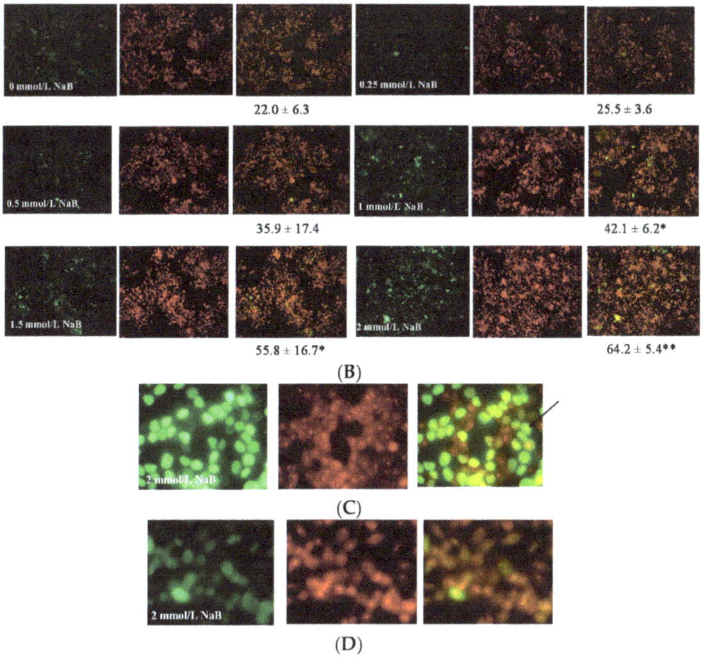

Figure 5. Effect of sodium butyrate (NaB) treatment for 15 h on p21 protein level and distribution at cellular level in HCT116 and NCM460 colon cells. Each sample consists three images: image 1, cells were labeled with anti-p21 antibody, and followed by anti-Rabbit IgG (H and L), $F(ab')_2$ Fragment (Alexa Fluor® 488 Conjugate) (green signals); image 2, cells were mounted by fluoroshield with PI as counter staining for overall cell morphology-background (red signals); image 3, the p21 protein image was superimposed on the respective overall cell morphology-background image to generate the composite image (orange signals). (**A**) HCT cells at 200× magnification; (**B**) NCM460 cells at 200× magnification; (**C**) HCT116 cells with intense p21 expression around the nucleus (arrow) at 1000× magnification; (**D**) NCM460 cells at 1000× magnification. For panel (**A**,**B**) composite images, the area of p21 protein level (green signals) in percentage when compared with that of overall cell morphology-background (red signals). Values are means ± SD, $n = 4$. There was a significant interaction between cell type and concentration ($p < 0.001$) by two-way ANOVA. * Different from control (0 mmol/L NaB); * $p < 0.05$, ** $p < 0.0001$.

4. Discussion

Butyrate has been shown to abrogate the S-phase cell cycle checkpoint, and exhibits colon cancer preventive effects through cell proliferation regulation [5,6,28–30]. As there are few reports concerning the apoptotic potential, we propose that butyrate plays differential roles in the cell proliferation of noncancerous NCM460 cell and cancerous HCT116 colon cells through cellular signaling modulation. Thus, examining molecular effects of butyrate on cell proliferation/apoptosis in cancerous and noncancerous colon cells is expected to shed light on butyrate's anticancer mechanism.

It has been reported that butyrate at mmol/L levels in the colon is well within physiological concentrations [7,8]. Our data showed that butyrate (0.25 to 2 mmol/L) was much more effective on inhibiting cell proliferation in cancerous (HCT116) colon cells than in noncancerous (NCM460) colon cells (Figure 1). Similarly, we found, for the first time, that butyrate was effective in inducing apoptosis/DNA fragmentation in HCT116 cells but not NCM460 cells (Figures 2 and 3). This observation suggests that the stronger DNA fragmentation and apoptotic potential may confer the increased sensitivity of cancerous colon cells to butyrate in terms of cell proliferation when compared with that of noncancerous colon cells. In our present apoptosis assay, 7-AAD was excluded from live, healthy cells and early apoptotic cells, but permeated late apoptotic or necrotic cells [27]. It has been demonstrated that secondary necrosis is a natural outcome of the complete apoptotic program (e.g., late apoptotic cells) [31]. Although lactate dehydrogenase (LDH), a cytoplasmic enzyme, is widely used to detect necrosis and secondary necrosis based on plasma membrane leakage, the measurement of 7-AAD positive cells is a powerful approach to directly detect leaky membrane cells [31,32]. As our results showed that the late apoptotic cell population (including necrosis and possible secondary necrosis) was greatly increased in HCT116 cells but to a lesser extent in NCM460 cells due to butyrate treatment, it is conceivable that necrotic cell death may evoke inflammatory responses [32,33]. In the future, clinical samples from patients are needed to examine the impact of inflammatory responses on host pathogenesis in the context of high or low exposure to butyrate.

The other important aspect is that the cellular signaling molecules underlying the differential effect of butyrate remain to be determined. The ERK1/2 pathway plays a pivotal role in cell proliferation as it is an important cellular signaling component that translates various extracellular signals into intracellular responses through phosphorylation cascades [18,34–36]. Moreover, cell-cycle arrest by PD184352 or U0126 requires inhibition of ERK1/2 activation [37]. Thus, the ERK1/2 pathway is recognized as a pro-survival signal and often activated by growth factors [18,34,35]. In this study, butyrate up-regulated ERK1/2 phosphorylation in NCM460 cells (Figure 4). In contrast, butyrate inhibited ERK1/2 phosphorylation in HCT116 cells, which is consistent with the previous report [38] (Figure 4). The opposing effect of butyrate on cell survival signals provides an important mechanistic insight into the observed differential efficacy of cell proliferation and apoptosis in cancerous and noncancerous colon cells.

Appropriate control over cell cycle and proliferation depends on many factors. Cyclin-dependent kinase (CDK) inhibitor p21 (also known as p21 (WAF1/Cip1)) is one of these factors that promotes both cell cycle arrest and proliferation in response to a variety of stimuli [39–41]. To provide further mechanistic insights, we examined p21 protein expression, which is known to be the most critical effector of butyrate-induced growth arrest in colon cancer cells [39,42] (Figure 4). Butyrate is known to induce general histone acetylation, specifically, hyperacetylation of the H3 and other species through inhibition of the histone deacetylase enzyme [42,43]. Previous studies have shown that histone hyperacetylation is at least partly responsible for the induction of p21 [42,44]. In addition, the nuclear protein c-Myc, a central regulator of cellular proliferation, activates a multitude of pathways to repress p21 at the transcriptional and post-transcriptional levels [19,20]. We found that butyrate increased histone H3 acetylation at 1.5 and 15 h while it decreased c-Myc expression only at 15 h in NCM460 cells (Figure 4). However, p21 expression was increased at 1.5 and 15 h in NCM460 cells. Therefore, our results suggest that butyrate-related histone acetylation (compared with c-Myc) plays a major role in p21 expression because we could only detect the increase of histone H3 acetylation and p21 but not c-Myc expression in NCM460 cells in early molecular events at 1.5 h.

The other important aspect of p21 function is that, depending on intracellular localization, p21 is involved in different signaling cascades [39–41]. It is generally believed that nuclear p21 is a negative regulator of cell proliferation and a tumor suppressor while cytoplasmic p21 facilitates cell proliferation and inhibits apoptosis [39–41]. In addition to high p21 levels in HCT116 cells (Figure 5A,B), our cellular immunofluorescent staining data demonstrated that butyrate-induced p21 protein was located in or surrounding the nuclei of HCT116 cells to a greater extent when compared with that of NCM460 cells (Figure 5C,D). This observation indicates that butyrate induces p21 expression, and may exacerbate the negative role of p21 in HCT116 cell proliferation when compared with that of NCM460 cells. Therefore, butyrate treatment leads to the significant induction of apoptosis and inhibition of cell proliferation in cancerous HCT116 colon cells, but to a lesser extent in the noncancerous NCM460 colon cells. To extrapolate these mechanistic data to all colon cancer cell types and disease stages, we are planning to test other pairs of noncancerous and cancerous colon cell lines. However, there are very limited noncancerous colon cell lines available, which is a challenge. The other approach would be to evaluate clinical samples from patients with possible high or low exposure to butyrate.

Colon carcinogenesis consists of initiation, promotion, and progression phases [45,46]. Suppression of apoptosis and promotion of colonocyte proliferation are key cellular carcinogenic events as a consequence of dysregulation of molecular signal cascades [46]. Taken together, our findings on the differential roles of butyrate in cell proliferation and the activation of ERK1/2, histone hyperacetylation, and c-Myc, p21 protein abundance and intracellular location in cancerous HCT116 and noncancerous NCM460 colon cells may, at least in part, account for the selective potential of butyrate's anticancer colon cancer action.

Acknowledgments: We greatly appreciate Emily Fair, Mary Briske-Anderson, Brenda Skinner, Kay Keehr, Bryan Safratowich, and Laura Idso for the technical support. This work was funded by the US Department of Agriculture, Agricultural Research Service, Research Project 3062-51000-050-00D.

Author Contributions: H.Z., W.-H.C. and R.H. conceived and designed the experiments; H.Z. and D.P.T. performed the experiments; H.Z. and L.K.J. analyzed the data; H.Z., W.-H.C. and R.H. wrote the paper.

Conflicts of Interest: The authors declare no conflict of interest.

References

1. American Cancer Society. *Cancer Facts & Figures*; American Cancer Society: Atlanta, GA, USA, 2016.
2. Simon, K. Colorectal cancer development and advances in screening. *J. Clin. Interv. Aging* **2016**, *11*, 967–976.
3. Perrin, P.; Pierre, F.; Patry, Y.; Champ, M.; Berreur, M.; Pradal, G.; Bornet, F.; Meflah, K.; Menanteau, J. Only fibres promoting a stable butyrate producing colonic ecosystem decrease the rate of aberrant crypt foci in rats. *Gut* **2001**, *48*, 53–61. [CrossRef] [PubMed]
4. Zeng, H.; Lazarova, D.L.; Bordonaro, M. Mechanisms linking dietary fiber, gut microbiota and colon cancer prevention. *World J. Gastrointest. Oncol.* **2014**, *6*, 41–51. [CrossRef] [PubMed]
5. Lazarova, D.L.; Bordonaro, M. Vimentin, colon cancer progression and resistance to butyrate and other HDACis. *J. Cell. Mol. Med.* **2016**, *20*, 989–993. [CrossRef] [PubMed]
6. Bultman, S.J. The microbiome and its potential as a cancer preventive intervention. *Semin. Oncol.* **2016**, *43*, 97–106. [CrossRef] [PubMed]
7. Fleming, S.E.; O'Donnell, A.U.; Perman, J.A. Influence of frequent and long-term bean consumption on colonic function and fermentation. *Am. J. Clin. Nutr.* **1985**, *41*, 909–918. [PubMed]
8. Fleming, S.E.; Marthinsen, D.; Kuhnlein, H. Colonic function and fermentation in men consuming high fiber diets. *J. Nutr.* **1983**, *113*, 2535–2544. [PubMed]
9. Leonel, A.J.; Alvarez-Leite, J.I. Butyrate: Implications for intestinal function. *Curr. Opin. Clin. Nutr. Metab. Care* **2012**, *15*, 474–479. [CrossRef] [PubMed]
10. Brown, D.G.; Rao, S.; Weir, T.L.; O'Malia, J.; Bazan, M.; Brown, R.J.; Ryan, E.P. Metabolomics and metabolic pathway networks from human colorectal cancers, adjacent mucosa, and stool. *Cancer Metab.* **2016**, *4*, 11. [CrossRef] [PubMed]
11. Zeng, H.; Davis, C.D. Down-regulation of proliferating cell nuclear antigen gene expression occurs during cell cycle arrest induced by human fecal water in colonic HT-29 cells. *J. Nutr.* **2003**, *133*, 2682–2687. [PubMed]
12. Hu, G.X.; Chen, G.R.; Xu, H.; Ge, R.S.; Lin, J. Activation of the AMP activated protein kinase by short-chain fatty acids is the main mechanism underlying the beneficial effect of a high fiber diet on the metabolic syndrome. *Med. Hypotheses* **2010**, *74*, 123–126. [CrossRef] [PubMed]
13. Ocker, M.; Schneider-Stock, R. Histone deacetylase inhibitors: Signalling towards $p21^{cip1/waf1}$. *Int. J. Biochem. Cell Biol.* **2007**, *39*, 1367–1374. [CrossRef] [PubMed]
14. Bi, G.; Jiang, G. The molecular mechanism of HDAC inhibitors in anticancer effects. *Cell. Mol. Immunol.* **2006**, *3*, 285–290. [PubMed]
15. Chen, H.P.; Zhao, Y.T.; Zhao, T.C. Histone deacetylases and mechanisms of regulation of gene expression. *Crit. Rev. Oncog.* **2015**, *20*, 35–47. [CrossRef] [PubMed]
16. Jones, S.M.; Kazlauskas, A. Growth-factor-dependent mitogenesis requires two distinct phases of signalling. *Nat. Cell Biol.* **2001**, *3*, 165–172. [CrossRef] [PubMed]

17. Karslioglu, E.; Kleinberger, J.W.; Salim, F.G.; Cox, A.E.; Takane, K.K.; Scott, D.K.; Stewart, A.F. cMyc is a principal upstream driver of beta-cell proliferation in rat insulinoma cell lines and is an effective mediator of human beta-cell replication. *Mol. Endocrinol.* **2011**, *25*, 1760–1772. [CrossRef] [PubMed]
18. Sun, Y.; Liu, W.Z.; Liu, T.; Feng, X.; Yang, N.; Zhou, H.F. Signaling pathway of MAPK/ERK in cell proliferation, differentiation, migration, senescence and apoptosis. *J. Recept. Signal Transduct. Res.* **2015**, *35*, 600–604. [CrossRef] [PubMed]
19. Gartel, A.L.; Ye, X.; Goufman, E.; Shianov, P.; Hay, N.; Najmabadi, F.; Tyner, A.L. Myc represses the p21(WAF1/CIP1) promoter and interacts with Sp1/Sp3. *Proc. Natl. Acad. Sci. USA* **2001**, *98*, 4510–4515. [CrossRef] [PubMed]
20. Wang, Z.; Liu, M.; Zhu, H.; Zhang, W.; He, S.; Hu, C.; Quan, L.; Bai, J.; Xu, N. Suppression of p21 by c-Myc through members of miR-17 family at the post-transcriptional level. *Int. J. Oncol.* **2010**, *37*, 1315–1321. [PubMed]
21. Moyer, M.P.; Manzano, L.A.; Merriman, R.L.; Stauffer, J.S.; Tanzer, L.R. NCM460, a normal human colon mucosal epithelial cell line. *In Vitro Cell. Dev. Biol. Anim.* **1996**, *32*, 315–317. [CrossRef] [PubMed]
22. Brattain, M.G.; Fine, W.D.; Khaled, F.M.; Thompson, J.; Brattain, D.E. Heterogeneity of malignant cells from a human colonic carcinoma. *Cancer Res.* **1981**, *41*, 1751–1756. [PubMed]
23. Megna, B.W.; Carney, P.R.; Nukaya, M.; Geiger, P.; Kennedy, G.D. Indole-3-carbinol induces tumor cell death: Function follows form. *J. Surg. Res.* **2016**, *204*, 47–54. [CrossRef] [PubMed]
24. De Meij, T.G.; Larbi, I.B.; van der Schee, M.P.; Lentferink, Y.E.; Paff, T.; Terhaar Sive Droste, J.S.; Mulder, C.J.; van Bodegraven, A.A.; de Boer, N.K. Electronic nose can discriminate colorectal carcinoma and advanced adenomas by fecal volatile biomarker analysis: Proof of principle study. *Int. J. Cancer* **2014**, *134*, 1132–1138. [CrossRef] [PubMed]
25. Zhao, D.; Keates, A.C.; Kuhnt-Moore, S.; Moyer, M.P.; Kelly, C.P.; Pothoulakis, C. Signal transduction pathways mediating neurotensin-stimulated interleukin-8 expression in human colonocytes. *J. Biol. Chem.* **2001**, *276*, 44464–44471. [CrossRef] [PubMed]
26. Chen, T.R. In situ detection of mycoplasma contamination in cell cultures by fluorescent Hoechst 33258 stain. *Exp. Cell Res.* **1977**, *104*, 255–262. [CrossRef]
27. Schmid, I.; Krall, W.J.; Uittenbogaart, C.H.; Braun, J.; Giorgi, J.V. Dead cell discrimination with 7-amino-actinomycin D in combination with dual color immunofluorescence in single laser flow cytometry. *Cytometry* **1992**, *13*, 204–208. [CrossRef] [PubMed]
28. Zeng, H.; Briske-Anderson, M. Prolonged butyrate treatment inhibits the migration and invasion potential of HT1080 tumor cells. *J. Nutr.* **2005**, *135*, 291–295. [PubMed]
29. Saldanha, S.N.; Kala, R.; Tollefsbol, T.O. Molecular mechanisms for inhibition of colon cancer cells by combined epigenetic-modulating epigallocatechin gallate and sodium butyrate. *Exp. Cell Res.* **2014**, *324*, 40–53. [CrossRef] [PubMed]
30. Gospodinov, A.; Popova, S.; Vassileva, I.; Anachkova, B. The inhibitor of histone deacetylases sodium butyrate enhances the cytotoxicity of mitomycin C. *Mol. Cancer Ther.* **2012**, *11*, 2116–2126. [CrossRef] [PubMed]
31. Silva, M.T. Secondary necrosis: The natural outcome of the complete apoptotic program. *FEBS Lett.* **2010**, *584*, 4491–4499. [CrossRef] [PubMed]
32. Chan, F.K.; Moriwaki, K.; De Rosa, M.J. Detection of necrosis by release of lactate dehydrogenase activity. *Methods Mol. Biol.* **2013**, *979*, 65–70. [PubMed]
33. Kono, H.; Rock, K.L. How dying cells alert the immune system to danger. *Nat. Rev. Immunol.* **2008**, *8*, 279–289. [CrossRef] [PubMed]
34. Meloche, S.; Pouysségur, J. The ERK1/2 mitogen-activated protein kinase pathway as a master regulator of the G1- to S-phase transition. *Oncogene* **2007**, *26*, 3227–3239. [CrossRef] [PubMed]
35. Xia, Z.; Dickens, M.; Raingeaud, J.; Davis, R.J.; Greenberg, M.E. Opposing effects of ERK and JNK-p38 MAP kinases on apoptosis. *Science* **1995**, *270*, 1326–1331. [CrossRef] [PubMed]
36. Park, J.I. Growth arrest signaling of the Raf/MEK/ERK pathway in cancer. *Front. Biol. (Beijing)* **2014**, *9*, 95–103. [CrossRef] [PubMed]
37. Squires, M.S.; Nixon, P.M.; Cook, S.J. Cell-cycle arrest by PD184352 requires inhibition of extracellular signal-regulated kinases (ERK) 1/2 but not ERK5/BMK1. *Biochem. J.* **2002**, *366*, 673–680. [CrossRef] [PubMed]

38. Davido, D.J.; Richter, F.; Boxberger, F.; Stahl, A.; Menzel, T.; Lührs, H.; Löffler, S.; Dusel, G.; Rapp, U.R.; Scheppach, W. Butyrate and propionate downregulate ERK phosphorylation in HT-29 colon carcinoma cells prior to differentiation. *Eur. J. Cancer Prev.* **2001**, *10*, 313–321. [CrossRef] [PubMed]
39. Karimian, A.; Ahmadi, Y.; Yousefi, B. Multiple functions of p21 in cell cycle, apoptosis and transcriptional regulation after DNA damage. *DNA Repair* **2016**, *42*, 63–71. [CrossRef] [PubMed]
40. Romanov, V.S.; Pospelov, V.A.; Pospelova, T.V. Cyclin-dependent kinase inhibitor p21(Waf1): Contemporary view on its role in senescence and oncogenesis. *Biochemistry (Mosc.)* **2012**, *77*, 575–584. [CrossRef] [PubMed]
41. Parveen, A.; Akash, M.S.; Rehman, K.; Kyunn, W.W. Dual Role of p21 in the Progression of Cancer and Its Treatment. *Crit. Rev. Eukaryot. Gene Expr.* **2016**, *26*, 49–62. [CrossRef] [PubMed]
42. Archer, S.Y.; Meng, S.; Shei, A.; Hodin, R.A. p21(WAF1) is required for butyrate-mediated growth inhibition of human colon cancer cells. *Proc. Natl. Acad. Sci. USA* **1998**, *95*, 6791–6796. [CrossRef] [PubMed]
43. Pham, T.X.; Lee, J. Dietary regulation of histone acetylases and deacetylases for the prevention of metabolic diseases. *Nutrients* **2012**, *4*, 1868–1886. [CrossRef] [PubMed]
44. Nian, H.; Delage, B.; Pinto, J.T.; Dashwood, R.H. Allyl mercaptan, a garlic-derived organosulfur compound, inhibits histone deacetylase and enhances Sp3 binding on the P21WAF1 promoter. *Carcinogenesis* **2008**, *29*, 1816–1824. [CrossRef] [PubMed]
45. Gatenby, R.A.; Vincent, T.L. An evolutionary model of carcinogenesis. *Cancer Res.* **2003**, *63*, 6212–6220. [PubMed]
46. Rajamanickam, S.; Agarwal, R. Natural products and colon cancer: Current status and future prospects. *Drug Dev. Res.* **2008**, *69*, 460–471. [CrossRef] [PubMed]

nutrients

MDPI

Article

Analysis of the Anti-Cancer Effects of Cincau Extract (*Premna oblongifolia* Merr) and Other Types of Non-Digestible Fibre Using Faecal Fermentation Supernatants and Caco-2 Cells as a Model of the Human Colon

Samsu U. Nurdin [1,2,3], Richard K. Le Leu [3,4], Graeme P. Young [3], James C. R. Stangoulis [1], Claus T. Christophersen [4,5] and Catherine A. Abbott [1,3,*]

1 School of Biological Sciences, Flinders University, Adelaide, SA 5042, Australia; samsu.udayana@fp.unila.ac.id (S.U.N.); james.stangoulis@flinders.edu.au (J.C.R.S.)
2 Department of Agricultural Product Technology, Lampung University, Bandar Lampung 35145, Indonesia
3 Flinders Centre for Innovation in Cancer, Adelaide, SA 5042, Australia; Richard.LeLeu@sa.gov.au (R.K.L.L.); graeme.young@flinders.edu.au (G.P.Y.)
4 CSIRO Food and Nutrition, Adelaide, SA 5000, Australia; c.christophersen@ecu.edu.au
5 School of Medical and Health Sciences, Edith Cowan University, Joondalup, WA 6027, Australia
* Correspondence: cathy.abbott@flinders.edu.au; Tel.: +61-8-8201-2078

Received: 15 December 2016; Accepted: 29 March 2017; Published: 3 April 2017

Abstract: Green cincau (*Premna oblongifolia* Merr) is an Indonesian food plant with a high dietary fibre content. Research has shown that dietary fibre mixtures may be more beneficial for colorectal cancer prevention than a single dietary fibre type. The aim of this study was to investigate the effects of green cincau extract on short chain fatty acid (SCFA) production in anaerobic batch cultures inoculated with human faecal slurries and to compare these to results obtained using different dietary fibre types (pectin, inulin, and cellulose), singly and in combination. Furthermore, fermentation supernatants (FSs) were evaluated in Caco-2 cells for their effect on cell viability, differentiation, and apoptosis. Cincau increased total SCFA concentration by increasing acetate and propionate, but not butyrate concentration. FSs from all dietary fibre sources, including cincau, reduced Caco-2 cell viability. However, the effects of all FSs on cell viability, cell differentiation, and apoptosis were not simply explainable by their butyrate content. In conclusion, products of fermentation of cincau extracts induced cell death, but further work is required to understand the mechanism of action. This study demonstrates for the first time that this Indonesian traditional source of dietary fibre may be protective against colorectal cancer.

Keywords: dietary fibre; colorectal cancer; fermentation; cincau; short chain fatty acids

1. Introduction

Colorectal cancer (CRC) incidence is rising significantly in most countries due to increasing prosperity [1]. Compounds such as short chain fatty acids (SCFAs), which are produced by bacterial fermentation of undigested dietary fibre, are capable of inhibiting cancer in vitro and in vivo [2–6]. The type of dietary fibre consumed influences the proportion and distribution of SCFAs in the gastrointestinal tract [7–10]. Rapidly fermentable dietary fibre is fermented in the proximal colon and results in increased SCFA levels in this region of the gut; conversely, slow fermentable dietary fibre will reach the distal colon and modulate SCFA production at this site [7,11].

Many researchers have shown mixtures of multiple dietary fibre types are more beneficial than a single dietary fibre [7,12–14]. Rats administered diets containing guar gum or pectin produced low proportions of butyrate in comparison to rats fed mixtures of both [12,13]. Compared with control or wheat bran diets alone, diets containing a combination of wheat bran and resistant starch produced higher wet and dry output, a lower pH and ammonia, as well as lower levels of phenol [13]. An in vitro fermentation study showed that a combination of Raftilose (oligofructose) and guar gum results in higher total SCFAs than individual guar gum [14]. Following 24 h culture, the SCFA production rate from individual Raftilose or guar gum fermentation decreased, but when these fibres were combined, the production rate kept increasing, indicating that a combination of fibre sources may be more beneficial.

The inulin-type compound fructan has also been well studied for its ability to protect against colorectal cancer when included in the diet [15–18]. In combination with lycopene and probiotics, inulin induced apoptosis, and inhibited cell proliferation and aberrant crypt formation (ACF) in rat colon when the chemical 1,2-dimethylhydrazine (DMH) was used to induce cancer [19]. Inulin intake reduced CRC levels in rats fed a high lipid diet or chemical-induced CRC through decreasing enzyme activity and bile acid concentration [20,21]. The dietary fibre pectin is fermentable by human faecal bacteria and produces high proportions of acetic acid in vitro and in vivo [22]. Fermentation supernatant from incubation of human faecal slurry with apple pectin was found to be rich in butyrate and inhibited histone deacetylase in nucleus extracted from tumour cell lines [23].

Green cincau (*Premna oblongifolia* Merr) is a tropical plant belonging to the Verbenaceae family which is a traditional food source in Indonesia. Extracts from green leaf of the cincau plant contain about 20% pectin and have free radical scavenging activity [24]. Research on cincau extracts indicates they have the ability to induce cell-mediated immune responses in vitro [25]. As a dietary fibre, cincau extracts have laxative properties and can effectively induce the growth of lactic acid producing bacteria in the colon [26]. This study aimed to compare the efficacy of cincau extracts as a traditional source of dietary fibre with other dietary fibre combinations known to be protective against CRC. Our study found that, when fermented, cincau extracts were able to reduce Caco-2 cell viability, but the mechanism was unclear. In addition, this study found that when two different dietary fibres were combined, the benefits were not always additive.

2. Materials and Methods

2.1. Green Cincau Extracts

Green cincau leaves (*Premna oblongifolia* Merr.) were collected from traditional farmers in Indonesia. The fresh leaves were dried in an oven at 50 °C (water content around 12%), ground into fine powder, and imported into Australia using an AQIS permit (IP07024278). To prepare extracts for this study, 5 g of dried cincau leaf powder was placed in a glass beaker, then boiled water was added until the final volume was 100 mL, and the mixture was stirred for 5 min at maximum speed. The mixture was then filtered and allowed to set at room temperature [24]. The resulting jelly like extract was then freeze dried (Dynavac) and ground with mortar and pestle before use. Table 1 shows the freeze dried cincau extract composition as determined by CSIRO analytical tests (Adelaide, South Australia), as described in Belobrajdic [27]. A modification of the AOACI Method 994.13 [28] was used to determine dietary fibre composition as soluble and insoluble non-starch polysaccharides (NSPs) [27].

Table 1. Composition of dried green cincau extract (g/100 g dry weight).

Dietary Component	Concentration
Moisture	4.4
Fat	4.4
Protein	13.3
Ash	12.2
Starch	1.8
Resistant starch	0.5
Soluble NSP	5.8
Insoluble NSP	46.3
Total non-starch polysaccharides (NSPs)	52.1

2.2. *In Vitro Fermentation of Dietary Fibre*

Seven substrates as a single or a mixture of two dietary fibres (50:50) were tested following a CSIRO protocol (Adelaide, Australia): pectin, inulin, cellulose, pectin-cellulose mixture, inulin-cellulose, pectin-inulin, and green cincau extract (Table 2). The anaerobic batch fermentation was carried out as described in Charoendsiddhi et al. [29] and was adapted from Zhou et al. [30]. Briefly, 150 mg of each dietary fibre source or a 50:50 mixture was placed in a 15 mL capped tube, then 9 mL of sterile fermentation media was added. The media contained 0.25% (*w*/*v*) Tryptone, 125 ppm (*v*/*v*) micro-mineral solution (containing $CaCl_2{\cdot}H_2O$ 13.2%, $MnCl_2{\cdot}4H_2O$ 10%, $CoCl_2{\cdot}6H_2O$ 1%, and $FeCl_3{\cdot}6H_2O$ 8%), 25% (*v*/*v*) carbonate buffer solution (0.4% NH_4HCO_3 and 3.5% $NaHCO_3$), 25% (*v*/*v*) macro-mineral solution (containing Na_2HPO_4 0.57%, KH_2PO_4 0.62%, and $MgSO_4{\cdot}7H_2O$ 0.06%), and 3.35% (*v*/*v*) reducing solution (containing cysteine hydrochloride 0.625%, $Na_2S{\cdot}9H_2O$ 0.625%, and NaOH 0.04 M). After addition of the dietary fibre/s to the fermentation media, the pH was adjusted to pH 7.0. For inoculums, fresh faecal slurry from three healthy volunteers was pooled and diluted in phosphate buffer to produce 10% (*w*/*v*) inoculums. Signed consent was obtained from staff volunteers for the collection of fresh faecal samples. The faecal collection process was approved by the CSIRO Human Ethics Committee. Final concentration of inoculums was 1% (*w*/*v*) after mixing of 1 mL of 10% inoculums with 9 mL of media containing dietary fibre/s. A negative control containing only fermentation media and inoculum was prepared as a faecal blank (FB). All processes were carried out in anaerobic chamber with rocking (SL Bactron IV, Cornelius, OR, USA) to maintain anaerobic conditions set at 37 °C for 24 h. To help monitor that the chamber was maintained under anaerobic conditions, 1.25 ppm (*w*/*v*) of resazurine solution (Sigma-Aldrich, St Louis, MO, USA) was added to the initial fermentation media. Supernatants were sterilized by filtration (pore size 0.22 μm) (Minisart®, Sartorius AG, Dandenong South, Victoria, Australia) and stored at −80 °C until use.

Table 2. Type of dietary fibre and combinations used for batch in vitro fermentation.

Dietary Fibre	Ratio (%)
Pectin	100
Inulin	100
Cellulose	100
Pectin + cellulose	50:50
Pectin + inulin	50:50
Inulin + cellulose	50:50
Cincau extract	100
Faecal blank (FB)	-

2.3. *Cell Culture*

Human colorectal carcinoma cells Caco-2 were obtained from the American Type Culture Collection (ATCC Number CCL-247). Experiments were conducted on Caco-2 cells passage number 76 to 85 and were performed three to four passages post thawing. Cultures were maintained in Dulbecco's modified Eagle's medium (DMEM) (Sigma-Aldrich) supplemented with 10% fetal bovine serum (Bovogen, Victoria, Australia), 100 U/mL penicillin-streptomycin (Sigma-Aldrich), 1% nonessential amino acids (Sigma-Aldrich), and 20 mM 4-(2-hydroxyethyl)-1-piperazineethanesulfonic acid (HEPES, Sigma-Aldrich) in a CO_2 incubator (37 °C and 5% CO_2). For each assay, cells were seeded so that following the 24 h attachment and 48 h experimental time, cells reached 80%–90% confluence.

2.4. SCFA Analysis

Fermentation supernatant (FS) samples were homogenized in three volumes of internal standard solution (heptanoic acid, 1.68 mmol/L) (Sigma-Aldrich) and centrifuged at 3000× *g* for 10 min. The supernatant was then distilled and 0.3 µL was injected into a gas chromatograph (Hewlett-Packard 5890 Series II A, Wilmington, DE, USA) equipped with a flame ionization detector and a capillary column (Zebron ZB-FFAP, 30 m × 0.53 mm i.d., 1-µm film, SGE, Phenomenex, Torrance, CA, USA). Helium was used as the carrier gas; the initial oven temperature was 120 °C and was increased at 30 °C/min to 190 °C; the injector temperature was 210 °C and the detector temperature was 210 °C. A standard SCFA mixture containing acetate, propionate, and butyrate (Sigma-Aldrich) was used for calculations, and the results are expressed as µmol/g of sample [31].

2.5. MTT Proliferation Assay

Caco-2 cells were seeded into a 96-well plate (Costar®, Corning incorporated, Corning, NY, USA) at a density of 1.5×10^4 cells per well 24 h before treatment with FS (day 0) to allow adherence, then incubated for 48 h in media containing 20% FS. For standard curves, 1:2 serial dilutions were prepared to generate a standard curve of 5000–80,000 cells per well, in final volume of 100 µL [32].

After 48 h treatment, media was removed and 100 µL of medium containing 0.5 mg/mL 3-4,5-dimethylthiazol-2-yl)2,5-diphenyl-tetrazolium bromide (MTT) (Sigma-Aldrich) solution was added to each well and incubated (37 °C, 5% CO_2) for 1 h (to allow MTT to be metabolized). The formazan (MTT metabolic product) was resuspended in 80 µL of 20% sodium dodecyl sulfate (SDS, Amresco, Solon, OH, USA) in 0.02 M HCl (Sigma-Aldrich), and the plate was incubated in the dark for 1 h at room temperature. The optical density was read at 570 nm with background absorbance at 630 nm (FLUOstar omega, BMG Labtech GmbH, Ortenberg, Germany). Optical densities were converted to a total number of live cells using a linear regression plot. Results were expressed as the number of live cells in wells containing treatment compared with the number of cells in control wells (medium alone).

2.6. Alkaline Phosphatase (AP) Activity Assay

For the AP assay, 3.0×10^5 cells were seeded into each well of a six-well plate with supplemented media (as described above) and allowed to adhere for 24 h. The medium was removed and replaced with media containing 20% FS. After 48 h incubation, the medium was removed and cells were detached by incubation with 1× Trypsin-EDTA solution (Sigma-Aldrich) for 5 min at 37 °C. Detached cells were resuspended in 50 mM Tris-HCl buffer, pH 10.0, and homogenized by sonification. The homogenized cells were centrifuged at 100,000 rpm for 30 min to remove cell debris.

AP activity was measured by hydrolysis of *p*-nitro phenol phosphate (5 mM) (Sigma-Aldrich) and expressed in units (the number of µmol *p*-nitrophenol liberated in 1 min measured at 400 nm per mg protein). *p*-nitrophenol (0–200 µM) was used to generate a standard curve [33].

2.7. Caspase 3–7 and Lactate Dehydrogenase (LDH) Assay

Caco-2 cells were seeded into 96-well white plates (Costar®) at a density of 1.5×10^4 cells per well in supplemented media. The cells were incubated 24 h to allow the cells to adhere prior to treatment with 20% FS or control. After FS treatment, the cells were incubated for 48 h. Staurosporine 5 µM (Sigma) was used as a positive control to induce apoptosis (data not shown). The CytoTox-ONE™ Homogeneous Membrane Integrity assay kit (Promega, Madison, WI, USA) was employed to quantify the LDH enzyme activity, where 70 μL of cell culture supernatant was mixed with 70 μL CytoTox-ONE™ Reagent and shaken for 30 s, then incubated for 10 min. The stop solution (35 μL) was added to each well, and fluorescence was measured at excitation wavelength of 560 nm and an emission wavelength of 590 nm. In parallel, quantification of caspase-3/7 activities was carried out using the Caspase-GloR 3/7 assay kit (Promega). The FS treatments were also applied to separate Caco-2 cells cultured in 96-well plates for determination of cell proliferation using the MTT assay.

To confirm the role of caspase 3/7 in the cell death mechanism, FS from the inulin, cincau extract, and faecal blank fermentation were applied to the Caco-2 cells in combination with 10 μM caspase inhibitor (Ac-DEVD-CHO, Promega). Cells were seeded in 96-well plates as outlined above and the inhibitor was added 1 h preceding FS treatment.

2.8. Statistical Analysis

All cell culture experiments were performed on three different occasions, and the results are expressed as the mean ± standard error of mean (SEM). Statistical analysis was carried out with the statistical program SPSS version 19. One way-ANOVA with Least Significant Difference test was used. Results were considered significant if $p < 0.05$.

3. Results

3.1. SCFA Content of Dietary Fibre Fermentation Supernatant

Fermentation with cellulose alone had no significant effect on SCFA production. In contrast, fermentation of all other dietary fibres, individually or in combination, increased the yields of total SCFA, acetate, and propionate levels in the FS in comparison to the FB ($p < 0.05$) (Figure 1A–C). Cincau as the dietary fibre source significantly increased total SCFA, acetate, and propionate, but not butyrate levels. Butyrate levels were only significantly increased in the FS after fermentation with inulin, inulin-cellulose, and inulin-pectin (Figure 1D).

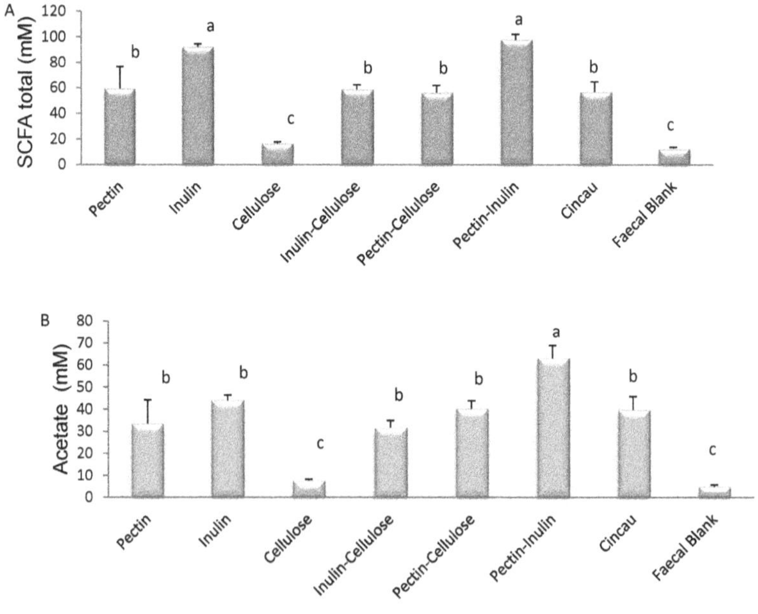

Figure 1. *Cont.*

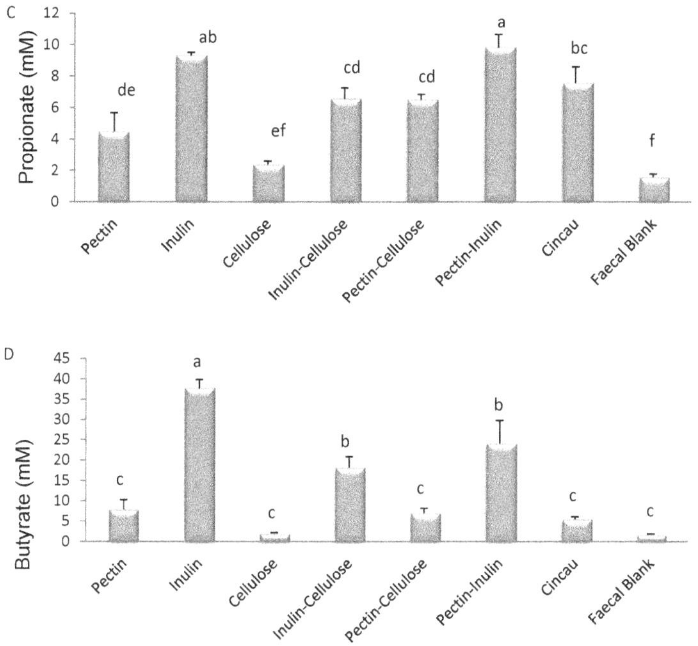

Figure 1. Effect of dietary fibre on the concentration of short chain fatty acid (SCFA) total (**A**), acetate (**B**), propionate (**C**), and butyrate (**D**) in fermentation supernatants. Dietary fibre/s were fermented with human faecal bacteria at 37 °C for 24 h in anaerobic conditions. The bars represent the mean, and the lines are SEM of four replicates. Data points denoted by different superscripts (letters above the bar) differ significantly when $p < 0.05$.

3.2. *Effect of Dietary Fibre FS on Caco-2 Cell Viability*

Due to the increased production of SCFA in the FS from the different fibre fermentations, we examined the effects of the FS on Caco-2 cell viability. As cellulose alone had no effect on SCFA production and inhibited SCFA production when mixed with inulin, no further studies were performed on FS from these two dietary fibre groups. In addition, as SCFA production was no different between the faecal blank (FB) and the cellulose group, for the remaining studies the blank served as the negative control. Treatment of Caco-2 cells with the remaining five FSs affected cell viability. Caco-2 cell number was significantly reduced after incubation of cells with 20% FS after incubation with cincau and with other dietary fibre/s compared to control FB (Figure 2, $p < 0.05$). Incubation with inulin FS inhibited cell growth the most when compared to FB. Combining pectin with inulin in the FS had no significant effect on the ability of inulin or pectin to inhibit cell growth.

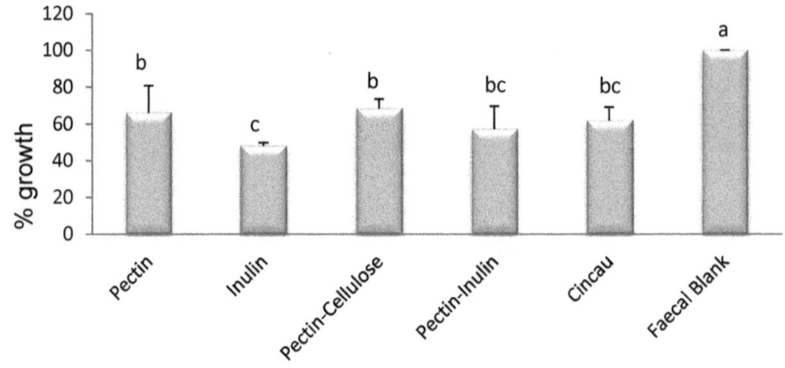

Figure 2. All dietary fibre sources reduced Caco-2 cell viability. Cells were seeded 1 day before the treatment with (fermentation supernatant) FS (day 0), then incubated for 48 h in media containing 20% FS. The bars represent the mean, and the lines are SEM of three independent experiments each performed in triplicate. Data points denoted by different superscripts (letters above the bar) differ significantly with $p < 0.05$.

3.3. *Effect of Dietary Fibre FS on Cell Differentiation*

Cell differentiation was assessed by measuring cellular levels of the enzyme alkaline phosphatase (AP) [34]. FSs from all dietary fibre sources, including cincau, failed to increase alkaline phosphatase enzyme levels but unexpectedly some caused significant decreases in alkaline phosphatase levels (Figure 3, $p < 0.05$). Cells that were incubated in FS after fermentation with inulin and mixtures of pectin and inulin had significantly lower alkaline phosphatase activity compared to FB, whereas cells incubated with FS from pectin, mixture of pectin-cellulose, and cincau displayed similar alkaline phosphatase activities to FB ($p < 0.05$).

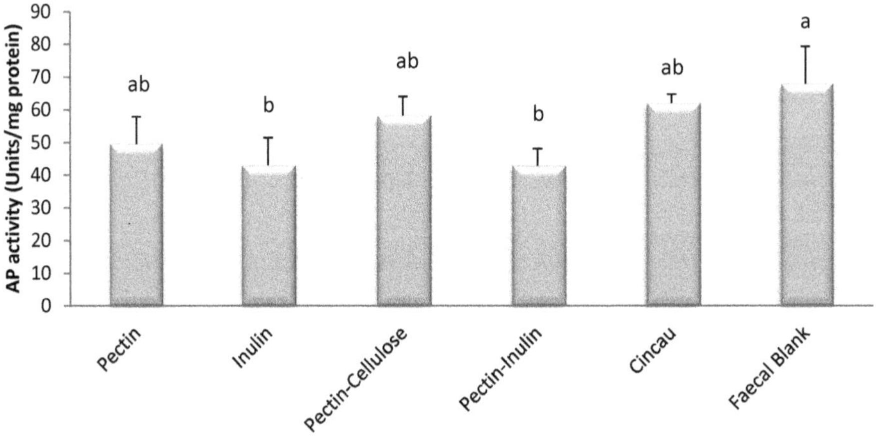

Figure 3. Effect of dietary fibre FS on alkaline phosphatase (AP) enzyme levels. AP enzyme activity was measured by hydrolysis of *p*-nitro phenol phosphate (5 mM) and expressed in units (the number of µmol *p*-nitrophenol liberated in 1 min measured at 400 nm per mg protein). The bars represent the mean, and the lines are SEM of three independent experiments each performed in triplicates. Data points denoted by different superscripts (letters above the bar) differ significantly with $p < 0.05$.

3.4. *Effect of Dietary Fibre FS on Caspase 3/7 Activity*

SCFAs have been shown to reduce proliferation and induce apoptosis in colorectal cell lines [2]. Caspase 3 and 7 are key effectors of apoptosis, therefore their activity was measured in Caco-2 cells after incubation with FS. Caspase 3/7 activity was affected by the type of dietary fibre fermented by colon microbiota (Figure 4, $p < 0.05$). Pectin, individually or in combination with inulin, induced higher caspase 3/7 activity compared to no treatment (control). In contrast, cincau extracts and the faecal blank suppressed caspase 3/7 activity ($p < 0.05$).

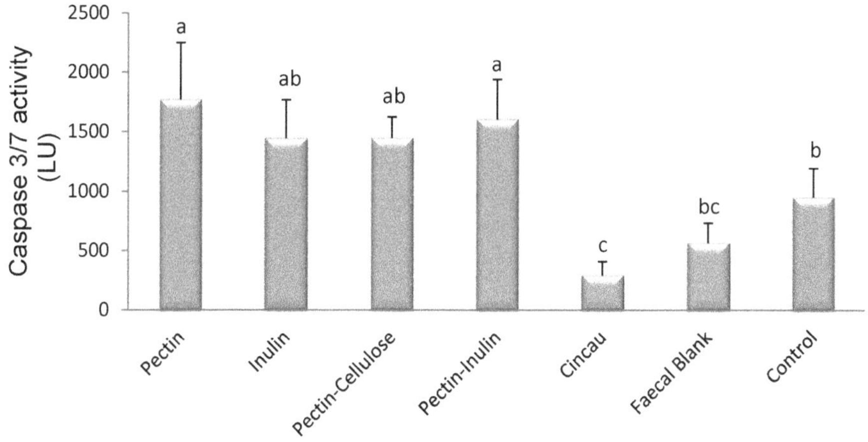

Figure 4. Effects of dietary fibre/s FS on caspase 3/7 activity. Cells were seeded 1 day before the treatment with FS (day 0), then incubated for 48 h in media containing 20% FS. Caspase-3 and -7 activities were measured using the Caspase-GloR 3/7 assay kit (Promega, USA). Control is cells incubated in media without FS. The bars represent the mean, and the lines are SEM of three independent experiments each performed in triplicate. Data points denoted by different superscripts (letters above the bar) differ significantly with $p < 0.05$. LU, Luminescence units.

3.5. *Mechanism of Cell Death Induced by FSs Containing SCFAs*

To further examine the increase in caspase 3/7 activity triggered by FSs from different dietary fibres above, a caspase inhibitor was utilised. Extracellular release of lactate dehydrogenase (LDH) was utilised as an additional measure of Caco-2 cell death. The caspase inhibitor significantly inhibited the ability of FSs from both inulin and the faecal blank to induce caspase 3/7 activity. In contrast, when cells were incubated with FS from cincau fermentation, very little caspase activity was detected and the inhibitor had no significant effect on this activity (Figure 5A; $p < 0.05$). LDH release in cells treated with FS when cincau was the fibre source was lower compared to that from inulin FS and FB (Figure 5B; $p < 0.05$). LDH release was not affected by the addition of the caspase inhibitor. Both inulin and cincau FS inhibited cell growth compared to the FB, and the caspase inhibitor was able to partially prevent this inhibition when inulin was the dietary fibre (Figure 5C; $p < 0.05$).

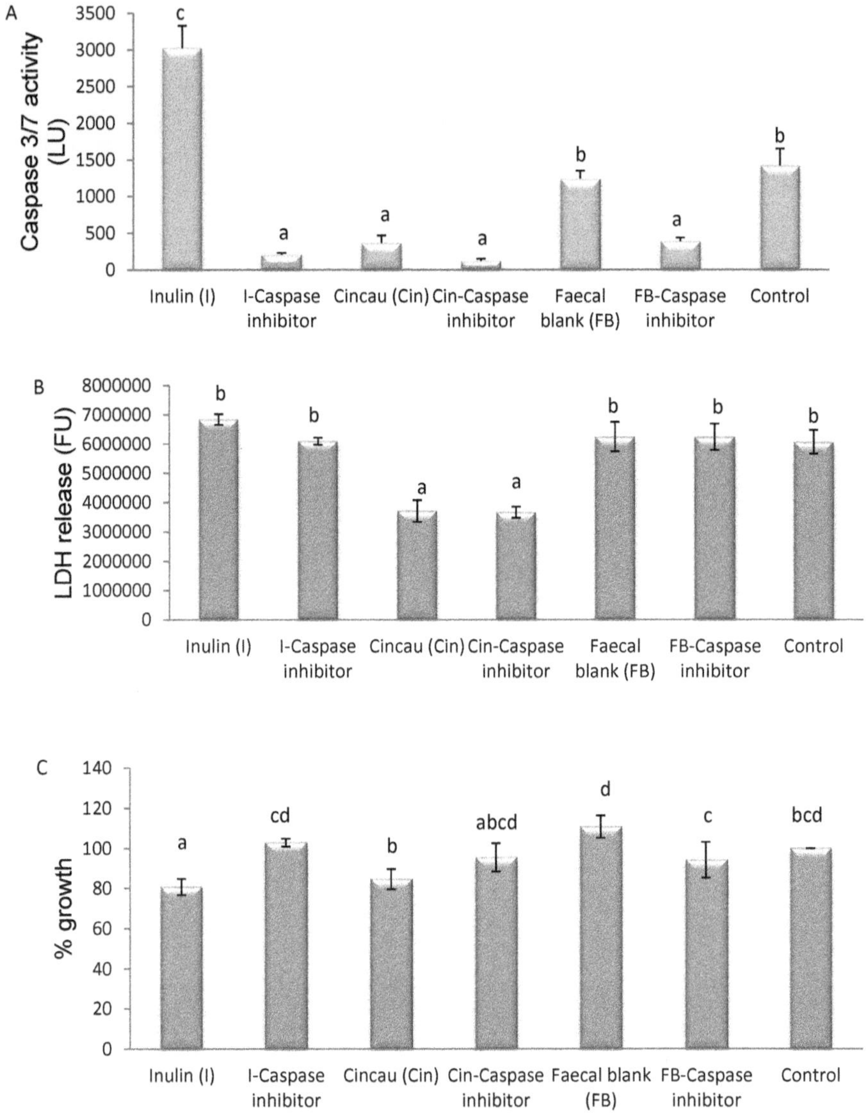

Figure 5. Effect of inulin and cincau on caspase 3/7 activity (**A**), LDH release (**B**), and Caco-2 cell viability (**C**) with or without caspase inhibitor. Cells were seeded 1 day before the treatment with FS (day 0), then incubated for 48 h in media containing 20% FS. Caspase inhibitor (10 μM) was added 1 h preceding FS treatment. Caspase 3–7 activity was measured using the Caspase-GloR 3/7 assay kit (Promega), the LDH activity was quantified using the CytoTox-ONE™ Homogeneous Membrane Integrity assay kit (Promega), and cell viability was measured using the MTT (dimethylthiazol-2-yl)2,5-diphenyl-tetrazolium bromide) assay and expressed as % growth against control. Control is cells incubated in media without FS. The bars represent the mean, and the lines are SEM of three independent experiments performed in triplicates. Data points denoted by different superscripts (letters above the bar) differ significantly with $p < 0.05$. LU, Luminescence units; FU, fluorescence units.

4. Discussion

This work demonstrates for the first time that green cincau, a traditional food that is indigenous to Indonesia, can be fermented to produce SCFAs which, when tested on colon cancer cells, can inhibit cell growth in vitro. In particular, cincau fermentation resulted in increased acetate and propionate production as assessed by their concentrations, but not butyrate. Furthermore, this study demonstrates that pectin and inulin alone, or in combination, had the greatest influence on individual and total SCFA production after fermentation by gut microbiota. Inulin produced the highest concentration of butyrate among the dietary fibres tested. Butyrate levels in FS from cellulose and pectin increased significantly if these dietary fibres were mixed with inulin. Inulin is known to stimulate butyrate-producing bacteria (*Roseburia intestinalis*, *Eubacterium rectale*, *Anaerostipes caccae*), which in turn leads to higher concentrations and proportions of butyrate [35].

The concentration of total SCFA, acetate, and butyrate produced in culture from the cincau extract was very similar to that produced when pectin or pectin-cellulose was added as the dietary fibre. Cellulose is a non-fermentable fibre and as a result has little effect on SCFA concentrations. Given that cincau extracts are known to contain 20% pectin [24], the increases in SCFA concentrations observed may be produced by the fermentation of the pectin component of this extract. However, when analysed these hot water extracts contained 5.8% soluble NSPs and 46.3% insoluble NSPs, thus it appears that the heating, cooling, and freeze drying process may have modified chemical and physical properties of the non-starch polysaccharides including pectin to form insoluble NSPs [36]. These now insoluble NSPs may also contribute to SCFA production during the in vitro fermentation.

SCFAs, and particularly butyrate, are well known for their ability to inhibit proliferation and induce apoptosis of colorectal cancer cells [2,3], but in this study high levels of butyrate in FS did not always affect cell viability. The butyrate content in pectin-inulin FS was nearly two-fold higher than pectin alone FS, while the propionate and acetate content from pectin-inulin FS was nearly double of pectin FS, however, the effect on Caco-2 cell growth when cultured in media containing these fermentation supernatants was no different. This indicates that butyrate or combinations of butyrate with propionate or acetate are not the main factors in fermentation supernatant that affect cell growth, and that non-SCFA compounds also contained in the FS may be involved [33]. Interestingly, cincau extract and pectin-cellulose FSs which had lower concentrations of total or individual SCFAs than pectin-inulin FS, inhibited Caco- 2 cell growth to the same extent as pectin-inulin FS.

Cell differentiation is one of the mechanisms by which SCFAs act in order to slow cancer cell growth [37]. This process requires cells to enter G1/G0 phase arrest, and cell proliferation is then inhibited [38]. Our results indicate that FS from pectin, inulin, pectin-cellulose mixture, pectin-inulin mixture, or cincau extract do not induce alkaline phosphatase, a marker of cell differentiation. Surprisingly, FS from blank (FB) induced higher alkaline phosphatase levels than pectin, inulin, or pectin-inulin, even though all of these dietary fibre FSs had high SCFA concentrations. There are some possibilities to explain these observations. First, the effect of butyrate on cell differentiation is dose dependent. It was previously observed that butyrate induced cell differentiation of Caco-2 cells at a concentration of 0.1 mM, but when the butyrate level was increased to 5 mM, activity of this enzyme decreased [39]. In the present study, the inulin and pectin-inulin FSs contained 37.7 and 24.2 mM of butyrate, respectively. When 20% of these FSs were added to the media, the final concentration of butyrate in the media would be 7.5 and 4.8 mM, respectively, whereas the final concentration of butyrate in media containing pectin, pectin-cellulose, and cincau was only 1.6, 1.4, and 1.1 mM, respectively. It is suggested that high levels of butyrate in inulin and pectin-inulin FSs may have led to the downregulation of AP activity. However, this explanation is not likely, as the blank (FB) which contains very little SCFA, elicited higher AP levels. Therefore, a second possibility needs to be considered to rationally explain the effects of FB. Previous researchers have also found that FB had an effect that was unexplainable by SCFA content in FS [16,33,40]. For example, Sauer et al. found that metabolic activity of HT-29 cells was increased by 15% by FB supplementation, with levels increasing similarly to those from inulin FS [16]. Moreover, these authors also found that FB enhanced gene expression of GSTA4, but inulin FS or SCFA mixture had no effects on this gene. GSTA4 is a gene encoding a glutathione S-transferase belonging to the alpha class 4 that has high catalytic efficiency with 4-hydroxyalkenals and other cytotoxic and mutagenic products of radical reactions and lipid peroxidation [41]. Taking this into account, data from this study indicate that the effect of FSs from dietary fibre on cell differentiation may depend on several factors including SCFA pattern and unidentified products formed during the fermentation process or that originally exist in the fresh faecal sample as a source of inoculums.

The ability of pectin, inulin, pectin-inulin, and pectin-cellulose FSs to induce apoptosis was confirmed by their ability to increase caspase 3/7 activity compared to control (Figure 4; $p < 0.05$). In contrast, cincau and FB, when compared to control, decreased levels of caspase 3/7. Previous research has shown that inulin induced apoptosis in HT-29 cells [42] or in a colon cancer rat model [43]. Our results support that inulin or pectin-inulin FSs are able to induce apoptosis through caspases, as caspase 3/7 activity increased in Caco-2 cells incubated with these FSs (Figure 4, $p < 0.05$).

Pectin or pectin-cellulose mixtures also increased caspase 3/7 activity (Figure 4, $p < 0.05$), and this may support a role for pectin via its increase in SCFAs as a dietary fibre that can affect the apoptosis process. Butyrate or other SCFAs produced by the fermentation of pectin may be able to inhibit histone deacetylase activity in order to induce gene transcription of caspase 3 and induce apoptosis [6,44–46].

Butyrate is the most potent SCFA for modulating colorectal cancer growth, including the induction of apoptosis [6,47]. However, our data indicate that modulation of apoptosis is not always dependant on butyrate content. The effect of FSs on caspase 3/7 activity was also unexplainable by total SCFA content of FS. Therefore, some factors other than SCFAs might be involved in modulating caspase 3/7 activity [23,42].

FSs from inulin, cincau, and FB were chosen to further elucidate the role of caspase 3/7 on cell death using the caspase inhibitor (Ac-DEVD-CHO) before the application of FS. LDH is an accurate method to assay cell death with membrane damage such as necrosis, while the MTT assay can measure differences in cell viability, but it cannot tell whether cells are being killed via apoptosis or necrosis [45]. The FS from inulin induced cell death through a caspase 3/7-dependent pathway, as the release of caspase 3/7 could be inhibited by the addition of the caspase inhibitor, and this led to an observed increase in Caco-2 cell viability. Cincau extract FS suppressed Caco-2 cell growth compared to FB (Figure 5C, $p < 0.05$), but the mechanism appeared to be different to that observed with inulin. Compared to FB, cincau did not induce caspase 3/7 activity (Figure 5A, $p < 0.05$), and indeed less LDH was released from cells treated with either cincau or cincau and caspase inhibitor (Figure 5B, $p < 0.05$), suggesting that cincau could protect cells from necrotic cell death. However, these cells were less viable than the control cells. Previously, Huang et al. [48] found that *Solanum nigrum* Linn leaf extract, rich in polyphenols and anthocyanidin, caused cell death due to the induction of autophagy and apoptosis. Acetone and ethyl acetate extracts from *Eupatorium odoratum* induced autophagic cell death in MCF-7 and Vero cell lines [49]. Cincau was extracted from green cincau leaves (*Premna oblongifolia* Merr.). The extract contains alkaloids, saponins, phenol hydroquinones, molisch, benedict, and tannins [50]. Supernatants collected after the non-digestible fraction of cooked common bean (*Phaseolus vulgaris* L.), when fermented with gut microbes, were able to induce apoptosis of HT-29 colon cells, and this was thought to be due to the participation of other phenolic fatty acid derivatives and biopeptides and not the SCFA contained in the supernates [51] Therefore, it may be possible that the phytochemical compounds from cincau or cincau fermentation induce autophagic cell death which cannot be measured by either the caspase or LDH assay, but would be worth investigating in future studies.

Our research implies that the beneficial effects of mixed dietary fibre as experienced in most human diets will depend on how each dietary fibre consumed interacts with the colon microbiota, and suggests the important role of unidentified compounds produced during fermentation by gut microbes in modulation of the effect of dietary fibre on CRC carcinogenesis. Furthermore, for the first time we show that Green cincau, a traditional Indonesian food, is not only able to inhibit colon cancer cell growth, but by an apoptosis-independent pathway. Further work should be conducted to assess the ability of this novel traditional dietary fibre as a chemopreventative.

Acknowledgments: This work was partially funded by an anonymous Philanthropic grant to Graeme P. Young (G.P.Y.) and by a Ph.D. scholarship from the Indonesian government to support Samsu U. Nurdin (S.U.N.). We would also like to thank Samsul Rizal from the University of Lampung, Indonesia for supplying the green cincau.

Author Contributions: S.U.N., R.K.L.L., G.P.Y., J.C.R.S. and C.A.A. all contributed to the design of this study. S.U.N. conducted all of the research and analysed all data. C.T.C. and R.K.L.L. helped S.U.N with setting up the in vitro fermentation and the SCFA measurements. S.U.N., R.K.L.L., G.P.Y. and C.A.A. contributed to the writing of the paper.

Conflicts of Interest: The authors declare no conflicts of interest.

References

1. Center, M.M.; Jemal, A.; Ward, E. International trends in colorectal cancer incidence rates. *Cancer Epidemiol. Biomarkers Prev.* **2009**, *18*, 1688–1694. [CrossRef] [PubMed]
2. Fung, K.Y.; Cosgrove, L.; Lockett, T.; Head, R.; Topping, D.L. A review of the potential mechanisms for the lowering of colorectal oncogenesis by butyrate. *Br. J. Nutr.* **2012**, *108*, 820–831. [CrossRef] [PubMed]
3. Encarnacao, J.C.; Abrantes, A.M.; Pires, A.S.; Botelho, M.F. Revisit dietary fiber on colorectal cancer: Butyrate and its role on prevention and treatment. *Cancer Metastasis Rev.* **2015**, *34*, 465–478. [CrossRef] [PubMed]
4. Scharlau, D.; Borowicki, A.; Habermann, N.; Hofmann, T.; Klenow, S.; Miene, C.; Munjal, U.; Stein, K.; Glei, M. Mechanisms of primary cancer prevention by butyrate and other products formed during gut flora-mediated fermentation of dietary fibre. *Mutat. Res.* **2009**, *682*, 39–53. [CrossRef] [PubMed]
5. Whitehead, R.H.; Young, G.P.; Bhathal, P.S. Effects of short chain fatty acids on a new human colon carcinoma cell line (lim1215). *Gut* **1986**, *27*, 1457–1463. [CrossRef] [PubMed]
6. Medina, V.; Edmonds, B.; Young, G.P.; James, R.; Appleton, S.; Zalewski, P.D. Induction of caspase-3 protease activity and apoptosis by butyrate and trichostatin a (inhibitors of histone deacetylase): Dependence on protein synthesis and synergy with a mitochondrial/cytochrome c-dependent pathway. *Cancer Res.* **1997**, *57*, 3697–3707. [PubMed]
7. Juskiewicz, J.; Zdunczyk, Z. Effects of cellulose, carboxymethylcellulose and inulin fed to rats as single supplements or in combinations on their caecal parameters. *Comp. Biochem. Phys. A* **2004**, *139*, 513–519. [CrossRef] [PubMed]
8. Pompei, A.; Cordisco, L.; Raimondi, S.; Amaretti, A.; Pagnoni, U.M.; Matteuzzi, D.; Rossi, M. In vitro comparison of the prebiotic effects of two inulin-type fructans. *Anaerobe* **2008**, *14*, 280–286. [CrossRef] [PubMed]
9. Nilsson, U.; Nyman, M.; Ahrne, S.; Sullivan, E.O.; Fitzgerald, G. Bifidobacterium lactis bb-12 and lactobacillus salivarius ucc500 modify carboxylic acid formation in the hindgut of rats given pectin, inulin, and lactitol. *J. Nutr.* **2006**, *136*, 2175–2180. [PubMed]
10. McIntyre, A.; Young, G.P.; Taranto, T.; Gibson, P.R.; Ward, P.B. Different fibers have different regional effects on luminal contents of rat colon. *Gastroenterology* **1991**, *101*, 1274–1281. [CrossRef]
11. Pluske, J.R.; Durmic, Z.; Pethick, D.W.; Mullan, B.P.; Hampson, D.J. Confirmation of the role of rapidly fermentable carbohydrates in the expression of swine dysentery in pigs after experimental infection. *J. Nutr.* **1998**, *128*, 1737–1744. [PubMed]
12. Henningsson, A.M.; Bjorck, I.M.; Nyman, E.M. Combinations of indigestible carbohydrates affect short-chain fatty acid formation in the hindgut of rats. *J. Nutr.* **2002**, *132*, 3098–3104. [PubMed]
13. Muir, J.G.; Yeow, E.G.; Keogh, J.; Pizzey, C.; Bird, A.R.; Sharpe, K.; O'Dea, K.; Macrae, F.A. Combining wheat bran with resistant starch has more beneficial effects on fecal indexes than does wheat bran alone. *Am. J. Clin. Nutr.* **2004**, *79*, 1020–1028. [PubMed]
14. Khan, K.M.; Edwards, C.A. In vitro fermentation characteristics of a mixture of raftilose and guar gum by human faecal bacteria. *Eur. J. Nutr.* **2005**, *44*, 371–376. [CrossRef] [PubMed]

15. Pool-Zobel, B.L. Inulin-type fructans and reduction in colon cancer risk: Review of experimental and human data. *Br. J. Nutr.* **2005**, *93*, S73–S90. [CrossRef] [PubMed]
16. Pool-Zobel, B.L.; Sauer, J. Overview of experimental data on reduction of colorectal cancer risk by inulin-type fructans. *J. Nutr.* **2007**, *137*, 2580s–2584s. [PubMed]
17. Qamar, T.R.; Syed, F.; Nasir, M.; Rehman, H.; Zahid, M.N.; Liu, R.H.; Iqbal, S. Novel combination of prebiotics galacto-oligosaccharides and inulin-inhibited aberrant crypt foci formation and biomarkers of colon cancer in wistar rats. *Nutrients* **2016**, *8*. [CrossRef] [PubMed]
18. Wu, W.T.; Yang, L.C.; Chen, H.L. Effects of konjac glucomannan, inulin and cellulose on acute colonic responses to genotoxic azoxymethane. *Food Chem.* **2014**, *155*, 304–310. [CrossRef] [PubMed]
19. Dias, M.C.; Vieiralves, N.F.; Gomes, M.I.; Salvadori, D.M.; Rodrigues, M.A.; Barbisan, L.F. Effects of lycopene, synbiotic and their association on early biomarkers of rat colon carcinogenesis. *Food Chem. Toxicol.* **2010**, *48*, 772–780. [CrossRef] [PubMed]
20. Wu, W.T.; Chen, H.L. Effects of konjac glucomannan on putative risk factors for colon carcinogenesis in rats fed a high-fat diet. *J. Agric. Food Chem.* **2011**, *59*, 989–994. [CrossRef] [PubMed]
21. Bertkova, I.; Hijova, E.; Chmelarova, A.; Mojzisova, G.; Petrasova, D.; Strojny, L.; Bomba, A.; Zitnan, R. The effect of probiotic microorganisms and bioactive compounds on chemically induced carcinogenesis in rats. *Neoplasma* **2010**, *57*, 422–428. [CrossRef] [PubMed]
22. Rao, C.V.; Chou, D.; Simi, B.; Ku, H.; Reddy, B.S. Prevention of colonic aberrant crypt foci and modulation of large bowel microbial activity by dietary coffee fiber, inulin and pectin. *Carcinogenesis* **1998**, *19*, 1815–1819. [CrossRef] [PubMed]
23. Waldecker, M.; Kautenburger, T.; Daumann, H.; Veeriah, S.; Will, F.; Dietrich, H.; Pool-Zobel, B.L.; Schrenk, D. Histone-deacetylase inhibition and butyrate formation: Fecal slurry incubations with apple pectin and apple juice extracts. *Nutrition* **2008**, *24*, 366–374. [CrossRef] [PubMed]
24. Nurdin, S.U.; Zuidar, S.A.; Suharyono. Dried extract from green cincau leaves as potential fibre sources for food enrichment. *Afr. Crop. Sci. J.* **2005**, *7*, 655–658.
25. Nurdin, S.U.; Hwang, J.K.; Hung, P. Effect of green cincau leaf (*Premna oblongifolia* merr.) water extracts on cytokines production in whole cell culture of mouse splenocytes. *Indo Food Nutr. Prog.* **2003**, *10*, 70–74.
26. Nurdin, S.U. Evaluation of laxative effect and fermentability of gel forming component of green cincau leaves (*Premna oblongifolia* merr.). *Teknologi dan Industri Pangan* **2007**, *18*, 10–16.
27. Belobrajdic, D.P.; Hino, S.; Kondo, T.; Jobling, S.A.; Morell, M.K.; Topping, D.L.; Morita, T.; Bird, A.R. High wholegrain barley beta-glucan lowers food intake but does not alter small intestinal macronutrient digestibility in ileorectostomised rats. *Int. J. Food Sci. Nutr.* **2016**, *67*, 678–685. [CrossRef] [PubMed]
28. Association of Official Analytical Chemists (AOAC). *Official Methods of Analysis, Method 994.13, Supplement Total Dietary Fibre (Determined as Neutral Sugar Residues, Uronic Acid Residues and Klason Lignin)*; AOAC: Arlington, VA, USA, 1995.
29. Charoensiddhi, S.; Conlon, M.A.; Vuaran, M.S.; Franco, C.M.M.; Zhang, W. Impact of extraction processes on prebiotic potential of the brown seaweed ecklonia radiata by in vitro human gut bacteria fermentation. *J. Funct. Foods* **2016**, *24*, 221–230. [CrossRef]
30. Zhou, Z.; Cao, X.; Zhou, J.Y.H. Effect of resistant starch structure on short-chain fatty acids production by human gut microbiota fermentation in vitro. *Starch Stärke* **2013**, *65*, 509–516. [CrossRef]
31. Le Leu, R.K.; Brown, I.L.; Hu, Y.; Bird, A.R.; Jackson, M.; Esterman, A.; Young, G.P. A synbiotic combination of resistant starch and bifidobacterium lactis facilitates apoptotic deletion of carcinogen-damaged cells in rat colon. *J. Nutr.* **2005**, *135*, 996–1001. [PubMed]
32. Young, F.M.; Phungtamdet, W.; Sanderson, B.J. Modification of mtt assay conditions to examine the cytotoxic effects of amitraz on the human lymphoblastoid cell line, wil2ns. *Toxicol. In Vitro* **2005**, *19*, 1051–1059. [CrossRef] [PubMed]
33. Beyer-Sehlmeyer, G.; Glei, M.; Hartmann, E.; Hughes, R.; Persin, C.; Bohm, V.; Rowland, I.; Schubert, R.; Jahreis, G.; Pool-Zobel, B.L. Butyrate is only one of several growth inhibitors produced during gut flora-mediated fermentation of dietary fibre sources. *Br. J. Nutr.* **2003**, *90*, 1057–1070. [CrossRef] [PubMed]
34. Matsumoto, H.; Erickson, R.H.; Gum, J.R.; Yoshioka, M.; Gum, E.; Kim, Y.S. Biosynthesis of alkaline-phosphatase during differentiation of the human colon cancer cell-line caco-2. *Gastroenterology* **1990**, *98*, 1199–1207. [CrossRef]

35. Van den Abbeele, P.; Gerard, P.; Rabot, S.; Bruneau, A.; El Aidy, S.; Derrien, M.; Kleerebezem, M.; Zoetendal, E.G.; Smidt, H.; Verstraete, W.; et al. Arabinoxylans and inulin differentially modulate the mucosal and luminal gut microbiota and mucin-degradation in humanized rats. *Environ. Microbiol.* **2011**, *13*, 2667–2680. [CrossRef] [PubMed]
36. Lovegrove, A.; Edwards, C.H.; De Noni, I.; Patel, H.; El, S.N.; Grassby, T.; Zielke, C.; Ulmius, M.; Nilsson, L.; Butterworth, P.J.; et al. Role of polysaccharides in food, digestion, and health. *Crit. Rev. Food Sci. Nutr.* **2017**, *57*, 237–253. [CrossRef] [PubMed]
37. Lanneau, D.; de Thonel, A.; Maurel, S.; Didelot, C.; Garrido, C. Apoptosis versus cell differentiation: Role of heat shock proteins hsp90, hsp70 and hsp27. *Prion* **2007**, *1*, 53–60. [CrossRef] [PubMed]
38. Ding, Q.M.; Ko, T.C.; Evers, B.M. Caco-2 intestinal cell differentiation is associated with g(1) arrest and suppression of cdk2 and cdk4. *Am. J. Physiol.* **1998**, *275*, C1193–C1200. [PubMed]
39. Orchel, A.; Dzierzewicz, Z.; Parfiniewicz, B.; Weglarz, L.; Wilczok, T. Butyrate-induced differentiation of colon cancer cells is pkc and jnk dependent. *Dig. Dis. Sci.* **2005**, *50*, 490–498. [CrossRef] [PubMed]
40. Kiefer, J.; Beyer-Sehlmeyer, G.; Pool-Zobel, B.L. Mixtures of scfa, composed according to physiologically available concentrations in the gut lumen, modulate histone acetylation in human ht29 colon cancer cells. *Br. J. Nutr.* **2006**, *96*, 803–810. [CrossRef] [PubMed]
41. Hubatsch, I.; Ridderstrom, M.; Mannervik, B. Human glutathione transferase a4-4: An alpha class enzyme with high catalytic efficiency in the conjugation of 4-hydroxynonenal and other genotoxic products of lipid peroxidation. *Biochem. J.* **1998**, *330 Pt 1*, 175–179. [CrossRef] [PubMed]
42. Munjal, U.; Glei, M.; Pool-Zobel, B.L.; Scharlau, D. Fermentation products of inulin-type fructans reduce proliferation and induce apoptosis in human colon tumour cells of different stages of carcinogenesis. *Br. J. Nutr.* **2009**, *102*, 663–671. [CrossRef] [PubMed]
43. Hughes, R.; Rowland, I.R. Stimulation of apoptosis by two prebiotic chicory fructans in the rat colon. *Carcinogenesis* **2001**, *22*, 43–47. [CrossRef] [PubMed]
44. Anh, T.D.; Ahn, M.Y.; Kim, S.A.; Yoon, J.H.; Ahn, S.G. The histone deacetylase inhibitor, trichostatin a, induces g2/m phase arrest and apoptosis in yd-10b oral squamous carcinoma cells. *Oncol. Rep.* **2012**, *27*, 455–460. [PubMed]
45. Hwang, J.J.; Kim, Y.S.; Kim, M.J.; Jang, S.J.; Lee, J.H.; Choi, J.; Ro, S.; Hyun, Y.L.; Lee, J.S.; Kim, C.S. A novel histone deacetylase inhibitor, cg0006, induces cell death through both extrinsic and intrinsic apoptotic pathways. *Anti-Cancer Drug* **2009**, *20*, 815–821. [CrossRef] [PubMed]
46. Wallace, D.M.; Donovan, M.; Cotter, T.G. Histone deacetylase activity regulates apaf-1 and caspase 3 expression in the developing mouse retina. *Investig. Ophth. Vis. Sci.* **2006**, *47*, 2765–2772. [CrossRef] [PubMed]
47. Matthews, G.M.; Howarth, G.S.; Butler, R.N. Short-chain fatty acids induce apoptosis in colon cancer cells associated with changes to intracellular redox state and glucose metabolism. *Chemotherapy* **2012**, *58*, 102–109. [CrossRef] [PubMed]
48. Huang, H.C.; Syu, K.Y.; Lin, J.K. Chemical composition of solanum nigrum linn extract and induction of autophagy by leaf water extract and its major flavonoids in au565 breast cancer cells. *J. Agric. Food Chem.* **2010**, *58*, 8699–8708. [CrossRef] [PubMed]
49. Harun, F.B.; Jamalullail, S.M.S.S.; Yin, K.B.; Othman, Z.; Tilwari, A.; Balaram, P. Autophagic cell death is induced by acetone and ethyl acetate extracts from eupatorium odoratum in vitro: Effects on mcf-7 and vero cell lines. *Sci. World J.* **2012**, *2012*, 1–9. [CrossRef] [PubMed]
50. Aryudhani, N. Mechanism of Antitumor Activity of Powdered Leaf Green Grass Jelly (*Premna blongifolia* merr.) in Mice Transplanted c3h Breast Tumor Cells. Master's Thesis, Bogor Agricultural University, Bogor, Indonesia, 2011.
51. Cruz-Bravo, R.K.; Guevara-Gonzalez, R.G.; Ramos-Gomez, M.; Oomah, B.D.; Wiersma, P.; Campos-Vega, R.; Loarca-Pina, G. The fermented non-digestible fraction of common bean (*Phaseolus vulgaris* L.) triggers cell cycle arrest and apoptosis in human colon adenocarcinoma cells. *Genes Nutr.* **2014**, *9*, 359. [CrossRef] [PubMed]

nutrients

MDPI

Article

Short- and Long-Term Effects of Wholegrain Oat Intake on Weight Management and Glucolipid Metabolism in Overweight Type-2 Diabetics: A Randomized Control Trial

Xue Li [1,2], Xiaxia Cai [1,3], Xiaotao Ma [1,4], Lulu Jing [1], Jiaojiao Gu [1], Lei Bao [1,5], Jun Li [6], Meihong Xu [1], Zhaofeng Zhang [1] and Yong Li [1,*]

1 Department of Nutrition and Food Hygiene, School of Public Health, Peking University, Beijing 100191, China; xue.li@ed.ac.uk (X.L.); shuiruoran8886@126.com (X.C.); maxt2008@sina.com (X.M.); jingll_wit@bjmu.edu.cn (L.J.); jiaojiaogu442@gmail.com (J.G.); baolei6230@163.com (L.B.); xumeihong@bjmu.edu.cn (M.X.); zzfeng1104@bjmu.edu.cn (Z.Z.)
2 Centre for Population Health Sciences, University of Edinburgh, Edinburgh EH8 9AG, UK
3 Department of Nutrition and Food Hygiene, School of Public Health, Capital Medical University, Beijing 100191, China
4 Department of Clinical Nutrition, China-Japan Friendship Hospital, Peking University, Beijing 100191, China
5 Department of Clinical Nutrition, International Hospital, Peking University, Beijing 100191, China
6 The 153 Hospital of People's Liberation Army, Zhengzhou 450001, China; pla153ywc@163.com
* Correspondence: liyongbmu@163.com; Tel./Fax: +86-10-8280-1177

Received: 21 June 2016; Accepted: 1 September 2016; Published: 7 September 2016

Abstract: Glycemic control and weight reduction are primary goals for the management of overweight and obese type 2 diabetes mellitus (T2DM). Effective management cannot be achieved without an appropriate diet. Our study aimed to evaluate the short- and long-term effects of oat intake and develop a reasonable dietary plan for overweight T2DM patients. A randomized control trial, registered under ClinicalTrials.gov (Identification code: NCT01495052), was carried out among adult T2DM patients. A subgroup of 298 overweight subjects was selected and received a 30-day centralized intervention and 1-year free-living follow-up. Participants were randomly allocated to one of the following four groups. The usual care group (n = 60) received no intervention; the healthy diet group (n = 79) received a low-fat and high-fiber diet ("healthy diet"); the 50 g-oats group (n = 80) and 100 g-oats group (n = 79) received the "healthy diet" with the same amount of cereals replaced by 50 g and 100 g oats respectively. Anthropometric, blood glycemic and lipid variables were measured. For the 30-day intervention, significant differences in the changes of FPG (fasting plasma glucose), PPG (postprandial plasma glucose), HbA1c (glycosylated hemoglobin), HOMA-IR (homeostasis model assessment of insulin resistance), TC (total cholesterol), TG (total triglycerides), and LDL-c (low-density lipoprotein cholesterol) were observed among the four groups. Compared to the healthy diet group, the 50 g-oats group had a bigger reduction in PPG (mean difference (MD): −1.04 mmol/L; 95% CI: −2.03, −0.05) and TC (MD: −0.24 mmol/L; 95% CI: −0.47, −0.01); the 100 g-oats group had a bigger reduction in PPG (MD: −1.48 mmol/L; 95% CI: −2.57, −0.39), HOMA-IR (MD: −1.77 mU·mol/L^2; 95% CI: −3.49, −0.05), TC (MD: −0.33 mmol/L; 95% CI: −0.56, −0.10) and LDL-c (MD: −0.22 mmol/L; 95% CI: −0.41, −0.03). In the 1-year follow-up, greater effects in reducing weight (MD: −0.89 kg; 95% CI: −1.56, −0.22), HbA1c (MD: −0.64%; 95% CI: −1.19, −0.09) and TG (MD: −0.70 mmol/L; 95% CI: −1.11, −0.29) were observed in the 100 g-oats group. In conclusion, short- and long-term oat intake had significant effects on controlling hyperglycemia, lowering blood lipid and reducing weight. Our study provided some supportive evidence for recommending oat as a good whole grain selection for overweight diabetics.

Keywords: type 2 diabetes; obesity; whole grain; oats; fiber

1. Introduction

Type 2 diabetes (T2DM) and obesity are both major global health problems, which have been linked with an increased risk of life-threatening comorbidities and enormous economic burdens [1,2]. Epidemiological studies report that most of the patients with T2DM are overweight or obese and, similarly, a significant number of obese individuals have diabetes [3]. This parallel prevalence indicates a strong association between T2DM and obesity. It has been further estimated that every 1 kilogram increase in body weight is associated with a 9% relative increase in diabetes prevalence [4]. Identification of this association has changed the primary goal of diabetes management in obese and overweight T2DM patients, and now controlling the blood glucose and reducing weight are both promoted [5].

Effective management of diabetes cannot be achieved without an appropriate diet, especially for type 2 diabetics who are overweight or obese. The recommended diet for controlling diabetes should be rich in dietary fiber, preferably provided by nature and less processed whole grains [6]. A Harvard study of health professionals found that high intake of whole grains was associated with lower incidence of T2DM [7] and therefore its benefit could be an important part of a diet which can help to improve diabetic control.

Wholegrain foods can be found in a variety of cereals, but the content and solubility of fiber can vary significantly [8]. People with diabetes are often advised to select a good source of whole grains. Oat, with the advantage of having a high concentration of β-glucan, can be used for the management of diabetes [9]. The effects of oat intake have been investigated in several aspects [10–12]. Soluble fiber from oats has been found to be effective in lowering total cholesterol and low-density lipoprotein (5%–10% reduction with 3 g β-glucan intake per day), and thus oat and oat-products have already been recommended to patients with hyperlipidemia [13]. Besides, it has been suggested that oat intake can improve insulin response and decrease postprandial hyperglycemia [11,14]. Although these effects have been supported in many studies, others failed to replicate these. In particular, the effects of oat intake on fasting glucose concentration and weight control remain conflicting [11,14]. Therefore, further work is needed to determine whether oat intake has the reported benefits and whether these benefits could be observed similarly in specific populations, particularly in overweight T2DM patients.

To develop a reasonable dietary plan, which includes wholegrain oats, a randomized control trail was conducted among adults with T2DM in Baotou, Inner Mongolia, China. This study aimed to compare the short- and long-term integrative effects of oat intake with a low-fat and high-fiber diet ("healthy diet") on weight management, blood glucose control and lipid-profile improvement in overweight T2DM patients.

2. Methods

2.1. Participants

A subgroup of 298 subjects, meeting the Chinese criteria of overweight (body mass index $\geq$ 24 kg/m^2), was selected from 445 adult patients with T2DM, who had participated in the 30-day centralized management of a dietary program and the 1-year free-living follow-up in Baotou, China. The sample size of the original study was calculated based on an estimated standard deviation (SD) of 2.7 mmol/L in HbA1c. A total of 420 participants were required to detect a difference of 0.80 SD of HbA1c with 90% power and allowing for 10% missing data. Individuals who were heavy smokers (smoking more than or equal to 25 cigarettes per day) or heavy drinkers (drinking more than 25 mL alcohol per day), or had recent changes (less than 3 months) in diet and physical activities, or had severe cardiovascular, renal or hepatic complications, mental illness or other serious diseases, or recently accepted glucocorticoid treatment, or had already been eating oats or oat products as part of their diet, were excluded. At the end of recruitment, a total of 445 individuals were included and randomized, of which 298 overweight participants were selected for this subgroup analysis.

Eleven patients dropped out during the 1-year follow-up due to personal reasons with no difference in drop-out rates among the four groups (p = 0.774) (Figure 1).

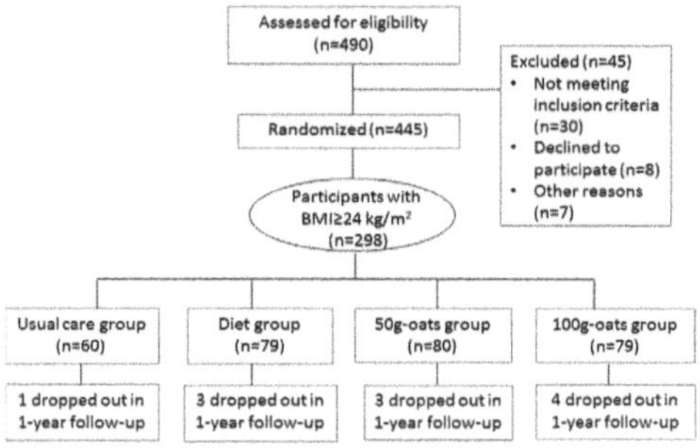

Figure 1. Flow chart for subject enrollment, allocation, intervention and follow-up.

2.2. Ethics

This study was approved by the ethic review board of China-Japan Friendship Hospital of Health Ministry China in December 2011 and registered under ClinicalTrials.gov (Identification code: NCT01495052 available at https://clinicaltrials.gov/). Written and oral information of the study protocol was given prior to the study initiation. Informed consent was signed by every participant.

2.3. Study Design

During the 30-day centralized intervention, all participants were arranged to live in a hotel and have meals together under the supervision of 12 qualified dietitians and 18 well trained investigators. Food intake and compliance of participants were recorded every day by the investigators. Physical activities were assessed and categorized using the recommendations of the international physical activity questionnaire (IPAQ). Participants were required to record uncomfortable symptoms and maintain their normal physical activities and medications. After a one-week run-in period, participants were randomly allocated to one of the following four groups by computer-generated random numbers. The usual care group (n = 60) served as the control group and received no dietry intervention. They took meals depending on their own eating habits. The healthy diet group (n = 79) received a low-fat and high-fiber diet ("healthy diet"). A 7-day cyclical menu (Supplementary Materials Table S1) was designed according to the China Food Composition [15], the Dietary Guidelines for Chinese Resident [16] and the China Medical Nutrition Therapy Guideline for Diabetes [17] to provide a low-fat and high-fiber diet. Each participant was provided with three meals a day, which contained 2275 kcal for men and 1890 kcal for women (60% from carbohydrate, 22% from fat, 18% from protein) and 30 g of dietary fiber. In addition, a maximum of an extra 10% of daily kcal intake was allowed according to the individual need of participants. For the 50 g and 100 g-oats groups, participants received the "healthy diet" with the same amount of cereals replaced by 50 g and 100 g of wholegrain oats respectively. The daily intake of energy and macronutrients for each group is shown in Table 1. Apart from the dietary intervention, the study dieticians gave nutritional education and training to the three intervention groups six times per week to encourage the participants to have a general healthy diet in daily life.

After the centralized management, all participants returned home and were asked to continue with their intervention and record their daily diet, uncomfortable symptoms and medication changes. Wholegrain oats were continuously provided for the 50 g and 100 g-oats groups. Investigators continued to give diet recommendations and supervise the daily life of participants by monthly group interviews through network-chat, telephone or face-to-face interviews. Scheduled clinical checks were performed every three months. The follow-up lasted for one year.

Table 1. The daily intake of energy and macronutrients (one day's intake).

Dietary Components	Usual Care Group	Treatment Diet		
		Healthy Diet Group	50 g-oats Group	100 g-oats Group
Energy (kcal) *	2441 (478)	2279 (196)	2281 (185)	2233 (204)
Carbohydrate (% of total energy)	50	60	59	58
Fat (% of total energy)	31	22	23	23
Protein (% of total energy)	19	18	18	19
Total fiber (g) *	22.1 (4.0)	33.0 (5.8)	36.1 (4.2)	39.0 (4.8)
Oat β-glucan (g)	0	0	2.65	5.30

* Variables are presented as mean with (SD (standard deviation)).

2.4. Wholegrain Oats

The wholegrain oats used in this study were provided by Inner Mongolia Sanzhuliang Natural Oats Industry Corporation (IMSNOIC) (Hohhot, Inner Mongolia, China). The oats were grown in northwest China and were processed by a peeling technology which retained the necessary ingredients and beneficial nutrients of the whole grain [18]. The nutrient composition of this product was analyzed by the laboratory of the School of Life Sciences, Sun Yat-sen University, according to a standard procedure (GB/T 5009). Each 100 g of wholegrain oats contained 63.5 g carbohydrate, 7.6 g fat, 13.7 g protein, and 8.7 g fiber, of which approximately 5.3 g was β-glucan.

2.5. Outcome Measurement

Physical examinations were performed at baseline, at the end of the 30-day intervention and at the end of the 1-year follow-up. Anthropometric measurements were carried out for weight, height, waist and hip circumference, and blood pressure. Body fat percent and visceral fat index (VFI) were measured using bioelectrical impedance scales (Tanita BF-622W, Tanita Corporation of the United State). Venus blood samples were collected after an overnight fast for testing fasting plasma glucose (FPG), 2-h postprandial plasma glucose (PPG), glycosylated hemoglobin (HbA1c), fasting plasma insulin, 2-h postprandial plasma insulin, total triglycerides (TG), total cholesterol (TC), low-density lipoprotein cholesterol (LDL-c), and high-density lipoprotein cholesterol (HDL-c). Insulin resistance was calculated by the formula: HOMA-IR = fasting serum insulin (μU/mL) × FPG (mmol/L)/22.5. All measurements were conducted with standard procedures by the same clinical staff in the third hospital of Inner Mongolia medical college, who were blinded to the group allocation.

2.6. Statistical Analyses

Categorical and continuous variables were analyzed by either Chi-squared test or sample *t*-test. Responses to interventions were assessed by the changes in anthropometric and metabolic variables, determined at baseline and at the end of the intervention. A generalized linear model (GLM) was applied to estimate the changes after adjusting for potential confounding factors including sex, age, drinking, smoking, physical activity level, education level, family history of diabetes, diabetic medications and the duration of diabetes. The mean differences (MD) of changes among groups were calculated to compare the effects of different interventions. We performed multiple imputations to account for missing data (SAS Institute, Inc., Cary, NC, USA). Results are presented as means with standard deviation (SD) or 95% confidence intervals (95% CI). All tests were two-sided and $p < 0.05$ was considered to be statistically significant. Analyses were conducted with the IBM SPSS Statistics 22 (IBM Corp., Armonk, NY, USA, 2013), unless otherwise stated.

3. Results

The main characteristics of the participants in each group are shown in Table 2. Among the four groups, there were no significant differences in the baseline characteristics of sex, age, drinking, smoking, physical activity, education level, the duration of diabetes, family history of diabetes, diabetic medications and blood pressure.

Table 2. The baseline characteristics of the study participants *.

Variables	Usual Care Group (n = 60)	Healthy Diet Group (n = 79)	50 g-oats Group (n = 80)	100 g-oats Group (n = 79)	p-Value
Male/female	39/21	42/37	41/39	33/46	0.059
Age (years)	59.00 (3.94)	59.73 (6.53)	59.72 (6.10)	59.44 (6.78)	0.886
Mild drinking	15 (25.0%)	20 (25.3%)	17 (21.3%)	16 (20.3%)	0.838
Mild smoking	14 (23.3%)	16 (20.3%)	14 (17.5%)	11 (13.9%)	0.523
Physical activity level	-	-	-	-	0.541
Low	13 (21.7%)	18 (22.8%)	17 (21.2%)	22 (27.8%)	-
Moderate	30 (50.0%)	42 (53.1%)	45 (56.3%)	46 (58.2%)	-
High	17 (28.3%)	19 (24.1%)	18 (22.5%)	11 (13.9%)	-
Education level	-	-	-	-	0.473
Less than primary school	9 (15.0%)	9 (11.4%)	15 (18.8%)	8 (10.1%)	-
Middle and high school	39 (65.0%)	56 (70.9%)	47 (58.8%)	49 (62.0%)	-
College or more	12 (20.0%)	14 (17.7%)	18 (22.5%)	22 (27.8%)	-
Duration of diabetes (month)	79.00 (36.52)	74.87 (61.92)	100.08 (75.73)	94.71 (76.63)	0.060
Family history of diabetes	19 (31.7%)	24 (30.4%)	36 (45.0%)	38 (48.1%)	0.051
Diabetic medications	-	-	-	-	0.999
No diabetic medication	5 (8.3%)	7 (8.9%)	6 (7.5%)	6 (7.6%)	-
Oral diabetic medication	32 (53.3%)	45 (57.0%)	43 (53.8%)	47 (59.5%)	-
Insulin injection	12 (20.0%)	14 (17.7%)	16 (20.0%)	12 (15.2%)	-
Combined treatment	11 (18.3%)	13 (16.4%)	15 (18.7%)	14(17.7%)	-
Systolic blood pressure (mmHg)	143.71 (15.83)	147.23 (21.31)	144.90 (19.18)	147.19 (17.68)	0.613
Diastolic blood pressure (mmHg)	84.43 (16.05)	84.63 (11.78)	82.93 (9.39)	83.10 (10.20)	0.737

* Continuous variables are presented as mean with (SD) and categorical variables are presented as a number (with percentage).

Changes in variables, and the mean differences of changes among the four groups after the 30-day intervention, are presented in Table 3. When compared to the baseline values of the anthropometric variables, the three intervention groups had a significant reduction in weight, BMI and waist circumference, while significant reduction in visceral fat index (VFI) was only observed in the 50 g oats group (adjusted change: −0.48; 95% CI: −0.69, −0.27) and the 100 g oats group (adjusted change: −0.44; 95% CI: −0.78, −0.10). When comparing the mean differences between groups, there were no statistically significant differences in the changes of anthropometric variables between the healthy diet group and the oats groups.

For the glycemic variables, a significant reduction in FPG, PPG and HbA1c from baseline was observed in the three intervention groups, while a significant decrease in HOMA-IR was observed in 50 g oats group (adjusted change: −1.80 mU·mol/L^2; 95% CI: −3.48, −0.12) and 100 g oats group (adjusted change: −2.65 mU·mol/L^2; 95% CI: −4.72, −0.58). When comparing the changes between groups (the healthy diet group was the reference), the 50 g oats group showed a bigger reduction in PPG (MD: −1.04 mmol/L; 95% CI: −2.03, −0.05), and the 100 g oats group showed a bigger reduction in PPG (MD: −1.48 mmol/L; 95% CI: −2.57, −0.39) and HOMA-IR (MD: −1.77 mU·mol/L^2; 95% CI: −3.49, −0.05).

Compared to the baseline values of the lipid variables, the three intervention groups had a significant reduction in TC and LDL-c. When comparing between groups, the 50 g oats group had a bigger reduction in TC (MD: −0.24 mmol/L; 95% CI: −0.47, −0.01) and the 100 g oats group had a bigger reduction in TC (MD: −0.33 mmol/L; 95% CI: −0.56, −0.10) and LDL-c (MD: −0.22 mmol/L; 95% CI: −0.41, −0.03) than the healthy diet group. For TG, no statistically significant difference in the reduction was observed in the two oats groups when compared to the healthy diet group.

The changes and mean differences of changes in variables between the baseline and the end of the 1-year intervention are shown in Table 4. Compared with the baseline values, the three intervention groups had significant reduction in FPG, PPG, HbA1c, TC, and LDL-c, while the significant decrease in weight, BMI and TG was only observed in the 50 g and 100 g oats groups. Comparing the oats groups to the healthy diet group, the 50 g oats group had a bigger reduction in TG (MD: −0.42 mmol/L; 95% CI: −0.83, −0.01) and LDL-c (MD: −0.27 mmol/L; 95% CI: −0.49, −0.05), and the 100 g oats group had a bigger reduction in weight (MD: −0.89 kg; 95% CI: −1.56, −0.22), PPG (MD: −1.17 mmol/L; 95% CI: −2.27, −0.07), HbA1c (MD: −0.64%; 95% CI: −1.19, −0.09), TC (MD: −0.30 mmol/L; 95% CI: −0.57, −0.03), TG (MD: −0.70 mmol/L; 95% CI: −1.11, −0.29), and LDL-c (MD: −0.37 mmol/L; 95% CI: −0.59, −0.15).

Table 3. Changes in variables and mean differences (MD) in changes among groups after 30-day intervention *.

Variables	Usual Care Group (*n* = 60)	Healthy Diet Group (*n* = 79)	50 g-oats Group (*n* = 80)	100 g-oats Group (*n* = 79)	*p*-Value
Weight (kg)					
Baseline	71.54 (5.82)	73.77 (8.58)	72.60 (8.67)	74.44 (7.63)	0.141
30-day intervention	71.45 (6.00)	72.59 (7.94)	71.74 (8.50)	72.70 (7.21)	-
Adjusted changes	−0.18 (−1.39, 1.02)	−1.20 (−2.22, −0.19)	−1.67(−2.69, −0.65)	−1.74 (−2.76, −0.71)	0.178
MD (vs. usual care group)	-	−1.02 (−2.56, 0.52)	−1.49 (−3.03, 0.05)	−1.56 (−3.14, 0.02)	-
MD (vs. diet group)	-	-	−0.47 (−1.89, 0.96)	−0.54 (−1.97, 0.89)	-
BMI (kg/m^2)					
Baseline	25.17 (0.89)	27.19 (2.82)	26.91 (2.69)	27.39 (2.42)	0.000
30-day intervention	25.14 (0.94)	26.77 (2.66)	26.28 (3.86)	26.77 (2.33)	-
Adjusted changes	−0.08 (−0.49, 0.33)	−0.43 (−0.78, −0.08)	−0.60(−0.95, −0.25)	−0.63 (−0.98, −0.28)	0.160
MD (vs. usual care group)	-	−0.35 (−0.88, 0.18)	−0.52 (−1.05, 0.01)	−0.55 (−1.10, 0.00)	-
MD (vs. diet group)	-	-	−0.17 (−0.66, 0.32)	−0.20 (−0.69, 0.29)	-
Waist circumference (cm)					
Baseline	92.69 (7.94)	94.81 (7.01)	93.38 (6.79)	94.86 (7.65)	0.210
30-day intervention	91.92 (8.22)	92.02 (8.63)	91.08 (3.98)	92.07 (7.27)	-
Adjusted changes	−0.78 (−2.92, 1.36)	−2.79 (−3.85, −1.73)	−2.32 (−3.37, −1.27)	−2.77 (−3.83, −1.70)	0.028
MD (vs. usual care group)	-	−2.01 (−3.54, −0.48)	−1.54 (−3.08, 0.00)	−1.99 (−3.48, −0.50)	-
MD (vs. diet group)	-	-	0.47 (−1.01, 1.95)	0.02 (−1.47, 1.50)	-
Waist-to-hip ratio(WHR)					
Baseline	0.91 (0.05)	0.92 (0.05)	0.91 (0.05)	0.92 (0.05)	0.398
30-day intervention	0.90 (0.05)	0.91(0.07)	0.90 (0.05)	0.90 (0.05)	-
Adjusted changes	−0.01(−0.02, 0.01)	−0.01 (−0.02, 0.01)	−0.01 (−0.02, 0.01)	−0.02 (−0.03, −0.01)	0.259
MD (vs. usual care group)	-	0.00 (−0.02, 0.02)	0.00 (−0.02, 0.02)	−0.01 (−0.03, 0.01)	-
MD (vs. diet group)	-	-	0.00 (−0.02, 0.02)	0.00 (−0.02, 0.02)	-
Body fat percent (%)					
Baseline	32.46 (5.49)	31.58 (6.11)	31.54 (5.87)	33.31 (5.12)	0.162
30-day intervention	32.21 (5.88)	31.05 (6.23)	31.37 (5.75)	32.78 (5.34)	-
Adjusted changes	−0.25 (−1.09, 0.59)	−0.59 (−1.20, 0.02)	−0.52 (−1.12, 0.08)	−0.52 (−1.13, 0.08)	0.878
MD (vs. usual care group)	-	−0.34 (−1.06, 0.36)	−0.27 (−0.85, 0.31)	−0.27 (−0.81, 0.26)	-
MD (vs. diet group)	-	-	0.07 (−0.51, 0.65)	0.07 (−0.51, 0.65)	-
Visceral fat index (VFI)					
Baseline	12.37 (3.64)	12.38 (3.86)	12.53 (4.14)	12.33 (3.59)	0.988
30-day intervention	12.13 (3.77)	12.13 (3.53)	12.06 (4.42)	11.87 (3.47)	-
Adjusted changes	−0.25 (−0.55, 0.05)	−0.27 (−0.62, 0.07)	−0.48 (−0.69, −0.27)	−0.44 (−0.78, −0.10)	0.380

Table 3. *Cont.*

Variables	Usual Care Group (n = 60)	Healthy Diet Group (n = 79)	50 g-oats Group (n = 80)	100 g-oats Group (n = 79)	p-Value
MD (vs. usual care group)	-	−0.02 (−0.44, 0.40)	−0.24 (−0.74, 0.26)	−0.19 (−0.73, 0.35)	-
MD (vs. diet group)	-	-	−0.22 (−0.70, 0.27)	−0.17 (−0.64, 0.31)	-
Fasting plasma glucose (mmol/L)					
Baseline	9.38 (2.81)	9.52 (2.87)	9.87 (2.83)	9.70 (3.30)	0.719
30-day intervention	9.40 (0.75)	8.16 (2.53)	8.67 (2.49)	8.03 (2.56)	-
Adjusted changes	−0.20 (−0.91, 0.52)	−1.27 (−1.88, −0.67)	−1.23 (−1.84, −0.62)	−1.70 (−2.31, −1.10)	0.002
MD (vs. usual care group)	-	−1.07 (−1.99, −0.15)	−1.03 (−1.94, −0.11)	−1.50 (−2.42, −0.58)	-
MD (vs. diet group)	-	-	0.04 (−0.81, 0.89)	−0.43 (−1.28, 0.42)	-
2-h postprandial plasma glucose (mmol/L)					
Baseline	19.10 (3.22)	17.58 (4.87)	18.23 (4.84)	17.89 (5.45)	0.284
30-day intervention	18.66 (3.07)	15.42 (4.31)	14.97 (4.10)	14.08 (4.62)	-
Adjusted changes	−0.53 (−1.45, 0.39)	−2.14 (−2.92, −1.36)	−3.18 (−3.95, −2.41)	−3.62 (−4.39., −2.84)	0.001
MD (vs. usual care group)	-	−1.61 (−2.79, −0.43)	−2.65 (−3.82, −1.47)	−3.09 (−4.27, −1.91)	-
MD (vs. diet group)	-	-	−1.04 (−2.03, −0.05)	−1.48 (−2.57, −0.39)	-
HbA1c (%)					
Baseline	8.05 (1.52)	8.10 (1.77)	8.37 (1.44)	8.28 (1.35)	0.463
30-day intervention	8.07 (1.52)	7.88 (1.82)	7.71 (1.94)	7.65 (1.93)	-
Adjusted changes	0.10 (−0.34, 0.54)	−0.61 (−0.98, −0.24)	−0.76 (−1.13, −0.39)	−0.71 (−1.09, −0.34)	0.001
MD (vs. usual care group)	-	−0.71 (−1.29, −0.13)	−0.86 (−1.43, −0.29)	−0.81 (−1.37, −0.24)	-
MD (vs. diet group)	-	-	−0.14 (−0.67, 0.39)	−0.10 (−0.63, 0.43)	-
HOMA-IR (mU·mol/L^2)					
Baseline	5.49 (4.99)	5.48 (5.40)	4.68 (3.78)	6.20 (5.78)	0.312
30-day intervention	5.31 (3.16)	4.50 (4.89)	3.41 (3.23)	3.76 (4.75)	-
Adjusted changes	−0.25 (−2.66, 2.16)	−0.89 (−3.52, 1.74)	−1.80 (−3.48, −0.12)	−2.65 (−4.72, −0.58)	0.010
MD (vs. usual care group)	-	−0.64 (−2.40, 1.12)	−1.55 (−3.30, 0.20)	−2.41 (−4.59, −0.23)	-
MD (vs. diet group)	-	-	−0.91 (−1.93, 0.11)	−1.77 (−3.49, −0.05)	-
TC (total cholesterol) (mmol/L)					
Baseline	5.84 (1.83)	4.98 (0.86)	5.04 (0.98)	5.24 (1.03)	0.000
30-day intervention	5.82 (1.88)	4.81 (0.87)	4.66 (0.87)	4.72 (0.85)	-
Adjusted changes	−0.07 (−0.26, 0.12)	−0.18 (−0.34, −0.02)	−0.42 (−0.59, −0.26)	−0.51 (−0.67, −0.35)	0.000
MD (vs. usual care group)	-	−0.11 (−0.35, 0.14)	−0.35 (−0.60, −0.10)	−0.44 (−0.69, −0.19)	
MD (vs. diet group)	-	-	−0.24 (−0.47, −0.01)	−0.33 (−0.56, −0.10)	-

Table 3. *Cont.*

Variables	Usual Care Group (*n* = 60)	Healthy Diet Group (*n* = 79)	50 g-oats Group (*n* = 80)	100 g-oats Group (*n* = 79)	*p*-Value
TG (total triglycerides) (mmol/L)					
Baseline	1.92 (0.94)	1.83 (0.88)	2.06 (1.06)	1.98 (1.00)	0.510
30-day intervention	1.95 (1.02)	1.57 (0.84)	1.98 (1.65)	1.56 (0.77)	-
Adjusted changes	0.01 (−0.25, 0.27)	−0.25 (−0.47, −0.03)	−0.09 (−0.31, 0.13)	−0.43 (−0.65, −0.21)	0.003
MD (vs. usual care group)	-	−0.26 (−0.60, 0.08)	−0.10 (−0.43, 0.23)	−0.44 (−0.78, −0.10)	-
MD (vs. diet group)	-	-	0.16 (−0.26, 0.58)	−0.17 (−0.59, 0.26)	-
LDL-c (low-density lipoprotein cholesterol) (mmol/L)					
Baseline	3.20 (1.05)	2.96 (0.71)	2.90 (0.77)	3.15 (0.85)	0.128
30-day intervention	3.18 (1.05)	2.85 (0.74)	2.70 (0.70)	2.79 (0.63)	-
Adjusted changes	−0.06 (−0.21, 0.10)	−0.12 (−0.25, 0.01)	−0.23 (−0.36, −0.10)	−0.34 (−0.47, −0.21)	0.001
MD (vs. usual care group)	-	−0.06 (−0.26, 0.14)	−0.17 (−0.37, 0.02)	−0.28 (−0.48, −0.08)	-
MD (vs. diet group)	-	-	−0.10 (−0.28, 0.08)	−0.22 (−0.41, −0.03)	-
HDL-c (high-density lipoprotein cholesterol) (mmol/L)					
Baseline	1.41 (0.45)	1.30 (0.24)	1.25 (0.21)	1.36 (0.36)	0.022
30-day intervention	1.39 (0.42)	1.22 (0.24)	1.20 (0.22)	1.28 (0.26)	-
Adjusted changes	−0.02 (−0.07, 0.04)	−0.08 (−0.19, 0.03)	−0.07 (−0.11, −0.02)	−0.08 (−0.13, −0.03)	0.635
MD (vs. usual care group)	-	−0.06 (−0.14, 0.01)	−0.05 (−0.12, 0.02)	−0.06 (−0.14, 0.02)	-
MD (vs. diet group)	-	-	0.01 (−0.05, 0.07)	0.00 (−0.07, 0.07)	-

* All values were presented as means (SD) or means (95% CI). Changes from the baseline were adjusted for potential confounding variables (sex, age, drinking, smoking, physical activity level, education level, family history of diabetes, diabetic medications and duration of diabetes) in the analysis of covariance model.

Table 4. Changes in variables and mean differences (MD) in changes among groups after 1-year follow-up *.

Variables	Usual Care Group (n = 59)	Healthy Diet Group (n = 76)	50 g-oats Group (n = 77)	100 g-oats Group (n = 75)	p-Value
Weight (kg)					
Baseline	71.54 (5.82)	73.77 (8.58)	72.60 (8.67)	74.44 (7.63)	0.141
1-year follow-up	71.47 (7.35)	72.76 (8.70)	71.39 (8.68)	72.43 (7.58)	-
Adjusted changes	−0.11 (−0.68, 0.46)	−1.08 (−2.31, 0.16)	−1.44 (−2.74, −0.15)	−1.97 (−3.06, −0.88)	0.012
MD (vs. usual care group)	-	−0.97 (−2.23, 0.29)	−1.33 (−2.69, 0.03)	−1.86 (−3.25, −0.47)	-
MD (vs. diet group)	-	-	−0.36 (−1.10, 0.38)	−0.89 (−1.56, −0.22)	-
BMI (kg/m^2)					
Baseline	25.17 (0.89)	27.19 (2.82)	26.91 (2.69)	27.39 (2.42)	0.000
1-year follow-up	25.13 (1.25)	26.80 (2.91)	26.48 (2.33)	26.64 (2.74)	-
Adjusted changes	−0.05 (−0.39, 0.29)	−0.37 (−0.74, 0.00)	−0.50 (−0.91, −0.09)	−0.73 (−1.08, −0.39)	0.128
MD (vs. usual care group)	-	−0.33 (−1.05, 0.39)	−0.45 (−1.19, 0.29)	−0.68 (−1.43, 0.07)	-
MD (vs. diet group)	-	-	−0.12 (−0.64, 0.40)	−0.33 (−0.83, 0.17)	-
Fasting plasma glucose (mmol/L)					
Baseline	9.38 (2.81)	9.52 (2.87)	9.87 (2.83)	9.70 (3.30)	0.719
1-year follow-up	9.52 (1.44)	7.94 (2.14)	8.19 (2.01)	7.74 (2.43)	-
Adjusted changes	0.08 (−0.63, 0.46)	−1.65 (−2.21, −1.10)	−1.62 (−2.17, −1.07)	−1.87 (−2.44, −1.31)	0.000
MD (vs. usual care group)	-	−1.57 (−2.36, −0.78)	−1.54 (−2.33, −0.75)	−1.79 (−2.58, −1.00)	-
MD (vs. diet group)	-	-	0.03 (−0.76, 0.82)	−0.22 (−1.02, 0.58)	-
2-h postprandial plasma glucose (mmol/L)					
Baseline	19.10 (3.22)	17.58 (4.87)	18.23 (4.84)	17.89 (5.45)	0.284
1-year follow-up	19.69 (3.27)	15.01 (3.63)	14.98 (3.02)	14.22 (3.78)	-
Adjusted changes	0.63 (−0.36, 1.63)	−2.41 (−3.40, −1.42)	−3.16 (−4.16, −2.16)	−3.58 (−4.63, −2.53)	0.000
MD (vs. usual care group)	-	−3.04 (−4.48, −1.60)	−3.79 (−5.22, −2.36)	−4.21 (−5.67, −2.75)	-
MD (vs. diet group)	-	-	−0.75 (−1.91, 0.41)	−1.17 (−2.27, −0.07)	-
HbA1c (%)					
Baseline	8.05 (1.52)	8.10 (1.77)	8.37 (1.44)	8.28 (1.35)	0.463
1-year follow-up	8.47 (1.86)	7.63 (1.89)	7.41 (1.18)	7.27 (1.72)	-
Adjusted changes	0.35 (−0.01, 0.71)	−0.42 (−0.79, −0.06)	−0.90 (−1.27, −0.54)	−1.06 (−1.44, −0.69)	0.000
MD (vs. usual care group)	-	−0.77 (−1.31, −0.23)	−1.25 (−1.79, −0.71)	−1.41 (−1.95, −0.87)	-
MD (vs. diet group)		-	−0.48 (−1.02, 0.06)	−0.64 (−1.19, −0.09)	-
TC (mmol/L)					
Baseline	5.84 (1.83)	4.98 (0.86)	5.04 (0.98)	5.24 (1.03)	0.000
1-year follow-up	6.01 (1.87)	4.8 (1.04)	4.69 (0.95)	4.76 (0.97)	-
Adjusted changes	0.12 (0.07, 0.31)	−0.19 (−0.38, −0.01)	−0.37 (−0.56, −0.18)	−0.49 (−0.68, −0.29)	0.000

Table 4. *Cont.*

Variables	Usual Care Group (n = 59)	Healthy Diet Group (n = 76)	50 g-oats Group (n = 77)	100 g-oats Group (n = 75)	p-Value
MD (vs. usual care group)	-	−0.31 (−0.62, 0.00)	−0.49 (−0.75, −0.23)	−0.61 (−0.88, −0.34)	-
MD (vs. diet group)	-	-	−0.18 (−0.45, 0.09)	−0.30 (−0.57, −0.03)	-
TG (mmol/L)					
Baseline	1.92 (0.94)	1.83 (0.88)	2.06 (1.06)	1.98 (1.00)	0.510
1-year follow-up	2.13 (1.41)	2.00 (1.91)	1.83 (1.19)	1.55 (0.97)	-
Adjusted changes	0.21 (−0.08, 0.50)	0.17 (−0.12, 0.46)	−0.27 (−0.56, 0.02)	−0.45 (−0.75, −0.16)	0.005
MD (vs. usual care group)	-	−0.04 (−0.45, 0.38)	−0.46 (−0.87, −0.05)	−0.66 (−1.07, −0.25)	-
MD (vs. diet group)	-	-	−0.42 (−0.83, −0.01)	−0.70 (−1.11, −0.29)	-
LDL-c (mmol/L)					
Baseline	3.20 (1.05)	2.96 (0.71)	2.90 (0.77)	3.15 (0.85)	0.128
1-year follow-up	3.35 (0.99)	2.84 (0.88)	2.50 (0.79)	2.64 (0.75)	-
Adjusted changes	0.16 (−0.01, 0.33)	−0.14 (−0.30, 0.01)	−0.41 (−0.56, −0.26)	−0.51 (−0.67, −0.35)	0.000
MD (vs. usual care group)	-	−0.30 (−0.51, −0.09)	−0.57 (−0.78, −0.36)	−0.67 (−0.89, −0.45)	-
MD (vs. diet group)	-	-	−0.27 (−0.49, −0.05)	−0.37 (−0.59, −0.15)	-
HDL-c (mmol/L)					
Baseline	1.41 (0.45)	1.30 (0.24)	1.25 (0.21)	1.36 (0.36)	0.022
1-year follow-up	1.39 (0.34)	1.34 (0.57)	1.29 (0.40)	1.39 (0.41)	-
Adjusted changes	−0.02 (−0.11, 0.07)	0.06 (−0.15, 0.03)	0.06 (−0.03, 0.15)	0.01 (−0.09, 0.10)	0.636
MD (vs. usual care group)	-	0.08 (−0.09, 0.26)	0.09 (−0.08, 0.26)	0.03 (−0.15, 0.21)	-
MD (vs. diet group)	-	-	0.00 (−0.17, 0.18)	−0.05 (−0.23, 0.12)	-

* All values were presented as means (SD) or means (95% CI). Changes from the baseline were adjusted for potential confounding variables (sex, age, drinking/smoking, physical activity level, education level, family history, medications and duration of diabetes) in the analysis of covariance model.

4. Discussion

The present study showed that a low-fat and high-fiber diet ("healthy diet") had beneficial effects on glucolipid metabolism in overweight T2DM patients, and these effects were more evident when combined with oat intake. In particular, the combination of short-term (30 days) oat intake with the "healthy diet" had greater effects on lowering the PPG, HOMA-IR, TC and LDL-c than that of merely having a low-fat and high-fiber diet. The 1-year follow-up showed that the reduction of PPG, HOMA-IR, TC and LDL-c can be maintained for long time, and significantly greater effects in decreasing weight, HbA1c and TG were observed.

The primary finding of this study was the significant effect of oat intake on hyperglycemia control. A growing number of studies have suggested that oats and oat-enriched products can significantly decrease the postprandial hyperglycemia [11,14]. Consistently, our study provided supportive evidence for the PPG lowering effect of oat intake in overweight T2DM patients. Although the mechanism of lowering PPG has not been fully understood, at least parts of the contribution could be attributed to the property of oat β-glucan. Oat β-glucan can increase the viscosity in the intestine, slow the absorption of carbohydrates, and thus reduce the PPG [19,20]. Research findings on the FPG lowering effects of oat intake are less consistent. A few human trials and diabetic mice laboratory studies have found that oat intake can significantly decrease the FPG concertation [14,21,22], but this finding was not supported by the majority of randomized control trials (RCTs) [11]. Although a subgroup analysis of high quality RCTs in a meta-analysis indicated that oat intake can slightly lower FPG concentration in the long-term intervention [11], our study did not find any FPG lowering effect that could be attributed to either short-term or long-term oat intake. The long-term oat intake had a significant effect in reducing HbA1c, but short-term oat intake did not. This finding is not totally unexpected. Considering that HbA1c levels usually reflect the blood glucose levels for the period of 8–12 weeks, the duration of a 30-day intervention may not be long enough to have significant changes in HbA1c, whereas a significant reduction in HbA1c could be shown in the longer 1-year follow-up. So far, a few studies have evaluated the effect of oat intake on HOMA-IR. A meta-analysis of three RCTs reported that oat intake had no effect on the improvement of HOMA-IR [11]. In contrast, our study suggested a significant effect on decreasing HOMA-IR. Our finding was consistent with a recent published RCT, which suggested oats consumption can significantly decrease the HOMA-IR index [23]. These varying results may be partly due to the different characteristics of study populations, probably because overweight and obese T2DM patients are likely to result in more severe insulin resistance, and insulin resistance is more likely to be modifiable in this population [24].

Furthermore, this study confirmed the serum lipid lowering effect of oat intake in overweight T2DM patients. The effect of oat intake on lowering TC and LDL-c has been supported in most published studies [10,13]. The main controversy is the magnitude of the effect. In some studies, the reduction of TC and LDL-c could be more than 10% [25,26], while in others, the reduction was less than 5% [27,28]. In our study, the decrease of TC and LDL-c was around 10%. However, the effect size in this study was not comparable with others, considering the study population, the dose of oats and oat processing were different from other studies. Comparing the duration of the intervention, the long-term oat intake had a significant effect on the reduction of TG. The mechanism of serum lipid-lowering effect also seems to be related to the increased viscosity attributed to the oat β-glucan, which can lead to the reduction in cholesterol absorption [20].

Another finding which is important for overweight T2DM patients is the weight loss effect of long-term oat intake. During the 30-day intervention, the three intervention groups had a significant decrease in body weight and the weight reduction was similar among the three diet groups. However, during the 1-year follow-up, the 100 g oats group had a significantly greater decrease in weight than the healthy diet group. Considering that oat intake was combined with the "healthy diet", it is possible that the moderate weight-reducing effect of a short-term (30 days) oat intake was covered up by the weight reduction due to the low-fat and high-fiber diet; or the duration of a 30-day oat intake was too short to have changes on weight. The bigger weight reduction observed in the 1-year oat intake was unlikely to be caused by the poorly controlled blood glucose level, since a significant reduction in FPG, PPG and HbA1c was also observed. The weight reduction effect is probably related to the oat β-glucan, which may enhance the viscosity of meals, decrease the starch digestion and reduce the food intake by increasing satiety [29]. In addition to our studies, a few other studies also indicated a weigh-reducing effect of oats in certain populations [23,29,30], but these findings were not consistently in agreement, as some studies found no decrease in weight [12,25,31]. Further research is needed to verify the weight-reducing effect of oat intake.

The predominant effect of oats on diabetic management is most likely to be attributed to the bioactivity of β-glucan. Although, compared to other cereals, wholegrain oats have distinct bioactive composition in lipids and phenolics, the most significant difference is in the high content of β-glucan, especially when considering that the effective dose of the other two components is not likely to be achieved through 50 g or 100 g wholegrain oats consumption [30,31]. As mentioned above, β-glucan has been reported to increase the intestinal viscosity, decrease the absorption of carbohydrates and lipids, and reduce food intake to control hyperglycemia, lower lipid and reduce weight. In addition, another important role of β-glucan involves the impact on gut microbiota. Specifically, the bacterial metabolism of β-glucan can increase the production of short-chain fatty acids and drive the release of bioactive compounds, which may interact with host biology to affect the risk of obesity and associated disorders [32,33]. Oat β-glucan has been shown to decrease the protein fermentation and thus reduce the detrimental metabolites produced [34]. Furthermore, the fermentation of β-glucan has also been reported to increase the diversity of gut microbiota, which is a potential benefit, considering that the reduced microbiota diversity is associated with obesity [35,36]. Studies exploring the mechanisms behind the health benefits of β-glucan and gut microbiota may provide more evidence to encourage an increase in oat intake and to maximize the health benefits derived from oats.

Strengths and limitations of the study design should be noted. In the first phase, a 30-day centralized management of intervention was designed to improve the compliance of participants. Potential dietary confounding factors for assessing the effects of oat intake were homogenized among groups by providing a general "healthy diet" to the intervention groups of oat intake and using a healthy diet group as the reference group. To estimate the beneficial effects due to the "healthy diet", a usual care group, with no dietry intervention, was established as a control group. To provide information for recommending a proper dose of daily oat intake (or oat β-glucan), we designed two intervention groups with different doses (50 g and 100 g) of oat intake. Considering that the duration of a 30-day intervention is probably too short for some variables, such as HbAc1 and weight, to have significant changes, a 1-year follow-up was designed to investigate the long-term changes of the variables and to determine if the significant changes observed in the 30-day intervention could be maintained for a long time. However, in this subgroup analysis, we only reported that the anthropometric and blood biochemical variables, cardiovascular events and other diabetic complications were not presented, which led us to consider that the duration of a 1-year intervention was relatively short for evaluating the diabetic complications. Another limitation was that the subjects were not fully blinded because of the different taste of oats and other cereals. Furthermore, the benefits of oat intake were assessed in comparison to an already healthy diet, and as discussed above, it is possible that the moderate beneficial effects of oat intake were covered up or magnified by the healthy reference diet. However, in either case, it should be emphasized that the whole grain oat intake should be recommended with a healthy diet.

5. Conclusions

In conclusion, our study provided some supportive evidence that oats can be a good selection of whole grains for overweight diabetics, but further larger scale studies are needed to evaluate these findings further.

Supplementary Materials: The following is available online at http://www.mdpi.com/2072-6643/8/9/549/s1, Table S1: A sample menus of the general healthy diet provided for intervention groups (average consumption per day).

Acknowledgments: The authors would like to thank the Beijing Nutrition Society for the consistent support in the field study and data collection herein. The authors would also like to thank the Third Hospital of Inner Mongolia Medical College for helping with the clinical examinations.

Author Contributions: Y.L. conceived the idea for the study. X.L. performed the statistical analysis and drafted the manuscript. All authors participated in the design of the study, study supervision, data collection and interpretation, revised and approved the final version of the manuscript.

Conflicts of Interest: The authors declare no conflict of interest. This study was sponsored by the Inner Mongolia Sanzhuliang Natural Oats Industry Corporation (IMSNOIC). The sponsor had no impact on the results and manuscript.

References

1. Series, W.T. Obesity: Preventing and managing the global epidemic. Report of a WHO consultation. *World Health Organ. Tech. Rep. Ser.* **2000**, *894*, 1–253.
2. NCD Risk Factor Collaboration. Effects of diabetes definition on global surveillance of diabetes prevalence and diagnosis: A pooled analysis of 96 population-based studies with 331,288 participants. *Lancet Diabetes Endocrinol.* **2015**, *3*, 624–637.
3. Yaturu, S. Obesity and type 2 diabetes. *J. Diabetes Mellit.* **2011**, *1*, 79–95. [CrossRef]
4. Mokdad, A.H.; Ford, E.S.; Bowman, B.A.; Nelson, D.E.; Engelgau, M.M.; Vinicor, F.; Marks, J.S. Diabetes trends in the U.S.: 1990–1998. *Diabetes Care* **2000**, *23*, 1278–1283. [CrossRef] [PubMed]
5. American Diabetes Association. Standards of medical care in diabetes-2015 abridged for primary care providers. *Clin. Diabetes* **2015**, *33*, 97–111.
6. American Diabetes Association. Evidence-based nutrition principles and recommendations for the treatment and prevention of diabetes and related complications. *Diabetes Care* **2002**, *25*, 202–212.
7. Fung, T.T.; Hu, F.B.; Pereira, M.A.; Liu, S.; Stampfer, M.J.; Colditz, G.A.; Willett, W.C. Whole-grain intake and the risk of type 2 diabetes: A prospective study in men. *Am. J. Clin. Nutr.* **2002**, *76*, 535–540. [PubMed]
8. Brennan, C.S.; Cleary, L.J. The potential use of cereal (1→3,1→4)-β-D-glucans as functional food ingredients. *J. Cereal Sci.* **2005**, *42*, 1–13. [CrossRef]
9. Clemens, R.; van Klinken, B.J. Oats, more than just a whole grain: An introduction. *Br. J. Nutr.* **2014**, *112* (Suppl. S2), S1–S3. [CrossRef] [PubMed]
10. Whitehead, A.; Beck, E.J.; Tosh, S.; Wolever, T.M. Cholesterol-lowering effects of oat beta-glucan: A meta-analysis of randomized controlled trials. *Am. J. Clin. Nutr.* **2014**, *100*, 1413–1421. [CrossRef] [PubMed]
11. Bao, L.; Cai, X.; Xu, M.; Li, Y. Effect of oat intake on glycaemic control and insulin sensitivity: A meta-analysis of randomised controlled trials. *Br. J. Nutr.* **2014**, *112*, 457–466. [CrossRef] [PubMed]
12. Saltzman, E.; Das, S.K.; Lichtenstein, A.H.; Dallal, G.E.; Corrales, A.; Schaefer, E.J.; Greenberg, A.S.; Roberts, S.B. An oat-containing hypocaloric diet reduces systolic blood pressure and improves lipid profile beyond effects of weight loss in men and women. *J. Nutr.* **2001**, *131*, 1465–1470. [PubMed]
13. Othman, R.A.; Moghadasian, M.H.; Jones, P.J. Cholesterol-lowering effects of oat beta-glucan. *Nutr. Rev.* **2011**, *69*, 299–309. [CrossRef] [PubMed]
14. Shen, X.L.; Zhao, T.; Zhou, Y.; Shi, X.; Zou, Y.; Zhao, G. Effect of oat beta-glucan intake on glycaemic control and insulin sensitivity of diabetic patients: A meta-analysis of randomized controlled trials. *Nutrients* **2016**, *8*, 39. [CrossRef] [PubMed]
15. Institute of Nutrition and Food Safety. *China CDC 2005 China Food Composition*; Peking University Medical Press: Beijing, China, 2005.
16. Chinese Nutrition Society. *Dietary Guidelines for Chinese Residents*; Tibet People's Publishing House: Lhasa, China, 2010.
17. Chinese Diabetes Society. China Medical Nutrition Therapy Guideline for Diabetes. Available online: http://www.cdschina.org/news_show.jsp?id=509.html (accessed on 16 October 2012).
18. Sun, Z. Process for Dehulling Oats without Removing Plumules. CN101264459 17 September 2008.

19. Hlebowicz, J. Postprandial blood glucose response in relation to gastric emptying and satiety in healthy subjects. *Appetite* **2009**, *53*, 249–252. [CrossRef] [PubMed]
20. Wang, Q.; Ellis, P.R. Oat beta-glucan: Physico-chemical characteristics in relation to its blood-glucose and cholesterol-lowering properties. *Br. J. Nutr.* **2014**, *112* (Suppl. S2), S4–S13. [CrossRef] [PubMed]
21. Pick, M.E.; Hawrysh, Z.J.; Gee, M.I.; Toth, E.; Garg, M.L.; Hardin, R.T. Oat bran concentrate bread products improve long-term control of diabetes: A pilot study. *J. Am. Diet. Assoc.* **1996**, *96*, 1254–1261. [CrossRef]
22. Shen, R.L.; Cai, F.L.; Dong, J.L.; Hu, X.Z. Hypoglycemic effects and biochemical mechanisms of oat products on streptozotocin-induced diabetic mice. *J. Agric. Food Chem.* **2011**, *59*, 8895–8900. [CrossRef] [PubMed]
23. Schuster, J.; Beninca, G.; Vitorazzi, R.; Morelo Dal Bosco, S. Effects of oats on lipid profile, insulin resistance and weight loss. *Nutr. Hosp.* **2015**, *32*, 2111–2116. [PubMed]
24. Qatanani, M.; Lazar, M.A. Mechanisms of obesity-associated insulin resistance: Many choices on the menu. *Genes Dev.* **2007**, *21*, 1443–1455. [CrossRef] [PubMed]
25. Charlton, K.E.; Tapsell, L.C.; Batterham, M.J.; O'Shea, J.; Thorne, R.; Beck, E.; Tosh, S.M. Effect of 6 weeks' consumption of beta-glucan-rich oat products on cholesterol levels in mildly hypercholesterolaemic overweight adults. *Br. J. Nutr.* **2012**, *107*, 1037–1047. [CrossRef] [PubMed]
26. Ma, X.; Gu, J.; Zhang, Z.; Jing, L.; Xu, M.; Dai, X.; Jiang, Y.; Li, Y.; Bao, L.; Cai, X.; et al. Effects of avena nuda l. On metabolic control and cardiovascular disease risk among Chinese patients with diabetes and meeting metabolic syndrome criteria: Secondary analysis of a randomized clinical trial. *Eur. J. Clin. Nutr.* **2013**, *67*, 1291–1297. [CrossRef] [PubMed]
27. Torronen, R.; Kansanen, L.; Uusitupa, M.; Hanninen, O.; Myllymaki, O.; Harkonen, H.; Malkki, Y. Effects of an oat bran concentrate on serum lipids in free-living men with mild to moderate hypercholesterolaemia. *Eur. J. Clin. Nutr.* **1992**, *46*, 621–627. [PubMed]
28. Kerckhoffs, D.A.; Hornstra, G.; Mensink, R.P. Cholesterol-lowering effect of beta-glucan from oat bran in mildly hypercholesterolemic subjects may decrease when beta-glucan is incorporated into bread and cookies. *Am. J. Clin. Nutr.* **2003**, *78*, 221–227. [PubMed]
29. Lyly, M.; Liukkonen, K.H.; Salmenkallio-Marttila, M.; Karhunen, L.; Poutanen, K.; Lahteenmaki, L. Fibre in beverages can enhance perceived satiety. *Eur. J. Nutr.* **2009**, *48*, 251–258. [CrossRef] [PubMed]
30. Rose, D.J. Impact of whole grains on the gut microbiota: The next frontier for oats? *Br. J. Nutr.* **2014**, *112* (Suppl. S2), S44–S49. [CrossRef] [PubMed]
31. Viscidi, K.A.; Dougherty, M.P.; Briggs, J.; Camire, M.E. Complex phenolic compounds reduce lipid oxidation in extruded oat cereals. *Food Sci. Technol.* **2004**, *37*, 789–796. [CrossRef]
32. El Khoury, D.; Cuda, C.; Luhovyy, B.L.; Anderson, G.H. Beta glucan: Health benefits in obesity and metabolic syndrome. *J. Nutr. Metab.* **2012**, *2012*, 851362. [CrossRef] [PubMed]
33. Den Besten, G.; van Eunen, K.; Groen, A.K.; Venema, K.; Reijngoud, D.J.; Bakker, B.M. The role of short-chain fatty acids in the interplay between diet, gut microbiota, and host energy metabolism. *J. Lipid Res.* **2013**, *54*, 2325–2340. [CrossRef] [PubMed]
34. Ross, A.B.; Pere-Trepat, E.; Montoliu, I.; Martin, F.P.; Collino, S.; Moco, S.; Godin, J.P.; Cleroux, M.; Guy, P.A.; Breton, I.; et al. A whole-grain-rich diet reduces urinary excretion of markers of protein catabolism and gut microbiota metabolism in healthy men after one week. *J. Nutr.* **2013**, *143*, 766–773. [CrossRef] [PubMed]
35. Martinez, I.; Lattimer, J.M.; Hubach, K.L.; Case, J.A.; Yang, J.; Weber, C.G.; Louk, J.A.; Rose, D.J.; Kyureghian, G.; Peterson, D.A.; et al. Gut microbiome composition is linked to whole grain-induced immunological improvements. *ISME J.* **2013**, *7*, 269–280. [CrossRef] [PubMed]
36. De Vos, W.M.; de Vos, E.A. Role of the intestinal microbiome in health and disease: From correlation to causation. *Nutr. Rev.* **2012**, *70* (Suppl. S1), S45–S56. [CrossRef] [PubMed]

nutrients

MDPI

Article

Soluble Fiber with High Water-Binding Capacity, Swelling Capacity, and Fermentability Reduces Food Intake by Promoting Satiety Rather Than Satiation in Rats

Chengquan Tan [1], Hongkui Wei [1], Xichen Zhao [1], Chuanhui Xu [1], Yuanfei Zhou [1,*] and Jian Peng [1,2,*]

1 Department of Animal Nutrition and Feed Science, College of Animal Science and Technology, Huazhong Agricultural University, Wuhan 430070, China; cooper2005@163.com (C.T.); weihongkui@mail.hzau.edu.cn (H.W.); FenziYY@126.com (X.Z.); xuchuanhui001@hzau.edu.cn (C.X.)
2 The Cooperative Innovation Center for Sustainable Pig Production, Wuhan 430070, China
* Correspondence: zhuoyuanfei@mail.hzau.edu.cn (Y.Z.); pengjian@mail.hzau.edu.cn (J.P.); Tel.: +86-27-8728-0122 (Y.Z.); +86-27-8728-6912 (J.P.)

Received: 31 July 2016; Accepted: 26 September 2016; Published: 2 October 2016

Abstract: To understand whether soluble fiber (SF) with high water-binding capacity (WBC), swelling capacity (SC) and fermentability reduces food intake and whether it does so by promoting satiety or satiation or both, we investigated the effects of different SFs with these properties on the food intake in rats. Thirty-two male Sprague-Dawley rats were randomized to four equal groups and fed the control diet or diet containing 2% *konjac* flour (KF), pregelatinized waxy maize starch (PWMS) plus guar gum (PG), and PWMS starch plus xanthan gum (PX) for three weeks, with the measured values of SF, WBC, and SC in the four diets following the order of PG > KF > PX > control. Food intake, body weight, meal pattern, behavioral satiety sequence, and short-chain fatty acids (SCFAs) in cecal content were evaluated. KF and PG groups reduced the food intake, mainly due to the decreased feeding behavior and increased satiety, as indicated by decreased meal numbers and increased inter-meal intervals. Additionally, KF and PG groups increased concentrations of acetate acid, propionate acid, and SCFAs in the cecal contents. Our results indicate that SF with high WBC, SC, and fermentability reduces food intake—probably by promoting a feeling of satiety in rats to decrease their feeding behavior.

Keywords: guar gum; water binding capacity; meal pattern; food intake; satiety

1. Introduction

Satiation and satiety are part of the body's appetite control system involved in limiting food intake. Satiation is reflected in meal size and meal duration, while satiety is reflected in meal number and inter-meal intervals [1]. Modulation of food intake by consuming foods with a high satiety or satiation value may be one of the approaches to help reduce obesity. The efficacy by which different types of dietary fibers promote satiety or satiation is varied [2,3]. This issue can be explored first by using laboratory animals due to the advantages of a complete control over the diet, facile collection of gut samples, and systematic observation of behaviors.

Growing evidence showed that the physicochemical properties of dietary fiber such as viscosity, water-binding capacity, and fermentability may contribute to decrease the food intake in human beings and rodents [3–5]. Viscous fibers increase chewing activity and saliva production in the mouth [6], which could result in early satiation and reduced food intake [7,8]. However, dietary fiber with high water-binding capacity may increase gastric distension by expanding their volume up to eight-fold in the stomach [9], which will increase feelings of satiety [10], probably via afferent vagal signals of fullness [6]. Moreover, a delay in gastric emptying accompanied by an increase in gastric distension is often associated with enhanced satiety between meals [11]. In addition, dietary fiber is also fermented by intestinal microbiota, contributing to the increase of short-chain fatty acids (SCFAs). Furthermore, SCFAs could stimulate the release of satiety-related peptides, such as peptide tyrosine-tyrosine (PYY) and glucagon-like peptide-1 (GLP-1) from entero-endocrine cells, which may promote feelings of satiety [12].

Konjac flour (KF) is a water soluble, viscous dietary fiber with a high water-binding capacity (15.5 mL H_2O/g) [13,14]. KF mainly contains *konjac* glucomannan (KGM), which is composed of β-1,4-linked D-mannosyl and D-glucosyl residues at a molar ratio of 1.6:1.0 as the main chain with a small number of branches through β-1,3 mannosyl units [15]. KGM is considered a functional fiber of food ingredient and has been consumed in the form of rubbery jelly, noodles, and other food products by humans in Asia for centuries [16]. KGM has been known to be helpful in lowering cholesterol levels, reducing weight in human beings [17], and modifying intestinal microbial metabolism in sows [18,19]. Our previous study indicated that dietary inclusion of KF with higher water-binding capacity (1.97 vs. 1.78 g/g) and swelling capacity (2.14 vs. 1.62 mL/g) than inclusion of wheat bran promoted the satiety of gestating sow [20]. However, the tuber is usually grown in Asian countries and the resources for commercial production are limited, suggesting the necessity to develop novel dietary fibers with functional properties similar to those of KF, as well as similar effects on food intake reduction by promoting satiety or satiation.

Pregelatinized waxy maize starch, a fermentable resistant starch composed mainly of highly branched amorphous amylopectin, has many specific food attributes [21]. Dietary supplementation with modified waxy maize starch lowers glucose-dependent insulinotropic polypeptides and has beneficial implications in weight management [22]. Guar and xanthan gums with high viscosity and hydrating properties are used as stabilizer and thickener in various food products [23,24]. A previous study reported that the digesta viscosity of subjects was increased after consuming cookies containing 2.5% guar gum alone for 42 days, without any effect on their food intake [3]. The consumption of beverages enriched with dietary fibers and xanthan gum (0.22%) for one week also had no influence on the appetite sensations in healthy men [25]. Our previous results showed that the combined fiber materials (pregelatinized waxy maize starch plus guar gum (PG) and pregelatinized waxy maize starch plus xanthan gum (PX)) had higher or similar water-binding capacity or swelling capacity than the KF [26]. Therefore, we hypothesized that the combination of pregelatinized waxy maize starch with guar gum or xanthan gum inclusion in diet may have a similar effect to that of KF on physicochemical properties (water-binding capacity and swelling capacity) and fermentability, as well as food intake reduction by promoting satiety or satiation. The objective of the present study was to investigate whether dietary fibers with high water-binding capacity, swelling capacity, and fermentability reduce food intake by promoting satiety or satiation as well as the mechanism underlying it by evaluating their effects on plasma concentrations of GLP-1 and PYY, SCFAs in cecal contents, meal pattern, feeding behavior, food intake, and body weight in rats.

2. Experimental Section

2.1. Animals and Diets

A total of 32 male Sprague-Dawley rats (average initial body weight of 377.10 ± 3.43 g; 10 weeks of age) (Hunan SJA Laboratory Animal Co., Ltd., Changsha, China) were housed individually in standard cages that allowed recording of food intake. The cages were placed in a temperature-and humidity-controlled room (21 ± 2 °C, 55% ± 10% humidity) with a 12:12 light/dark cycle (lights off at 8:30 p.m.). The animals were acclimatized for one week with the control diet fed prior to the experiment. Rats were given free access to water and food. All the experiment protocols were approved by the animal care and use committee of Huazhong Agriculture University and were in accordance with the

National Research Council's Guide for the Care and Use of Laboratory Animals. Sprague-Dawley rats were used because they are reported to have a good consistency in meal patterns [27].

Rats were divided randomly to four dietary treatment groups (8 rats/treatment): the control fed control diet with wheat bran as a fiber source (Control); a positive control fed the control diet with 2% *konjac* flour (Qingjiang Konjac Products Co., Ltd., Wuhan, China) to replace 2% wheat bran (KF); a treatment fed the control diet with 2% pregelatinized waxy maize starch (Hangzhou Puluoxiang Starch Corp., Ltd., Hangzhou, China) plus guar gum (Shangdong Yunzhou Science and Technology Corp., Ltd., Yunzhou, China) to replace 2% wheat bran (PG) (PG; 85.7% pregelatinized waxy maize starch and 14.3% guar gum); and a treatment fed the control diet with 2% pregelatinized waxy maize starch plus xanthan gum (Shangdong Yunzhou Science and Technology Corp., Ltd., Yunzhou, China) to replace 2% wheat bran (PX) (PX; 95% pregelatinized waxy maize starch and 5% xanthan gum). The ingredient and chemical composition of the diets are listed in Table 1. The experiment lasted 21 days, during which food intake was determined daily and body weights were measured.

Table 1. Ingredient and composition of experimental diets.

Ingredient (% *w/w*)	**Control [1]**	**KF [1]**	**PG [1]**	**PX [1]**
Corn	52.2	52.2	52.2	52.2
Soybean meal	15.9	15.9	15.9	15.9
Fish meal	10.0	10.0	10.0	10.0
Wheat bran	12.0	10.0	10.0	10.0
Sucrose	5.0	5.0	5.0	5.0
Fiber source		2.0	2.0	2.0
AIN-93 Mineral mix [2]	3.5	3.5	3.5	3.5
AIN-93 Vitamin mix [3]	1.0	1.0	1.0	1.0
Composition				
Crude protein (%)	20.04	19.94	19.78	19.90
Energy (kcal/g)	3.81	3.83	3.76	3.74
Soluble fiber (%)	1.91	2.89	3.09	2.57
Insoluble fiber (%)	10.46	10.58	10.61	11.10
Viscosity (mPa/s)	1.53	1.66	1.60	1.57
Swelling (mL/g)	1.81	2.63	3.03	2.18
Water-binding capacity (g/g)	2.05	2.58	2.87	2.26

[1] Diets were control or supplemented with 2% fiber of *konjac* flour (KF), 2% pregelatinized waxy maize starch plus guar gum (PG) or 2% pregelatinized waxy maize starch plus xanthan gum (PX); [2] AIN-93 Mineral mix according to Reeves (1997), per kg mix: Calcium carbonate, 357.00; Potassium phosphate, 196.00; Potassium citrate, 70.78; Sodium chloride, 74.00; Potassium sulfate, 46.60; Magnesium oxide, 24.00; Ferric citrate, 6.06; Zinc carbonate, 1.65; Sodium meta-silicate, 1.45; Manganous carbonate, 0.63; Cupric carbonate, 0.30; Chromium potassium sulfate, 0.28; Boric acid, 0.08; Sodium fluoride, 0.06; Nickel carbonate, 0.03; Lithium chloride, 0.02; Sodium selenate, 0.01; Potassium iodate, 0.01; Ammonium paramolybdate, 0.008; Ammonium vanadate, 0.007; Powdered sucrose, 221.03; [3] AIN-93 Vitamin mix according to Reeves (1997). Vitamin (mg/kg) (except as noted): Nicotinic acid, 3.00; Ca pantothenate, 1.60; Pyridoxine, 0.70; Thiamin, 0.60; Folic acid, 0.20; Biotin, 0.02; Vitamin B_{12}, 2.50; Vitamin E (500 IU/g), Vitamin A (500,000 IU/g), 0.80; Vitamin D_3 (400,000 IU/g), 0.25; Vitamin K, 0.08; Powdered sucrose, 974.65.

2.2. Behavioral Satiety Sequence

The analysis of the behavioral satiety sequence was performed on day 15 of dietary treatment essentially as described by Halford et al. [28]. Rats were housed individually in transparent observational cages and fasted overnight for 12 h. Water was available ad libitum. The following morning (8:30–9:30), rats were given a pre-weighed amount of food and their behaviors were monitored. For all rats, behavior was recorded every 30 s for 1 h as reported previously [29] and food intake was calculated. Feeding and non-feeding behaviors were continuously scored using a video system connected with a computer in a nearby room by a highly trained experimenter blind to the dietary treatment of the animals. Behaviors were categorized as: feeding (animal at hopper trying to obtain food, chewing, gnawing, or holding food in paws), drinking (animal licking spout of water bottle), grooming (animal scratching, licking, or biting any part of its anatomy), activity (including locomotion, sniffing, or rearing), inactivity (immobility when aware, or signs of sickness behavior), resting (animal curled up, resting head with eyes closed). Data were collated into 5-min period bins for display. With time spent in each of the behaviors as % of the total behavior.

2.3. Meal Pattern Analysis

On day 17 of dietary treatment, the rats were housed individually in transparent observational cages that allowed continuous recording of food intake for three days. The first two days served as the adaptation period, and the meal pattern and food intake were analyzed on the third day. The measurements were performed similar to previous studies [30]. Rats were fasted overnight for 12 h before the meal pattern analysis. Meal patterns of the nocturnal (from 8:30 p.m. to 8:30 a.m.) and diurnal (from 8:30 a.m. to 8:30 p.m.) periods were analyzed and recorded. Rats were fed respective diets ad libitum during the meal pattern analysis. The results were collected as total food intake (g), feeding rate (mg/s), meal size (g), meal duration (s), meal number, and inter-meal interval (min). A meal was defined as an intake larger than 0.3 g lasting a period longer than 13 s, and two distinct meals needed to be separated by >10 min [27]. The meal patterns for rats were recorded using monitoring equipment in a computer-based data acquisition system (Shenzhen Quick Zoom Technology Co., Ltd., N5063 960P, Shenzhen, China).

2.4. Samples Collection

On day 20 of dietary treatment, rats were fasted overnight and then given food ad libitum the following morning. Two hours after the meal presentation, the rats were anesthetized (ethylene oxide) and opened by laparotomy. Blood samples were collected by cardiac puncture and placed into tubes containing ethylene diamine tetraacetic acid (EDTA) and a peptidase inhibitor cocktail containing general protease inhibitor (Roche Diagnostics Ltd., Burgess Hill, West Sussex, UK), followed by centrifugation at 3000× *g* for 10 min at 4 °C and storage at −80 °C until GLP-1 and PYY analysis. The gut was removed to sample the contents from cecum and tissue from distal ileum. Cecal contents were stored at −80 °C until analysis of short chain fatty acids (SCFAs). Tissues from distal ileum were immersed in RNAlater (QIAGEN, Crawley, UK) for 5 days at 4 °C and then stored at −80 °C until analysis.

2.5. Chemical Analysis

Diet samples were analyzed for crude protein according to the Association of Analytical Communities (AOAC) [31]. Gross energy was determined by bomb calorimetry using a LECO Ac 300 automated calorimeter system 789-500 (Parr Instrument Co., Moline, IL, USA). Soluble dietary fiber and insoluble fiber were determined by AOAC Method 991.43 [31]. Viscosity in extracts of diets was measured as reported by Johansen et al. [32]. The water-binding capacity and swelling capacity of diets were measured as described by Serena et al. [33].

The concentrations of GLP-1 and PYY in plasma were analyzed using an ultrasensitive rat GLP-1 and PYY enzyme-linked immunosorbent assay (ELISA) kit (Biosource Inc., Sunnyvale, CA, USA) according to the instructions. The SCFAs concentration of cecal contents was analyzed by gas chromatography (Varian CP-3800, Shimadzu Co., Kyoto, Japan), as described by Bosch et al. [34]. Total SCFAs was determined as the sum of analyzed acetate, propionate, and butyrate. All procedures were performed in duplicate.

2.6. Quantitative PCR (QPCR)

QPCR technology was employed to verify changes in the mRNA levels of GLP-1 and PYY genes. Total RNA was isolated from the distal ileum tissue using TRIZOL reagent (Invitrogen, Life Technologies Co., Carlsbad, CA, USA) according to the manufacturer's recommendations. Briefly, 2.5 μg of RNA was reverse transcribed using a First-strand cDNA synthesis kit (TOYOBO, Kyoto, Japan) and cDNAs were stored at −20 °C. After 10-fold dilution, cDNA was used for the relative quantification of gene amplification. Primer sets for all genes were designed using Primer 6.0 Software (Applied Biosystems, Foster City, CA, USA) and synthesized commercially by Sangon (Shanghai, China). The primers sequences for rat PYY were sense 5′ CCGTTATGGTCGCAATGCT 3′, antisense 5′ TCTCGCTGTCGTCTGTGAA 3′. The primers sequences for rat GLP-1 were: sense 5′ CGGAAGAAGTCGCCATAGC 3′, antisense 5′ CAGCCAGTTGATGAAGTCTCT 3′. Rat β-*actin* was selected as the internal control gene for all QPCR reactions by using the following primers sequences: 5′ CTTTCTACAATGAGCTGCGTGTG 3′, antisense 5′ GTCAGGATCTTCATGAGGTAGTCTGTC 3′. cDNA was amplified by QPCR using a Bio-Rad CFX Connect™ Real-Time PCR Detection System (Bio-Rad, Richmond, CA, USA) under the following conditions: 95 °C for 3 min for enzyme activation, followed by denaturing at 95 °C for 20 s and annealing at 59 °C for 20 s and elongation at 72 °C for 20 s, repeated for a total of 40 cycles. Gene expression levels were calculated after normalization to the standard housekeeping gene β-*actin* using the $\Delta\Delta C_t$ method. Briefly, the mean values of the triplicate cycle thresholds (CT) of the target genes (PYY and GLP-1) were normalized to the mean values of triplicate CT of the reference β-*actin* using the calculation formula "$2^{CT_{\beta\text{-}actin} - CT_{\text{target gene}}}$", which indicated a relative value as a fraction of PYY or GLP-1.

2.7. Statistical Analysis

Data were compared by repeated ANOVA measures plus Tukey's post-hoc test, using the "PROC MIXED" function of the SAS software program (SAS 9.1, SAS Institute Inc., Cary, NC, USA). Data were examined to ensure patterns of constant variance and a normal distribution. The results that did not meet these conditions were transformed to appropriate data using logarithms or square roots. Data were presented as means ± SEM, and significant differences were accepted at a probability of $p < 0.05$.

3. Results

3.1. Food Intake and Body Weight

Average daily food intake throughout the experiment was affected by the dietary treatment in the decreasing magnitude order of control > PX > PG > KF ($p < 0.05$). Accordingly, cumulative food intake was significantly lower for rats fed the KF and PG diets than their control counterparts ($p < 0.05$), but with no significant difference between control and PX groups (Figure 1B). Compared with the control group, the final body weight and body weight gain showed a lower tendency in the KF and PG groups, but was not statistically significant ($p > 0.05$) (Figure 1C,D).

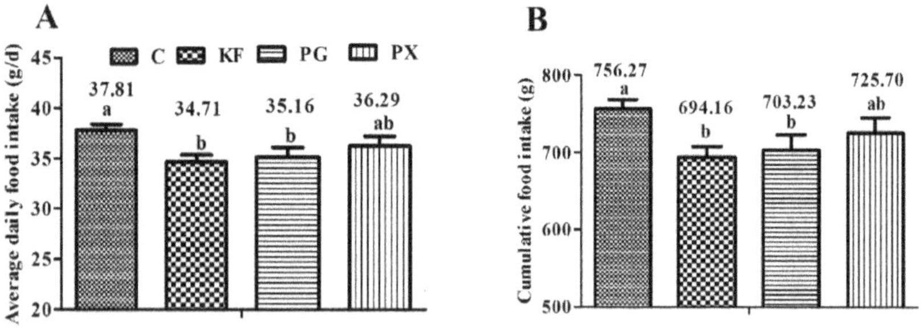

Figure 1. *Cont.*

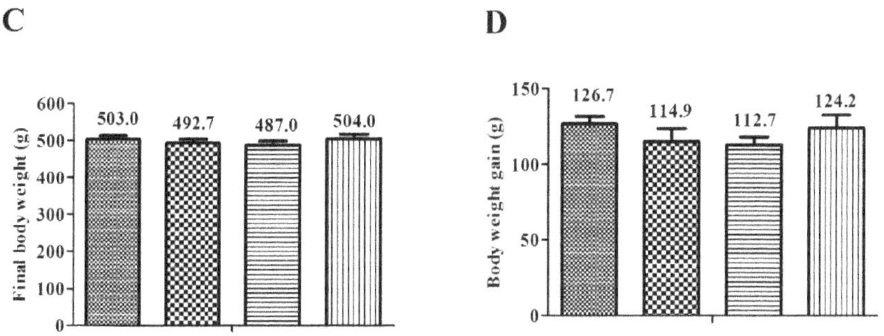

Figure 1. Food intake and body weight. (**A**) Average daily food intake; (**B**) cumulative food intake; (**C**) final body weight; and (**D**) body weight gain in rats given diets containing different dietary fibers for three weeks. Diets were control (C) or supplemented with 2% fiber of *konjac* flour (KF), pregelatinized waxy maize starch plus guar gum (PG) or pregelatinized waxy maize starch plus xanthan gum (PX); Values are mean ± SEM of $n = 8$ per group. Bars with different letters indicate a significant difference ($p < 0.05$).

3.2. Behavioral Satiety Sequence

The behavioral satiety sequence (feeding, drinking, activity, inactivity, grooming, and resting) of rats is shown in Table 2 and Figure 2. The overall pattern of behaviors was similar among all the dietary treatments. Quantification of individual behaviors indicated that the KF and PG groups spent significantly less time on feeding than the control group ($p < 0.05$; Table 2). When compared with other groups, the control group showed the feeding peak in the second time bin (control 91.88%, KF 84.38%, PG 74.38%, and PX 78.75%, respectively, $p = 0.07$; Figure 2). Furthermore, compared with bin 7 in the control group (Figure 2F–I), the KF, PG, and PX groups showed the transition from eating to resting in time bins 6, 5, and 6, respectively, which was consistent with the result that KF and PG groups had a lower food intake than the control group during the 1 h observation period ($p < 0.05$; Figure 2A).

Table 2. Behavioral satiety sequence of rats given diets containing different dietary fibers on day 15 [1].

Item	Control [2]	KF [2]	PG [2]	PX [2]	*p*-Value
Behavior (% time)					
Feeding	44.69 ± 3.45 ^{a}	34.53 ± 3.06 ^{b}	30.83 ± 3.19 ^{b}	35.94 ± 2.94 ^{a,b}	0.03
Drinking	6.04 ± 0.69	6.88 ± 0.70	5.47 ± 0.48	5.36 ± 0.80	0.38
Activity	21.15 ± 2.75	24.11 ± 3.54	21.82 ± 3.99	20.78 ± 2.12	0.88
Inactivity	10.42 ± 0.87	8.85 ± 1.52	10.73 ± 1.30	11.51 ± 2.01	0.64
Grooming	3.49 ± 0.47	4.53 ± 0.91	4.32 ± 1.09	4.11 ± 0.31	0.79
Resting	14.22 ± 4.08	21.09 ± 4.06	26.82 ± 4.28	22.29 ± 5.28	0.21

[1] After a 12-h fast, rats were given food, and their behaviors monitored for 1 h. The percentage of time spent in each behavior was calculated and represented as mean ± SEM of $n = 8$ per group. Rows with different superscript letters indicate a significant difference ($p < 0.05$); [2] Diets were control or supplemented with 2% fiber of *konjac* flour (KF), pregelatinized waxy maize starch plus guar gum (PG), or pregelatinized waxy maize starch plus xanthan gum (PX).

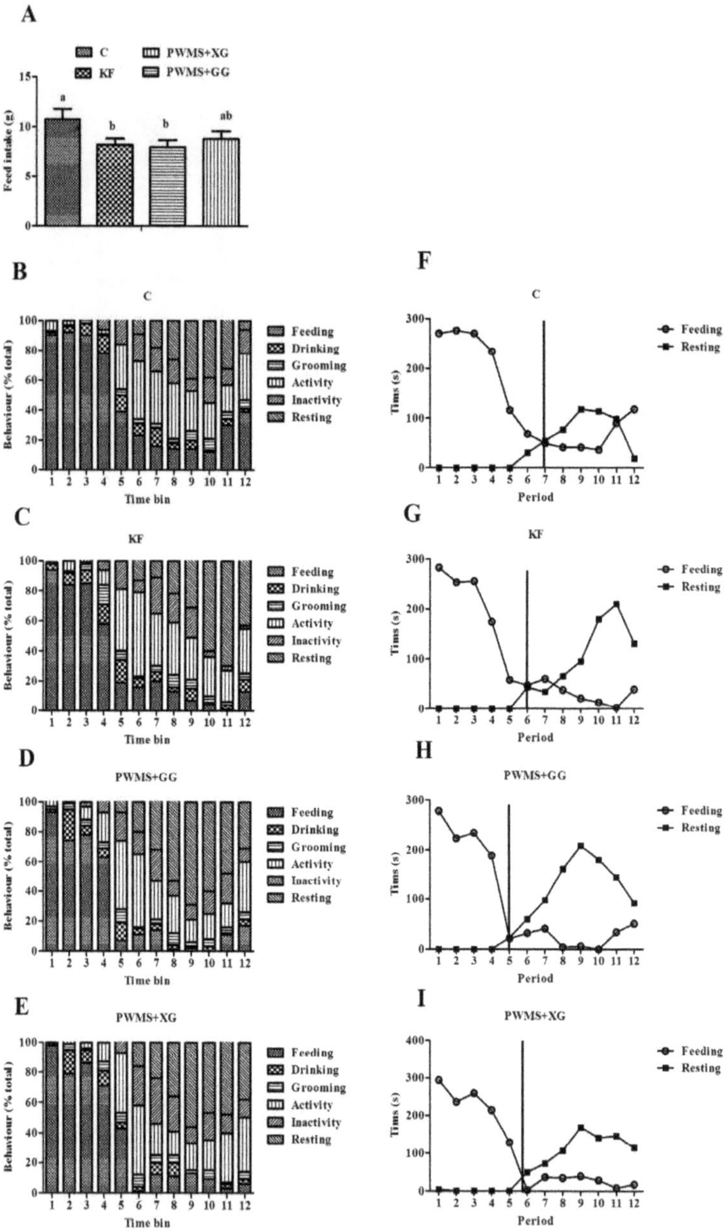

Figure 2. Food intake (**A**) in rats was calculated at 1 h and is presented as mean ± SEM for $n = 8$ per group. Bars with different letters indicate a significant difference ($p < 0.05$). Periods 1–12 correspond to the twelve 5-min time bins comprising the 60 min test session; (**B–E**) Frequency data within each behavioral category are expressed as a proportion of the total number of observations per time bin; (**F–I**) correspond to crossover graphs illustrating the point of transition from eating to resting. The perpendicular line indicates satiety point. Diets were control (C) or supplemented with 2% fiber of *konjac* flour (KF), pregelatinized waxy maize starch plus guar gum (PG), or pregelatinized waxy maize starch plus xanthan gum (PX).

3.3. Meal Pattern Parameters

Meal pattern parameters are presented in Table 3. Although the diurnal and nocturnal food intakes were similar among the four groups, the PG, KF, and PX groups were significantly lower than the control group in total food intake ($p < 0.01$). The feeding rate, meal size and meal duration (total, diurnal, and nocturnal) were similar among all the groups. However, the total and nocturnal meal numbers of the KF and PG groups were significantly lower than those of the control group ($p < 0.05$). As expected, the PG group was obviously higher than the control group in total inter-meal interval ($p < 0.05$), and the KF and PX groups were also higher, but not statistically significant.

Table 3. Meal pattern parameters of rats given diets containing different dietary fibers for three weeks [1].

Item	Control [2]	KF [2]	PG [2]	PX [2]	*p*-Value
Food intake (g/day)					
Total	51.68 ± 1.50 [a]	46.58 ± 0.86 [b]	46.01 ± 1.07 [b]	48.47 ± 0.79 [b]	<0.01
Nocturnal	23.40 ± 1.20	20.55 ± 1.04	20.79 ± 0.96	20.18 ± 1.53	0.24
Diurnal	28.29 ± 0.67	26.03 ± 1.33	25.22 ± 0.64	28.29 ± 1.62	0.16
Feeding rate (mg/s)					
Total	6.59 ± 0.93	6.54 ± 0.68	8.41 ± 1.29	5.89 ± 0.57	0.26
Nocturnal	5.67 ± 0.88	6.04 ± 0.44	7.09 ± 0.52	5.37 ± 0.62	0.26
Diurnal	6.59 ± 1.08	7.38 ± 1.25	8.47 ± 0.85	6.32 ± 0.60	0.45
Meal size (g/day)					
Total	3.12 ± 0.20	3.21 ± 0.13	3.39 ± 0.19	2.92 ± 0.19	0.33
Nocturnal	2.36 ± 0.14	2.53 ± 0.16	2.52 ± 0.15	2.20 ± 0.10	0.30
Diurnal	4.36 ± 0.41	4.22 ± 0.33	4.89 ± 0.47	3.73 ± 0.30	0.22
Meal duration (s)					
Total	507.45 ± 39.86	517.79 ± 41.60	437.35 ± 35.27	517.51 ± 41.47	0.43
Nocturnal	449.70 ± 38.00	440.70 ± 49.95	365.73 ± 28.00	437.96 ± 37.82	0.35
Diurnal	584.90 ± 49.69	620.19 ± 51.21	591.17 ± 40.64	612.64 ± 49.50	0.94
Meal number (meals/day)					
Total	16.88 ± 0.74 [a]	14.63 ± 0.50 [b]	13.88 ± 0.83 [b]	17.00 ± 0.89 [a]	0.01
Nocturnal	10.00 ± 0.38 [a]	8.25 ± 0.41 [b]	8.38 ± 0.50 [b]	9.25 ± 0.70 [a,b]	0.07
Diurnal	6.88 ± 0.61a [b]	6.38 ± 0.50 [a,b]	5.50 ± 0.53 [b]	7.75 ± 0.41 [a]	0.03
Inter-meal interval (min)					
Total	73.49 ± 4.57 [b]	87.72 ± 4.16 [a,b]	98.23 ± 9.48 [a]	76.53 ± 4.03 [b]	0.03
Nocturnal	58.34 ± 4.70	73.24 ± 6.40	70.90 ± 6.68	65.10 ± 4.74	0.27
Diurnal	106.65 ± 13.23	113.15 ± 9.48	133.19 ± 13.33	93.65 ± 5.61	0.09

[1] Values are mean ± SEM of $n = 8$, rows with different superscript letters indicate a significant difference ($p < 0.05$); [2] Diets were control or supplemented with 2% fiber of *konjac* flour (KF), pregelatinized waxy maize starch plus guar gum (PG), or pregelatinized waxy maize starch plus xanthan gum (PX).

3.4. Plasma Concentrations of GLP-1/PYY, mRNA Abundance in Distal Ileum of GLP-1/PYY, and Concentrations of SCFAs in Cecal Contents

There was no significant difference in the plasma concentrations of GLP-1 and PYY, and the mRNA abundance of GLP-1 and PYY in ileum tissue among the four dietary treatments (Figure 3). Compared with the control group, the concentrations of acetic acid and SCFAs in cecal contents were increased in the KF and PG groups ($p < 0.05$; Figure 4). Additionally, the KF, PG, and PX groups had higher concentrations of the propionic acid in cecal contents than the control group ($p < 0.05$).

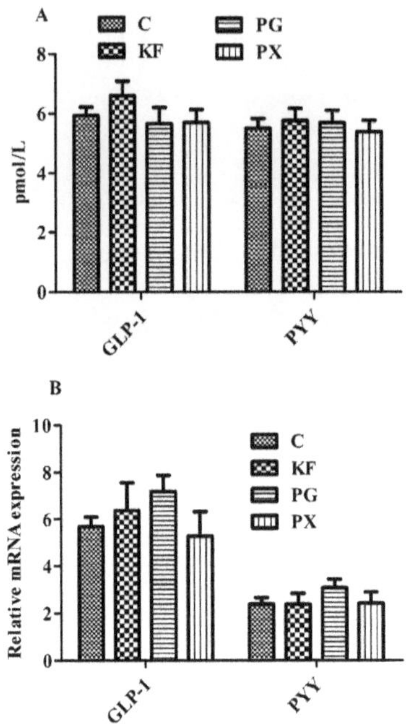

Figure 3. Plasma concentrations (**A**) and mRNA abundance in distal ileum (**B**) of GLP-1 and PYY in rats given diets containing different dietary fibers for three weeks; Diets were control (C) or supplemented with 2% fiber of *konjac* flour (KF), pregelatinized waxy maize starch plus guar gum (PG), or pregelatinized waxy maize starch plus xanthan gum (PX); Values are mean ± SEM, n = 6–8 per group. GLP-1, glucagon-like peptide-1; PYY, peptide tyrosine-tyrosine.

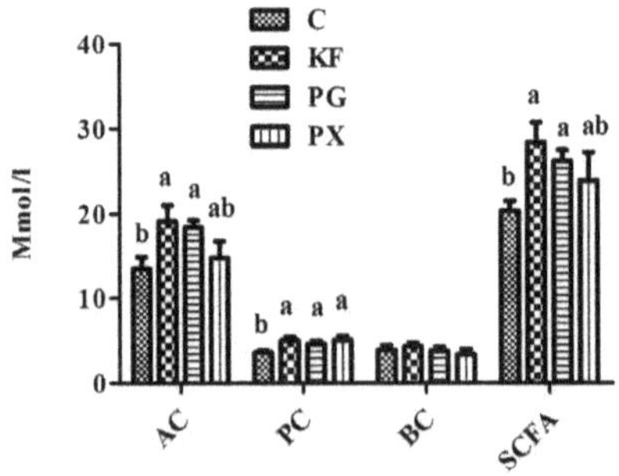

Figure 4. Concentration of SCFAs in cecal contents of rats given diets containing different dietary fibers for three weeks. Diets were control (C) or supplemented with 2% fiber of *konjac* flour (KF), pregelatinized waxy maize starch plus guar gum (PG) or pregelatinized waxy maize starch plus xanthan gum (PX); Values are mean ± SEM of n = 6–8 per group. Bars with different letters indicate a significant difference ($p < 0.05$). SCFAs, short-chain fatty acids; AC, acetate acid; PC, propionate acid; BC, butyrate acid.

4. Discussion

The present study aimed to explore whether dietary fibers regulate appetite by promoting satiety or satiation, and to this end, behavioral satiety sequence and meal pattern were monitored.

Detailed analysis of the behavioral satiety sequence revealed that the overall pattern of the behavioral response to fast-induced food intake in rats was normal. However, we observed a decrease in short-term (1 h) food intake, accompanied by reduced feeding behavior in rats fed the KF and PG diets. Furthermore, the transition from eating to resting occurred in early time bins in the PG, PX, and KF groups, indicating that satiety was induced in the three groups [35]. To our knowledge, this is probably the first report so far about a detailed analysis of the behavioral satiety sequence following dietary fiber treatments in rats.

The present results are consistent with our previous study in that supplementation of KF reduced the non-feeding oral behavior and promoted the satiety of sows [20]. In the current study, there was no significant difference in the feeding rates of rats among all the dietary treatments. Based on the association of taste and flavor aversions with a decrease in feeding rate [36], the consistent feeding rates indicated that dietary fiber supplementation did not produce a significant effect on food palatability, implying that the changes in the meal pattern observed here might be attributed to physiological factors rather than changes in diet palatability or flavor.

In the present study, dietary supplementation of KF and PG reduced the total food intake, mainly due to the increased satiety, as indicated by decreased meal numbers and increased inter-meal intervals. This is in agreement with a previous study that reported the suppression of food intake 2 h after the administration of the mixture of guar gum and fructo-oligosaccharide, due to decreased meal numbers and increased inter-meal intervals [37]. It is worth noting that the current result contrasted with a most recent study about diets supplemented with guar gum or fructo-oligosaccharide alone [30]. Although both of them reduced the food intake immediately after dietary fiber ingestion, the result was mainly attributed to a decrease of meal size and meal duration but not meal number and inter-meal intervals, indicating that the decrease in food intake is associated with increased satiation rather than satiety. In the current study, the rats consumed such a high proportion of their daily intake during the light phase, probably due to their 12-h fast overnight before the meal pattern analysis.

Pregelatinized waxy maize starch and fructo-oligosaccharide are highly fermentable fibers [38,39], and guar gum is a viscous fiber with high water-binding capacity [3]. This suggests that the combination of fibers with different physicochemical properties may affect the physiological processes (satiation or satiety) of appetite regulation. In the present study, dietary treatments were similar in insoluble fiber and viscosity, but their soluble fiber, water-binding capacity, and swelling capacity followed the sequence of PG > KF > PX > control.

The addition of a small amount of hydrocolloids resulted in a large enhancement in water-binding capacity and swelling capacity of starch pastes, but a reduction of syneresis in starch gels, indicating that the magnitude of such changes in paste rheology and texture depends on the type of starch and gum used [40,41]. The current results (PG group with highest water-binding capacity and swelling capacity) could be explained by a previous study which showed that the most pronounced effect has been the retardation of gelation kinetics of waxy maize starch plus the guar gum, rather than the combination with other gums [42].

Gelatinized waxy maize starch was subjected to different time and temperature conditions of storage to obtain samples with different extents of amylopectin retrogradation. Increased retrogradation extents reduced the enzyme susceptibilities to pancreatic alpha amylase and amyloglucosidase at 37 °C [43]. The pregelatinized starch produced more satiety than the raw potato starch, probably because this starch was digested too slowly to increase the postprandial blood glucose concentrations to any appreciable extent [44,45].

Soluble fiber with high water-binding capacity and viscosity may slow gastric emptying and small bowel transit [46,47], and several of the aforementioned signals generated in the gastrointestinal tract cooperate to promote satiety by activating vagal afferents and/or by acting directly on the brain [48,49]. Thus, the increased satiety by dietary supplementation of KF and PG is associated with decreased food intake in rats, which may be attributed to the high water-binding capacity and swelling capacity in those diets.

In the current study, supplementation of KF and PG significantly increased the concentrations of acetic acid, propionate acid, and SCFAs in the cecal content of rats. A number of factors—including chemical structure, particle size, surface area, and solubility of the fiber—affect the fermentation in the gut and the nature of the SCFAs produced [50,51]. Carbohydrates containing glucomannan or alpha-galacturonic acid residues are generally more susceptible to fermentation [51]. A comparison of *konjac* gum, guar gum, xanthan gum, and pectin in human fecal inoculum in a 48-h static fermentation culture system showed that all the gums increased the SCFAs level, and *konjac* and guar gum had the strongest acid-reducing ability among gum dietary fibers [52]. Resistant starch is completely degraded in the large bowel, and thus long-term consumption of fermentable fiber could produce satiety benefits [53].

It has been suggested that SCFAs stimulate the production and secretion of satiety-related hormones, such as GLP-1 and PYY, possibly via G-protein coupled receptors [54]. However, in the current study, dietary treatments did not alter the GLP-1 and PYY either in plasma concentration or mRNA abundance in distal ileum two hours after feeding, which is not consistent with a previous report that dietary supplementation of fructooligosaccharide increased the plasma concentration of PYY in the fasted state of rats [37]. It can be inferred that dietary fiber effect on satiety hormones (GLP-1/PYY) is associated with fed or fasted state. PYY and GLP-1 are both synthesized and released from L-cells located in the small intestine and large intestine [55]. They showed no increased expression here in distal ileum, probably due to an overall increase in L-cell number along the enlarged intestines, which was not detectable here since the real time PCR method measures expression per mg tissue. Slowly digestible starch inclusion in pig diet decreased distal ileum SCFAs transporter mRNA abundance [56]. This is why we selected the distal ileum for anatomical analysis.

The SCFAs produced via bacterial fermentation directly suppresses appetite via central hypothalamic mechanisms in rodents [57]. Recent findings from human study suggest that propionate production may play an important role in attenuating reward-based eating behavior via striatal pathways, independent of changes in plasma PYY and GLP-1 [58]. It is well known that SCFAs serve as an additional energy source, especially at the moment when glucose absorption is decreasing (or completed) in the small intestine, which helps to stabilize glucose levels in blood [59,60]. Delayed postprandial glucose transient declines could delay the onset of the ensuing meal and induce inter-meal satiety [61].

In the current study, dietary treatments had no effect on final body weight and body weight gain in the rats. At 10 weeks of age, the tested rats were young adults. The adult rats might continue to gain body mass at a slower rate, but the juvenile rapid growth phase ceased [62]. Therefore, the similarity in the body weight gain of rats among all the dietary treatments can be explained from the analysis of short-term effects.

The slight but not significant variation in feeding behavior, meal number, and SCFAs yield in PX group may result in an overall reduction trend but not in notable changes in food intake, probably due to the reason that the PX diet did not reach the level of KF and PG diets in the physicochemical properties (water-binding capacity and swelling capacity) and fermentability (SCFAs), thus it could not produce a significant effect on the satiety and food intake in rats.

In the current study, the daily dosage of soluble fiber per kilogram of body weight in rats was 1.4 g/kg (35 g (daily food intake) × 2% (dosage)/0.5 kg (body weight) = 1.4 g/kg body weight). Based on the dose translation formula (Human equivalent doses (mg/kg) = Animal dose (mg/kg) × (Animal Km/Human Km)) from animal to human studies revisited [63,64], the corresponding soluble fiber dose for humans was estimated to be 0.23 g/kg (1.4 g/kg (Animal dose) × 6 (Animal Km)/37 (Human Km) = 0.23 g/kg), which means the soluble fiber dose for a 60 kg person is 13.8 g (0.23 g/kg × 60 kg = 13.8 g). Further work is required to translate the findings to humans.

5. Conclusions

KF and PG reduce the food intake, probably by promoting the satiety, which was supported by decreased meal numbers and increased inter-meal intervals, but without a reduction in body weight gain. Additionally, dietary soluble fibers with high levels of physicochemical properties (water-binding capacity and swelling capacity) and fermentability (SCFAs) have a more significant effect on food intake, meal pattern, and feeding behavior in rats.

Author Contributions: All authors contributed to the paper in the following ways: conception and design of the study (J.P., Y.F.Z.), acquisition of data (C.Q.T., X.C.Z., C.H.X.), analysis and interpretation of the data (J.P., C.Q.T., H.K.W.), drafting the article (C.Q.T.), and final approval (J.P., C.Q.T., Y.F.Z.).

Conflicts of Interest: The authors declare no conflict of interest.

References

1. Raghad, A.; Hala, G.; Mohamad, A.; Omar, O. Meal pattern of male rats maintained on amino acid supplemented diets: The effect of tryptophan, lysine, arginine, proline and threonine. *Nutrients* **2014**, *6*, 2509–2522.
2. Schroeder, N.; Marquart, L.F.; Gallaher, D.D. The role of viscosity and fermentability of dietary fibers on satiety- and adiposity-related hormones in rats. *Nutrients* **2013**, *5*, 2093–2113. [CrossRef] [PubMed]
3. Wanders, A.J.; Jonathan, M.C.; van den Borne, J.J.; Mars, M.; Schols, H.A.; Feskens, E.J.; de Graaf, C. The effects of bulking, viscous and gel-forming dietary fibres on satiation. *Br. J. Nutr.* **2013**, *109*, 1330–1337. [CrossRef] [PubMed]
4. Bortolotti, M.; Levorato, M.; Lugli, A.; Mazzero, G. Effect of a balanced mixture of dietary fibers on gastric emptying, intestinal transit and body weight. *Ann. Nutr. Metab.* **2008**, *52*, 221–226. [CrossRef] [PubMed]
5. Rendon-Huerta, J.A.; Juarez-Flores, B.; Pinos-Rodriguez, J.M.; Aguirre-Rivera, J.R.; Delgado-Portales, R.E. Effects of different sources of fructans on body weight, blood metabolites and fecal bacteria in normal and obese non-diabetic and diabetic rats. *Plant Foods Hum. Nutr.* **2012**, *67*, 64–70. [CrossRef] [PubMed]
6. Howarth, N.C.; Saltzman, E.; Roberts, S.B. Dietary fiber and weight regulation. *Nutr. Rev.* **2001**, *59*, 129–139. [CrossRef] [PubMed]
7. Li, J.; Zhang, N.; Hu, L.; Li, Z.; Li, R.; Li, C.; Wang, S. Improvement in chewing activity reduces energy intake in one meal and modulates plasma gut hormone concentrations in obese and lean young Chinese men. *Am. J. Clin. Nutr.* **2011**, *94*, 709–716. [CrossRef] [PubMed]
8. Zijlstra, N.; Mars, M.; de Wijk, R.A.; Westerterp-Plantenga, M.S.; de Graaf, C. The effect of viscosity on ad libitum food intake. *Int. J. Obes.* **2008**, *32*, 676–683. [CrossRef] [PubMed]
9. Dabin, B. Fibres for fertility: The inclusion of raw fibre in sow diets has many positive effects. In *Feed Mix*; Misset International: Doetinchem, The Netherlands, 2006; pp. 18–21.
10. Bergmann, J.F.; Chassany, O.; Petit, A.; Triki, R.; Caulin, C.; Segrestaa, J.M. Correlation between echographic gastric emptying and appetite: Influence of psyllium. *Gut* **1992**, *33*, 1042–1043. [CrossRef] [PubMed]
11. Phillips, R.J.; Powley, T.L. Tension and stretch receptors in gastrointestinal smooth muscle: Re-evaluating vagal mechanoreceptor electrophysiology. *Brain Res. Brain Res. Rev.* **2000**, *34*, 1–26. [CrossRef]
12. Heijboer, A.C.; Pijl, H.; van den Hoek, A.M.; Havekes, L.M.; Romijn, J.A.; Corssmit, E.P.M. Gut-brain axis: Regulation of glucose metabolism. *J. Neuroendocrinol.* **2006**, *18*, 883–894. [CrossRef] [PubMed]
13. Silva, E.; Birkenhake, M.; Scholten, E.; Sagis, L.M.C.; Linden, E.V.D. Controlling rheology and structure of sweet potato starch noodles with high broccoli powder content by hydrocolloids. *Food Hydrocoll.* **2013**, *30*, 42–52. [CrossRef]
14. Sun, H.Q.; Zhou, Y.F.; Tan, C.Q.; Zheng, L.F.; Peng, J.; Jiang, S.W. Effects of konjac flour inclusion in gestation diets on the nutrient digestibility, lactation feed intake and reproductive performance of sows. *Animal* **2014**, *8*, 1089–1094. [CrossRef] [PubMed]
15. Katsuraya, K.; Okuyama, K.; Hatanaka, K.; Oshima, R.; Sato, T.; Matsuzaki, K. Constitution of konjac glucomannan: Chemical analysis and 13 C NMR spectroscopy. *Carbohydr. Polym.* **2003**, *53*, 183–189. [CrossRef]
16. Chua, M.; Baldwin, T.C.; Hocking, T.J.; Chan, K. Traditional uses and potential health benefits of *Amorphophallus konjac* K. Koch ex NEBr. *J. Ethnopharmacol.* **2010**, *128*, 268–278. [CrossRef] [PubMed]

17. Shah, B.R.; Li, B.; Wang, L.; Liu, S.; Li, Y.; Wei, X.; Jin, W.; Li, Z. Health benefits of konjac glucomannan with special focus on diabetes. *Bioact. Carbohydr. Diet. Fibre* **2015**, *5*, 179–187. [CrossRef]
18. Tan, C.Q.; Wei, H.K.; Sun, H.Q.; Long, G.; Ao, J.T.; Jiang, S.W.; Peng, J. Effects of supplementing sow diets during two gestations with konjac flour and *Saccharomyces boulardii* on constipation in peripartal period, lactation feed intake and piglet performance. *Anim. Feed Sci. Technol.* **2015**, *210*, 254–262. [CrossRef]
19. Tan, C.Q.; Wei, H.K.; Ao, J.T.; Long, G.; Peng, J. Inclusion of konjac flour in the gestation diet changes the gut microbiota, alleviates oxidative stress, and improves insulin sensitivity in sows. *Appl. Environ. Microbiol.* **2016**, *82*, 5899–5909. [CrossRef] [PubMed]
20. Sun, H.; Tan, C.; Wei, H.; Zou, Y.; Long, G.; Ao, J.; Xue, H.; Jiang, S.; Peng, J. Effects of different amounts of konjac flour inclusion in gestation diets on physio-chemical properties of diets, postprandial satiety in pregnant sows, lactation feed intake of sows and piglet performance. *Anim. Reprod. Sci.* **2015**, *152*, 55–64. [CrossRef] [PubMed]
21. Copeland, L.; Blazek, J.; Salman, H.; Tang, M.C.M. Form and functionality of starch. *Food Hydrocoll.* **2009**, *23*, 1527–1534. [CrossRef]
22. Shimotoyodome, A.; Suzuki, J.; Kameo, Y.; Hase, T. Dietary supplementation with hydroxypropyl-distarch phosphate from waxy maize starch increases resting energy expenditure by lowering the postprandial glucose-dependent insulinotropic polypeptide response in human subjects. *Br. J. Nutr.* **2011**, *106*, 96–104. [CrossRef] [PubMed]
23. Fuongfuchat, A.; Seetapan, N.; Makmoon, T.; Pongjaruwat, W.; Methacanon, P.; Gamonpilas, C. Linear and non-linear viscoelastic behaviors of crosslinked tapioca starch/polysaccharide systems. *J. Food Eng.* **2012**, *109*, 571–578. [CrossRef]
24. Mandala, I.G.; Bayas, E. Xanthan effect on swelling, solubility and viscosity of wheat starch dispersions. *Food Hydrocoll.* **2004**, *18*, 191–201. [CrossRef]
25. Paquet, É.; Bédard, A.; Lemieux, S.; Turgeon, S.L. Effects of apple juice-based beverages enriched with dietary fibres and xanthan gum on the glycemic response and appetite sensations in healthy men. *Bioact. Carbohydr. Diet. Fibre* **2014**, *4*, 39–47. [CrossRef]
26. Tan, C.Q.; Wei, H.K.; Zhao, X.C.; Xu, C.H.; Peng, J. Effects of Water Binding Capacity and Swelling Capacity of Soluble Fibers on Physicochemical Properties of Gastrointestinal Digesta and Food Intake in Rats. *Food Nutr. Res.* **2015**, in press.
27. Glendinning, J.I.; Smith, J.C. Consistency of meal patterns in laboratory rats. *Physiol. Behav.* **1994**, *56*, 7–16. [CrossRef]
28. Halford, J.C.; Wanninayake, S.C.; Blundell, J.E. Behavioral satiety sequence (BSS) for the diagnosis of drug action on food intake. *Pharmacol. Biochem. Behav.* **1998**, *61*, 159–168. [CrossRef]
29. Lira, L.A.; Almeida, L.C.A.; Silva, A.A.M.D.; Cavalcante, T.C.F.; Melo, D.D.C.B.D.; Souza, J.A.D.; Campina, R.C.F.; Souza, S.L.D. Perinatal undernutrition increases meal size and neuronal activation of the nucleus of the solitary tract in response to feeding stimulation in adult rats. *Int. J. Dev. Neurosci.* **2014**, *38*, 23–29. [CrossRef] [PubMed]
30. Hadri, Z.; Chaumontet, C.; Fromentin, G.; Even, P.C.; Darcel, N.; Bouras, A.D.; Tome, D.; Rasoamanana, R. Long term ingestion of a preload containing fructo-oligosaccharide or guar gum decreases fat mass but not food intake in mice. *Physiol. Behav.* **2015**, *147*, 198–204. [CrossRef] [PubMed]
31. Association of Official Analytical Chemists. *Official Methods of Analysis*, 16th ed.; AOAC International: Arlington, VA, USA, 1999.
32. Johansen, H.N.; Bach Knudsen, K.E.; Wood, P.J.; Fulcher, R.G. Physico-Chemical Properties and the Degradation of Oat Bran Polysaccharides in the Gut of Pigs. *J. Sci. Food Agric.* **1997**, *73*, 81–92. [CrossRef]
33. Serena, A.; Jorgensen, H.; Knudsen, K.E.B. Digestion of carbohydrates and utilization of energy in sows fed diets with contrasting levels and physicochemical properties of dietary fiber. *J. Anim. Sci.* **2008**, *86*, 2208–2216. [CrossRef] [PubMed]
34. Bosch, G.; Pellikaan, W.F.; Rutten, P.G.P.; van der Poel, A.F.B.; Verstegen, M.W.A.; Hendriks, W.H. Comparative in vitro fermentation activity in the canine distal gastrointestinal tract and fermentation kinetics of fiber sources. *J. Anim. Sci.* **2008**, *86*, 2979–2989. [CrossRef] [PubMed]
35. Orozco-Solis, R.; Lopes-de-Souza, S.; Barbosa Matos, R.J.; Grit, I.; Le-Bloch, J.; Nguyen, P.; Manhaes-de-Castro, R.; Bolanos-Jimenez, F. Perinatal undernutrition-induced obesity is independent of the developmental programming of feeding. *Physiol. Behav.* **2009**, *96*, 481–492. [CrossRef] [PubMed]

36. Labouré, H.; Saux, S.; Nicolaidis, S. Effects of food texture change on metabolic parameters: Short- and long-term feeding patterns and body weight. *Am. J. Physiol. Regul. Integr. Comp. Physiol.* **2001**, *280*, R780–R789. [PubMed]
37. Rasoamanana, R.; Even, P.C.; Darcel, N.; Tomé, D.; Fromentin, G. Dietary fibers reduce food intake by satiation without conditioned taste aversion in mice. *Physiol. Behav.* **2013**, *17*, 13–19. [CrossRef] [PubMed]
38. Alles, M.S.; de Roos, N.M.; Bakx, J.C.; van de Lisdonk, E.; Zock, P.L.; Hautvast, G.A. Consumption of fructooligosaccharides does not favorably affect blood glucose and serum lipid concentrations in patients with type 2 diabetes. *Am. J. Clin. Nutr.* **1999**, *69*, 64–69. [PubMed]
39. Da Silva, C.S.; Bosch, G.; Bolhuis, J.E.; Stappers, L.J.N.; van Hees, H.M.J.; Gerrits, W.J.J.; Kemp, B. Effects of alginate and resistant starch on feeding patterns, behaviour and performance in ad libitum-fed growing pigs. *Animal* **2014**, *8*, 1917–1927. [CrossRef] [PubMed]
40. Eidam, D.C.D.; Kuhn, K.; Stute, R. Formation of Maize Starch Gels Selectively Regulated by the Addition of Hydrocolloids. *Starch Stärke* **1995**, *47*, 378–384. [CrossRef]
41. Sudhakar, V.; Singhal, R.S.; Kulkarni, P.R. Effect of salts on interactions of starch with guar gum. *Food Hydrocoll.* **1996**, *10*, 329–334. [CrossRef]
42. Biliaderis, C.G.; Arvanitoyannis, I.; Izydorczyk, M.S.; Prokopowich, D.J. Effect of Hydrocolloids on Gelatinization and Structure Formation in Concentrated Waxy Maize and Wheat Starch Gels. *Starch Stärke* **1997**, *49*, 278–283. [CrossRef]
43. Eerlingen, R.C.; Jacobs, H.; Delcour, J.A. Enzyme-resistant starch. V. Effect of retrogradation of waxy maize starch on enzyme susceptibility. *Cereal Chem.* **1994**, *71*, 351–355.
44. Liljeberg, H.G.; Akerberg, A.K.; Björck, I.M. Effect of the glycemic index and content of indigestible carbohydrates of cereal-based breakfast meals on glucose tolerance at lunch in healthy subjects. *Am. J. Clin. Nutr.* **1999**, *69*, 647–655. [PubMed]
45. Raben, A.; Tagliabue, A.; Christensen, N.J.; Madsen, J.; Holst, J.J.; Astrup, A. Resistant starch: The effect on postprandial glycemia, hormonal response, and satiety. *Am. J. Clin. Nutr.* **1994**, *60*, 544–551. [PubMed]
46. Burton-Freeman, B. Dietary fiber and energy regulation. *J. Nutr.* **2000**, *130*, 272S–275S. [PubMed]
47. Kristensen, M.; Jensen, M.G. Dietary fibres in the regulation of appetite and food intake. Importance of viscosity. *Appetite* **2011**, *56*, 65–70. [CrossRef] [PubMed]
48. Moran, T.H.; Ladenheim, E.E.; Schwartz, G.J. Within-meal gut feedback signaling. *Int. J. Obes. Relat. Metab. Disord.* **2001**, *25*, S39–S41. [CrossRef] [PubMed]
49. Schwartz, G. Integrative capacity of the caudal brainstem in the control of food intake. *Philos. Trans. R. Soc. B Biol. Sci.* **2006**, *361*, 1275–1280. [CrossRef] [PubMed]
50. Blackwood, A.D.; Salter, J.; Dettmar, P.W.; Chaplin, M.F. Dietary fibre, physicochemical properties and their relationship to health. *J. R. Soc. Promot. Health* **2000**, *120*, 242–247. [CrossRef] [PubMed]
51. Slavin, J.; Savarino, V.; Paredes-Diaz, A.; Fotopoulos, G. A review of the role of soluble fiber in health with specific reference to wheat dextrin. *J. Int. Med. Res.* **2009**, *37*, 1–17. [CrossRef] [PubMed]
52. Fiszman, S.; Varela, P. The role of gums in satiety/satiation. A review. *Food Hydrocoll.* **2013**, *32*, 147–154. [CrossRef]
53. Yang, H.-F.; Chen, H.-L. Utilization of Gum Dietary Fibers by the Human Fecal Inoculum in the Static Fermentation Culture System. *Taiwan J. Agric. Chem. Food Sci.* **2008**, *46*, 183–189.
54. Tilg, H.; Moschen, A.R. Microbiota and diabetes: An evolving relationship. *Gut* **2014**, *63*, 1513–1521. [CrossRef] [PubMed]
55. Del, P.A.; Iadevaia, M.; Loguercio, C. The role of gut hormones in controlling the food intake: What is their role in emerging diseases? *Endocrinol. Nutr.* **2012**, *59*, 197–206.
56. Woodward, A.D.; Regmi, P.R.; Gänzle, M.G.; van Kempen, T.A.; Zijlstra, R.T. Slowly digestible starch influences mRNA abundance of glucose and short-chain fatty acid transporters in the porcine distal intestinal tract. *J. Anim. Sci.* **2012**, *90*, 80–82. [CrossRef] [PubMed]
57. Frost, G.; Sleeth, M.L.; Sahuri-Arisoylu, M.; Lizarbe, B.; Cerdan, S.; Brody, L.; Anastasovska, J.; Ghourab, S.; Hankir, M.; Shuai, Z. The short-chain fatty acid acetate reduces appetite via a central homeostatic mechanism. *Nat. Commun.* **2014**, *5*, 3611. [CrossRef] [PubMed]
58. Byrne, C.S.; Chambers, E.S.; Alhabeeb, H.; Chhina, N.; Morrison, D.J.; Preston, T.; Tedford, C.; Fitzpatrick, J.; Irani, C.; Busza, A. Increased colonic propionate reduces anticipatory reward responses in the human striatum to high-energy foods123. *Am. J. Clin. Nutr.* **2016**, *188*, 724–732.

59. Higgins, J.A. Resistant starch: Metabolic effects and potential health benefits. *J. AOAC Int.* **2004**, *87*, 761–768. [CrossRef] [PubMed]
60. Leeuw, J.A.D.; Jongbloed, A.W.; Spoolder, H.A.M.; Verstegen, M.W.A. Effects of hindgut fermentation of non-starch polysaccharides on the stability of blood glucose and insulin levels and physical activity in empty sows. *Livest. Prod. Sci.* **2005**, *96*, 165–174. [CrossRef]
61. De Leeuw, J.A.; Jongbloed AWVerstegen, M.W. Dietary Fiber Stabilizes Blood Glucose and Insulin Levels and Reduces Physical Activity in Sows (Sus scrofa). *J. Nutr.* **2004**, *134*, 1481–1486. [PubMed]
62. Sengupta, P. The Laboratory Rat: Relating Its Age With Human's. *Int. J. Prev. Med.* **2013**, *4*, 624–630. [PubMed]
63. Food and Drug Administration. *Guidance for Industry: Estimating the Maximum Safe Starting Dose in Initial Clinical Trials for Therapeutics in Adult Healthy Volunteers*; Food and Drug Administration: Washington, DC, USA, 2005.
64. Reagan-Shaw, S.; Nihal, M.; Ahmad, N. Dose translation from animal to human studies revisited. *FASEB J.* **2008**, *22*, 659–661. [CrossRef] [PubMed]

nutrients MDPI

Article

Effect of Fibre Supplementation on Body Weight and Composition, Frequency of Eating and Dietary Choice in Overweight Individuals

Vicky A. Solah [1,*], Deborah A. Kerr [1], Wendy J. Hunt [1], Stuart K. Johnson [1], Carol J. Boushey [2], Edward J. Delp [3], Xingqiong Meng [4], Roland J. Gahler [5], Anthony P. James [1,6], Aqif S. Mukhtar [1,7], Haelee K. Fenton [1] and Simon Wood [1,8,9]

1 School of Public Health, Faculty of Health Sciences, Curtin University, Perth WA 6845, Australia; d.kerr@curtin.edu.au (D.A.K.); w.hunt@curtin.edu.au (W.J.H.); s.johnson@curtin.edu.au (S.K.J.); T.P.James@curtin.edu.au (A.P.J.); Aqif.Mukhtar@curtin.edu.au (A.S.M.); h.fenton@curtin.edu.au (H.K.F.); simonwood@shaw.ca (S.W.)
2 Epidemiology Program, University of Hawaii Cancer Center, Honolulu, HI 96813, USA; cjboushey@cc.hawaii.edu
3 Video and Image Processing Laboratory, School of Electrical and Computer Engineering, Purdue University, West Lafayette, IN 47907, USA; ace@ecn.purdue.edu
4 Flinders Centre for Innovation in Cancer, School of Medicine, Flinders University, Adelaide 5001, Australia; rosie.meng@flinders.edu.au
5 Factors Group R & D, Burnaby, BC V3N4S9, Canada; rgahler@naturalfactors.com
6 Curtin Health Innovation Research Institute, Faculty of Health Sciences, Curtin University, Perth WA 6845, Australia
7 Centre for Population Health Research, Faculty of Health Sciences, Curtin University, Perth WA 6845, Australia
8 InovoBiologic Inc., Calgary, AB Y2N4Y7, Canada
9 Food, Nutrition and Health Program, University of British Columbia, Vancouver, BC V6T1Z4, Canada
* Correspondence: v.solah@curtin.edu.au; Tel.: +61-8-9266-2771; Fax: +61-8-9266-2958

Received: 12 December 2016; Accepted: 13 February 2017; Published: 16 February 2017

Abstract: Fibre supplementation can potentially reduce energy intake and contribute to weight loss. The mechanism may be reduced frequency of eating, resulting in reduced food consumption. The objective of this research was to determine the effectiveness of fibre supplementation with PolyGlycopleX® (PGX®), on body weight and composition, frequency of eating and dietary intake in 118 overweight adults. In a three-arm, parallel, blind, randomised controlled trial participants were randomised to one of three groups; 4.5 g PGX as softgels (PGXS), 5 g PGX granules (PGXG) or 5 g rice flour (RF) control. Prior to supplementation and at 12 weeks, participants captured before and after images of all food and beverages consumed within 4 days using a mobile food record app (mFR). The mFR images were analysed for food group serving sizes and number of eating occasions. In the PGXG group, per-protocol analysis showed there was a significant reduction in waist circumference (2.5 cm; $p = 0.003$). Subgroup analysis showed that PGXG supplementation at the recommended dose resulted in a reduction in body weight (-1.4 ± 0.10 kg, $p < 0.01$), body mass index (BMI) reduction (-0.5 ± 0.10, $p < 0.01$), reduced number of eating occasions (-1.4 ± 1.2, $p < 0.01$) and a reduced intake of grain food (-1.52 ± 1.84 serves, $p = 0.019$). PGXG at the recommended dose resulted in a reduction in weight and BMI which was significantly greater than that for RF ($p = 0.001$). These results demonstrate the potential benefits of PGX fibre in controlling frequency of eating and in weight loss.

Keywords: fibre; weight; waist circumference; frequency; eating; PolyGlycopleX® (PGX)

1. Introduction

The burden of chronic disease in many countries is increasing concomitant with the percentage of the population with a high body mass index (BMI) [1]. Providing tools to improve the healthiness of the food environment and assisting people to make healthy food choices are important in the prevention of excessive weight gain [1].

Dietary pattern evidence has shown that higher dietary quality i.e. consumption of mainly whole grains, vegetables, fruit, nuts, legumes, seafood, plant protein and low-fat dairy leads to marked reductions in all-cause, cardiovascular disease and cancer mortality [2,3]. Similarly, a healthy dietary pattern which includes consumption of fruits, vegetables, grains, combined with a lower intake of sweets, red meat and processed meat, lowers the risk of developing colorectal cancer [4].

Evidence supports the role of dietary fibre in improving metabolic health. A higher intake of fibre is associated with increased satiety and reduced energy intake and therefore may be important in obesity management [5–11].

Total fibre is the sum of both dietary fibre (complete, intrinsic non-digestible plant carbohydrates, lignin) and functional fibres (non-digestible carbohydrates that have been isolated but still have beneficial physiological effects) [12]. What constitutes a 'beneficial physiological effect' and the level of evidence required for this to be substantiated remains unspecified [13]. Solubility or the ability of a fibre to dissolve in water will affect water holding capacity, viscosity and fermentability [11]. The properties of fibre that are associated with appetite, energy intake and body weight include solubility [11]. Solubility remains a common classification technique, although it has been suggested that fibres should be categorised according to functional properties such as viscosity and fermentability [14], since not all fibre is equal in delivering a beneficial physiological effect.

PolyGlycopleX (PGX) is a commercial functional fibre complex, manufactured by a proprietary process (EnviroSimplex®) from three dietary fibres: konjac glucomannan, sodium alginate, and xanthan gum [9]. PGX is a soluble viscous non-starch polysaccharide complex that has been identified as contributing to improved satiety, lipidaemia and glycaemia [8–10,15,16].

In the modern food environment both portion size and frequency of eating have increased in the population [17]. Mattes [17] has suggested that increased frequency of eating is a major factor in weight gain and is linked to the increased energy intake and rising BMI trends. In addition to frequency of eating, the types and amount of food and beverages consumed at an eating occasion may influence energy intake. Aljuraiban et al. [18] suggest that modifying eating behaviour through more frequent meals of low energy density and high nutrient quality may be an important approach to controlling obesity.

A challenge for understanding the contribution of dietary factors is our ability to measure diet. This is even more difficult in overweight and obese participants who are more prone to misreporting or underreporting their energy intake [19,20]. In addition, details such as time of eating is important in examining eating frequency and are difficult to accurately capture with paper-based methods. Advancement in technology has made available new image-based food recording systems such as those using a mobile food record app (mFR) [21–25]. Among the advantages of mFRs is the provision of real-time data capture which allows for the extraction of information from the images on the timing and location of the eating occasion, without relying on individuals to report these details [22,23]. Thus the mFR app allows for more accurate capture of time of eating while reducing the burden to the participant of reporting food consumption [23,24]. A unique aspect of this study was the use of the mFR to capture frequency of eating and dietary intake.

The objective of this research was to determine the effectiveness of diet supplementation with the viscous and gel-forming fibre, PolyGlycopleX (PGX), on body weight and composition and to determine if frequency of eating and diet can explain subsequent changes in 118 overweight adults.

2. Materials and Methods

2.1. Study Design

A three-arm, parallel, blind, randomised control trial was conducted to determine whether PGX supplementation would promote weight loss and reduce waist circumference and BMI, change dietary patterns and reduce the frequency of eating or number of eating occasions. Participants (118 in total) were divided between three groups, 4.5 g PGX as softgels (PGXS), 5 g PGX granules (PGXG) and 5 g rice flour (RF) control, (Figure 1) and were assessed at baseline and 12 weeks. This trial was registered with the Australian New Zealand Clinical Trials Registry (reference ACTRN12614000701628).

The food images sent via the mFR were stored by a participant identification number (ID) only. No personal information was stored with the images. The research was conducted in accordance with the principles proposed by the Australian Association for Research in Education (AARE), the Australian Vice-Chancellor's Committee (AVCC) and the National Health and Medical Research Council (NHMRC). The study was conducted in accordance with the Declaration of Helsinki and ethics approval was granted by the Human Research Ethics Committee, Curtin University (reference HR170/2014).

2.2. Study Participants

Participants, aged 25–70 years and with BMI 25–35 kg/m^2 were recruited through advertisements on Curtin University radio, as well as email communication systems. Individuals that expressed interest were screened for eligibility by completing a screening questionnaire. Participants were excluded if they were: (a) pregnant; (b) unable to complete the 12-week study; (c) undertaking extreme forms of exercise or dieting; (d) unable to attend the study centre; or (e) had an allergy to any food ingredient used in the study; (f) had previous or current renal, liver or respiratory failure; (g) had previous gastric or weight-loss surgery; (h) had any malabsorption conditions or (i) had current or recent dietary fibre supplementation. The participant flow diagram (Figure 1) lists the reasons for exclusion. Once assessed as eligible, further details of the study were provided and informed consent obtained.

2.3. Baseline Assessments

Participants who met the selection criteria had height, weight and waist circumference anthropometric measurements taken at baseline. A portable stadiometer was used to measure height; weight was measured using a pre-calibrated digital scale and waist was measured as described by Norton and Olds [26]. To electronically record food consumption, iPods with mFR application installed were given to the participants, who were asked to keep a 4-day mFR at baseline and during the twelfth week of the study.

Before beginning their baseline image-based 4-day food record, all participants received a 30-minute interactive training session by a single researcher who conducted individual or small group training sessions using PowerPoint slides on how to connect the iPod to the Wi-Fi and how to use the mFR app. Training sessions were held at Curtin University in a room with Wi-Fi access. The inclusion of a fiducial marker (a checkerboard pattern of known shape, size and colour) in all food record images gave a known reference of dimension and markings to assist with food identification and portion size estimation [25]. During training, participants were able to practice taking before and after images using food models. Collected food record images were automatically uploaded from the iPod touch, when in Wi-Fi range. The iPods were coded with the participant ID ensuring each image was tagged with the participant ID, date and time of eating occasion. Participant ID was used to identify the images on the server. The server was accessible by researchers only via password.

Prior to the commencement of supplementation and during the twelfth week of the study, participants took before and after images of all foods and drinks (excluding water) consumed over four consecutive days. Food consumption during the entire study was ad libitum.

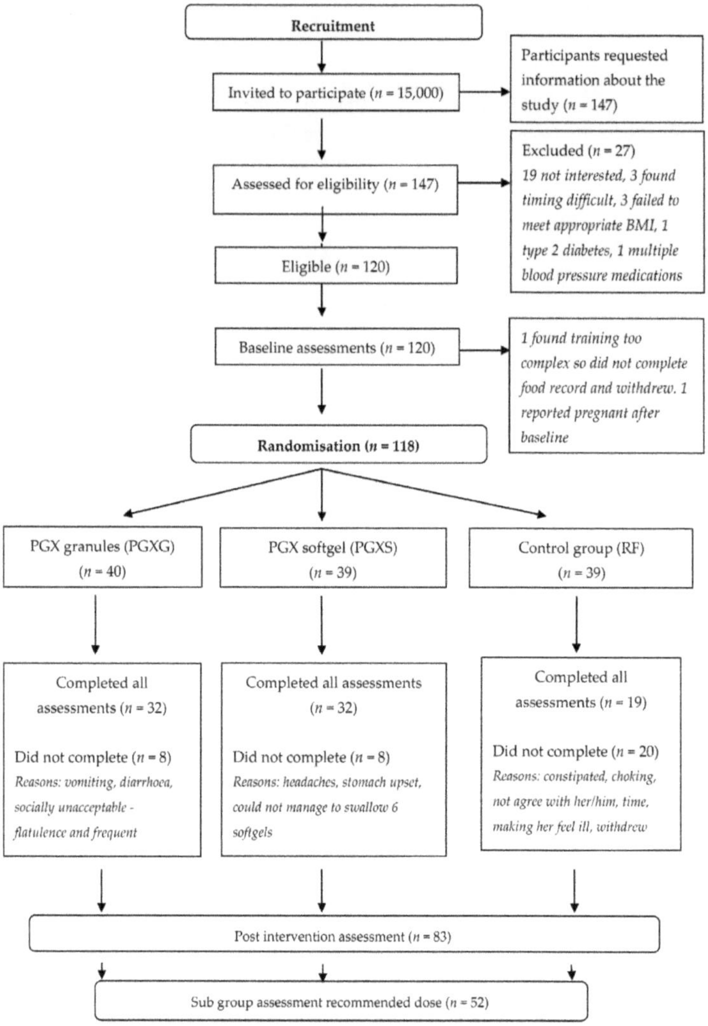

Figure 1. Participant flow diagram. RF: rice flour.

2.4. PGX Supplementation

The PGXS, PGXG and RF control supplements were provided to participants in a carry bag containing a 12-week supply labelled with a three-digit code. PGXG and the control were provided as 5 g individual doses in identical foil sachets and PGXS was provided in plain white jars each containing one month's supply. Research staff were blinded to the treatment allocation until all analyses were completed.

In Arm 1 (PGXS) instructions were provided in writing and verbally to the participants: "Take 1–2 softgels three times a day in week 1, 2–4 softgels three times a day in week 2 and 4–6 softgels, three times a day in week 3 to week 12". The recommended dose was four (4) to six (6) softgels containing 0.64 g fibre each, three times a day. This represented a supplement of dietary of between 7.6–11.4 g/day. Participants were also asked to consume 500 mL water with every softgel dose. Participants in Arm 2 were instructed to consume 5 g of PGXG containing 4.4 g fibre provided in a single dose foil sachet taken three times a day just before or with meals over the 12-week intervention period. This represented a supplement of dietary fibre of 12.2 g/day. Those in Arm 3 were provided with 5 g of RF containing 4 g fibre in the same dose format as the PGXG, representing 12 g fibre/day. RF was selected due to its neutral taste and hypoallergenicity, and it has a similar dietary fibre content, energy, colour and texture to PGX [7]. The recommended dose was 1 sachet, three times per day. Directions were "Stir 1 sachet into your meal or in a drink and consume immediately. You must consume 500mL of water each time you take a sachet." Participants were also advised that "If you have any discomfort, reduce the dose to 1 sachet a day for week 1, 2 sachets for week 2 and 3 sachets week 3 to week 12. Contact the researcher to discuss any issues." Participants were informed of the importance of consuming water with the supplement as well as the possible gastrointestinal effects of fibre such as diarrhoea, bloating and flatulence as described in research by Kacinik et al. [7]. All participants were instructed to record their daily sachet or softgel intake and report in person to the researcher at the end of week 12 of the intervention.

2.5. Post-Intervention Assessments

At the end of the 12-week intervention period, measurement of participants' height, weight and waist circumference were repeated, along with the 4-day mFR being repeated during week 12. At the end of the 12-week intervention, during the final meeting participants reported the number of doses to the interviewer and data were recorded in participant files.

2.6. Dietary Analysis

A researcher reviewed the 4-day food record images and as needed, confirmed the content of images with participants. Eating occasions were defined as all food and beverages (except water) and were taken from the image metadata and any additional notes supplied by the participant. Eating occasions were categorised as beverage only, food only, single item, food and beverage or fibre only. The images of fibre also allowed dose of fibre taken to be determined. Analysis was conducted to measure any change in eating occasions from baseline to study week 12.

Images were analysed and eating occasions, types of foods and serving sizes were entered into a database specifically designed to capture the number of eating occasions and food groups according to the Australian Guide to Healthy Eating food group serves (vegetables, fruit, grain (cereal) foods, mostly wholegrain and/or high cereal fibre varieties, lean meats and poultry, fish, eggs, tofu, nuts and seeds and legumes/beans, milk, yoghurt cheese and/or alternatives, mostly reduced fat) (NHMRC 2013) plus junk food (Table 1).

The primary outcome variables measured at baseline and at the end of the intervention were: changes in weight, waist circumference and BMI; eating occasions and foods consumed each day classified as serves of junk food (energy-dense nutrient poor), grain (cereal), meat, dairy, fruits and vegetables for the three intervention groups. Within each intervention group, participants were further categorised into fibre dose compliance level and number of eating occasions and the primary outcomes for this subgroup were also evaluated.

2.7. Statistical Analysis

Per-protocol analyses were performed and reported. The distribution of all outcome variables, weight, waist and BMI were checked by construction of histograms to check normality. A mixed effect model with clustering of participants' ID and robust variance-covariance estimation were used to assess outcome variables. For per-protocol analysis, only those who completed the study at week 12 were included and missing values were not imputed. Further analysis of subgroups by actual dose consumed was performed and reported. All tests were two tailed and a p value < 0.05 was regarded as statistically significant. All analyses were performed using Stata MP 14.1 (Stata Corp., College Station, TX, USA).

Table 1. Serve size in g or mL National Health and Medical Research Council (NHMRC), 2013 [27]. Fibre is 1 serve (g), with 2.5 serves daily minimum recommended dose.

Grains				**Vegetable**	**Fruit**	**Meats**			**Dairy**		**Junk Food**		**Fibre ***	
Bread	Porridge cooked	Muesli/Oats raw	Rice Pasta cooked			Beef Lamb Pork	Chicken	Fish	Milk	Cheese	Meat pie	Donut or Cake	PGXSPGXG	
40	120	30	75–120 (1/2 cup)	75	150	65	80	100	250 mL	40	60	40	3.8	4.4

* Dose determined by study. PGXS = PGX softgel, PGXG = PGX granules.

3. Results

3.1. Baseline Characteristics

3.1.1. Per-Protocol Analysis

Baseline measurements showing of all recruited participant characteristics according to treatment group are shown in Table 2. There were 92 females and 28 males, evenly distributed across the three treatment groups. In total 83 of the 118 participants (63% retention) completed the 12-week study. Greater attrition was observed in the first two weeks of the supplementation for participants who reported stomach upsets and diarrhoea after PGXG consumption (attrition = 6); who reported diarrhoea, headaches, difficulty swallowing recommended PGXS dose (attrition = 6) and during the first six weeks of supplementation in the RF group (attrition = 15) due to constipation and feeling ill.

Baseline data (Table 2) shows the characteristics of study participants randomised (n = 118) and shows that at baseline there were no significant differences ($p > 0.05$) in age, height, weight, waist circumference, BMI and food group servings across three groups. At baseline PGXS participants had similar baseline frequency of eating (number of eating occasions) to the PGXG and RF participants but those allocated to the PGXG intervention had a significantly greater number of eating occasions per day than those allocated to the RF intervention ($p = 0.04$) (Table 2).

Table 2. Characteristics of all recruited study participants randomised at baseline (n = 120) comparing groups.

All Participants	PGXS (n = 40)	PGXG (n = 40)	RF (n = 40)
Men	9	10	9
Women	31	30	31
Mean ± SD			
Age (years)	42.2 ± 16.0	46.5 ± 14.0	43.3 ± 16.8
Height (cm)	167.4 ± 9.1	167.3 ± 9.0	166.4 ± 7.9
Weight (kg)	82.7 ± 16.8	80.9 ± 16.6	81.3 ± 17.7
Waist (cm)	89.8 ± 12.8	90.7 ± 12.1	88.4 ± 14.3
Body Mass Index (BMI, kg/m^2)	29.4 ± 4.8	28.7 ± 4.4	29.2 ± 4.8
Eating occasions per day	5.4 ± 2.8	6.3 ± 2.0	4.8 ± 2.1
Food group servings (mean daily serves ± SD)			
Fruit (150 g)	0.8 ± 0.8	1.0 ± 1.0	1.1 ± 1.2
Vegetable (75 g)	2.4 ± 1.5	2.6 ± 1.4	2.5 ± 1.1
Grain (cereal) (40 g bread, 75–120 g cooked rice, pasta etc. or 500 kJ)	3.8 ± 1.8	4.3 ± 2.2	4 .0 ± 1.5
Dairy (250 mL milk, 40 g cheese or 500–600 kJ)	1.3 ± 0.9	1.6 ± 0.8	1.3 ± 0.8
Junk food (60 g meat pie or hot chips, 40 g donut or cake)	3.5 ± 1.9	3.1 ± 1.6	3.0 ± 1.7
Meat (65 g meat, 100 g fish or 500–699 kJ)	1.0 ± 0.7	1.6 ± 0.8	1.4 ± 0.7
Alcohol (150 mL)	0.5 ± 0.8	0.4 ± 0.5	0.1 ± 0.2

PGXS = PGX softgel, PGXG = PGX granules, RF = Rice Flour. SD = Standard Deviation.

3.1.2. Subgroup Analysis

Baseline measurements according to treatment group showing participant characteristics of all who consumed the recommended dose of fibre supplements are shown in Table 3. Baseline data (Table 3) shows the characteristics of study participants (n = 54) and shows that at baseline there were no significant differences ($p > 0.05$) in weight, waist circumference and BMI across three groups. PGXG and RF intervention sub-group numbers of eating occasions per day were not significantly different to each other or to the baseline group but the PGXS subgroup number of eating occasions was 7.4 times per day (Table 3).

Table 3. Characteristics of study participants randomised at baseline (n = 54) comparing subgroups who consumed the recommended dose of fibre supplements.

All Participants	PGXS (n = 17)	PGXG (n = 18)	RF (n = 17)	p Value
Body weight (kg)	76.5 ± 15.9	87.7 ± 20.2	78.3 ± 15.0	0.62
BMI (kg/m^2)	27.2 ± 4.5	28.7 ± 5.2	28.3 ± 5.2	0.64
Waist (cm)	84.8 ± 12.2	89.2 ± 20.4	87.1 ± 13.8	0.59
Eating occasions per day	7.4 ± 2.5	6.0 ± 2.0	5.5 ± 2.6	$p > 0.05$

PGXS = PGX softgel, PGXG = PGX granules, RF = Rice Flour.

3.2. *Effect of Intervention on Body Weight and Body Composition*

3.2.1. Per-Protocol Analysis

Per-protocol analysis revealed a significant reduction in waist circumference at week 12 of minus 2.5cm (Confidence Interval = −3.9, −0.8, p = 0.003) for those in the PGXG group (Table 4). No effect was seen on waist circumference for the PGXS and RF groups ($p > 0.05$). There was no effect of the PGXS or PGXG interventions on weight and BMI.

3.2.2. Subgroup Analysis

Analyses of the subgroup who consumed the recommended dose of fibre supplements showed a significant weight loss and reduction in BMI in the PGXG intervention compared to baseline (Table 5). However, the PGXS subgroup did not show a significant weight change during the intervention period. Compared to effect of the intervention on weight seen in the RF subgroup, that of the PGXG subgroup was significantly greater (p = 0.001).

Table 4. Change in participant characteristics from baseline to week 12 of the interventions of all participants who completed the interventions (per-protocol analysis).

All Participants	PGXS (n = 32)	PGXG (n = 32)	RF (n = 19)
Body weight (kg)	0.47 ± 1.85	−0.49 ± 0.34	−0.03 ± 0.58
BMI (kg/m^2)	0.15 ± 0.65	−0.17 ± 0.13	0.01 ± 0.20
Waist (cm)	−0.17 ± 2.92	**−2.50 ± 0.60 p = 0.03**	−1.3 ± 1.0
Eating occasions per day	−0.60 ± 1.5	**−0.82 ± 1.28 p = 0.01**	−0.22 ± 1.72
Food group servings (mean daily serves ± SD)			
Fruit (150 g) [1]	−0.2 ± 0.76	0.08 ± 0.7	−0.18 ± 0.75
Vegetable (75 g) [1]	−0.07 ± 1.11	−0.34 ± 1.22	−0.23 ± 0.64
Grain (cereal)	0.21 ± 1.73	−0.79 ± 1.66	−0.51 ± 1.23
Dairy	0.11 ± 0.63	−0.22 ± 0.64	0.07 ± 0.35
Junk food	−0.14 ± 2.00	−0.57 ± 1.29	0.28 ± 2.12
Meat	0.08 ± 0.59	0.01 ± 0.79	−0.09 ± 0.78
Alcohol	−0.22 ± 0.73	0.17 ± 0.99	−0.02 ± 0.26
Fibre (3.8–4.4 g) [1]	1.89 ± 0.91	2.17 ± 0.71	2.35 ± 0.58

Bold values denote significant within treatment effect. PGXS = PGX softgel, PGXG = PGX granules, RF = Rice Flour.
[1] 1 serve of fruit = 150 g, 1 serve vegetable = 75 g, 1 serve fibre = 3.8 to 4.4 g.

Table 5. Change in participant characteristics from baseline to week 12 of the PGXS, PGXG and RF interventions in the subgroup analysis of those who consumed the recommended dose of fibre supplements.

All Participants	PGXS (n = 17)	PGXG (n = 18)	RF (n = 17)
Body weight (kg)	0.22 ± 1.61	**−1.4 ± 0.10 p < 0.01**	−0.03 ± 0.58
BMI (kg/m^2)	0.07 ± 0.59	**−0.5 ± 0.10 p < 0.01**	0.01 ± 0.20
Waist (cm)	−1.04 ± 2.28	−1.2 ± 1.00	−1.3 ± 1.0
Eating occasions per day	−1.3 ± 1.9	**−1.4 ± 1.20 p < 0.01**	−0.22 ± 1.72
Food group servings (mean daily serves ± SD)			
Fruit (150 g)	−0.43 ± 0.59	**−0.63 ± 0.57 p = 0.022**	−0.18 ± 0.75
Vegetable (75 g)	−0.35 ± 0.96	−0.82 ± 1.31	−0.23 ± 0.64
Grain (cereal)	−0.93 ± 1.47	**−1.52 ± 1.84 p = 0.019**	−0.51 ± 1.23
Dairy	−0.05 ± 0.56	**−0.59 ± 0.50 p = 0.012**	0.07 ± 0.35
Junk food	−0.17 ± 1.48	−0.76 ± 0.85	0.28 ± 2.12
Meat	−0.06 ± 0.62	0.18 ± 0.90	−0.09 ± 0.78
Alcohol	−0.50 ± 0.98	0.11 ± 0.32	−0.02 ± 0.26
Fibre supplement serves (serving size 4.5–5 g)	2.6 ± 0.47	2.82 ± 0.24	2.35 ± 0.58

Bold values denote significant within treatment effect. PGXS = PGX softgel, PGXG= PGX granules, RF = Rice Flour. SD = standard deviation.

3.3. *Number of Eating Occasions and Food Group Servings*

Collection of mFR images required participants to use the iPod provided by the study to record images before and after each eating occasion during the 4-day food record (Figure 2).

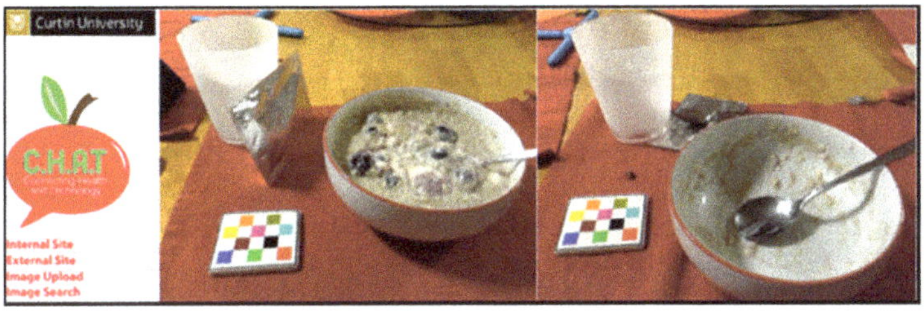

Figure 2. Before and after images of an eating occasion with foil sachet containing PGXG and fiducial marker captured with the mobile food record App on an iPod.

3.3.1. Per-Protocol Analysis

Analysis was conducted to measure change in number of eating occasions from baseline to week 12 of the interventions. The number of eating occasions was significantly reduced in the PGXG group (p = 0.01) during the intervention (Table 4). No significant differences in number of eating occasions between baseline and week 12 were observed in the groups PGXS and RF or in food group servings in any of the intervention groups (Table 4) in per-protocol analyses.

3.3.2. Subgroup Analysis

For the subgroup analysis, the participants who consumed PGXG at the recommended dose of 2.5 to 3 times per day, significantly reduced their eating occasions by 1.4 ± 1.2 (CI −2.1, −0.6, p < 0.01) during the intervention period (Table 5).

Likewise, the participants who consumed PGXG at the recommended dose significantly reduced their daily intake of fruit (−0.63 ± 0.57 serves, p = 0.02), dairy (−0.59 ± 0.50 serves, p = 0.01) and grain food (−1.52 ± 1.84 serves, p = 0.02) during the intervention (Table 5). Analysis of types of foods in the mFR showed that 1.6 to 2 serves of the grain food consumed at baseline were white bread for these participants. This consumption of white bread for the PGXG group also dropped significantly to 0.74 serves per day at 12 weeks of intervention.

3.4. *Adverse Events*

Adverse effects reported by the participants were mild and agreed with common reported reactions to increased fibre, for example those reported by Kacinik et al. (2011) [7] where for PGX supplementation, 30.9 % of participants reported diarrhoea, bloating and flatulence whereas for rice flour consumption 7.8% reported constipation.

4. Discussion

This 12 week randomised controlled study showed that when consumed at the recommended dose (subgroup), the PGXG intervention gave a reduction in BMI and body weight, the number of eating occasions per day and consumption of servings of grain food.

The weight loss and BMI reduction observed for the PGXG intervention is most likely a result of compliance to the recommended dose, resulting in 64% of participants who consumed PGXG at the recommended dose losing weight and reducing BMI. The average 1.4-kg weight loss found in our study of overweight adults for the PGX per-protocol intervention is in agreement with previous research by Lyon et al. [28] who found a weight loss in women of 1.6 kg with 12 weeks PGX supplementation. Pal et al. [29] reported obese adults on 12-week supplementation of both artificially sweetened and flavoured PGX and psyllium lost weight (1.6 kg and 1.1 kg respectively).

On an individual basis, the highest weight loss in the PGXS group (per-protocol) was 4.4 kg, with a waist circumference decrease of 5.5 cm. However, in this group a weight gain of 6.3 kg and waist circumference increase was 9.6 cm was also recorded in one participant. This high variance in change in weight and waist circumference resulted in a non-significant weight loss for this group. Data collected by personal communication at the 6-week visit showed five participants in the PGXS group reporting that they expected PGXS to be a "magic bullet" for weight loss, which was an unexpected issue that requires consideration in future research. Protocol in future research may involve education of participants on using PGX to control appetite.

The significant reduction in waist circumference observed in the present study for PGXG per-protocol group of 2.5 cm was similar in magnitude to that reported in a study by Reimer et al. [8] where PGX consumption over 14 weeks resulted in a significant reduction of 1.96 cm in waist circumference. The significant reduction in BMI of 0.5 observed in the present study for PGXG sub-group was in contrast to Reimer [8] who found no significant differences in BMI compared to baseline.

The findings from our study that PGXS and PGXG consumption (per-protocol groups) did not affect weight is similar to research on PGX consumption by Kacinik et al. [7] who reported no significant differences in weight loss between PGX and the placebo groups in a study involving a low-calorie diet of 1000 kcal/day for both treatments. There was also no weight loss recorded in a three-week study by Reimer et al. [30] where PGX was pre-mixed with breakfast cereal and consumed with yogurt. In our study participants were not on an energy restricted diet nor were the PGX and RF doses mixed with other products.

The use of the mFR allowed our research to determine level of compliance to the recommended dose of the PGXG subgroup by reviewing the images collected. The mFR image analysis of the foods eaten, serving sizes and number of eating occasions per day enabled important information about the dietary pattern of the overweight participants to be collected. The reduced number of eating occasions found with the PGXG subgroup, translated into reduced consumption of grain food of 1.52 serves ($p = 0.019$), mainly being a reduction in consumption of white bread.

Research by Kerr et al. [23] reported a reduction in consumption of energy-dense nutrient-poor (EDNP) foods as a result of tailored dietary feedback using the mFR. In the present study there was a non-significant reduction in junk food consumption of 0.57 in the PGXG per-protocol group and 0.76 serves in the PGXG subgroup. Pollard et al. [31] also found overweight people were more likely than those who were a healthy weight to decrease their intake grain food when trying to lose weight, supporting the reduced grain food trend found in this research. Small reductions in conscious or mindful energy intake can improve weight gain [32] and the choice to reduce grain food intake found in this research may have been the contributor to weight loss. Although we observed a reduction in daily intake of fruit and dairy, which is not desirable based on dietary guidelines [27], the magnitude of this change was minor.

Data from the mFR showed participants in all groups, other than the PGXG subgroup, appeared to make no changes to their eating pattern, as after 12 weeks of intervention, food group servings were not significantly different to baseline. This finding is supported by previous studies [32–34] where it was reported that humans tend to consume a consistent weight or volume of food from day to day. While participants reported feeling full in previous PGXS and PGXG research [9,10,35,36], most participants in this study did not appear to use appetite to change their eating patterns, except in the PGXG subgroup who consumed the recommended dose, most likely resulting reduced appetite and reduced food intake.

Dietary feedback using the mFR indicated a reduction of 1 serve white bread, each day, which may have been a contributor to the reduction of 40 g in weight daily in the PGXG per-protocol group [27]. In a previous study, a reduction of 31.5 g carbohydrate per day was recorded at 12 weeks after PGX supplementation using a 3-day food and drink diary [29]. The 3-day food and drink diary does not provided details on type carbohydrates foods, whereas the mFR reports provided detail of types of foods and serving sizes. Dietary intake records collected using the mFR can reduce the bias found in auto-assessment [24].

In the present study, PGXG was taken with 500 mL water immediately before or with a meal. The PGXG was mixed in the water, in juice or mixed into the meal. The mechanism for weight loss in the PGXG sub-group in the present study may have been as a result of reducing dietary energy density of the meals with which it was consumed by increasing the fibre and water content of meals while maintaining the volume of food eaten [37,38]. Decreasing dietary energy density has been shown to be useful in long-term weight loss [39].

The detailed dietary feedback from the mFR enabled this research to determine weight loss was possible when PGXG at the recommended dose was consumed and the reduction in the number of eating occasions may be part of the mechanism for this effect. Previous research indicates that a possible mechanism behind the appetite and body weight reduction effects of PGX may be related to circulating gut hormones [30]. Reimer et al. [30] reported increased peptide YY, which can slow gastric emptying and decreased ghrelin (an appetite stimulant) on consumption of PGX. More work is required to confirm the physiological mechanisms controlling these effects of PGX.

The detailed dietary feedback from the mFR enabled this research to more accurately determine food group changes after 12 weeks. The reason the PGXS, and PGXG per-protocol groups did not reduce their weight may be because they did not reduce the number of eating occasions or change their daily intake of the foods and continued to consume the amount and type of food usually eaten. In addition, research by Polidori et al. [40] reports that weight loss leads to increased appetite, and appetite increases by approximately 100 kcal/day per kg of lost weight. The reason fibre such as PGXG helps some individuals in the control of appetite and not others requires more research.

Limitation

Meals and consumption of test products were self-administered; the possibility of non-compliance could not be avoided. In the current study misreporting of intake may have occurred due to participants not taking images of all food and beverages consumed. In addition, the assessment of food group serves by a trained analyst may not be sensitive enough to detect changes in dietary intake.

5. Conclusions

Supplementation with PGX at the recommended dose resulted in a reduction in body weight (kg), BMI (kg/m^2), reduced frequency of eating and reduced intake of white bread. The weight loss and BMI reduction from baseline to 12 weeks was significantly greater for PGXG at the recommended dose than for the RF treatment. Dietary assessment using the mFR provided detailed information enabling accurate analysis of the number of eating occasions and changes to food group servings per day. Further research on reducing the frequency eating of specific foods, such as junk food is warranted. These results demonstrate the potential benefits of PGX fibre in controlling frequency of eating and in weight loss.

Acknowledgments: PGX® and PolyGlycopleX® are registered trademarks of InovoBiologic Inc., Calgary, AB, Canada. Financial support for the submitted work was provided by Factors Group, Australia Pty Ltd. RJG owns the Factors Group of Companies, which retains an interest in PGX. SW receives consulting fees from InovoBiologic Inc.

Author Contributions: V.A.S., D.A.K., W.J.H., X.M., S.K.J. and S.W. designed and conducted the research; C.J.B., D.A.K. and E.J.D. developed the mFR part of this research; R.J.G. critically reviewed the study design; X.M., V.A.S., A.S.M. and D.A.K. analysed the data; V.A.S., D.A.K., W.J.K., S.K.J., C.J.B., E.J.D., X.M., A.P.J., A.S.M., H.K.F. and S.W. wrote the paper; all authors read and approved the final manuscript.

Conflicts of Interest: The authors declare no conflict of interest.

References

1. Swinburn, B.; Kraak, V.; Rutter, H.; Vandevijvere, S.; Lobstein, T.; Sacks, G.; Gomes, F.; Marsh, T.; Magnusson, R. Strengthening of accountability systems to create healthy food environments and reduce global obesity. *Lancet* **2015**, *385*, 2534–2545. [CrossRef]
2. Liese, A.D.; Krebs-Smith, S.M.; Subar, A.F.; George, S.M.; Harmon, B.E.; Neuhouser, M.L.; Boushey, C.J.; Schap, T.E.; Reedy, J. The Dietary Patterns Methods Project: Synthesis of findings across cohorts and relevance to dietary guidance. *J. Nutr.* **2015**, *145*, 393–402. [CrossRef] [PubMed]
3. Reedy, J.; Krebs-Smith, S.M.; Miller, P.E.; Liese, A.D.; Kahle, L.L.; Park, Y.; Subar, A.F. Higher diet quality is associated with decreased risk of all-cause, cardiovascular disease, and cancer mortality among older adults. *J. Nutr.* **2014**, *144*, 881–889. [CrossRef] [PubMed]
4. Tayyem, R.F.; Bawadi, H.A.; Shehadah, I.; Agraib, L.M.; AbuMweis, S.S.; Al-Jaberi, T.; Al-Nusairr, M.; Bani-Hani, K.E.; Heath, D.D. Dietary patterns and colorectal cancer. *Clin. Nutr.* **2016**, in press. [CrossRef] [PubMed]
5. Delzenne, N.M.; Cani, P.D. A place for dietary fiber in the management of the metabolic syndrome. *Curr. Opin. Clin. Nutr. Metab. Care* **2005**, *8*, 636–640. [CrossRef] [PubMed]
6. Kristensen, M.; Jensen, M.G. Dietary fibres in the regulation of appetite and food intake. Importance of viscosity. *Appetite* **2011**, *56*, 65–70. [CrossRef] [PubMed]
7. Kacinik, V.; Lyon, M.; Purnama, M.; Reimer, R.A.; Gahler, R.; Green, T.J.; Wood, S. Effect of PGX, a novel functional fibre supplement, on subjective ratings of appetite in overweight and obese women consuming a 3-day structured, low-calorie diet. *Nutr. Diabetes* **2011**, *1*, 1–8. [CrossRef] [PubMed]
8. Reimer, R.A.; Yamaguchi, H.; Eller, L.K.; Lyon, M.R.; Gahler, R.J.; Kacinik, V.; Juneja, P.; Wood, S. Changes in visceral adiposity and serum cholesterol with a novel viscous polysaccharide in Japanese adults with abdominal obesity. *Obesity* **2013**, *21*, E379–E387. [PubMed]
9. Solah, V.; Brand-Miller, J.; Atkinson, F.; Gahler, R.; Kacinik, V.; Lyon, M.; Wood, S. Dose-response effect of a novel functional fibre, PolyGlycopleX, PGX, on satiety. *Appetite* **2014**, *77*, 72–76. [CrossRef] [PubMed]
10. Solah, V.A.; O'Mara-Wallace, B.; Meng, X.; Gahler, R.J.; Kerr, D.A.; James, A.P.; Fenton, H.K.; Johnson, S.K.; Wood, S. Consumption of the Soluble Dietary Fibre Complex PolyGlycopleX® Reduces Glycaemia and Increases Satiety of a Standard Meal Postprandially. *Nutrients* **2016**, *8*, 268. [CrossRef] [PubMed]
11. Wanders, A.J.; Van Den Borne, J.J.G.C.; De Graaf, C.; Hulshof, T.; Jonathan, M.C.; Kristensen, M.; Mars, M.; Schols, H.A.; Feskens, E.J.M. Effects of dietary fibre on subjective appetite, energy intake and body weight: A systematic review of randomized controlled trials. *Obes. Rev.* **2011**, *12*, 724–739. [CrossRef] [PubMed]
12. Slavin, J.; Green, H. Dietary fibre and satiety. *Nutr. Bull.* **2007**, *32*, 32–42. [CrossRef]

13. Mann, J.I.; Cummings, J.H. Possible implications for health of the different definitions of dietary fibre. *Nutr. Metab. Cardiovasc. Dis.* **2009**, *19*, 226–229. [CrossRef] [PubMed]
14. Slavin, J.L. Dietary fibre and body weight. *Nutrition* **2005**, *21*, 411–418. [CrossRef] [PubMed]
15. Brand-Miller, J.C.; Atkinson, F.S.; Gahler, R.J.; Kacinik, V.; Lyon, M.R; Wood, S. Effects of PGX, a novel functional fibre, on acute and delayed postprandial glycaemia. *Eur. J. Clin. Nutr.* **2010**, *64*, 1488–1493. [CrossRef] [PubMed]
16. Brand-Miller, J.C.; Atkinson, F.S.; Gahler, R.J.; Kacinik, V.; Lyon, M.R.; Wood, S. Effects of added PGX®, a novel functional fibre, on the glycaemic index of starchy foods. *Br. J. Nutr.* **2012**, *108*, 245–248. [CrossRef] [PubMed]
17. Mattes, R. Energy intake and obesity: Ingestive frequency outweighs portion size. *Physiol. Behav.* **2015**, *134*, 110–118. [CrossRef] [PubMed]
18. Aljuraiban, G.S.; Chan, Q.; Griep, L.M.O.; Brown, I.J.; Daviglus, M.L.; Stamler, J.; Van Horn, L.; Elliott, P.; Frost, G.S.; INTERMAP Research Group. The impact of eating frequency and time of intake on nutrient quality and Body Mass Index: The INTERMAP Study, a Population-Based Study. *J. Acad. Nutr. Diet.* **2015**, *115*, 528–536. [CrossRef] [PubMed]
19. Thompson, F.E.; Subar, A.F. Dietary Assessment Methodology. In *Nutrition in the Prevention and Treatment of Disease*, 3rd ed.; Coulston, A.M., Boushey, C.J., Ferruzzi, M.G., Eds.; Elsevier Academic Press: San Diego, CA, USA, 2013.
20. Meng, X.; Kerr, D.A.; Zhu, K.; Devine, A.; Solah, V.A.; Wright, J.; Binns, C.W.; Prince, R.L. Under-reporting of energy intake in elderly Australian women is associated with a higher body mass index. *J. Nutr. Health Aging* **2013**, *17*, 112–118. [CrossRef] [PubMed]
21. Bosch, M.; Zhu, F.; Khanna, N.; Boushey, C.J.; Delp, E.J. Combining global and local features for food identification in dietary assessment. *IEEE Trans. Image Process.* **2011**, *2011*, 1789–1792. [PubMed]
22. Harray, A.J.; Boushey, C.J.; Pollard, C.M.; Delp, E.J.; Ahmad, Z.; Dhaliwal, S.S.; Mukhtar, S.A.; Kerr, D.A. A novel dietary assessment method to measure a healthy and sustainable diet using the Mobile Food Record: Protocol and methodology. *Nutrients* **2015**, *7*, 5375–5395. [CrossRef] [PubMed]
23. Kerr, D.A.; Pollard, C.M.; Howat, P.; Delp, E.J.; Pickering, M.; Kerr, K.R.; Dhaliwal, S.S.; Pratt, I.S.; Wright, J.; Boushey, C.J. Connecting Health and Technology (CHAT): Protocol of a randomized controlled trial to improve nutrition behaviours using mobile devices and tailored text messaging in young adults. *BMC Public Health* **2012**, *12*, 477. [CrossRef] [PubMed]
24. Kerr, D.A.; Harray, A.J.; Pollard, C.M.; Dhaliwal, S.S.; Delp, E.J.; Howat, P.A.; Pickering, M.R.; Ahmad, Z.; Meng, X.; Pratt, I.S.; et al. The connecting health and technology study: A 6-month randomized controlled trial to improve nutrition behaviours using a mobile food record and text messaging support in young adults. *Int. J. Behav. Nutr. Phys. Act.* **2016**, *13*, 52. [CrossRef] [PubMed]
25. Zhu, F.; Bosch, M.; Khanna, N.; Boushey, C.J.; Delp, E.J. Multiple hypotheses image segmentation and classification with application to dietary assessment. *IEEE J. Biomed. Health Inform.* **2015**, *19*, 377–388. [CrossRef] [PubMed]
26. Norton, K.; Olds, T. *Anthropometrica*; University of New South Wales Press: Sydney, Australia, 2000.
27. National Health and Medical Research Council. Eat for Health. Australian Dietary Guidelines Summary. Canberra: Australian Government, Department of Health and Ageing. 2013. Available online: http://www.nhmrc.gov.au/_files_nhmrc/publications/attachments/n55a_australian_dietary_guidelines_susumma_131014.pdf (accessed on 2 February 2015).
28. Lyon, M.; Wood, S.; Pelletier, X.; Donazzolo, Y.; Gahler, R.; Bellisle, F. Effects of a 3-month supplementation with a novel soluble highly viscous polysaccharide on anthropometry and blood lipids in nondieting overweight or obese adults. *J. Hum. Nutr. Diet.* **2011**, *24*, 351–359. [CrossRef] [PubMed]
29. Pal, S.; Ho, S.; Gahler, R.J.; Wood, S. Effect on body weight and composition in overweight/obese Australian adults over 12 months consumption of two different types of fibre supplementation in a randomized trial. *Nutr. Metab.* **2016**, *13*, 82. [CrossRef] [PubMed]
30. Reimer, R.A.; Pelletier, X.; Carabin, I.G.; Lyon, M.; Gahler, R.; Parnell, J.A.; Woods, S. Increased plasma PYY levels following supplementation with functional fiber PolyGlycopleX in healthy adults. *Eur. J. Clin. Nutr.* **2010**, *64*, 1186–1191. [CrossRef] [PubMed]

31. Pollard, C.M.; Pulker, C.; Meng, X.; Denham, F.; Solah, V.; Scott, J.A.; Kerr, D.A. Cereal foods consumption trends and factors associated with changing intake, among Western Australian adults, 1995 to 2012. *FASEB J.* **2016**, *30*, 409.
32. Hill, J.O. Can a small-changes approach help address the obesity epidemic? A report of the Joint Task Force of the American Society for Nutrition, Institute of Food Technologists, and International Food Information Council. *Am. J. Clin. Nutr.* **2009**, *89*, 477–484. [CrossRef] [PubMed]
33. Bell, E.A.; Castellanos, V.H.; Pelkman, C.L.; Thorwart, M.L.; Rolls, B.J. Energy density of foods affects energy intake in normal-weight women. *Am. J. Clin. Nutr.* **1998**, *67*, 412–420.
34. Bell, E.A.; Rolls, B.J. Energy density of foods affects energy intake across multiple levels of fat content in lean and obese women. *Am. J. Clin. Nutr.* **2001**, *73*, 1010–1018. [PubMed]
35. Solah, V.A.; Meng, X.; Wood, S.; Gahler, R.J.; Kerr, D.A.; James, A.P.; Pal, S.; Fenton, H.K.; Johnson, S.K. Effect of training on the reliability of satiety evaluation and use of trained panellists to determine the satiety effect of dietary fibre: A randomised controlled trial. *PLoS ONE* **2015**, *10*, e012. [CrossRef] [PubMed]
36. Yong, M.K.; Solah, V.A.; Johnson, S.K.; Meng, X.; Kerr, D.A.; James, A.P.; Fenton, H.K.; Gahler, R.J.; Wood, S. Effects of a viscous-fibre supplemented evening meal and the following un-supplemented breakfast on post-prandial satiety responses in healthy women. *Physiol. Behav.* **2016**, *154*, 34–39. [CrossRef] [PubMed]
37. Rolls, B.J.; Castellanos, V.H.; Halford, J.C.; Kilara, A.; Panyam, D.; Pelkman, C.L.; Smith, G.P.; Thorwart, M.L. Volume of food consumed affects satiety in men. *Am. J. Clin. Nutr.* **1998**, *67*, 1170–1177. [PubMed]
38. Rolls, B.J. The relationship between dietary energy density and energy intake. *Physiol. Behav.* **2009**, *97*, 609–615. [CrossRef] [PubMed]
39. Ello-Martin, J.A.; Roe, L.S.; Ledikwe, J.H.; Beach, A.M.; Rolls, B.J. Dietary energy density in the treatment of obesity: A year-long trial comparing 2 weight-loss diets. *Am. J. Clin. Nutr.* **2007**, *85*, 1465–1477. [PubMed]
40. Polidori, D.; Sanghvi, A.; Seeley, R.J.; Hall, K.D. How strongly does appetite counter weight loss? Quantification of the feedback control of human energy intake. *Obesity* **2016**, *24*, 2289–2295. [CrossRef] [PubMed]

nutrients

MDPI

Article

Intake and Dietary Food Sources of Fibre in Spain: Differences with Regard to the Prevalence of Excess Body Weight and Abdominal Obesity in Adults of the ANIBES Study

Liliana G. González-Rodríguez [1,2], José Miguel Perea Sánchez [1,2], Javier Aranceta-Bartrina [3,4], Ángel Gil [4,5], Marcela González-Gross [4,6], Lluis Serra-Majem [4,7], Gregorio Varela-Moreiras [8,9] and Rosa M. Ortega [2,10,*]

1 Department of Nutrition and Dietetics, Faculty of Health Sciences, University Alfonso X El Sabio, Madrid 28691, Spain; liligoro@uax.es (L.G.G.-R.); josepesa@uax.es (J.M.P.S.)
2 VALORNUT Research Group, Department of Nutrition, Faculty of Pharmacy, Complutense University, Madrid 28040, Spain
3 Department of Preventive Medicine and Public Health, University of Navarra, Pamplona, Navarra 31008, Spain; jaranceta@unav.es
4 Biomedical Research Networking Center for Physiopathology of Obesity and Nutrition (CIBEROBN), Carlos III Health Institute, Madrid 28029, Spain; agil@ugr.es (A.G.); marcela.gonzalez.gross@upm.es (M.G.-G.); lluis.serra@ulpgc.es (L.S.-M.)
5 Department of Biochemistry and Molecular Biology II and Institute of Nutrition and Food Sciences, University of Granada, Granada 18100, Spain
6 ImFINE Research Group, Department of Health and Human Performance, Technical University of Madrid, Madrid 28040, Spain
7 Research Institute of Biomedical and Health Sciences, University of Las Palmas de Gran Canaria, Faculty of Health Sciences, c/Doctor Pasteur s/n Trasera del Hospital, Las Palmas de Gran Canaria, 35016 Las Palmas, Spain
8 Department of Pharmaceutical and Health Sciences, Faculty of Pharmacy, CEU San Pablo University, Madrid 28668, Spain; gvarela@ceu.es
9 Spanish Nutrition Foundation (FEN), Madrid 28010, Spain
10 Department of Nutrition, Faculty of Pharmacy, Madrid Complutense University, Madrid 28040, Spain
* Correspondence: rortega@ucm.es; Tel.: +34-913-941-837; Fax: +34-913-941-810

Received: 8 December 2016; Accepted: 21 March 2017; Published: 25 March 2017

Abstract: The aim was to study the intake and food sources of fibre in a representative sample of Spanish adults and to analyse its association with excess body weight and abdominal obesity. A sample of 1655 adults (18–64 years) from the ANIBES ("Anthropometric data, macronutrients and micronutrients intake, practice of physical activity, socioeconomic data and lifestyles") cross-sectional study was analysed. Fibre intake and dietary food sources were determined by using a three-day dietary record. Misreporters were identified using the protocol of the European Food Safety Authority. Mean (standard deviation) fibre intake was 12.59 (5.66) g/day in the whole sample and 15.88 (6.29) g/day in the plausible reporters. Mean fibre intake, both in the whole sample and the plausible reporters, was below the adequate intake established by European Food Safety Authority (EFSA) and the Institute of Medicine of the United States (IOM). Main fibre dietary food sources were grains, followed by vegetables, fruits, and pulses. In the whole sample, considering sex, and after adjusting for age and physical activity, mean (standard error) fibre intake (adjusted by energy intake) was higher in subjects who had normal weight (NW) 13.40 (0.184) g/day, without abdominal obesity 13.56 (0.192) g/day or without excess body weight and/or abdominal obesity 13.56 (0.207) g/day compared to those who were overweight (OW) 12.31 (0.195) g/day, $p < 0.001$ or obese (OB) 11.83 (0.266) g/day, $p < 0.001$, with abdominal obesity 12.09 (0.157) g/day, $p < 0.001$ or with excess body weight and/or abdominal obesity 12.22 (0.148) g/day, $p < 0.001$. There were no significant differences in relation with the fibre intake according to the body mass index (BMI), presence or absence of abdominal obesity or excess body weight and/or abdominal obesity in the plausible reporters. Fibre from afternoon snacks was higher in subjects with NW (6.92%) and without abdominal obesity (6.97%) or without excess body weight and/or abdominal obesity (7.20%), than those with OW (5.30%), $p < 0.05$ or OB (4.79%), $p < 0.05$, with abdominal obesity (5.18%), $p < 0.01$, or with excess body weight and/or abdominal obesity (5.21%), $p < 0.01$, in the whole sample. Conversely, these differences were not observed in the plausible reporters. The present study demonstrates an insufficient fibre intake both in the whole sample and in the plausible reporters and confirms its association with excess body weight and abdominal obesity only when the whole sample was considered.

Keywords: fibre; food sources; obesity; abdominal obesity; misreporting; adults; Spain; ANIBES

---

1. Introduction

In recent decades, there has been a significant increase in the prevalence of overweight (OW) and obesity (OB) in children and adults, in both developed and developing countries [1]. Excess body weight increases the risk of developing various diseases, such as cardiovascular disease, type 2 diabetes, some types of cancers, musculoskeletal disorders, and neurodegenerative diseases, which have an important health and social impact [1–3].

Diet and physical activity are the main factors that influence the development of OW and OB [1,4]. In this respect, several studies have shown that the intake of dietary fibre may have a positive effect on body weight control; however, the available results are inconsistent [5–8]. There are several possible mechanisms to explain the anti-obesogenic effect of dietary fibre. Among the most documented mechanisms is the one that refers to the benefits of the fibre capacity (mainly soluble fibre) to form viscous gels that delay the gastric emptying, which helps, on the one hand, to increase the satiety sensation and consequently reduces energy intake [9] and, secondly, to control the postprandial glycaemia by delaying the intestinal absorption [10]. Another possible mechanism is associated with short-chain fatty acid produced during fermentation of fibre in the gastrointestinal tract [11] since it has been shown that this can contribute to regulating the secretion of some gastrointestinal hormones, such as glucagon-like peptide-1 (GLP-1), involved in satiety, and ghrelin, involved in appetite control [12,13], and to increase the oxidation of fatty acids and energy expenditure and to regulate glucose metabolism [11].

In addition, there are few recent studies regarding the intake of fibre in a representative Spanish adults sample and none of these studies have analysed the relation between the fibre intake, fibre from different meals of the day and food sources and the problematic of excess body weight and abdominal obesity [14,15]. Additionally, it is the first Spanish study that takes into account the dietary misreporting of the participants.

Therefore, the aim of the present work was to study the intake and dietary food sources of fibre in a representative sample of the Spanish adults from the ANIBES ("Anthropometric data, macronutrients and micronutrients intake, practice of physical activity, socioeconomic data and lifestyles") study and to analyse the differences in fibre intake between people with different body weight and with or without abdominal obesity. The present work shows the analysed data for the total sample and plausible reporters of the study.

2. Materials and Methods

2.1. Study Design and Sampling Procedure

The complete design, protocol, and methodology of the ANIBES study have been already described in detail elsewhere [16,17]. In summary, the ANIBES study was carried out to analyse anthropometric data, physical activity, intake of food and beverages, and dietary habits in the Spanish population (9–75 years old, *n* = 2009). The participants were randomly selected from the Northeast, East, Southwest, North-Central, Barcelona, Madrid, Balearic, and Canary Islands areas of Spain, including rural, semi-urban and urban populations [16,17]. The present study is focused on 1655 adults (779 men and 858 women) with ages ranging 18–64.

The following exclusion criteria were applied:

- Those individuals living in an institutional setting (e.g., colleges, nursing homes, hospitals, and others);
- Individuals following a therapeutic diet owing to recent surgery or taking any medical prescriptions;
- Potential participants with a transitory illness (i.e., flu, gastroenteritis) at the time of the fieldwork; and
- Individuals employed in areas related to consumer science, marketing, or the media [16,17].

The fieldwork for the ANIBES study was carried out from mid-September 2013 to mid-November 2013. The final protocol was approved by the Ethical Committee for Clinical Research of the Region of Madrid (Spain) (code FEN 2013/31, May 2013). All participants were informed of the protocol and risks and benefits of their participation in the study and a written informed consent was obtained from all the study's participants.

2.2. *Anthropometric Data*

Weight, height, and waist circumference (WC) were measured by trained interviewers following standardized procedures [18]. Weight was measured once with a Seca® model 804 weighing scale (Medizinische Messsysteme und Waagen seit 1840, Hamburg, Germany; range: 70–205 cm, precision: 1 mm). Height was assessed in triplicate using a Seca® model 206 stadiometer (Medizinische Messsysteme und Waagen seit 1840, Hamburg, Germany; range: 0.1–150 kg, precision: 100 g). WC was measured in triplicate using a Seca® 201 tape measure (Seca, Hamburg, Germany; range: 0–150 cm, precision: 1 mm).

Excess body weight was assessed using the body mass index (BMI) and abdominal obesity by the waist to height ratio (WHtR). BMI was calculated as weight (kg)/height (m)^2 and WHtR as WC (cm)/height (cm). Participants were classified into the following categories using the BMI: underweight (UW) (BMI <18.5 kg/m^2), normal weight (NW) (BMI 18.5–24.9 kg/m^2), OW (BMI 25–29.9 kg/m^2), and OB (BMI $\geq$30 kg/m^2), based on the World Health Organization classification [19], and using the WHtR respondents were classified into two categories: "non-abdominal obesity" (WHtR <0.5) and those with "abdominal obesity" (WHtR $\geq$0.5) [20–23]. BMI and WHtR were combined into one category called "excess body weight and/or abdominal obesity" (BMI $\geq$25 kg/m^2 and/or WHtR $\geq$0.5) for subsequent analysis [19,21–23].

2.3. *Physical Activity*

To obtain physical activity data of the studied participants, a detailed interview using the International Physical Activity Questionnaire (IPAQ) for adults was performed [24]. In addition, different physical activity measurements were obtained with an accelerometer ActiGraph (model GT3x and GT3x+; ActiGraph, Pensacola, FL, USA) in a subsample of 167 adults. Individuals were asked to wear the ActiGraph on a belt above the right hip, for three consecutive full days. This previous information was used to validate the physical activity questionnaire administered to the whole sample.

There were calculated the following indicators of physical activity in the participants of the present study:

- Total physical activity expressed as minutes of activity per week;
- Time spent in vigorous physical activity expressed as minutes of activity per week.

Subjects were classified into two levels of physical activity based on two questions of the IPAQ [24]:

"Sedentary activity level" as those subjects who have performed less than 30 min per day of physical activity of daily life and less than 2 h per week of structured physical exercise.

"Active activity level" as those subjects who have performed at least 30 min per day of physical activity of daily life or have performed at least 2 h per week of structured physical exercise.

2.4. Food and Beverage Record

Study participants were provided with a tablet device (Samsung Galaxy Tab 2 7.0, Samsung Electronics, Suwon, South Korea) and trained in how to record information by taking photos of all food and beverages consumed during the three days of the study, both at home and outside the home. Photos had to be taken before beginning to eat and drink, and again after finishing, so as to record the actual intake. Additionally, a brief description of meals (including the type of food), recipes, brands, and the use of dietary supplements were recorded using the device.

Energy and fibre intake were calculated from food consumption records using VD-FEN 2.1 software (Dietary Evaluation Programme, Spanish Nutrition Foundation, Madrid, Spain) which was newly developed for the ANIBES study by the Spanish Nutrition Foundation and is based mainly on Spanish food composition tables [25], with several expansions and updates. Data obtained from food manufacturers and nutritional information provided on food labels were also included. A food photographic atlas was also used to assist in assigning gram weights to serving sizes [26].

The present study was focused on the intake of fibre expressed in grams per day (g/day) raw (before the energy intake adjustment) and after the energy intake adjustment by the residual methods [27,28] and the intake of fibre expressed in grams per 1000 kcal per day. The mean intake of fibre of the studied participants was compared with the adequate intake set out by European Food Safety Authority (EFSA): 25 g/day in adults [29], and by the Institute of Medicine of the United States (IOM): 38 g/day for men and 25 g/day for women of 19–50 years and 30 g/day for men and 21 g/day for women of 51–70 years (14 g/1000 kcal/day) [30].

Once fibre intake has been established, the percentage of fibre from each one of the meal times (breakfast, mid-morning snack, lunch, afternoon snack, and dinner) was calculated.

The contribution of each food to total fibre intake has been calculated by adding the amount of fibre provided by each specific food and dividing by the total intake of fibre, all multiplied by 100 [31].

2.5. Evaluation of Misreporting

The assessment of dietary intake based on self-reported or self-recorded data by the study subjects is often prone to bias. One of the main sources of error is misreporting, including both under- and over-reporting, which are often influenced by age, sex, and other individual characteristics, including BMI [32]. The magnitude of misreporting of the intake of food may lead to biased interpretation of the results. In the present study the protocol of the EFSA was used to identify misreporters [33,34]. This method is based mainly on the Goldberg [35] and Black [36,37] work. This method evaluates the reported energy intake (EIrep) against the presumed energy requirements. EIrep is expressed as a multiple of the mean basal metabolic rate estimated (BMRest) (from formulas), and it is compared with the presumed energy expenditure of the studied population. Then the ratio EIrep:BMRest is referred to as the physical activity levels (PAL) [33,34]. The PAL is established for adults ($\geq$18 years) in three levels: low, 1.4; moderate, 1.6; and vigorous, 1.8. Additionally, the protocol indicates that analyses should be performed at two levels, group and individual. The group level determines the overall bias to the reported energy intake, and the individual level shows the rate of under and over reporters. The BMRest was calculated using the Schöfield equations [38]. Misreporting cut-offs at group and individual levels for the ANIBES study has been described in a previous paper [39]. Subjects were classified into two categories:

"Plausible reporters" as those subjects with estimated values of the ratio EIrep:BMRest ranging between calculated lower cut-off and upper cut-off values for the studied population allocated to the different category of physical activity [33,34].

"Misreporters" as those subjects with estimated values of EIrep:BMRest below the calculated lower cut-off value (under-reporters) and those subjects with estimated values of EIrep:BMRest above the upper calculated cut -off value (over-reporters) [33,34].

In the present study, the results are showed in the total sample (before the exclusion of the non-plausible reporters) and in the plausible reporters.

2.6. *Statistical Analysis*

Descriptive data were presented as mean and standard deviation (SD), median and interquartile range (IQR) (both without any adjustment), and frequencies (%) stratified by sex, BMI, presence of abdominal obesity, and excess body weight and/or abdominal obesity. The normality of the data and equality of the variances were tested using the Kolmogorov–Smirnov and Levene's test, respectively.

The statistical differences of the studied quantitative variables by sex were assessed using Student's *t*-test when data were normally distributed, and using the Mann–Whitney test, otherwise. A two-way ANOVA test was used to assess the differences within the studied variables using sex and the variables of BMI, abdominal obesity or excess body weight and/or abdominal obesity. Two-way ANOVA main effects for BMI, abdominal obesity, and excess body weight and/or abdominal obesity were obtained. The Bonferroni post hoc test for comparison for more than two groups was used. A two-way ANCOVA test was used to assess the differences within the studied variables using the previous ANOVA model taking into account the age and the physical activity (PA) of the participants as covariates to control their influence on the dependent variable. Two-way ANCOVA main effects and interactions were analysed and they are only reported in the text as estimated marginal means and the standard error (SE) when a significant inverse trend, significant changes, or an interaction with sex were observed. The level of significance was set at $p < 0.05$. All calculations were performed using IBM SPSS version 22.0 (IBM Corp., Armonk, NY, USA).

3. Results

3.1. *Study Population*

A sample of 1655 adults (48.2% men and 51.8% women) with ages ranging from 18 to 64 years was studied. In total, 26.16% ($n = 433$) (36.4% men and 63.5% women) of the studied adults were classified as plausible reporters. Table 1 shows the anthropometric and physical activity data of the whole sample and of the plausible reporters. The combined prevalence of OW and OB in the whole sample was 55.70% and 32.80% in the plausible reporters. The prevalence of abdominal obesity was 58.40% and 39.3% and the presence of excess body weight and/or abdominal obesity was 63.93% and 42.7% in the whole sample and in the plausible reporters, respectively. A 44.40% of the whole sample and 44.3% of the plausible reporters were sedentary.

3.2. *Fibre Intake and Dietary Food Sources in the Whole Sample and in the Plausible Reporters and by Sex*

Mean dietary fibre intake (raw) was 12.59 (SD 5.66) g/day, and adjusted by energy was 12.59 (SD 4.91) g/day, while the intake of fibre expressed as grams per 1000 kcal per day was 7.05 (SD 2.81) in the whole sample (Table 2). Fibre intake (raw) was significantly lower in women than in men, but when it was adjusted by energy intake or when was expressed as grams per 1000 kcal per day, it was significantly lower in men than in women in the whole sample (Table 2). Meanwhile, in the group of plausible reporters, the mean dietary fibre (raw) was 15.88 (SD 6.29) g/day, and it was also significantly lower in women than in men, however, there were no statistically significant differences in relation with the fibre intake adjusted by the energy intake or expressed as g/1000 kcal/day (Table 2). Lunch and dinner contributed the highest proportions of fibre to the total daily intake in the whole sample and in the plausible reporters (75.85% and 70.59%, respectively). It is noteworthy that the fibre from breakfast was quite low in the whole sample (13.04%) as well as in the plausible reporters (14.27%). The proportion of fibre from breakfast and afternoon snacks was higher in women and from dinner in men in the whole sample. No significant differences were observed regarding the fibre from the different meals in the plausible reporters (Table 2).

The main food sources of fibre in the whole studied population and in the plausible reporters were grains (39.13% and 39.14%), vegetables (24.17% and 20.99%), fruits (16.60% and 18.51%), pulses (9.28% and 9.14%), ready-to-eat-meals (4.50% and 4.99%), sauces and condiments (2.18% and 1.97%), appetizers (1.53% and 2.30%), sugars and sweets (0.67% and 1.15%), non-alcoholic beverages (0.49% and 0.53%), dairy products (0.39% and 0.28%), and supplements and meal replacers (0.14% and 0.09%, respectively).

3.3. Fibre Intake and Dietary Food Sources in the Whole Sample and in the Plausible Reporters by Body Mass Index Classification

Considering the whole sample, the fibre intake (raw) was higher in subjects who had NW compared to those who had OW or OB, taking into account sex and after adjusting for the age and PA (Table 3). When the interaction of sex by BMI was analysed, it was noted that the intake of fibre (raw) was slightly different according to sex. Men who presented NW 14.83 (SE 0.327) g/day had a higher intake compared to those who had OW 12.45 (SE 0.304) g/day ($p < 0.001$) or OB 11.67 (SE 0.413) g/day ($p < 0.001$). While women who were UW 14.52 (SE 1.077) g/day had a higher intake than those with OW 11.48 (SE 0.335) g/day ($p < 0.05$) or OB 11.33 (SE 0.455) g/day ($p < 0.05$).

Fibre intake adjusted by energy intake (considering sex) was similar for the different groups of BMI in the whole sample (Table 3). However, after adjusting for the age and the PA, it was observed that subjects with NW 13.29 (SE 0.183) g/day had a higher intake than subjects with OW 12.26 (SE 0.194) g/day ($p < 0.001$) or OB 11.79 (SE 0.265) g/day ($p < 0.001$). Analysing the interaction of sex at different levels of BMI, these differences were observed only in men. Thus, men who presented NW 13.46 (SE 0.279) g/day had a higher intake in comparison with those who had OW 11.81 (SE 0.260) g/day ($p < 0.001$) or OB 11.33 (SE 0.353) g/day ($p < 0.001$).

The intake of fibre per 1000 kcal per day (considering sex) was similar for the different groups of BMI in the whole sample (Table 3). However, after adjusting for the age and the PA, it was observed that subjects with NW 7.35 (SE 0.104) g/1000 kcal/day had a higher intake than subjects with OW 6.92 (SE 0.110) g/1000 kcal/day ($p < 0.05$) or OB 6.68 (SE 0.151) g/1000 kcal/day ($p < 0.01$).

No significant differences were observed regarding the fibre intake (raw, adjusted by the energy intake and expressed as grams per 1000 kcal/day) according with the BMI in the plausible reporters, considering sex and after adjusting for the age and the PA (Table 3).

The proportion of fibre from the lunch was higher in individuals with OW than those with NW taking into account sex, but this difference disappeared when an adjustment for age and PA was performed. Fibre from the afternoon snack was higher in individuals with NW than those with OW or OB (taking into account sex and even after adjusting for age and PA) (Table 3). While fibre from dinner was lower (after adjusting for the age and PA) in individuals who had OW 27.50% (SE 0.581) compared to those with OB 30.27% (SE 0.795) ($p < 0.05$). However, the proportion of fibre from the different meals was similar according the BMI in the plausible reporters (Table 3).

Regarding the fibre food sources according to the BMI in the whole sample, we observed that fibre from breakfast cereals and cereal bars was higher in individuals with NW than those with OW and fibre from vegetables was higher in individuals with OB than those with NW, but these differences disappeared when an adjustment for age and PA was performed (Table S1). Fibre from fruits (taking into account sex and after adjusting for the age and PA) was significantly higher in individuals with NW 18.36% (SE 0.574%) compared to subjects with OW 15.16% (SE 0.605%) ($p < 0.01$). In analysing the interaction of sex, it was observed that only in men, the fibre from fruits was higher in those with NW 18.50% (SE 0.881%) than those with OW 14.01% (SE 0.819%) ($p < 0.001$) or OB 12.92% (SE 1.094%) ($p < 0.001$).

After excluding misreporters, we observed that fibre from grains and flours was higher in subjects with NW than those subjects with OW, but this difference disappeared when an adjustment for age and PA was performed (Table S2). Fibre from pasta (taking into account sex and after adjusting for age and PA) was significantly higher individuals with UW 10.83 (SE 2.231%) compared to subjects with NW 4.72% (0.383%) ($p < 0.05$) or OW 4.59% (0.580%) ($p < 0.05$). In analysing the interaction of sex, it was observed that only in men, the fibre from pasta was higher in those with UW 17.98% (SE 4.207%) than in those with NW 4.71% (SE 0.616%) ($p < 0.05$) or OW 4.62% (SE 0.835%) ($p < 0.05$).

3.4. *Fibre Intake and Dietary Food Sources in the Whole Sample and in the Plausible Reporters by the Presence of Abdominal Obesity Determined by the Waist to Height Ratio*

Having into account the whole sample, fibre intake (raw) was higher in subjects without abdominal obesity (taking into account sex and even after adjusting for the age and PA) than those with abdominal obesity (Table 4). In analysing the interaction of sex was found that fibre intake in both men and women without abdominal obesity was higher 15.14 (SE 0.337) g/day and 12.76 (SE 0.276) g/day than those subjects with abdominal obesity 12.04 (SE 0.244) g/day ($p < 0.001$) and 11.47 (SE 0.264) g/day ($p < 0.01$), respectively.

Fibre intake (adjusted by energy intake) considering the sex of the participants was similar independently of the presence or absence of abdominal obesity in the whole sample (Table 4). However, after adjusting for the age and PA, subjects without abdominal obesity 13.43 (SE 0.191) g/day had significantly higher intake than subjects with abdominal obesity 12.05 (SE 0.157) g/day ($p < 0.001$). In analysing the interaction of sex was found that fibre intake in both men and women without abdominal obesity was higher 13.63 (SE 0.288) g/day and 13.24 (SE 0.236) g/day that those with abdominal obesity 11.57 (SE 0.208) g/day ($p < 0.001$) and 12.52 (SE 0.226) g/day ($p < 0.05$), respectively.

The intake of fibre per 1000 kcal per day (considering sex) was similar regardless the presence or absence of abdominal obesity in the whole sample (Table 4). However, after adjusting for the age and the PA, it was observed that the subjects without abdominal obesity 7.44 (SE 0.109) g/1000 kcal/day had a higher intake than subjects with abdominal obesity 6.79 (SE 0.089) g/1000 kcal/day ($p < 0.001$). An interaction of sex was found and it was observed that fibre intake only in men without abdominal obesity was higher 7.36 (SE 0.164) g/1000 kcal/day than in those men with abdominal obesity 6.40 (SE 0.119) g/1000 kcal/day ($p < 0.001$).

Nevertheless, no significant differences were observed regarding the fibre intake (raw, adjusted by the energy intake and expressed as grams per 1000 kcal/day) according with the presence or absence of abdominal obesity, considering sex and after adjusting for the age and the PA in the plausible reporters (Table 4).

Fibre from the mid-morning snack was higher in subjects without abdominal obesity than in subjects with abdominal obesity in the whole sample, but this difference disappeared when an adjustment for age and PA was performed (Table 4).

Considering sex and after adjusting for age and PA, the proportion of fibre from lunch was higher in subjects with abdominal obesity than those without abdominal obesity. In contrast, fibre from the afternoon snack was higher in individuals without abdominal obesity unlike those with abdominal obesity (Table 4). The proportion of fibre from the different meals was similar according the presence or absence of abdominal obesity in the plausible reporters (Table 4).

Concerning the fibre food sources according to the presence or absence of abdominal obesity in the whole sample, we observed that fibre from grains, breakfast cereals, and cereal bars, ready-to-eat meals, and sauces and condiments was higher in individuals without abdominal obesity than those with abdominal obesity and fibre from vegetables was higher in individuals with abdominal obesity than those subjects without abdominal obesity, but all of these differences disappeared when an adjustment for age and PA was performed (Table S3). We only found that fibre from bread (taking into account sex and after adjusting for the age and PA) was higher in subjects with abdominal obesity than those who did not have this problem (Table S3). Similarly, after adjusting for the age and the PA, it was observed that the fibre from pasta was higher in individuals with abdominal obesity 6.73% (SE 0.272%) unlike those participants without abdominal obesity 5.68% (SE 0.332%) ($p < 0.05$). In contrast, the fibre from fruits (taking into account sex and after adjusting for the age and PA) was higher in subjects without abdominal obesity 18.46% (SE 0.600%) than in subjects with abdominal obesity 15.46% (SE 0.491%) ($p < 0.001$). However, when the interaction with sex was analysed (Table S3), the previous result only was observed in men without abdominal obesity 19.15% (SE 0.902%) compared to those with abdominal obesity 13.78% (SE 0.654%) ($p < 0.001$). In relation to the group of sugars and sweets and specifically chocolates, individuals without abdominal obesity had a higher intake than subjects with abdominal obesity (Table S3).

In the plausible reporters, we observed that fibre from pasta was higher in subjects without abdominal obesity than those with abdominal obesity, but this difference disappeared when an adjustment for age and PA was performed (Table S4). Fibre from ready-to-eat-meals (taking into account sex and after adjusting for age and PA) was significantly higher in individuals with abdominal obesity 6.39% (SE 0.585%) compared to subjects without abdominal obesity 4.02% (0.484%) ($p < 0.01$).

3.5. Fibre Intake and Dietary Food Sources in the Whole Sample and in the Plausible Reporters by the Presence of Excess Body Weight and/or Abdominal Obesity Using the Body Mass Index and Waist to Height Ratio

Fibre intake (raw) was higher in individuals without excess body weight and/or abdominal obesity in the whole sample (taking into account sex and after adjusting for the age and PA) (Table 5). An interaction of sex was found and it was observed that fibre intake in both men and women without excess body weight and/or abdominal obesity was higher 15.22 (SE 0.371) g/day and 12.81 (SE 0.291) g/day than in those who had excess body weight and/or abdominal obesity 12.28 (SE 0.232) g/day ($p < 0.001$) and 11.55 (SE 0.252) g/day ($p < 0.01$), respectively.

Fibre intake (adjusted by energy intake) considering sex was similar according to the presence or absence of excess body weight and/or abdominal obesity in the whole sample (Table 5). However, after adjusting for the age and PA, it was found that subjects without excess body weight and/or abdominal obesity 13.43 (SE 0.206) g/day had significantly higher intake than subjects with excess body weight and/or abdominal obesity 12.18 (SE 0.148) g/day ($p < 0.001$). An interaction of sex was found and it was observed that fibre intake only in men without excess body weight and/or abdominal obesity was higher 13.68 (SE 0.317) g/day than in those men with excess body weight and/or abdominal obesity 11.74 (SE 0.198) g/day ($p < 0.001$).

The intake of fibre per 1000 kcal per day (considering sex) was similar regardless the presence or absence of excess body weight and/or abdominal obesity in the whole sample (Table 5). However, after adjusting for the age and the PA, it was observed that the subjects without excess body weight and/or abdominal obesity 7.43 (SE 0.117) g/1000 kcal/day had a higher intake than subjects with excess body weight and/or abdominal obesity 6.86 (SE 0.084) g/1000 kcal/day ($p < 0.001$). An interaction of sex was found and it was observed that fibre intake only in men without excess body weight and/or abdominal obesity was higher 7.36 (SE 0.180) g/1000 kcal/day than in those men with excess body weight and/or abdominal obesity 6.48 (SE 0.113) g/1000 kcal/day ($p < 0.001$).

No significant differences were observed regarding the fibre intake (raw, adjusted by the energy intake and expressed as grams per 1000 kcal/day) according with the presence or absence of excess body weight and/or abdominal obesity in the plausible reporters, considering sex and after adjusting for the age and the PA (Table 5).

Considering the sex and after adjusting for the age and the PA, the proportion of fibre from lunch was higher in subjects with excess body weight and/or abdominal obesity than those who did not have excess body weight and/or abdominal obesity. In contrast, the fibre from the afternoon snack was higher in individuals who had no excess body weight and/or abdominal obesity, unlike those with excess body weight and/or abdominal obesity (Table 5). The proportion of fibre from the different meals was similar according the presence or absence of excessive body weight and/or abdominal obesity in the plausible reporters (Table 5).

Table 1. Anthropometric and physical activity data in the whole sample and in plausible reporters of the ANIBES study of the Spanish adult population (18–64 years).

Personal, Anthropometric and Physical Activity Data	Statistical Data	Whole Sample	Plausible Reporters
n		1655	433
Age (years)	Mean (SD)	39.97 (12.19)	38.53 (11.67)
	P50 (IQR)	39.00 (20.00)	37.00 (17.00)
Weight (kg)	Mean (SD)	74.18 (16.47)	65.71 (13.06)
	P50 (IQR)	72.10 (21.80)	63.80 (17.2)
Height (cm)	Mean (SD)	167.67 (9.35)	165.98 (9.56)
	P50 (IQR)	167.00 (14.00)	165.00 (14.00)
Body mass index (kg/m^2)	Mean (SD)	26.31 (5.14)	23.78 (3.88)
	P50 (IQR)	25.60 (6.20)	23.10 (5.00)
Underweight	%	1.80	4.60
Normal	%	42.50	62.60
Overweight	%	35.80	25.20
Obesity	%	19.90	7.60
Waist circumference (cm)	Mean (SD)	88.06 (14.50)	81.42 (11.70)
	P50 (IQR)	86.83 (19.74)	79.73 (16.17)
Waist to height ratio	Mean (SD)	0.52 (0.08)	0.49 (0.07)
	P50 (IQR)	0.51 (0.11)	0.48 (0.09)
Non-abdominal obesity	%	41.60	60.70
Abdominal obesity	%	58.40	39.30
Non-excess body weight and/or abdominal obesity	%	36.07	57.30
Excess body weight and abdominal obesity	%	63.93	42.70
Physical activity (minutes/week)	Mean (SD)	856.60 (637.72)	889.22 (640.23)
	P50 (IQR)	735.00 (920.00)	800.00 (960.00)
Vigorous activity (minutes/week)	Mean (SD)	149.20 (264.15)	168.68 (275.13)
	P50 (IQR)	0 (180.00)	0 (260)
Sedentary activity level	%	44.40	44.30
Active activity level	%	55.60	55.70

SD: standard deviation; P50: 50th percentile; IQR: interquartile range; Abdominal obesity: waist to height ratio ≥ 0.5; Excess body weight and/or abdominal obesity: body mass index ≥ 25 kg/m^2 and/or waist to height ratio ≥ 0.5.

Table 2. Fibre intake in the whole sample and in plausible reporters of the ANIBES study of the Spanish adult population (18–64 years) by sex.

Whole Sample	Statistical Data	Total (n = 1655)	Men (n = 798)	Women (n = 857)	p
Energy (kcal/day)	Mean (SD)	1815.58 (511.96)	1966.22 (543.22)	1675.31 (436.85)	***
	P50 (IQR)	1758.00 (683)	1919.00 (770)	1648.00 (598)	
Total fibre (g/day) (raw)	Mean (SD)	12.59 (5.66)	13.09 (6.09)	12.13 (5.20)	**
	P50 (IQR)	11.63 (6.98)	12.15 (7.27)	11.27 (6.68)	
Total fibre (g/day) (adjusted by energy intake)	Mean (SD)	12.59 (4.91)	12.26 (5.14)	12.91 (4.67)	***
	P50 (IQR)	11.75 (6.01)	11.32 (5.79)	12.25 (6.00)	
Fibre per 1000 kcal/day	Mean (SD)	7.05 (2.81)	6.71 (2.66)	7.37 (2.91)	***
	P50 (IQR)	6.55 (3.53)	6.25 (3.24)	6.99 (3.78)	
Fibre from breakfast (%)	Mean (SD)	13.04 (11.59)	12.15 (11.68)	13.88 (11.44)	***
	P50 (IQR)	10.84 (15.02)	9.73 (15.68)	11.78 (14.48)	
Fibre from mid-morning snack (%)	Mean (SD)	5.16 (8.19)	4.99 (8.21)	5.31 (8.18)	NS
	P50 (IQR)	7.51 (11.69)	0.00 (8.01)	0.87 (8.20)	
Fibre from lunch (%)	Mean (SD)	47.46 (16.60)	48.00 (16.83)	46.96 (16.37)	NS
	P50 (IQR)	47.10 (22.74)	47.61 (23.11)	46.17 (22.50)	
Fibre from afternoon snack (%)	Mean (SD)	5.92 (8.67)	5.48 (8.94)	6.34 (8.39)	***
	P50 (IQR)	1.52 (9.66)	0 (8.55)	3.13 (10.62)	
Fibre from dinner (%)	Mean (SD)	28.39 (14.05)	29.35 (14.43)	27.49 (13.64)	*
	P50 (IQR)	27.03 (18.67)	27.82 (19.40)	26.53 (18.49)	
Plausible Reporters	**Statistical data**	**Total (n = 433)**	**Men (n = 158)**	**Women (n = 275)**	p
Energy (kcal/day)	Mean (SD)	2352 (425)	2712 (358)	2145 (306)	***
	P50 (IQR)	2297 (625)	2640 (490)	2095 (403)	
Total fibre (g/day) (raw)	Mean (SD)	15.88 (6.29)	17.97 (7.19)	14.68 (5.36)	***
	P50 (IQR)	14.89 (7.38)	16.63 (8.26)	14.10 (7.40)	
Total fibre (g/day) (adjusted by energy intake)	Mean (SD)	15.88 (5.81)	15.93 (6.87)	15.85 (5.12)	NS
	P50 (IQR)	14.78 (7.69)	14.26 (8.38)	14.94 (7.46)	
Fibre per 1000 kcal/day	Mean (SD)	6.79 (2.44)	6.64 (2.52)	6.87 (2.38)	NS
	P50 (IQR)	6.31 (3.36)	6.07 (3.03)	6.47 (3.46)	
Fibre from breakfast (%)	Mean (SD)	14.27 (11.39)	13.68 (10.89)	14.61 (11.66)	NS
	P50 (IQR)	12.04 (13.54)	11.75 (13.88)	12.45 (12.90)	
Fibre from mid-morning snack (%)	Mean (SD)	6.32 (8.35)	5.99 (7.91)	6.50 (8.60)	NS
	P50 (IQR)	3.38 (9.32)	2.53 (9.44)	3.78 (9.28)	
Fibre from lunch (%)	Mean (SD)	42.98 (14.84)	44.05 (15.06)	42.37 (14.70)	NS
	P50 (IQR)	42.22 (20.90)	43.32 (21.27)	41.05 (22.17)	
Fibre from afternoon snack (%)	Mean (SD)	8.81 (9.66)	8.16 (9.76)	9.19 (9.60)	NS
	P50 (IQR)	6.15 (13.72)	5.05 (12.22)	6.46 (13.25)	
Fibre from dinner (%)	Mean (SD)	27.61 (12.52)	28.12 (12.11)	27.32 (12.76)	NS
	P50 (IQR)	26.01 (17.25)	27.04 (16.31)	25.79 (18.58)	

SD: standard deviation; P50: 50th percentile; IQR: interquartile range; p: denotes statistical mean differences by sex. * $p < 0.05$. ** $p < 0.01$. *** $p < 0.001$. NS: non-significant.

Table 3. Fibre intake in the whole sample and in the plausible reporters of the ANIBES study of the Spanish adult population (18–64 years) by body mass index.

Whole Sample	Statistical Data	Underweight (n = 30)	Normal Weight (n = 704)	Overweight (n = 592)	Obesity (n = 329)	Two-Way ANOVA	Two-Way ANCOVA
Energy intake (kcal/day)	Mean (SD)	1930.90 (592.45)	1872.51 (526.97)	1773.45 (502.33) $_b$	1759.05 (475.65) $_b$	S ** BMI ***	S ** BMI ***
	P50 (IQR)	1857.00 (2114.00)	1827.00 (4018.00)	1712.50 (2843.00)	1676.00 (3109.00)		
Total fibre intake (g/day) (raw)	Mean (SD)	12.86 (6.35)	13.05 (5.98)	12.27 (5.40) $_b$	12.19 (5.33) $_b$	BMI ** I *	BMI *** I *
	P50 (IQR)	11.20 (22.98)	11.82 (40.66)	11.46 (34.16)	11.46 (35.71)		
Total fibre (g/day) (adjusted by energy) intake)	Mean (SD)	12.22 (4.56)	12.73 (5.13)	12.50 (4.71)	12.50 (4.83)	NS	BMI *** I *
	P50 (IQR)	11.19 (7.68)	11.86 (6.19)	11.90 (6.07)	11.57 (5.81)		
Fibre per 1000 kcal/day	Mean (SD)	6.58 (2.39)	7.06 (2.78)	7.05 (2.79)	7.08 (2.97)	S *	S * BMI **
	P50 (IQR)	6.15 (9.10)	6.56 (18.82)	6.64 (18.35)	6.42 (23.84)		
Fibre from breakfast (%)	Mean (SD)	10.51 (11.89)	13.25 (11.56)	13.16 (11.79)	12.65 (11.30)	NS	NS
	P50 (IQR)	7.34 (41.49)	11.01 (69.25)	10.94 (61.66)	10.37 (64.58)		
Fibre from mid-morning snack (%)	Mean (SD)	6.29 (9.91)	5.32 (8.00)	5.19 (8.48)	4.64 (7.93)	NS	NS
	P50 (IQR)	0.29 (35.40)	1.08 (58.11)	0 (58.29)	0 (63.99)		
Fibre from lunch (%)	Mean (SD)	47.19 (15.69)	45.83 (16.24	48.99 (16.87) $_b$	48.25 (16.71)	BMI **	NS
	P50 (IQR)	46.20 (57.35)	44.81 (93.52)	48.96 (88.61)	48.18 (97.88)		
Fibre from afternoon snack (%)	Mean (SD)	7.43 (5.93)	6.92 (9.11)	5.30 (8.49) $_b$	4.79 (7.99) $_b$	BMI **	BMI *
	P50 (IQR)	6.80 (19.78)	3.25 (52.26)	0.0 (66.44)	0.0 (60.28)		
Fibre from dinner (%)	Mean (SD)	28.58 (12.39)	28.66 (13.96)	27.35 (14.06)	29.65 (14.32)	NS	BMI *
	P50 (IQR)	29.00 (66.69)	27.95 (79.03)	25.80 (91.30)	27.64 (76.37)		
Plausible Reporters	**Statistical Data**	**Underweight (n = 20)**	**Normal Weight (n = 271)**	**Overweight (n = 109)**	**Obesity (n = 33)**	**Two-Way ANOVA**	**Two-Way ANCOVA**
Energy intake (kcal/day)	Mean (SD)	2153 (466)	2307 (425)	2443 (394) $_{a,b}$	2539 (395) $_{a,b}$	BMI **	S *** BMI ***
	P50 (IQR)	2070 (799)	2244 (619)	2405 (616)	2413 (459)		
Total fibre intake (g/day) (raw)	Mean (SD)	14.12 (6.35)	15.58 (6.35)	16.69 (5.86)	16.75 (6.97)	NS	NS
	P50 (IQR)	11.96 (10.08)	14.62 (7.13)	16.45 (8.34)	15.82 (6.45)		
Total fibre (g/day) (adjusted by energy) intake)	Mean (SD)	15.25 (4.93)	15.83 (5.81)	16.17 (5.84)	15.69 (6.41)	NS	NS
	P50 (IQR)	14.24 (8.93)	14.89 (7.09)	15.48 (8.71)	14.31 (7.62)		
Fibre per 1000 kcal/day	Mean (SD)	6.44 (2.19)	6.78 (2.44)	6.93 (2.46)	6.59 (2.48)	NS	NS
	P50 (IQR)	6.15 (4.26)	6.38 (3.12)	6.53 (3.96)	6.08 (3.26)		
Fibre from breakfast (%)	Mean (SD)	11.81 (13.33)	14.47 (11.63)	14.12 (10.64)	14.69 (10.81)	NS	NS
	P50 (IQR)	8.03 (19.27)	12.23 (14.34)	13.08 (12.56)	13.45 (14.12)		
Fibre from mid-morning snack (%)	Mean (SD)	9.07 (11.13)	6.47 (8.57)	6.10 (7.86)	4.14 (5.30)	NS	NS
	P50 (IQR)	6.05 (16.17)	3.78 (9.31)	2.64 (9.42)	1.71 (7.15)		
Fibre from lunch (%)	Mean (SD)	42.40 (15.06)	42.61 (15.11)	43.72 (14.52)	43.97 (14.00)	NS	NS
	P50 (IQR)	42.29 (29.63)	40.16 (20.22)	45.93 (21.66)	43.65 (22.68)		
Fibre from afternoon snack (%)	Mean (SD)	8.12 (6.06)	8.60 (9.28)	9.58 (11.37)	8.43 (8.50)	NS	NS
	P50 (IQR)	6.66 (10.27)	6.15 (13.48)	5.27 (14.07)	7.79 (12.94)		
Fibre from dinner (%)	Mean (SD)	28.61 (12.83)	27.85 (12.69)	26.48 (11.89)	28.77 (13.26)	NS	NS
	P50 (IQR)	26.64 (16.05)	26.68 (17.34)	25.48 (16.86)	26.58 (18.43)		

SD: standard deviation; P50: 50th percentile; IQR: interquartile range; Two-way ANOVA was performed taking into account sex (S) and body mass index (BMI); Two-way ANCOVA was performed taking into account S and BMI and age and physical activity as covariates; Two-way ANOVA significant differences between BMI classification: a: regarding underweight, b: regarding normal weight, c: regarding overweight; I: Interaction; * $p < 0.05$, ** $p < 0.01$, *** $p < 0.001$; NS: non-significant.

Table 4. Fibre intake in the whole sample and in plausible reporters of the ANIBES Study Spanish adult population (18–64 years) by the presence or absence of abdominal obesity using the waist to height ratio.

Whole Sample	Statistical Data	Non-Abdominal Obesity (*n* = 689)	Abdominal Obesity (*n* = 966)	Two-Way ANOVA	Two-Way ANCOVA
Energy intake (kcal/day)	Mean (SD)	1886.03 (543.28)	1765.33 (482.43)	S *** WHtR ***	S *** WHtR ***
	P50 (IQR)	1832.00 (701.00)	1705.00 (653.00)		
Total fibre intake (g/day) (raw)	Mean (SD)	12.96 (5.97)	12.33 (5.43)	S *** WHtR ** I **	S *** WHtR *** I **
	P50 (IQR)	11.94 (7.34)	11.46(6.52)		
Total fibre (g/day) (adjusted by energy intake)	Mean (SD)	12.58 (5.06)	12.61 (4.81)	I *	WHtR *** I **
	P50 (IQR)	11.71 (6.06)	11.81 (5.83)		
Fibre per 1000 kcal/day	Mean (SD)	6.97 (2.80)	7.11 (2.82)	S ***	S *** WHtR *** I *
	P50 (IQR)	6.46 (3.54)	6.59 (3.49)		
Fibre from breakfast (%)	Mean (SD)	13.15 (11.81)	12.97 (11.43)	S **	S *
	P50 (IQR)	10.75 (15.44)	10.87 (15.04)		
Fibre from mid-morning snack (%)	Mean (SD)	5.70 (8.59)	4.77 (7.88)	WHtR *	NS
	P50 (IQR)	1.44 (8.23)	0 (7.80)		
Fibre from lunch (%)	Mean (SD)	45.35 (16.26)	48.97 (16.67)	WHtR ***	WHtR **
	P50 (IQR)	44.29 (23.29)	48.81(22.57)		
Fibre from afternoon snack (%)	Mean (SD)	6.97 (8.96)	5.18 (8.38)	WHtR ***	WHtR **
	P50 (IQR)	3.31 (11.75)	0 (8.03)		
Fibre from dinner (%)	Mean (SD)	28.81 (14.26)	28.09 (13.91)	S **	S *
	P50 (IQR)	27.96 (18.71)	26.64 (18.59)		
Plausible Reporters	**Statistical Data**	**Non-Abdominal Obesity (*n* = 263)**	**Abdominal Obesity (*n* = 170)**	**Two-Way ANOVA**	**Two-Way ANCOVA**
Energy intake (kcal/day)	Mean (SD)	2319.06 (446.79)	2401.78 (384.418)	S ***	S ***
	P50 (IQR)	2244.00 (641.00)	2366.50 (558)		
Total fibre intake (g/day) (raw)	Mean (SD)	15.36 (6.28)	16.67 (6.23)	S ***	S ***
	P50 (IQR)	14.47 (7.36)	16.32 (7.67)		
Total fibre (g/day) (adjusted by energy intake)	Mean (SD)	15.54 (5.57)	16.39 (6.13)	NS	NS
	P50 (IQR)	14.65 (7.01)	15.27 (8.23)		
Fibre per 1000 kcal/day	Mean (SD)	6.63 (2.31)	7.03 (2.59)	NS	NS
	P50 (IQR)	6.22 (3.21)	6.52 (3.59)		
Fibre from breakfast (%)	Mean (SD)	14.36 (11.94)	14.12 (10.49)	NS	NS
	P50 (IQR)	11.89 (14.42)	13.16 (12.53)		
Fibre from mid-morning snack (%)	Mean (SD)	6.88 (9.00)	5.43 (7.14)	NS	NS
	P50 (IQR)	4.11 (10.44)	2.60 (8.64)		
Fibre from lunch (%)	Mean (SD)	41.97 (14.99)	44.54 (14.50)	NS	NS
	P50 (IQR)	39.91 (19.86)	45.79 (23.04)		
Fibre from afternoon snack (%)	Mean (SD)	8.57 (9.10)	9.18 (10.48)	NS	NS
	P50 (IQR)	6.28 (13.48)	6.03 (13.92)		
Fibre from dinner (%)	Mean (SD)	28.19 (12.64)	26.70 (12.31)	NS	NS
	P50 (IQR)	26.87 (17.32)	25.50 (16.84)		

SD: standard deviation; P50: 50th percentile; IQR: interquartile range; Two-way ANOVA was performed taking into account sex (S) and the waist to height ratio (WHtR); Two-way ANCOVA was performed taking into account S and the WHtR and the age and physical activity as covariates. I: interaction. * $p < 0.05$. ** $p < 0.01$. *** $p < 0.001$. NS: non-significant.

Table 5. Fibre intake in the whole sample and in plausible reporters of the ANIBES study of the Spanish adult population (18–64 years) by the presence or absence of excess body weight and/or abdominal obesity using the body mass index and the waist to height ratio.

Whole Sample	Statistical Data	Non-Excess Body Weight and/or Abdominal Obesity (n = 597)	Excess Body Weight and/or Abdominal Obesity (n = 1058)	Two-Way ANOVA	Two-Way ANCOVA
Energy intake (kcal/day)	Mean (SD)	1892.54 (539.47)	1772.15 (490.72)	S *** BMI_WHtR ***	S *** BMI_WHtR ***
	P50 (IQR)	1848.00 (686.00)	1707.00 (669.00)		
Total fibre intake (g/day) (raw)	Mean (SD)	13.00 (5.96)	12.36 (5.49)	S *** BMI_WHtR** I**	S *** BMI_WHtR *** I**
	P50 (IQR)	11.94 (7.25)	11.47 (6.54)		
Total fibre (g/day) (adjusted by energy intake)	Mean (SD)	12.58 (5.09)	12.60 (4.81)	I *	BMI_WHtR *** I **
	P50 (IQR)	11.71 (6.14)	11.79 (5.86)		
Fibre per 1000 kcal/day	Mean (SD)	6.97 (2.78)	7.1 (2.84)	S ***	S *** BMI_WHtR ** I *
	P50 (IQR)	6.47 (3.56)	6.59 (3.5)		
Fibre from breakfast (%)	Mean (SD)	13.21 (11.85)	12.96 (11.45)	S * I *	S * I *
	P50 (IQR)	10.76 (15.27)	10.85 (15.07)		
Fibre from mid-morning snack (%)	Mean (SD)	5.66 (8.31)	4.88 (8.13)	NS	NS
	P50 (IQR)	1.46 (8.31)	0 (7.76)		
Fibre from lunch (%)	Mean (SD)	45.17 (16.17)	48.76 (16.71)	BMI_WHtR ***	BMI_WHtR **
	P50 (IQR)	44.13 (22.98)	48.64 (22.37)		
Fibre from afternoon snack (%)	Mean (SD)	7.20 (9.09)	5.21 (8.35)	BMI_WHtR ***	BMI_WHtR **
	P50 (IQR)	3.61 (12.03)	0 (8.03)		
Fibre from dinner (%)	Mean (SD)	28.76 (13.84)	28.19 (14.18)	S **	S *
	P50 (IQR)	27.91 (18.71)	26.79 (18.62)		
Plausible Reporters	**Statistical Data**	**Non-Excess Body Weight and/or Abdominal Obesity (n = 248)**	**Excess Body Weight and/or Abdominal Obesity (n = 185)**	**Two-Way ANOVA**	**Two-Way ANCOVA**
Energy intake (kcal/day)	Mean (SD)	2296 (434)	2426 (402)	S ***	S *** BMI_WHtR **
	P50 (IQR)	2223 (623)	2385 (601)		
Total fibre intake (g/day) (raw)	Mean (SD)	15.16 (6.09)	16.85 (6.43)	S ***	S ***
	P50 (IQR)	14.42 (7.27)	16.36 (7.87)		
Total fibre (g/day) (adjusted by energy intake)	Mean (SD)	15.47 (5.47)	16.43 (6.20)	NS	NS
	P50 (IQR)	14.62 (6.84)	15.33 (8.33)		
Fibre per 1000 kcal/day	Mean (SD)	6.62 (2.31)	7.02 (2.58)	NS	NS
	P50 (IQR)	6.22 (3.10)	6.53 (3.71)		
Fibre from breakfast (%)	Mean (SD)	14.34 (12.12)	14.19 (10.35)	NS	NS
	P50 (IQR)	11.47 (14.64)	13.31 (12.24)		
Fibre from mid-morning snack (%)	Mean (SD)	6.98 (9.08)	5.43 (7.17)	NS	NS
	P50 (IQR)	4.22 (10.74)	2.63 (8.70)		
Fibre from lunch (%)	Mean (SD)	41.93 (14.99)	44.40 (14.56)	NS	NS
	P50 (IQR)	39.75 (20.10)	45.69 (22.85)		
Fibre from afternoon snack (%)	Mean (SD)	8.71 (9.22)	8.96 (10.25)	NS	NS
	P50 (IQR)	6.37 (13.86)	5.98 (13.44)		
Fibre from dinner (%)	Mean (SD)	28.05 (12.81)	27.02 (12.13)	NS	NS
	P50 (IQR)	26.71 (17.24)	25.64 (17.04)		

SD: standard deviation; P50: 50th percentile; IQR: interquartile range; Two-way ANOVA was performed taking into account sex (S) and the body mass index and/or waist to height ratio (BMI-WHtR); Two-way ANCOVA was performed taking into account S and the BMI-WHtR and the age and physical activity as covariates. I: interaction. * $p < 0.05$. ** $p < 0.01$. *** $p < 0.001$. NS: non-significant.

Relating to the fibre food sources, according to the presence or absence of excess body weight and/or abdominal obesity in the whole sample, we found that fibre from grains, breakfast cereals, and cereal bars, chocolates, ready-to-eat meals, sauces, and condiments, was higher in individuals without excess body weight and/or abdominal obesity than those with excess body weight and/or abdominal obesity, and fibre from vegetables was higher in individuals with excess body weight and/or abdominal obesity than those subjects without excess body weight and/or abdominal obesity, but all these differences disappeared when an adjustment for age and PA was performed (Table S5). Fibre from bread (taking into account sex and after adjusting for the age and PA) was higher in subjects who had excess body weight and/or abdominal obesity than in those who did not have this problematic (Table S5). Similarly, after adjusting for the age and the PA, it was observed that the fibre from the pasta was higher in individuals with excess body weight and/or abdominal obesity 6.65% (SE 0.256%) as opposed to those without it 5.63% (SE 0.358%) ($p < 0.05$). In contrast, fibre from fruits (taking into account sex and after adjusting for the age and PA) was higher in subjects without excess body weight and/or abdominal obesity 19.06% (SE 0.644%) than in subjects with excess body weight and/or abdominal obesity 15.45% (SE 0.462%) ($p < 0.001$). However, when analysing the interaction with sex (Table S5), this result was only observed in men without excess body weight and/or abdominal obesity 20.12% (SE 0.990%) compared to those with excess body weight and/or abdominal obesity 13.87% (SE 0.619%) ($p < 0.001$).

In the plausible reporters, we observed that fibre from the groups of grains and flours, pasta and juices and nectars was higher in subjects without excess body weight and/or abdominal obesity than those with excess body weight and/or abdominal obesity, but these differences disappeared when an adjustment for age and PA was performed (Table S6). Taking into account sex and after adjusting for age and PA, fibre from fruits was significantly higher in individuals without excess body weight and/or abdominal obesity 20.2% (SE 1.042%) compared to subjects with excess body weight and/or abdominal obesity 16.9% (1.144%) ($p < 0.05$). Conversely, the fibre from ready-to-eat-meals was higher in those subjects with excess body weight and/or abdominal obesity 6.41 (SE 0.558%) than those without excess body weight and/or abdominal obesity 3.81% (SE 0.508%) ($p < 0.01$).

4. Discussion

The present study provides updated information on fibre intake and dietary sources and their association with the condition of excess body weight and abdominal obesity in a representative sample of the Spanish adult population. It is highlighted the ANIBES is the first national diet and nutrition survey in Spain that has taken into account the plausible reporters in the analysis of the data, based on well-harmonised procedures [33,34].

A great proportion of participants of the whole sample and of the plausible reporters had OW or OB, which is in concordance with other studies performed in the Spanish population [40,41]. Nonetheless, it is highlighted the prevalence of OW or OB was lower in the plausible reporters in comparison with the whole sample. When comparing our results with the FANPE study (carried out in 2009 on a representative sample of the Spanish population), we found that the combined prevalence of OW and OB of the study (47.80%) was lower than that observed in our study in the whole sample (55.70%) and higher than that observed in the plausible reporters (32.80%) [41], while the combined prevalence observed in the ENPE study, conducted in 2014–2015, also in Spain, was higher (60.9%) than that observed in the present study both in the whole sample and in the plausible reporters [40].

Some studies have indicated that the WHtR is a better predictor of metabolic syndrome or cardiovascular disease and mortality than the WC or BMI [21,23]. Possibly, the most important advantage of using the WHtR resides in the fact that this ratio takes into account the height of the subject, which avoids the overestimation or underestimation of individuals who have a high or low height [21,23,42]. In our study, the mean WHtR in the whole sample was 0.52 (SD 0.08) and 0.49 (SD 0.07) in the plausible reporters. These values are in line to those indicated by the FANPE and ENPE studies [40,43]. Using this parameter, 58.4% of the whole sample and 39.30%

of the plausible reporters had abdominal obesity, lower than those indicated in the DARIOS Study (conducted in 2013 in Spanish population), in which 89% of men and 77% of women had abdominal obesity [44]. Moreover, when the presence of excess body weight and/or the presence of abdominal obesity were examined, it was found that 63.93% of the whole sample and 42.70% of the plausible reporters had one or both of these problems.

Furthermore, we found that a high proportion of the studied population was sedentary, which has been already discussed in detail in a previous paper [45].

The mean dietary fibre intakes (raw, adjusted by energy intake and expressed in grams per 1000 kcal per day) both in the whole sample and in the plausible reporters were very similar and were lower in comparison with the observed in other studies performed in population with similar ages and characteristics [14,15,46,47]. When comparing the results of our study with those observed by the ENIDE study (carried out in a representative sample of the Spanish population aged 18 to 64 years in 2011), the fibre intake of the participants of our study was lower than the results of such study (men: 20.94 (SD 11.38) g/day and women: 18.85 (SD 10.06) g/day) [14]. Likewise, the mean fibre intakes shown in other study also performed in Spain 20.2 (SD 7.8) g/day and in a study carried out in Irish population 25.7 (SD 8.1) g/day were higher than that observed in our study [15,46]. However, our results were more similar to those observed in the National Health and Nutrition Examination Survey (NHANES 2009–2010) performed in United States adults aged 19 years and older where the fibre intake was 17.0 g/day [47].

The mean intake of fibre (raw) both in men and women was below the adequate intake established by the EFSA and IOM [29,30] in the whole sample and in the plausible reporters. This situation was close to the results shown in various studies performing in similar population [14,46,48,49].

We observed only in the whole sample that the fibre intake after adjusting for energy intake and the fibre per 1000 kcal per day were significantly higher in women than in men. This may be explained because women are usually more concerned about following healthy eating habits and tend to include more healthy foods in their diet compared to men [50]. The analysis of the source of daily fibre intake depending on the different meals throughout the day, revealed that nearly half came from lunch (47.46% and 42.98%) and almost a third from dinner (28.39% and 27.61%) in the whole sample and plausible reporters, respectively. It is noteworthy that the fibre from breakfast was too low in the whole sample (13.04%) and in the plausible reporters (14.27%). The number of frequency of meals per day, including snacks, has been positively related to the intake of various nutrients including the fibre intake [51]. In our study, the mid-morning and afternoon snacks provided the 11.08% and the 15.13% of the daily fibre in the whole sample and in the plausible reporters, respectively. In contrast to our results, the 2001–2010 NHANES study observed that most of the daily fibre came from dinner (37% for adults 19–50 years) [52]. Furthermore, the pattern of fibre intake from the different meals of the day differs according to sex. The proportion of fibre from breakfast and afternoon snacks was higher in women and from dinner in men only in the whole sample. These differences in the pattern of fibre intake are probably due to the differences in the food choices made by the subjects at each meal of the day [52]. A better contribution of fibre from breakfast or afternoon snack, with respect to other meals, could help to reduce appetite and food intake at subsequent meals [6,9]. This could be related to the better situation observed in women compared to men in connection with the presence of excess body weight and abdominal obesity described in a previous paper in more detail for the ANIBES Spanish adult population [53].

Regarding dietary sources of fibre, the main sources in the studied sample were grains, followed by vegetables, fruits, and pulses and were very similar in both studied samples. Similar food groups were identified as the major contributors in the Belgian population [49]. Unlike our study, the main sources of fibre in the ENIDE study were fruits (30%), followed by legumes and nuts (26%), cereals (22%), and vegetables (14%) [14]. Differences were also observed when compared to the results of the 2001–2010 NHANES study, where it was observed that the main sources were the vegetables, followed by cereals and fruits [52].

Some studies performed on populations from the United States [5], the Netherlands [4], and Spain [54] have observed an inverse association between fibre intake and BMI. In accordance with this, in our study, taking into account sex, and after adjusting for the age and physical activity of the participants, fibre intake (raw, adjusted by energy intake and expressed as grams per 1000 kcal per day) was different according to the BMI only in the whole sample. Participants with NW had a significantly higher intake of fibre (raw and expressed as grams per 1000 kcal per day) than those subjects with OW or OB. However, the differences on fibre intake adjusted by the energy intake only were observed in the male sex, where men with NW had a greater intake than those who had OW or OB, which is consistent with what is stated in the study conducted in the Dutch population, where they have found an inverse association between fibre intake and BMI only in men [4]. Moreover, the pattern of fibre intake in the different meals during the day varied depending on the body weight situation only in the whole sample. Specifically, we found that the percentage of fibre that comes from the afternoon snack was higher in individuals with NW than those with OW or OB, while the fibre from dinner was higher in individuals who had OB than those who had OW. The difference found regarding the contribution of fibre from the afternoon snack according to BMI, as previously mentioned, could be related, on the one hand, to the fact that a higher fibre content may favour a reduced appetite which, in turn, can help to take in less food at subsequent meals, in this case during dinner, thus balancing the daily energy intake [6,9]. On the other hand, this also could be explained due to an afternoon snack that contains a higher amount of fibre, which could also include healthier foods with a lower content of energy or fat.

An inverse relation between dietary fibre from cereals and fruits and body weight gain has been described in a study performed in male adults (40–75 years old) from the United States [55]. Although the fibre from grains was the most important fibre food source in the present study, there were no significant differences according to BMI in the whole sample. Conversely, we found that the intake of fibre coming from fruits was higher in men with NW compared to those who had OW or OB in the whole sample. These differences may be explained due to fruits that are rich in soluble fibre, which may help control appetite, or because people who consume fruits and vegetables regularly also tend to have a healthier lifestyle [9,49].

We only observed in the men of the group of plausible reporters that fibre from pasta was higher in those with UW than in those with NW or OW. This may be due to subjects who have an excessive body weight try to control their weight by the reduction of carbohydrates of the diet reducing the intake of this type of food.

When the data were analysed according to the presence or absence of abdominal obesity using the WHtR, we found that the intake of fibre (raw, adjusted by energy intake and express per 1000 kcal per day) only in the whole sample was higher in those subjects without abdominal obesity. In this manner, it becomes clear that the fibre intake may help to avoid the appearance of abdominal obesity, which has also been described in a study performed in Chinese adults that observed subjects with a lower WHtR had a higher fibre intake [56].

On the other hand, the pattern of fibre intake in the different meals during the day varied depending on the presence or absence of abdominal obesity only in the whole sample. The proportion of fibre from lunch was higher in the participants with abdominal obesity compared to their normal counterparts, which could be due to the style of eating in Spain, since in general, lunch is characterized by the presence of an abundant amount of foods like cereals, pulses and vegetables that provide a great amount of fibre, respect to other meals of the day. This type of lunch is largely respected by the general population regardless of individual food habits. However, in relation to the snack and dinner, in Spain is observed that there is a much more marked difference in the composition depending on the food habits of each person. On the other hand, the proportion of fibre from afternoon snacks was higher in individuals without abdominal obesity than in those who had this problem. This finding suggests that a higher intake of fibre in the afternoon could have a beneficial effect in relation to the abdominal accumulation of body fat and not only with respect to the body weight situation described previously. Nevertheless, further studies are needed to clarify this aspect.

Some studies have indicated that the consumption of whole grain foods seems to have benefits regarding weight control and abdominal adiposity, emphasizing that the consumption of whole grain products seems to have not promote weight gain, while refined-grain products are directly associated with the excess of weight and abdominal fat [7,57]. In our study, the contribution to the intake of fibre from bread and pasta was higher only in subjects with abdominal obesity of the whole sample. However, the information about the type of bread or pasta consumed by the population was not available in our study. Moreover, various studies have found an inverse association between dietary fibre from fruits and the WC, insulin resistance, and metabolic syndrome [58–60]. In line with this, in our study, the fibre from fruits was higher only in men of the whole sample without abdominal obesity than in those with this problem. This difference, as previously noted, could be explained because of the beneficial effect of soluble fibre on the reduction of the appetite or due to a healthier lifestyle [9,49]. A similar trend was also observed in relation to the group of sugars and sweets and, in particular, with the subgroup of chocolates. However, because the food groups disaggregated by food items have not been analysed, it was not possible to give an explanation. However, it is assumed that this difference may be due to participants without abdominal obesity selecting and consuming some type of chocolate or similar healthier product with a higher content of fibre, unlike the group who has abdominal obesity.

We only observed in the group of plausible reporters that fibre from ready-to-eat-meals was higher in individuals with abdominal obesity compared to subjects without abdominal obesity, which is according with following an unhealthy diet rich in ready-to-eat-meals, which is common in individuals with obesity.

Likewise, when analysing the excess body weight and abdominal obesity individually, it was confirmed that there was a greater fibre intake in subjects without excess body weight and abdominal obesity compared with those who had one or two of these problems only in the whole sample.

It is noted that the fibre from the afternoon snack seems to play a major role in the body weight situation and abdominal obesity. Even when considering the presence or absence of both problems in the same individual, we also found that those subjects in the whole sample with excess body weight or abdominal obesity had a lower proportion of fibre from the afternoon snack and higher from lunch than their counterparts. This suggests that, probably, the meal of the day in which the fibre is consumed is of relevance to obtaining the benefits of the fibre in relation to excess body weight or abdominal obesity.

In relation to the dietary fibre sources according to the excess body weight and/or abdominal obesity, we found a consistent tendency when the sources were analysed according to the excess body weight and abdominal obesity separately. A higher proportion of fibre from bread and pasta (in men and woman), and less from fruit (only in men), is associated with excess body weight and/or abdominal obesity in comparison with subjects with NW and without abdominal obesity.

As in the whole sample, in the plausible reporters we also observed that fibre from fruits was significantly higher in individuals without excess body weight and/or abdominal obesity compared to subjects with excess body weight and/or abdominal obesity. However, only in the plausible reporters, the fibre from ready-to-eat-meals was higher in those subjects with excess body weight and/or abdominal obesity than those without excess body weight and/or abdominal obesity, which is consistent with the results when the fibre dietary sources were analysed according to the presence or absence of abdominal obesity individually.

A limitation of our study was the inability to analyse the types of fibre (soluble and insoluble) and the food groups disaggregated by food items, since such information was not available. Nonetheless, this did not represent an impediment to achieve the aim of our work that was to study the intake and dietary food sources of fibre and analyse the differences in the fibre intake between people with different body weight situations, and with or without abdominal obesity. In contrast, the main strengths of our study include the methodological design used in the ANIBES study, such as the fact that all anthropometric data were measured and they were not self-reported by the participants, which improves the validity of the study, and the possibility of extrapolating our results to the Spanish population because it was conducted in a representative sample. It is important to highlight that this is the first Spanish study at national level that analyses the data for the whole population and the plausible reporters.

The findings regarding the association between diet and the health outcomes analysed in the present study should be interpreted with caution given the discrepancy observed between both samples. Further studies considering different methods to address misreporting are needed to confirm the association between the fibre intake and the excess body weight and/or abdominal obesity. At the same time, the information derived from our study can be useful in designing nutrition intervention strategies to increase the intake of fibre in our country that it was low both in the whole sample and in the plausible reporters, which in turn could prevent and control some health problems such as excess body weight and abdominal obesity.

5. Conclusions

The present study demonstrates an insufficient fibre intake among the Spanish adult population, both in the whole sample and in the plausible reporters. The main dietary sources were grains, followed by vegetables, fruits, and pulses for both samples. This study observed an association between the fibre intake and excess body weight and abdominal obesity in the whole sample but not in the plausible reporters. Further studies are needed to confirm the association between the fibre intake and the excess body weight and/or abdominal obesity. Nonetheless, it is advisable to increase the intake of foods rich in fibre in order to prevent diseases related with a low intake.

Supplementary Materials: The following are available online at www.mdpi.com/1999-4907/9/04/325/s1, Table S1: Dietary food sources of total fibre (%) in the whole sample of the ANIBES study of the Spanish adult population (18–64 years) by body mass index., Table S2: Dietary food sources of total fibre (%) in the plausible reporters of the ANIBES study of the Spanish adult population (18–64 years) by body mass index, Table S3: Dietary food sources of total fibre (%) in the whole sample of the ANIBES Study Spanish adult population (18–64 years) by the presence or absence of abdominal obesity using the waist to height ratio, Table S4: Dietary food sources of total fibre (%) in the plausible reporters of the ANIBES Study Spanish adult population (18–64 years) by the presence or absence of abdominal obesity using the waist to height ratio, Table S5: Dietary food sources of total fibre (%) in the whole sample of the ANIBES study of the Spanish adult population (18–64 years) by the presence or absence of excess body weight and/or abdominal obesity using the body mass index and the waist to height ratio, Table S6: Dietary food sources of total fibre (%) in the plausible reporters of the ANIBES study of the Spanish adult population (18–64 years) by the presence or absence of excess body weight and/or abdominal obesity using the body mass index and the waist to height ratio.

Acknowledgments: The authors would like to thank Coca-Cola Iberia and IPSOS for its support and technical advice, particularly Rafael Urrialde and Javier Ruiz.

Author Contributions: L.G.G.-R., J.M.P.S and R.M.O. analysed the data. L.G.G.-R. also drafted and wrote the manuscript. J.M.P.S and R.M.O. contributed to the analysis and wrote the manuscript. J.A.-B., A.G., R.M.O., M.G.-G., and L.S.-M. are members of the Scientific Advisory Board of the ANIBES study and were responsible for careful review of the protocol, design, and methodology. These authors provided continuous scientific advice for the study and for the interpretation of results. These authors also critically reviewed the manuscript. G.V.-M., Principal Investigator of the ANIBES study, was responsible for the design, protocol, methodology, and follow-up checks of the study. All authors approved the final version of the manuscript.

Conflicts of Interest: The ANIBES study was financially supported by a grant from Coca Cola Iberia through an agreement with the Spanish Nutrition Foundation (FEN). The funding sponsors had no role in the design of the study, in the collection, analyses, or interpretation of the data; in the writing of the manuscript, and in the decision to publish the results. The authors declare no conflict of interest.

Abbreviations

ANIBES	Anthropometric data, macronutrients and micronutrients intake, practice of physical activity, socioeconomic data and lifestyles
BMI	Body Mass Index
EFSA	European Food Safety Authority
GLP-1	Glucagon-like peptide-1
IOM	Institute of Medicine of the United States

IPAQ	International Physical Activity Questionnaire
NHANES	National Health and Nutrition Examination Survey
NW	Normal weight
OB	Obesity
OW	Overweight
PA	Physical activity
UW	Underweight
WC	Waist circumference
WHtR	Waist to height ratio

1. Tucker, L.A.; Thomas, K.S. Increasing Total Fiber Intake Reduces Risk of Weight and Fat Gains in Women. *J. Nutr.* **2009**, *139*, 576–581. [CrossRef] [PubMed]
2. Buil-Cosiales, P.; Toledo, E.; Salas-Salvado, J.; Zazpe, I.; Farras, M.; Basterra-Gortari, F.J.; Diez-Espino, J.; Estruch, R.; Corella, D.; Ros, E.; et al. Association between Dietary Fibre Intake and Fruit, Vegetable Or Whole-Grain Consumption and the Risk of CVD: Results from the PREvencion Con DIeta MEDiterranea (PREDIMED) Trial. *Br. J. Nutr.* **2016**, *116*, 534–546. [CrossRef] [PubMed]
3. Lin, Y.; Huybrechts, I.; Vereecken, C.; Mouratidou, T.; Valtuena, J.; Kersting, M.; Gonzalez-Gross, M.; Bolca, S.; Warnberg, J.; Cuenca-Garcia, M.; et al. Dietary Fiber Intake and its Association with Indicators of Adiposity and Serum Biomarkers in European Adolescents: The HELENA Study. *Eur. J. Nutr.* **2015**, *54*, 771–782. [CrossRef] [PubMed]
4. Van de Vijver, L.P.; van den Bosch, L.M.; van den Brandt, P.A.; Goldbohm, R.A. Whole-Grain Consumption, Dietary Fibre Intake and Body Mass Index in the Netherlands Cohort Study. *Eur. J. Clin. Nutr.* **2009**, *63*, 31–38. [CrossRef] [PubMed]
5. King, D.E.; Mainous, A.G., 3rd; Lambourne, C.A. Trends in Dietary Fiber Intake in the United States, 1999–2008. *J. Acad. Nutr. Diet.* **2012**, *112*, 642–648. [CrossRef] [PubMed]
6. Hamedani, A.; Akhavan, T.; Samra, R.A.; Anderson, G.H. Reduced Energy Intake at Breakfast is Not Compensated for at Lunch if a High-Insoluble-Fiber Cereal Replaces a Low-Fiber Cereal. *Am. J. Clin. Nutr.* **2009**, *89*, 1343–1349. [CrossRef] [PubMed]
7. Serra-Majem, L.; Bautista-Castano, I. Relationship between Bread and Obesity. *Br. J. Nutr.* **2015**, *113*, S29–S35. [CrossRef] [PubMed]
8. Slavin, J.L. Dietary Fiber and Body Weight. *Nutrition* **2005**, *21*, 411–418. [CrossRef] [PubMed]
9. Guess, N.D.; Dornhorst, A.; Oliver, N.; Bell, J.D.; Thomas, E.L.; Frost, G.S. A Randomized Controlled Trial: The Effect of Inulin on Weight Management and Ectopic Fat in Subjects with Prediabetes. *Nutr. Metab. (Lond.)* **2015**, *12*, 36. [CrossRef] [PubMed]
10. Lupton, J.R. Sugar and Fiber Intake and Type of Adiposity: Are they Related? *Am. J. Clin. Nutr.* **2009**, *90*, 1119–1120. [CrossRef] [PubMed]
11. Barczynska, R.; Bandurska, K.; Slizewska, K.; Litwin, M.; Szalecki, M.; Libudzisz, Z.; Kapusniak, J. Intestinal Microbiota, Obesity and Prebiotics. *Pol. J. Microbiol.* **2015**, *64*, 93–100. [PubMed]
12. Sleeth, M.L.; Thompson, E.L.; Ford, H.E.; Zac-Varghese, S.E.; Frost, G. Free Fatty Acid Receptor 2 and Nutrient Sensing: A Proposed Role for Fibre, Fermentable Carbohydrates and Short-Chain Fatty Acids in Appetite Regulation. *Nutr. Res. Rev.* **2010**, *23*, 135–145. [CrossRef] [PubMed]
13. St-Pierre, D.H.; Rabasa-Lhoret, R.; Lavoie, M.E.; Karelis, A.D.; Strychar, I.; Doucet, E.; Coderre, L. Fiber Intake Predicts Ghrelin Levels in Overweight and Obese Postmenopausal Women. *Eur. J. Endocrinol.* **2009**, *161*, 65–72. [CrossRef] [PubMed]
14. Agencia Española de Seguridad Alimentaria y Nutrición (AESAN). Evaluación Nutricional De La Dieta Española. I Energía Y Macronutrientes. Sobre Datos De La Encuesta Nacional De Ingesta Dietética (ENIDE), 2011. Available online: http://www.Aesan.Msc.Es/AESAN/Docs/Docs/Notas_prensa/Presentacion_ENIDE.Pdf (accessed on 15 February 2016).
15. Moreno Franco, B.; Leon Latre, M.; Andres Esteban, E.M.; Ordovas, J.M.; Casasnovas, J.A.; Penalvo, J.L. Soluble and Insoluble Dietary Fibre Intake and Risk Factors for Metabolic Syndrome and Cardiovascular Disease in Middle-Aged Adults: The AWHS Cohort. *Nutr. Hosp.* **2014**, *30*, 1279–1288. [PubMed]
16. Ruiz, E.; Avila, J.M.; Castillo, A.; Valero, T.; del Pozo, S.; Rodriguez, P.; Bartrina, J.A.; Gil, A.; Gonzalez-Gross, M.; Ortega, R.M.; et al. The ANIBES Study on Energy Balance in Spain: Design, Protocol and Methodology. *Nutrients* **2015**, *7*, 970–998. [CrossRef] [PubMed]

17. Moreiras, G.V.; Avila, J.M.; Ruiz, E. Energy Balance, a New Paradigm and Methodological Issues: The ANIBES Study in Spain. *Nutr. Hosp.* **2015**, *31*, 101–112.
18. Marfell-Jones, M.; Olds, T.; Stewart, A.; Carter, L. *International Standards for Anthropometric Assessment*; International Society for the Advancement of Kinanthropometry: Potchefstroom, South Africa, 2006; pp. 1–137.
19. WHO. Obesity: Preventing and Managing the Global Epidemic. Report of a WHO Consultation. *World Health. Organ. Tech. Rep. Ser.* **2000**, *894*, 1–253.
20. Srinivasan, S.R.; Wang, R.; Chen, W.; Wei, C.Y.; Xu, J.; Berenson, G.S. Utility of Waist-to-Height Ratio in Detecting Central Obesity and Related Adverse Cardiovascular Risk Profile among Normal Weight Younger Adults (from the Bogalusa Heart Study). *Am. J. Cardiol.* **2009**, *104*, 721–724. [CrossRef] [PubMed]
21. Browning, L.M.; Hsieh, S.D.; Ashwell, M. A Systematic Review of Waist-to-Height Ratio as a Screening Tool for the Prediction of Cardiovascular Disease and Diabetes: 0.5 could be a Suitable Global Boundary Value. *Nutr. Res. Rev.* **2010**, *23*, 247–269. [CrossRef] [PubMed]
22. Ashwell, M.; Hsieh, S.D. Six Reasons Why the Waist-to-Height Ratio is a Rapid and Effective Global Indicator for Health Risks of Obesity and how its use could Simplify the International Public Health Message on Obesity. *Int. J. Food Sci. Nutr.* **2005**, *56*, 303–307. [CrossRef] [PubMed]
23. Schneider, H.J.; Friedrich, N.; Klotsche, J.; Pieper, L.; Nauck, M.; John, U.; Dorr, M.; Felix, S.; Lehnert, H.; Pittrow, D.; et al. The Predictive Value of Different Measures of Obesity for Incident Cardiovascular Events and Mortality. *J. Clin. Endocrinol. Metable* **2010**, *95*, 1777–1785. [CrossRef] [PubMed]
24. Craig, C.L.; Marshall, A.L.; Sjostrom, M.; Bauman, A.E.; Booth, M.L.; Ainsworth, B.E.; Pratt, M.; Ekelund, U.; Yngve, A.; Sallis, J.F.; et al. International Physical Activity Questionnaire: 12-Country Reliability and Validity. *Med. Sci. Sports Exerc.* **2003**, *35*, 1381–1395. [CrossRef] [PubMed]
25. Moreiras, O.; Carbajal, A.; Cabrera, L.; Cuadrado, C. *Tablas De Composición De Alimentos/Guía De Prácticas*, 16th ed.; Ediciones Pirámide: Madrid, Spain, 2013.
26. Hercberg, S.; Deheeger, M.; Preziosi, P. *Portions Alimentaires. Manuel Photos Pour L'estimation Des Quantités. SUVIMAX*; Polytechnica: Paris, France, 1994.
27. Willett, W.; Stampfer, M.J. Total Energy Intake: Implications for Epidemiologic Analyses. *Am. J. Epidemiol.* **1986**, *124*, 17–27. [CrossRef] [PubMed]
28. Willett, W.C.; Sampson, L.; Stampfer, M.J.; Rosner, B.; Bain, C.; Witschi, J.; Hennekens, C.H.; Speizer, F.E. Reproducibility and Validity of a Semiquantitative Food Frequency Questionnaire. *Am. J. Epidemiol.* **1985**, *122*, 51–65. [CrossRef] [PubMed]
29. EFSA Panel on Dietetic Products, Nutrition, and Allergies (NDA). Scientific Opinion on Dietary Reference Values for Carbohydrates and Dietary Fibre. *EFSA J.* **2010**, *8*, 1462.
30. Institute of Medicine. *Reference Intakes for Energy, Carbohydrate, Fiber, Fat, Fatty Acids, Cholesterol, Protein and Aminoacids*; The National Academies Press: Washington, DC, USA, 2005.
31. Krebs-Smith, S.M.; Kott, P.S.; Guenther, P.M. Mean Proportion and Population Proportion: Two Answers to the Same Question? *J. Am. Diet. Assoc.* **1989**, *89*, 671–676. [PubMed]
32. Rhee, J.J.; Sampson, L.; Cho, E.; Hughes, M.D.; Hu, F.B.; Willett, W.C. Comparison of Methods to Account for Implausible Reporting of Energy Intake in Epidemiologic Studies. *Am. J. Epidemiol.* **2015**, *181*, 225–233. [CrossRef] [PubMed]
33. Ambrus, Á.; Horváth, Z.; Farkas, Z.; Dorogházi, E.; Cseh, J.; Petrova, S.; Dimitrov, P.; Duleva, V.; Rangelova, L.; Chikova-Iscener, E. Pilot Study in the View of a Pan-European Dietary survey—Adolescents, Adults and Elderly. *EFSA Support. Publ.* **2013**, *EN-485*, 1–85.
34. European Food Safety Authority (EFSA). Example of a Protocol for Identification of Misreporting (Under- and Over-Reporting of Energy Intake) Based on the PILOT-PANEU Project. *EFSA J.* **2013**, *11*, 1–17. Available online: http://www.efsa.europa.eu/sites/default/files/efsa_rep/blobserver_assets/3944A-8-2-1.pdf (Accessed on 1 March 2017).
35. Goldberg, G.R.; Black, A.E.; Jebb, S.A.; Cole, T.J.; Murgatroyd, P.R.; Coward, W.A.; Prentice, A.M. Critical Evaluation of Energy Intake Data using Fundamental Principles of Energy Physiology: 1. Derivation of Cut-Off Limits to Identify Under-Recording. *Eur. J. Clin. Nutr.* **1991**, *45*, 569–581. [PubMed]
36. Black, A.E. Critical Evaluation of Energy Intake using the Goldberg Cut-Off for Energy Intake:Basal Metabolic Rate. A Practical Guide to its Calculation, use and Limitations. *Int. J. Obes. Relat. Metab. Disord.* **2000**, *24*, 1119–1130. [CrossRef] [PubMed]

37. Black, A.E. The Sensitivity and Specificity of the Goldberg Cut-Off for EI:BMR for Identifying Diet Reports of Poor Validity. *Eur. J. Clin. Nutr.* **2000**, *54*, 395–404. [CrossRef] [PubMed]
38. Schofield, W.N. Predicting Basal Metabolic Rate, New Standards and Review of Previous Work. *Hum. Nutr. Clin. Nutr.* **1985**, *39*, 5–41. [PubMed]
39. Olza, J.; Aranceta-Bartrina, J.; Gonzalez-Gross, M.; Ortega, R.M.; Serra-Majem, L.; Varela-Moreiras, G.; Gil, A. Reported Dietary Intake, Disparity between the Reported Consumption and the Level Needed for Adequacy and Food Sources of Calcium, Phosphorus, Magnesium and Vitamin D in the Spanish Population: Findings from the ANIBES Study Dagger. *Nutrients* **2017**. [CrossRef] [PubMed]
40. Aranceta-Bartrina, J.; Perez-Rodrigo, C.; Alberdi-Aresti, G.; Ramos-Carrera, N.; Lazaro-Masedo, S. Prevalence of General Obesity and Abdominal Obesity in the Spanish Adult Population (Aged 25–64 Years) 2014–2015: The ENPE Study. *Rev. Esp. Cardiol. (Engl. Ed.)* **2016**, *69*, 579–587. [CrossRef] [PubMed]
41. Ortega Anta, R.M.; Lopez-Solaber, A.M.; Perez-Farinos, N. Associated Factors of Obesity in Spanish Representative Samples. *Nutr. Hosp.* **2013**, *28*, 56–62. [PubMed]
42. Ashwell, M.; Gunn, P.; Gibson, S. Waist-to-Height Ratio is a Better Screening Tool than Waist Circumference and BMI for Adult Cardiometabolic Risk Factors: Systematic Review and Meta-Analysis. *Obes. Rev.* **2012**, *13*, 275–286. [CrossRef] [PubMed]
43. Navia, B.; Aparicio, A.; Perea, J.M.; Perez-Farinos, N.; Villar-Villalba, C.; Labrado, E.; Ortega, R.M. Sodium Intake may Promote Weight Gain; Results of the FANPE Study in a Representative Sample of the Adult Spanish Population. *Nutr. Hosp.* **2014**, *29*, 1283–1289. [PubMed]
44. Felix-Redondo, F.J.; Grau, M.; Baena-Diez, J.M.; Degano, I.R.; de Leon, A.C.; Guembe, M.J.; Alzamora, M.T.; Vega-Alonso, T.; Robles, N.R.; Ortiz, H.; et al. Prevalence of Obesity and Associated Cardiovascular Risk: The DARIOS Study. *BMC Public Health* **2013**, *13*, 542. [CrossRef] [PubMed]
45. Mielgo-Ayuso, J.; Aparicio-Ugarriza, R.; Castillo, A.; Ruiz, E.; Avila, J.M.; Aranceta-Batrina, J.; Gil, A.; Ortega, R.M.; Serra-Majem, L.; Varela-Moreiras, G.; et al. Physical Activity Patterns of the Spanish Population are mostly Determined by Sex and Age: Findings in the ANIBES Study. *PLoS ONE* **2016**, *11*, e0149969. [CrossRef] [PubMed]
46. Galvin, M.A.; Kiely, M.; Harrington, K.E.; Robson, P.J.; Moore, R.; Flynn, A. The North/South Ireland Food Consumption Survey: The Dietary Fibre Intake of Irish Adults. *Public Health Nutr.* **2001**, *4*, 1061–1068. [CrossRef] [PubMed]
47. Reicks, M.; Jonnalagadda, S.; Albertson, A.M.; Joshi, N. Total Dietary Fiber Intakes in the US Population are Related to Whole Grain Consumption: Results from the National Health and Nutrition Examination Survey 2009 to 2010. *Nutr. Res.* **2014**, *34*, 226–234. [CrossRef] [PubMed]
48. McGill, C.R.; Birkett, A.; Fulgonii Iii, V.L. Healthy Eating Index-2010 and Food Groups Consumed by US Adults Who Meet Or Exceed Fiber Intake Recommendations NHANES 2001–2010. *Food Nutr. Res.* **2016**, *60*, 29977. [CrossRef] [PubMed]
49. Lin, Y.; Huybrechts, I.; Vandevijvere, S.; Bolca, S.; De Keyzer, W.; De Vriese, S.; Polet, A.; De Neve, M.; Van Oyen, H.; Van Camp, J.; et al. Fibre Intake among the Belgian Population by Sex-Age and Sex-Education Groups and its Association with BMI and Waist Circumference. *Br. J. Nutr.* **2011**, *105*, 1692–1703. [CrossRef] [PubMed]
50. Grunert, K.G.; Wills, J.M.; Fernandez-Celemin, L. Nutrition Knowledge, and use and Understanding of Nutrition Information on Food Labels among Consumers in the UK. *Appetite* **2010**, *55*, 177–189. [CrossRef] [PubMed]
51. Kerver, J.M.; Yang, E.J.; Obayashi, S.; Bianchi, L.; Song, W.O. Meal and Snack Patterns are Associated with Dietary Intake of Energy and Nutrients in US Adults. *J. Am. Diet. Assoc.* **2006**, *106*, 46–53. [CrossRef] [PubMed]
52. McGill, C.R.; Fulgoni, V.L., 3rd; Devareddy, L. Ten-Year Trends in Fiber and Whole Grain Intakes and Food Sources for the United States Population: National Health and Nutrition Examination Survey 2001–2010. *Nutrients* **2015**, *7*, 1119–1130. [CrossRef] [PubMed]
53. Lopez-Sobaler, A.M.; Aparicio, A.; Aranceta-Bartrina, J.; Gil, A.; Gonzalez-Gross, M.; Serra-Majem, L.; Varela-Moreiras, G.; Ortega, R.M. Overweight and General and Abdominal Obesity in a Representative Sample of Spanish Adults: Findings from the ANIBES Study. *Biomed. Res. Int.* **2016**, *2016*, 8341487. [CrossRef] [PubMed]

54. Bes-Rastrollo, M.; Martinez-Gonzalez, M.A.; Sanchez-Villegas, A.; de la Fuente Arrillaga, C.; Martinez, J.A. Association of Fiber Intake and Fruit/Vegetable Consumption with Weight Gain in a Mediterranean Population. *Nutrition* **2006**, *22*, 504–511. [CrossRef] [PubMed]
55. Koh-Banerjee, P.; Franz, M.; Sampson, L.; Liu, S.; Jacobs, D.R., Jr.; Spiegelman, D.; Willett, W.; Rimm, E. Changes in Whole-Grain, Bran, and Cereal Fiber Consumption in Relation to 8-Y Weight Gain among Men. *Am. J. Clin. Nutr.* **2004**, *80*, 1237–1245. [PubMed]
56. Thompson, A.L.; Adair, L.; Gordon-Larsen, P.; Zhang, B.; Popkin, B. Environmental, Dietary, and Behavioral Factors Distinguish Chinese Adults with High Waist-to-Height Ratio with and without Inflammation. *J. Nutr.* **2015**, *145*, 1335–1344. [CrossRef] [PubMed]
57. Liu, S.; Willett, W.C.; Manson, J.E.; Hu, F.B.; Rosner, B.; Colditz, G. Relation between Changes in Intakes of Dietary Fiber and Grain Products and Changes in Weight and Development of Obesity among Middle-Aged Women. *Am. J. Clin. Nutr.* **2003**, *78*, 920–927. [PubMed]
58. Du, H.; van der, A.D.L.; Boshuizen, H.C.; Forouhi, N.G.; Wareham, N.J.; Halkjaer, J.; Tjonneland, A.; Overvad, K.; Jakobsen, M.U.; Boeing, H.; et al. Dietary Fiber and Subsequent Changes in Body Weight and Waist Circumference in European Men and Women. *Am. J. Clin. Nutr.* **2010**, *91*, 329–336. [CrossRef] [PubMed]
59. Hosseinpour-Niazi, S.; Mirmiran, P.; Mirzaei, S.; Azizi, F. Cereal, Fruit and Vegetable Fibre Intake and the Risk of the Metabolic Syndrome: A Prospective Study in the Tehran Lipid and Glucose Study. *J. Hum. Nutr. Diet.* **2015**, *28*, 236–245. [CrossRef] [PubMed]
60. McKeown, N.M.; Meigs, J.B.; Liu, S.; Saltzman, E.; Wilson, P.W.; Jacques, P.F. Carbohydrate Nutrition, Insulin Resistance, and the Prevalence of the Metabolic Syndrome in the Framingham Offspring Cohort. *Diabetes Care* **2004**, *27*, 538–546. [CrossRef] [PubMed]

nutrients

MDPI

Article

Effect of Consuming Oat Bran Mixed in Water before a Meal on Glycemic Responses in Healthy Humans—A Pilot Study

Robert E. Steinert [1,*], Daniel Raederstorff [1] and Thomas M. S. Wolever [2]

[1] DSM Nutritional Products Ltd., R & D Human Nutrition and Health, Basel 4057, Switzerland; daniel.raederstorff@dsm.com

[2] Glycemic Index Laboratories, Inc., Toronto, ON M5C 2N8, Canada; thomas.wolever@utoronto.ca

* Correspondence: robert.steinert@dsm.com

Received: 23 June 2016; Accepted: 19 August 2016; Published: 26 August 2016

Abstract: Background: Viscous dietary fibers including oat β-glucan are one of the most effective classes of functional food ingredients for reducing postprandial blood glucose. The mechanism of action is thought to be via an increase in viscosity of the stomach contents that delays gastric emptying and reduces mixing of food with digestive enzymes, which, in turn, retards glucose absorption. Previous studies suggest that taking viscous fibers separate from a meal may not be effective in reducing postprandial glycemia. Methods: We aimed to re-assess the effect of consuming a preload of a commercially available oat-bran (4.5, 13.6 or 27.3 g) containing 22% of high molecular weight oat β-glucan (O22 (OatWell®22)) mixed in water before a test-meal of white bread on glycemic responses in 10 healthy humans. Results: We found a significant effect of dose on blood glucose area under the curve (AUC) ($p = 0.006$) with AUC after 27.3 g of O22 being significantly lower than white bread only. Linear regression analysis showed that each gram of oat β-glucan reduced glucose AUC by 4.35% ± 1.20% ($r = 0.507$, $p = 0.0008$, $n = 40$) and peak rise by 6.57% ± 1.49% ($r = 0.582$, $p < 0.0001$). Conclusion: These data suggest the use of oat bran as nutritional preload strategy in the management of postprandial glycemia.

Keywords: postprandial glycemia; dietary fibre; blood glucose; type 2 diabetes mellitus; preload

1. Introduction

In current obesogenic societies with many people having mild or moderate hyperglycemia, postprandial blood glucose patterns account for the majority of variability of overall glycemic control [1,2]. This is not surprising considering that most individuals spend perhaps only about three to four hours before breakfast in a truly fasted state [1,3]. Dietary means to lower postprandial glycemic responses are, thus, urgently needed for the prevention of Type 2 Diabetes mellitus (T2DM). Viscous dietary fibers including high molecular weight (HMW) oat β-glucan are one of the most effective classes of functional food ingredients for reducing postprandial glucose [4]. The mechanism of action is thought to be their ability to increase the viscosity of the contents of the upper gastrointestinal (GI) tract and, hence, slow gastric emptying (GE) [5]. The rate of GE has a substantial impact on postprandial glycemia by determining glucose absorption and incretin hormone secretion [6,7]. In addition, an increase in viscosity of GI contents reduces the rate of digestion of starch by pancreatic amylase and the rate of absorption of glucose in the small intestine by increasing the thickness of the unstirred water layer [5].

Previous studies suggest that taking viscous fibers separate from a main meal may not be effective in reducing postprandial glycemia [8,9]. One potential solution to this problem may be to consume, before eating, a fiber "preload", which develops viscosity slowly, so that it can be consumed in a palatable form, and remains liquid in the stomach long enough to be able to mix effectively with the main meal, but becomes viscous by the time the stomach starts to empty the meal. OatWell®22 (O22) is a commercially available oat-bran including 44% dietary fiber and 22% HMW oat β-glucan, which forms a palatable drink when mixed with water and which becomes viscous after several minutes. Therefore, we evaluated the dose-response effect of O22 mixed in water and consumed before a white bread meal on glycemic responses in healthy humans.

2. Subjects and Methods

2.1. Subjects

Ten healthy normal-weight, overweight and obese subjects (5 male/5 female, mean age (years): 48.0 ± 15.3 (range 22–65), BMI (kg/m^2): 29.5 ± 4.4 (range 23.2–36.9)) were studied using an open-label, randomized block design. The study was performed according to accepted standards and the Declaration of Helsinki. Ethical approval was obtained from the Western Institutional Review Board, and the study was registered as a clinical trial with clinical trials.gov (registration number NCT02801916). Written informed consent was obtained from all participants.

2.2. Study Outline

Each subject underwent 4 treatments on separate days, with each subject performing up to 3 tests per week separated by at least one day. On each test day, subjects came to the laboratory in the morning after a 10–14 h overnight fast. Two fasting blood samples ($t = -5$ min and $t = 0$ min) were obtained by finger-prick. After the first fasting blood sample, subjects consumed a preload consisting of 200 mL water either alone or mixed with 4.5, 13.6 or 27.3 g of O22 containing 0.9, 2.6, and 5.3 g of oat β-glucan, respectively (DSM Nutritional Products, Table 1). After the second fasting blood sample ($t = 0$ min), subjects were asked to consume a test meal consisting of a portion (119 g) of white bread containing 50 g available carbohydrate (Table 1). The time taken to consume the bread was between 7 and 12 min. Further blood samples were obtained at 15, 30, 45, 60, 90 and 120 min after meal onset. Subjects remained seated quietly during the 2 h of the test. After the last blood sample was obtained, subjects were offered a snack and then permitted to leave.

Table 1. Nutrient content of test meal ingredients.

Test Meal	Energy (kcal)	Weight (g)	Protein (g)	Fat (g)	tCHO [1] (g)	Fibre (g)		avCHO [1] (g)
						Total	β-Glucan	
White Bread [1]	245	119	9.0	1.0	52.6	2.6	0	50.0
OatWell®22 [2]	13.1	4.5	1.0	0.2	3.0	2.2	0.9	0.8
	39.7	13.6	3.1	0.6	8.8	6.5	2.6	2.3
	79.7	27.3	6.2	1.1	17.7	13.1	5.3	4.6

[1] Baked at Glycemic Index Laboratories using an automatic bread maker; values represent the mean of 5 proximate analyses performed by Gelda Scientific, Mississauga, ON, Canada; [2] Nutritional analysis, including β-glucan content, was performed by SGS Institute Fresenius GmbH, Im Maisel, Taunusstein, Germany.

2.3. Measurements

After consuming the test meal, subjects rated the palatability of the test meal using a visual analogue scale consisting of a 100-mm line anchored at the left end by "very unpalatable" and at the right end by "very palatable". Subjects made a vertical mark along the line to indicate their perceived palatability. The distance from the left end of the line to the mark made by the subject is the palatability rating; the higher the value, the higher the perceived palatability.

Blood samples (2–3 drops each) were collected into 5 mL tubes containing ~500 μg sodium fluoride and 400 μg potassium oxalate. The samples were mixed and refrigerated immediately during the testing session. After completion of the test session, samples were stored at −20 °C prior to glucose analysis. Blood glucose analysis, using a YSI (Yellow Spring Instruments, Yellow Springs, OH, USA) analyzer, took place within five days of collection.

2.4. Data and Statistical Analysis

The primary endpoint was incremental area under the blood glucose curve (AUC) which was calculated using the trapezoid rule, ignoring area beneath the baseline. Baseline blood glucose was calculated as mean of values obtained at $t = -5$ min and $t = 0$ min. AUC and peak rise were analyzed using repeated-measures analysis of variance (RMANOVA) examining for the main effects of treatment dose. In case of significant heterogeneity, differences among different doses were tested using Tukey's test to adjust for multiple comparisons. AUC and peak rises for each dose of O22 were expressed relative to the AUC or peak rise after the test of white bread alone taken by the same subject. The glycemic response of 1 subject with a relative response after the 13.6 g dose of 2.55 × SD above the mean was considered to be an outlier and the data removed; the values were replaced using a procedure described by Snedecor and Cochran [10], and the error degrees of freedom in RMANOVA reduced by one. Blood glucose concentrations at each time were subjected to RMANOVA examining for the main effects of time and treatment and the time × treatment interaction; after demonstrating a highly significant time × treatment interaction ($p = 1.2 \times 10^{-17}$), blood glucose concentrations at each time were subjected to RMANOVA followed by Tukey's test, as described above for AUC. Differences were considered to be statistically significant if 2-tailed $p < 0.05$.

3. Results

There were significant differences in blood glucose concentration among doses at 15 ($p = 0.0015$), 30 ($p < 0.0001$), 45 ($p = 0.0003$) and 120 min ($p = 0.0004$). At 15 min, blood glucose concentration after 27.3 g was significantly lower than those after 0 g and 4.5 g. At 30 min, blood glucose after the 27.3 g dose was significantly lower than after 13.6 g, which, in turn, was significantly lower than the 0 and 4.5 g doses. At 45 min blood glucose concentration after 27.3 g of O22 was significantly lower than those after the 0, 4.5 and 13.6 g doses. At 120 min, blood glucose after 27.3 g of O22 was significantly higher than that after the 0 and 4.5 g doses (Figure 1A). There was a significant effect of dose on blood glucose AUC ($p = 0.006$) with AUC after 27.3 g of O22 (141 ± 21 mmol × min/L) being significantly lower than both the 4.5 g and 0 g doses (174 ± 1 7 and 185 ± 18 mmol × min/L, respectively) and the AUC after 13.6 g being intermediate (167 ± 19 mmol × min/L). When AUC was expressed relative to that of bread alone, the relative responses for the 4.5, 13.6 and 27.3 g doses of O22, respectively, were 95.0% ± 4.1%, 90.3% ± 4.7% and 76.3% ± 7.7% with the only significant reduction being seen with the highest dose. However, linear regression analysis showed that each gram of oat β-glucan reduced glucose AUC by 4.35% ± 1.20% ($r = 0.507$, $p = 0.0008$, $n = 40$; Figure 1B). There was also a significant effect of dose for blood glucose peak rise ($p < 0.0001$) with the peak rise after 27.3 g of O22, 1.96 ± 0.29 mmol/L, being significantly lower than that after all the other doses (3.07 ± 0.25, 2.83 ± 0.30 and 2.72 ± 0.30 g for the 0, 4.5 and 13.6 g doses of O22, respectively). When peak rise was expressed relative to that for bread alone, the relative responses for the 4.5, 13.6 and 27.3 g doses of O22, respectively, were 92.5% ± 6.8%, 88.5% ± 7.2% and 63.8% ± 7.1% with the only significant reduction being seen with the highest dose. However, linear regression analysis showed that each gram of oat β-glucan reduced glucose peak rise by 6.57% ± 1.49% ($r = 0.582$, $p < 0.0001$, $n = 40$; Figure 1C).

There was a significant main effect of dose on palatability, with all 3 doses of O22 rated as being less palatable than white bread alone (palatability in mm: 71 ± 7 for white bread alone; 38 ± 9 for 4.5 g O22; 33 ± 10 for 13.6 g O22; 31 ± 9 for 27.3 g O22; $p = 0.0003$). Although palatability tended to decrease as the dose increased, this difference was not significant. There was no significant relationship between palatability and glucose AUC (expressed as % of that after white bread) for 4.5 g ($r = 0.439$, $p = 0.20$, $n = 10$), 13.6 g ($r = 0.502$, $p = 0.14$, $n = 10$) or 27.3 g ($r = 0.398$, $p = 0.25$, $n = 10$) doses of O22.

No adverse effects were observed.

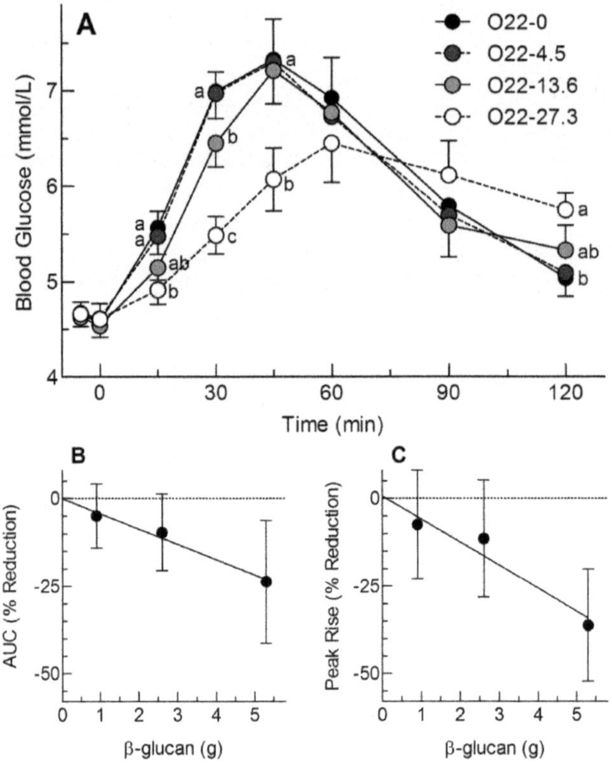

Figure 1. Panel (**A**): Blood glucose concentrations after taking 0, 4.5, 13.6 and 27.3 g, respectively, of OatWell®22 (O22-0, O22-4.5, O22-13.6 and O22-27.3) at −5 min followed by 50 g available carbohydrate from white bread at 0 min. Values are means ± SEM for $n = 10$ subjects. [a–c] Means at the same time containing different letters within the superscripts differ significantly by Tukey's test $p < 0.05$; (**B**,**C**): Percentage reduction from control in incremental areas under the curve (AUC); (**B**) and peak rise in blood glucose; (**C**) after taking 0, 4.5, 13.6 and 27.3 g of OatWell®22 (containing 0, 0.9, 2.6 and 5.3 g oat β-glucan, respectively) at −5 min followed by 50 g available carbohydrate from white bread at 0 min. Values are means ± 95% confidence interval for $n = 9$ or 10 subjects (after excluding outlying values).

4. Discussion

We demonstrated that consuming a commercially available oat-bran containing 22% of HMW oat β-glucan mixed in water before a white bread meal significantly lowers postprandial glycemia in a dose dependent manner with 27.3 g of O22 being significantly lower than white bread only. Linear regression analysis, in addition, showed that each gram of oat β-glucan reduced glucose AUC by ~4% and peak rise by ~7%. Given that the magnitude of this reduction would be similar in patients with T2DM, these data may have considerable implications for nutritional strategies in the management of diabetes, however, this concept warrants further investigation. The mechanism of action of oat beta-glucan to reduce postprandial glycemia is well established. In their native form, oat beta-glucan consists of very high molecular weight polysaccharides that exhibit high viscosities at low concentrations [11]. An increase in viscosity of a meal bolus in the stomach delays gastric emptying and reduces mixing of food with digestive enzymes. This retards absorption of glucose making oat β-glucan one of the most effective classes of functional food ingredients to reduce postprandial blood glucose and insulin responses [4,5].

Previous studies have suggested that taking viscous fibers, such as psyllium or guar gum, separate from a main meal may not be effective in reducing postprandial glycemia [12,13]. In contrast, the concept of a "preload" that refers to administration of a small load of nutrient at a fixed interval before a main meal to lower postprandial blood glucose via the slowing of GE has been confirmed several times [14–16]. While in the classical sense of the preload concept, the slowing of GE is related primarily to a nutrient-induced neuroendocrine feedback [14–16], the present findings suggest that the preload concept also applies to fibers such as oat beta-glucan that delay GE via increases in meal bolus viscosity. It requires consideration, however, that the oat bran also contained about 20% protein that may have contributed to the slowing of GE via neuroendocrine feedbacks. In addition, the protein may have lowered postprandial blood glucose independently of the preload effect because a reduction in postprandial blood glucose was observed also in studies with protein ingested simultaneously with carbohydrate-rich meals [17]. The discrepancy between the current results and those of previous investigations mentioned above suggests that proper control of method of administration of the preload such as timing (i.e., interval between preload administration and meal onset) and the physicochemical properties of the fiber at meal onset, as well as other macronutritional components, are important. Ideally the fiber preload remains liquid in the stomach long enough to be able to mix effectively with the meal, but becomes viscous by the time the stomach starts to empty the meal.

The present results are in line with the health claim that has previously been evaluated by the European Food Safety Authority (EFSA) and authorized by the European commission for β-glucans from oats and barley and reduction of postprandial glycemia [18]. The conditions of use state that in order to obtain the claimed effect, 4 g of beta-glucans for each 30 g of available carbohydrates should be consumed per meal. Our results further indicate that lower doses of HMW oat β-glucan may be sufficient to impact postprandial glycemia when consumed in a suitable manner (e.g., several smaller doses/day, correct timing/preload paradigm). This approach is in line with a recent systematic review by Tosh et al. [4], including 119 treatments from 34 publications that finds that the efficacy of oat and barley β-glucan in lowering postprandial blood glucose is more strongly related to β-glucan content alone than to the ratio of β-glucan/available carbohydrate. In addition, when authors actually calculated a ratio, 4 g of β-glucan per meal were found to be sufficient to reduce post-prandial blood glucose in a clinical relevant amount for meals with up to 80 g of available carbohydrate.

A limitation of this pilot trial that requires consideration is that it was not powered to detect small differences seen with the lower doses used here (i.e., 4.5 and 13.6 g). We only found a significant effect with 27.3 g of O22, however, the results show that the expected reduction in AUC and peak rise for the 13.6 g dose were 11.3% and 17.1%, respectively. Therefore, based on the results of this study, 27 subjects would be required to have 80% power to detect an 11.3% reduction in AUC and 14 subjects to detect a 17.1% reduction in peak rise. The additional energy intake associated with an oat bran preload should also be considered if using such a strategy over the long term, althoughsubjects usually tend to compensateat least in part, for extra energy by eating less at a subsequent ad libitum meal. There is good evidence for particularly viscous fibers to reduce appetite and eating. For example, a recent systematic review including 58 original studies by Wanders et al. [19] reports a reduction in appetite perception by 7.4% over a 4 h time interval when dietary fiber is added as part of a preload. Similarly, a recent meta-analysis including 6 human studies shows that polydextrose fiber as part of a mid-morning preload reduces energy intake at a subsequent ad libitum meal at lunch time by 12.5% [20]. Finally, there is evidence from epidemiological studies that show associations between high fiber intakes and weight loss [21,22].

In conclusion, consuming O22 mixed in water before a meal reduces glycemic response in a dose-dependent manner with each gram of oat β-glucan reducing glucose AUC by about 4%. This suggests the use of O22 as a nutritional preload strategy in the management of postprandial glycemia.

Author Contributions: Robert E. Steinert, Thomas M. S. Wolever and Daniel Raederstorff conceptualized the study. Thomas M. S. Wolever conducted the experiments and statistical analysis. Robert E. Steinert, Thomas M. S. Wolever and Daniel Raederstorff interpreted the data. Robert E. Steinert and Thomas M. S. Wolever drafted the manuscript. All authors reviewed and approved the manuscript.

Conflicts of Interest: The authors declare no conflict of interest. Robert E. Steinert and Daniel Raederstorff are employees of DSM Nutritional Products, Basel, Switzerland. Thomas M. S. Wolever is part owner, President and Medical Director of Glycemic Index Laboratories, Inc. (GI Labs) and his wife is also a part owner and Chief Financial Officer of GI Labs.

References

1. Monnier, L.; Lapinski, H.; Colette, C. Contributions of fasting and postprandial plasma glucose increments to the overall diurnal hyperglycemia of type 2 diabetic patients: Variations with increasing levels of HbA(1c). *Diabetes Care* **2003**, *26*, 881–885. [CrossRef] [PubMed]
2. Peter, R.; Dunseath, G.; Luzio, S.D.; Owens, D.R. Estimates of the relative and absolute diurnal contributions of fasting and post-prandial plasma glucose over a range of hyperglycaemia in type 2 diabetes. *Diabetes Metab.* **2013**, *39*, 337–342. [CrossRef] [PubMed]
3. Monnier, L.; Colette, C.; Owens, D. Postprandial and basal glucose in type 2 diabetes: Assessment and respective impacts. *Diabetes Technol. Ther.* **2011**, *13*, S25–S32. [CrossRef] [PubMed]
4. Tosh, S.M. Review of human studies investigating the post-prandial blood-glucose lowering ability of oat and barley food products. *Eur. J. Clin. Nutr.* **2013**, *67*, 310–317. [CrossRef] [PubMed]
5. Würsch, P.; Pi-Sunyer, F.X. The role of viscous soluble fiber in the metabolic control of diabetes: A review with special emphasis on cereals rich in beta-glucan. *Diabetes Care* **1997**, *20*, 1774–1780. [CrossRef] [PubMed]
6. Horowitz, M.; Edelbroek, M.A.; Wishart, J.M.; Straathof, J.W. Relationship between oral glucose tolerance and gastric emptying in normal healthy subjects. *Diabetologia* **1993**, *36*, 857–862. [CrossRef] [PubMed]
7. Marathe, C.S.; Rayner, C.K.; Jones, K.L.; Horowitz, M. Relationships between gastric emptying, postprandial glycemia, and incretin hormones. *Diabetes Care* **2013**, *36*, 1396–1405. [CrossRef] [PubMed]
8. Fuessl, S.; Adrian, T.E.; Bacarese-Hamilton, A.J.; Bloom, S.R. Guar in NIDD: Effect of different modes of administration on plasma glucose and insulin responses to a starch meal. *Pract. Diabetes Int.* **1986**, *3*, 258–260. [CrossRef]
9. Jenkins, D.J.; Nineham, R.; Craddock, C.; Craig-McFeely, P.; Donaldson, K.; Leigh, T.; Snook, J. Fibre in diabetes. *Lancet* **1979**, *1*, 434–435. [CrossRef]
10. Snedecor, G.W.; Cochran, W.G. *Statistical Methods*, 7th ed.; Iowa State University Press: Ames, IA, USA, 1980.
11. Ren, Y.; Ellis, P.R.; Sutherland, I.W.; Ross-Murphy, S.B. Dilute and semi-dilute solution properties of an exopolysaccharide from *Escherichia coli* strain S61. *Carbohydr. Polym.* **2003**, *52*, 189–195. [CrossRef]
12. Wolever, T.M.; Vuksan, V.; Eshuis, H.; Spadafora, P.; Peterson, R.D.; Chao, E.S.; Storey, M.L.; Jenkins, D.J. Effect of method of administration of psyllium on glycemic response and carbohydrate digestibility. *J. Am. Coll. Nutr.* **1991**, *10*, 364–371. [CrossRef] [PubMed]
13. Cohen, M.; Leong, V.W.; Salmon, E.; Martin, F.I. Role of guar and dietary fibre in the management of diabetes mellitus. *Med. J. Aust.* **1980**, *1*, 59–61. [PubMed]
14. Gentilcore, D.; Chaikomin, R.; Jones, K.L.; Russo, A.; Feinle-Bisset, C.; Wishart, J.M.; Rayner, C.K.; Horowitz, M. Effects of fat on gastric emptying of and the glycemic, insulin, and incretin responses to a carbohydrate meal in type 2 diabetes. *J. Clin. Endocrinol. Metab.* **2006**, *91*, 2062–2067. [CrossRef] [PubMed]
15. Ma, J.; Stevens, J.E.; Cukier, K.; Maddox, A.F.; Wishart, J.M.; Jones, K.L.; Clifton, P.M.; Horowitz, M.; Rayner, C.K. Effects of a protein preload on gastric emptying, glycemia, and gut hormones after a carbohydrate meal in diet-controlled type 2 diabetes. *Diabetes Care* **2009**, *32*, 1600–1602. [CrossRef] [PubMed]
16. Ma, J.; Jesudason, D.R.; Stevens, J.E.; Keogh, J.B.; Jones, K.L.; Clifton, P.M.; Horowitz, M.; Rayner, C.K. Sustained effects of a protein "preload" on glycaemia and gastric emptying over 4 weeks in patients with type 2 diabetes: A randomized clinical trial. *Diabetes Res. Clin. Pract.* **2015**, *108*, e31–e34. [CrossRef] [PubMed]
17. Lan-Pidhainy, X.; Wolever, T.M.S. The hypoglycemic effect of fat and protein is not attenuated by insulin resistance. *Am. J. Clin. Nutr.* **2010**, *91*, 98–105. [CrossRef] [PubMed]

18. Panel on Dietetic Products, Nutrition and Allergies (NDA). Scientific Opinion on the substantiation of health claims related to beta-glucans from oats and barley and maintenance of normal blood LDL-cholesterol concentrations (ID 1236, 1299), increase in satiety leading to a reduction in energy intake (ID 851, 852), reduction of post-prandial glycaemic responses (ID 821, 824), and "digestive function" (ID 850) pursuant to Article 13(1) of Regulation (EC) No 1924/2006. *EFSA J.* **2011**, *9*. [CrossRef]
19. Wanders, A.J.; van den Borne, J.J.G.C.; de Graaf, C.; Hulshof, T.; Jonathan, M.C.; Kristensen, M.; Mars, M.; Schols, H.A.; Feskens, E.J.M. Effects of dietary fibre on subjective appetite, energy intake and body weight: A systematic review of randomized controlled trials. *Obes. Rev. Off. J. Int. Assoc. Study Obes.* **2011**, *12*, 724–739. [CrossRef] [PubMed]
20. Ibarra, A.; Astbury, N.M.; Olli, K.; Alhoniemi, E.; Tiihonen, K. Effect of polydextrose on subjective feelings of appetite during the satiation and satiety periods: A systematic review and meta-analysis. *Nutrients* **2016**, *8*. [CrossRef] [PubMed]
21. Howarth, N.C.; Saltzman, E.; Roberts, S.B. Dietary fiber and weight regulation. *Nutr. Rev.* **2001**, *59*, 129–139. [CrossRef] [PubMed]
22. Alfieri, M.A.; Pomerleau, J.; Grace, D.M.; Anderson, L. Fiber intake of normal weight, moderately obese and severely obese subjects. *Obes. Res.* **1995**, *3*, 541–547. [CrossRef] [PubMed]

nutrients

MDPI

Article

Effect on Insulin, Glucose and Lipids in Overweight/Obese Australian Adults of 12 Months Consumption of Two Different Fibre Supplements in a Randomised Trial

Sebely Pal [1,*], Suleen Ho [1], Roland J. Gahler [2] and Simon Wood [3]

[1] School of Public Health, Curtin University, Perth 6845, Australia; suleen.ho@curtin.edu.au
[2] Factors Group Research, Burnaby, BC V3N 4S9, Canada; rgahler@naturalfactors.com
[3] Food, Nutrition and Health Program, University of British Columbia, Vancouver, BC V6T 1Z4, Canada; simonwood@shaw.ca
[*] Correspondence: s.pal@curtin.edu.au; Tel.: +61-8-9266-4755

Received: 30 September 2016; Accepted: 16 January 2017; Published: 29 January 2017

Abstract: Higher fibre intakes are associated with risk reduction for chronic diseases. This study investigated the effects of supplementation with PolyGlycopleX® (PGX), a complexed polysaccharide, on insulin, glucose and lipids in overweight and obese individuals. In this double-blind 12 months study, participants were randomised into three groups: control (rice flour); PGX or psyllium (PSY). Participants followed their usual lifestyle and diet but consumed 5 g of their supplement before meals. Insulin was significantly lower in the PGX and PSY groups compared to control at 3 and 6 months and in the PSY group compared to control at 12 months. Serum glucose was significantly lower in the PGX group at 3 months compared to control. Total cholesterol was significantly lower in the PGX and PSY groups compared to control at 3 and 6 months. High density lipoprotein (HDL) cholesterol was significantly increased in the PGX group compared to control at 12 months. low density lipoprotein (LDL) cholesterol was significantly lower in the PGX group at 3 and 6 months compared to control and in the PSY group at 3 months compared to control. A simple strategy of fibre supplementation may offer an effective solution to glucose, insulin and lipid management without the need for other nutrient modification.

Keywords: obesity; PGX; psyllium; cholesterol; insulin

1. Introduction

Previous studies have consistently shown that higher fibre intakes are correlated with lower body weight, body mass index (BMI), waist circumference [1,2] and improved plasma lipid profiles [3–12], glycaemia and insulinaemia [13], indicating benefits and risk reduction for metabolic syndrome, cardiovascular disease (CVD) and type 2 diabetes.

While the benefits of a high fibre diet are well known, increasing fruit and vegetable intake to meet the recommended intake of fibre is difficult for many [14]. Present estimations of dietary fibre intake in Australian, Canadian, European and American adults is approximately 15–25 g/day [3,15], which is below the current recommendations for adults in Australia, Canada, Europe and the USA of 25–30 g/day [16]. Therefore, fibre supplements can provide a cost effective and easy alternative method for increasing the fibre content of a diet without the need for other major nutrient modifications.

PolyGlycopleX (PGX) has been shown to have lipid lowering effects in healthy subjects [17] as well as in overweight and obese adults [18]. In a clinical trial with healthy subjects, 25 males and 29 females, mean age of 31.6 ± 10.5 years entered the study [17] and consumed 2.5 g of PGX twice a day as part of two main meals (breakfast and/or lunch, and/or dinner) for the first seven days, followed by 5 g PGX for the last 14 days of the study. The control product was a skimmed milk powder. PGX's effects on decreasing total and low density lipoprotein (LDL) cholesterol levels in the study concur with similar reports in the literature [19]. Studies are required to investigate if these benefits are sustainable over a longer duration and also in those who are overweight/obese. Another study with 29 overweight and obese adults, ages 20–65 with a BMI between 25–36 kg/m^2, consuming 5 g of PGX in 500 mL of water 5–10 min before each meal, 2–3 times a day for 14 days showed a significant reduction of total cholesterol (TC) and LDL levels of 19% and 25% respectively, compared to baseline [18]. However, the supplement was combined with advice for healthy eating, weight loss and exercise so it is difficult to evaluate the effect of the fibre alone on lipids. This was not a randomised controlled trial as there was no control group in this study. Recent human studies have shown that the addition of 2.5 to 5 g of PGX with a meal is highly effective in reducing postprandial glycaemia, lowering the glycaemic index of food [20] and modifying satiety hormones in healthy adults [21]. However, these studies have some limitations; they were acute or short term, mostly conducted in healthy, normal weight participants or combined with lifestyle changes.

Psyllium has been evaluated in various human studies for effects on glucose and insulin homeostasis, body weight, body composition and appetite as well as lipids and lipoproteins [22–30]. Psyllium was reviewed in 2012 for its effect on metabolic syndrome [31]. The authors concluded that "Collectively, research to date does support the notion that the consumption of psyllium may provide benefits to many components of the metabolic syndrome". Psyllium fibre decreased fat absorption in overweight and obese men, but had no effect on postprandial glucose and insulin concentrations [32]. In another study, simply adding a psyllium fibre supplement to a normal diet (10.2 g/day) was sufficient to see improvements in TC and LDL cholesterol but not fasting glucose or insulin concentrations when compared to the control group [22]. However, a meta-analysis [33] found that in type 2 diabetes patients, psyllium fibre significantly improved fasting blood glucose, proportional to loss of glycaemic control.

Apart from these few studies, limited research is available on the effect of PGX fibre on blood insulin, glucose and lipids. Randomised controlled clinical trials are required to verify whether PGX can be used for improving insulin, glucose and lipids in the long term and whether this fibre type is better than other soluble fibres, such as psyllium. Therefore the aim of this study was to investigate the effect of PGX on insulin, glucose and lipid concentrations. Given the effect of PGX on total and LDL cholesterol in healthy weight participants and its considerably higher viscosity, we hypothesise that PGX will have a greater health outcome than psyllium in overweight and obese individuals.

2. Materials and Methods

2.1. Subjects

Overweight and obese individuals with a body mass index (BMI) between 25–47 kg/m^2 and aged between 19 and 68 years, were recruited from the community in Perth, Australia (via newspaper and radio). Potential participants were screened by telephone or online questionnaire and attended Curtin University to assess suitability for the study, at which time the details of the study were explained. Exclusion criteria included smoking, lipid lowering medication, use of steroids and other agents that may influence lipid metabolism, use of warfarin, diabetes mellitus, hypo- and hyperthyroidism, cardiovascular events within the last 6 months, psychological unsuitability, major systemic diseases, gastrointestinal problems, proteinuria, liver, renal failure, weight fluctuations over the past 6 months, vegetarianism and participation in any other clinical trials within the last 6 months. This study was approved by and conducted in accordance with the ethical standards of Curtin Human Research Ethics Committee. Written consent was obtained from all participants. ANZCTR number: ACTRN12611000415909.

2.2. Study Design

This study is part of a larger trial, which was a randomised, double blind, parallel design study over a 52 week period. Study participants were randomised by the trial sponsors using a Web site (http://www.randomization.com) to one of the three groups (three randomly permuted blocks): the control group who consumed the placebo with their usual diet; the psyllium supplement group (PSY) who consumed a psyllium supplement with their usual diet and a PGX supplement group (PGX) who consumed a PGX supplement with their usual diet. Psyllium is a soluble fibre and PolyGlycopleX (PGX) is a novel, highly viscous functional non-starch polysaccharide complex, with developing viscosity, manufactured from konjac (glucomannan), sodium alginate and xanthan gum by a proprietary process (EnviroSimplex®). The fibre supplementation consisted of either 5 g of psyllium (a proprietary psyllium product with the trade name PgxSyl™) (InovoBiologic, Inc., Calgary, AB, Canada) or 5 g of PGX (InovoBiologic, Inc., Calgary, AB, Canada). Placebo consisted of 5 g rice flour. All supplements were artificially sweetened and flavoured. The rice flour provided an appropriate placebo due to its low energy and fibre content and similarity in texture and appearance to the psyllium and PGX supplement. Participants were instructed to take either 5 g of the fibre supplements or placebo, mixed with a minimum of 250 mL water followed by a further 250 mL water, three times daily, 5–10 min before breakfast, lunch and dinner. Extra water was allowed to be taken *ad libitum* during or after the meal if desired and subjects were encouraged to do this. The supplement packages (control, PGX and psyllium) were from a single batch provided by the manufacturer, and appeared identical so that the research assistants and participants were blinded to the type of supplement being consumed. Packages consisted of 5 g doses of the control, PGX or psyllium and were only marked by the participant ID, with the group allocation only known to the trial sponsors to ensure blinding. Quantities of rice flour and psyllium were determined by input, with the amounts weighed and checked by the dispensing and blending department while PGX was analysed according to USP Monograph FCC9 3rd Sup 2015 [34]. All identifiable information from participants was coded to ensure privacy.

The subjects attended a briefing session on how to consume the supplement, complete food records and comply with the study protocol as previously reported [35]. Briefly, the dietary intake over the course of the trial was monitored through the completion of 3-day food diaries at baseline, 12, 26 and 52 weeks. All participants in the control and the fibre supplement groups were asked to maintain their usual dietary intake for the duration of the study. To monitor compliance, all participants were required to complete a diary to record their supplement consumption and asked to return both the empty and unused sachets of the supplements at their visits.

2.3. Anthropometry and Body Composition

Measures of body weight, height, waist and hip circumference were undertaken at baseline, 3, 6 and 12 months. Body weight (HBF-514, Omron, Kyoto, Japan) was recorded in light clothing without shoes. Height was measured to the nearest 0.1 cm using a stadiometer without shoes. Waist circumference was measured in the standing position at the narrowest area between the lateral lower rib and the iliac crest. Hip measurement was taken at the largest circumference of the lower abdomen.

2.4. Diet and Physical Activity

Participants completed 3-day food and drink diaries at baseline, 3, 6 and 12 months to monitor for changes in food intake. Data were analysed with Foodworks 7 Professional (Xyris Software, Brisbane, Australia), based on data from the AUSNUT database. Participants also completed the International Physical Activity Questionnaire (IPAQ) at the same time points.

2.5. Measurements of Lipids, Glucose and Insulin Levels

Participants attended clinical rooms at Curtin University Bentley, after a 10–12 h fast, for baseline measurements. Fasting blood samples (20 mL) were drawn by venipuncture. The collection of fasting blood samples was repeated at 3, 6 and 12 months. Serum tubes were allowed to clot and blood samples were centrifuged at 2500 rpm at 4 °C for 10 min using a Hettich Rottina 48R centrifuge. Serum and plasma were then aliquoted and samples stored at −80 °C and analysed after study completion.

Serum triglyceride and total cholesterol was measured by enzymatic colorimetric kits (TRACE Scientific Ltd., Melbourne, Australia). Serum HDL cholesterol was determined after precipitation of apoB (apolipoprotein B)-containing lipoproteins with phosphotungstic acid and $MgCl_2$ (magnesium chloride); the supernatant containing the HDL cholesterol was determined by enzymatic colorimetry (TRACE Scientific Ltd., Melbourne, Australia). Serum LDL cholesterol was determined by using the Friedewald equation [36]. Non-esterified fatty acid (NEFA) was determined using WAKO NEFA C kit (Osaka, Japan). ApoB was analysed using an ELISA kit obtained from Mabtech AB (Nacka Strand, Stockholm, Sweden).

Plasma glucose concentrations were measured using the Randox glucose GOD-PAP kit (Antrim, UK), according to the manufacturer's instructions. Plasma insulin was measured by an ELISA kit (Alpha Diagnostics International, San Antonio, TX, USA). HOMA2-IR (homeostasis model assessment of insulin resistance) was used to assess insulin resistance from fasting glucose and insulin concentrations using a computer model [37].

2.6. Statistical Analysis

A sample size of 24 subjects per group was predicted to provide sufficient power (80%) to detect a 3% difference in weight before and after treatment within a group. We recruited a total of 53 subjects per group to accommodate for 50% dropouts. Calculations were based on an average mean weight of 80 kg and a standard deviation of 5% within a group on all eligible subjects. Statistical analysis was undertaken using SPSS 22 for Windows (SPSS Inc., Chicago, IL, USA). Data were expressed as mean (±SD or SEM) and assessed for normality to ensure that the assumptions of the analysis were met. Baseline differences between groups were analysed with one-way ANOVA. The data were analysed using general linear models with baseline value covariates. If significant between–groups effects were present, post hoc comparisons between the treatment groups was made using the least significant difference (LSD) method. Statistical significance was considered at $p < 0.05$. Intention–to–treat analysis was also carried out with missing data replaced with the last observation carried forward.

3. Results

3.1. Participants

The 159 participants (19 to 68 years) who met the eligibility criteria were randomised to one of three groups (Control, PSY, PGX) by assignment of an ID number and the corresponding numbered supplement. Participant flow through the study can be seen in Figure 1. Although the PGX group had the highest attrition rate, it was generally due to factors unrelated to the study. A total of 127 participants (54 male, 73 female) completed at least 3 months of the study and were included in the analysis (45 in Control (24 male), 43 in PSY (15 male) and 39 in PGX (15 male)). Thirty-two participants withdrew before 3 months and were excluded from analysis due to non-compliance, unrelated health issues, minor adverse effects and personal reasons. A total of 108 participants at 6 months (38 in Control, 39 in PSY and 31 in PGX) and 93 participants at 12 months (32 in Control, 36 in PSY and 25 in PGX) were analysed. Results for intention–to–treat analysis for the primary outcome variables can be found in supplementary files.

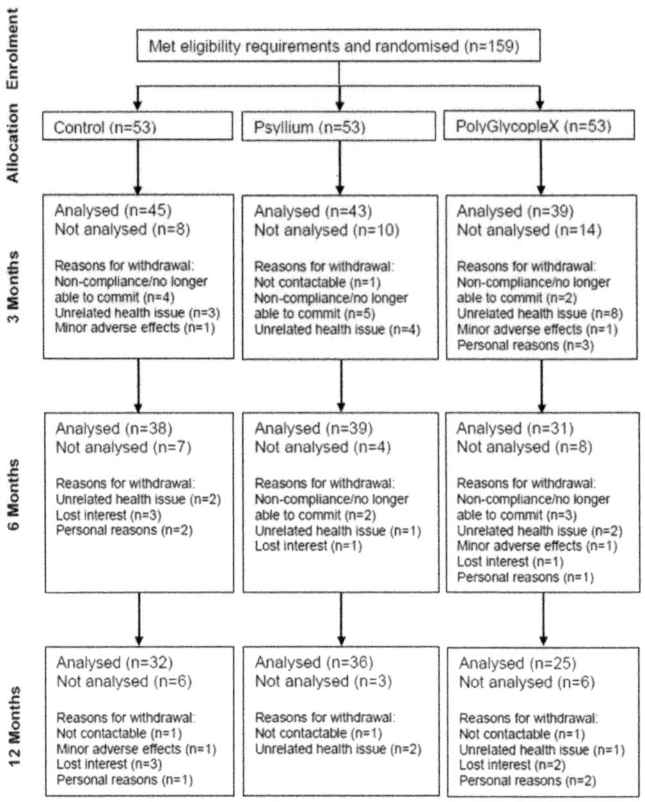

Figure 1. Participant flow diagram.

3.2. Baseline Characteristics

There were no significant differences at baseline between groups for major characteristics, energy intake, fibre intake, lipids, insulin or glucose (Table 1).

Table 1. Baseline characteristics.

	Control (n = 45)	PSY (n = 43)	PGX (n = 39)	p
Gender (Male/Female)	24/21	15/28	15/24	
Age (year)	49.82 ± 11.75	49.93 ± 11.04	47.87 ± 12.08	
Height (cm)	171.68 ± 10.04	169.16 ± 10.52	169.76 ± 10.51	
Weight (kg)	94.69 ± 17.05	91.17 ± 14.74	96.24 ± 18.02	0.365
BMI (kg/m^2)	32.01 ± 4.2	31.74 ± 3.22	33.25 ± 4.3	0.189
Waist (cm)	103.12 ± 11.02	101.17 ± 9.76	105.97 ± 12.72	0.154
Hip (cm)	112.87 ± 9.04	114.63 ± 8.63	115.71 ± 9.37	0.414
Waist Hip Ratio	0.91 ± 0.08	0.88 ± 0.08	0.92 ± 0.1	0.158
TC (mmol/L)	5 ± 0.85	4.93 ± 1.06	5.02 ± 0.85	0.904
HDL (mmol/L)	1.33 ± 0.37	1.36 ± 0.38	1.28 ± 0.26	0.563
LDL (mmol/L)	3.02 ± 0.87	3.04 ± 0.96	3.2 ± 0.77	0.592
TG (mmol/L)	1.44 ± 1.12	1.18 ± 0.67	1.2 ± 0.56	0.269
Insulin (μIU/mL)	6.11 ± 1.43	5.87 ± 1.64	6.56 ± 1.94	0.172
Glucose (mmol/L)	4.94 ± 0.73	4.79 ± 0.52	4.99 ± 0.56	0.302

Values are mean ± SD. PSY (Psyllium), PGX (PolyGlycopleX), TC (Total Cholesterol), TG (Triglyceride). p values are differences between groups.

3.3. *Diet*

The dietary analysis can be seen in Table 2. When examining differences between groups, energy intake was significantly lower compared to control at 3 months and 6 months in the PGX and PSY groups and at 12 months only the PGX group demonstrated significantly lower energy intake compared to the control. Carbohydrate intake was significantly lower at 3 months and 6 months in the PGX and PSY groups compared to control. Fat intake and protein intake were significantly lower compared to control at 3 months in the PGX and PSY groups and at 6 months in the PGX group compared to control.

Table 2. Dietary intake during 12 months of fibre supplementation.

Variable		3 Months	*n*	*P*	6 Months	*n*	*P*	12 Months	*n*	*p*
Energy (kJ/day)	CTR	9013.1 ± 223.6^{a}	39	0.641	8803.3 ± 282.9^{a}	34	0.928	8218 ± 295.4^{a}	31	0.111
	PSY	7272.3 ± 218^{b}	41	<0.001	7539.2 ± 278.8^{b}	35	<0.001	$7657.1 \pm 277.9^{a,b}$	35	0.001
	PGX	7556.3 ± 243.1^{b}	33	0.001	7453.7 ± 323.5^{b}	26	0.009	7315.3 ± 342.4^{b}	23	0.012
CHO (g/day)	CTR	212.6 ± 7.7^{a}	39	0.827	213.4 ± 10^{a}	34	0.787	200.5 ± 8.4	31	0.212
	PSY	181 ± 7.5^{b}	41	0.002	164.7 ± 9.8^{b}	35	0.002	183.9 ± 7.9	35	0.015
	PGX	175.3 ± 8.4^{b}	33	0.003	177.2 ± 11.4^{b}	26	0.032	176.3 ± 9.7	23	0.012
Fat (g/day)	CTR	83.8 ± 3.2^{a}	39	0.907	82.3 ± 4.3^{a}	34	0.887	73 ± 4	31	0.066
	PSY	66.9 ± 3.1^{b}	41	<0.001	$72.9 \pm 4.2^{a,b}$	35	0.147	73 ± 3.8	35	0.070
	PGX	72.2 ± 3.4^{b}	33	0.055	69.1 ± 4.9^{b}	26	0.047	66 ± 4.7	23	0.020
Total Fibre (g/day)	CTR	24.2 ± 1.2^{a}	39	0.599	22.1 ± 1^{a}	34	0.790	21.6 ± 1.3^{a}	31	0.613
	PSY	36.4 ± 1.2^{b}	41	<0.001	35.1 ± 0.9^{b}	35	<0.001	36.6 ± 1.3^{b}	35	<0.001
	PGX	36.6 ± 1.3^{b}	33	<0.001	34.1 ± 1.1^{b}	26	<0.001	36.1 ± 1.6^{b}	23	<0.001

Values are mean ± SEM with baseline as a covariate. Different letters in superscript represent significant differences between groups $p < 0.05$. *p* Values are within group differences compared to baseline. CHO (carbohydrate), CTR (control), PGX (PolyGlycopleX), PSY (psyllium).

3.4. *Physical Activity*

Physical activity levels did not significantly change from baseline within any groups and there were no significant differences between groups at any time point (Table 3).

Table 3. Physical activity during 12 months of fibre supplementation.

	3 Months	Mean Change	*n*	*P*	6 Months	Mean Change	*n*	*P*	12 Months	Mean Change	*n*	*p*
CTR	2802.4 ± 449.3	−130.5	29	0.837	2868.2 ± 454.7	−141.2	32	0.823	3294.5 ± 525.6	415.4	30	0.569
PSY	2933 ± 443.6	620.8	30	0.345	3009.3 ± 433.2	187	35	0.876	2879.1 ± 497.8	609.6	33	0.526
PGX	2181.7 ± 470.6	751.3	27	0.254	2681.1 ± 495.5	328.2	27	0.711	2684.9 ± 619.1	194.3	22	0.886

Values are mean kJ/day ± SEM with baseline as a covariate. Mean change from baseline. *p* Values are within group differences compared to baseline.

3.5. *Lipids*

Total cholesterol was significantly lower in the PGX group at 3 months (−8%, $p < 0.001$) and 6 months (−5.1%, $p = 0.048$) compared to baseline, as shown in Figure 2A. Total cholesterol was significantly lower in the PSY group at 3 months (−6.5%, $p < 0.001$) and 6 months (−4.8%, $p = 0.006$) compared to baseline. Total cholesterol was significantly lower at 3 months in the PGX (−8.2%, $p < 0.001$) and PSY (−7%, $p = 0.001$) groups and at 6 months in the PGX (−5.5%, $p = 0.047$) and PSY (−5.3%, $p = 0.042$) groups compared to control. There were no significant differences in total cholesterol between PSY and PGX groups at 3, 6 or 12 months.

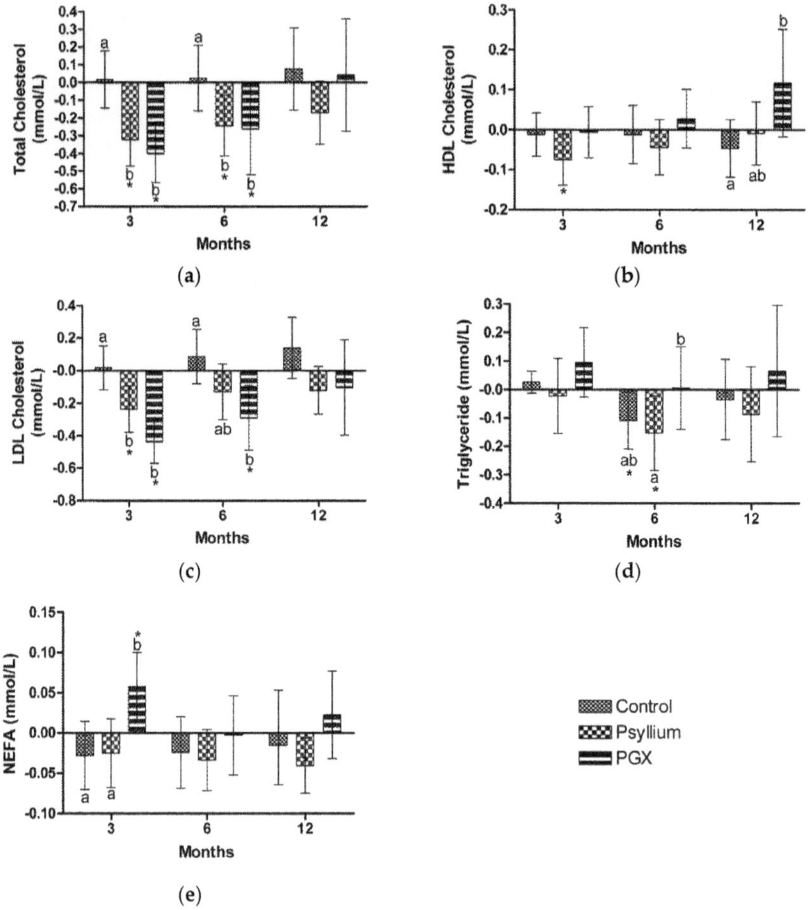

Figure 2. Changes in fasting blood lipids during 12 months of fibre supplementation (**a**) Total Cholesterol; (**b**) high density lipoprotein (HDL); (**c**) low density lipoprotein (LDL); (**d**) Triglyceride; (**e**) NEFA (non-esterified fatty acid). Values are mean ± 95% CI with baseline as a covariate. * indicates within group differences compared to baseline. Different letters represent significant differences between groups $p < 0.05$.

High density lipoprotein (HDL) cholesterol was significantly lower in the PSY group at 3 months (−5.5%, $p = 0.022$) compared to baseline, as shown in Figure 2B. HDL was significantly higher at 12 months in the PGX group (11.5%, $p = 0.019$) compared to control. There were no significant differences in HDL between control and PSY or between PSY and PGX groups at 3, 6 or 12 months.

LDL was significantly lower in the PGX group at 3 months (−13.7%, $p < 0.001$) and 6 months (−9.1%, $p = 0.006$) compared to baseline, shown in Figure 2C. LDL cholesterol was significantly lower in the PSY group at 3 months (−7.8%, $p = 0.002$) compared to baseline. LDL was significantly lower compared to control at 3 months in the PGX (−13.9%, $p < 0.001$) and PSY (−8.1%, $p = 0.007$) groups and at 6 months in the PGX (−11%, $p = 0.006$) group compared to control. There were no significant differences in LDL between PSY and PGX groups at 3, 6 or 12 months.

Triglyceride was significantly lower in the control group at 6 months (−7.6%, $p = 0.033$) compared to baseline (Figure 2D). TG was significantly lower in the PSY group at 6 months (−12.7%, $p = 0.023$) compared to baseline.

Non-esterified fatty acid (NEFA) was significantly lower in the PSY group at 12 months (−9.5%, $p = 0.021$) compared to baseline, as shown in Figure 2E. NEFA was significantly higher in the PGX group at 3 months (15.7%, $p = 0.009$) compared to baseline. NEFA was significantly higher in the PGX group compared to control (16.9%, $p = 0.027$) and PSY (18.2%, $p = 0.017$) at 3 months. There were no significant differences in NEFA between control and PSY at 3, 6 or 12 months.

ApoB did not significantly change within any of the study groups. There were no significant differences in apoB between control, PSY or PGX groups at 3, 6 or 12 months (data not shown).

3.6. Insulin

Insulin was significantly lower in the PGX group at 3 months (−7.6%, $p < 0.001$) compared to baseline (Figure 3A). Insulin was significantly lower in the PSY group at 3 months (−5.5%, $p = 0.032$) compared to baseline. Insulin was significantly lower compared to control at 3 months in the PGX (−9%, $p = 0.008$) and PSY (−9.4%, $p = 0.004$) groups, at 6 months in PGX (−9.8%, $p = 0.038$) and PSY (−9.1%, $p = 0.040$) groups compared to control and at 12 months in the PSY group (−9.4%, $p = 0.029$) compared to control. There were no significant differences in insulin between PSY and PGX groups at 3, 6 or 12 months.

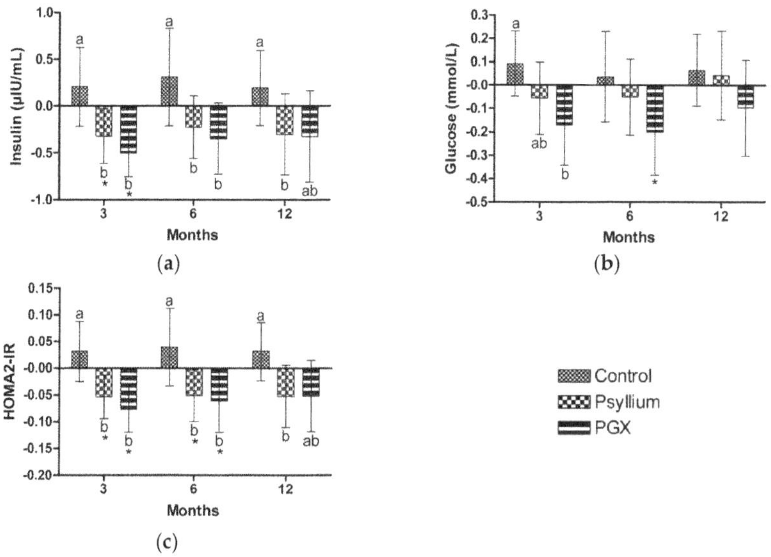

Figure 3. Changes in fasting blood parameters during 12 months of fibre supplementation (**a**) Insulin, (**b**) Glucose; (**c**) HOMA2-IR. Values are mean ± 95% CI with baseline as a covariate. * indicates within group differences compared to baseline. Different letters represent significant differences between groups $p < 0.05$.

3.7. Glucose

Glucose was significantly lower in the PGX group at 6 months (−3.9%, $p = 0.033$) compared to baseline, while the decrease at 3 months did not reach significance (−3.4%, $p = 0.053$) (Figure 3B). Glucose was significantly lower compared to control at 3 months in the PGX (−4.8%, $p = 0.019$) group. There were no significant differences in glucose between control and PSY or between PSY and PGX groups at 3, 6 or 12 months.

3.8. *Homeostasis Model Assessment of Insulin Resistance*

The HOMA2-IR score was significantly lower in the PGX group at 3 months (−9%, p = 0.001) and 6 months (−7.3%, p = 0.039) compared to baseline (Figure 3C). HOMA2-IR was significantly lower in the PSY group at 3 months (−7%, p = 0.011) and 6 months (−6.7%, p = 0.037) compared to baseline. HOMA2-IR was significantly lower compared to control at 3 months in the PGX (−10.8%, p = 0.005) and PSY (−10.8%, p = 0.001) groups, at 6 months in PGX (−11.9%, p = 0.033) and PSY (−11.9%, p = 0.018) groups compared to control and at 12 months in the PSY group (−11%, p = 0.011) compared to control. There was a trend for HOMA2-IR to be lower in the PGX group compared to control at 12 months but this was not significant (−8.5%, p = 0.068). There were no significant differences in HOMA2-IR score between PSY and PGX groups at 3, 6 or 12 months.

3.9. *Adverse Events*

Minor adverse events were gastrointestinal related (e.g., flatulence, diarrhoea) with four withdrawing from the study, two in the PGX group and two in the control group. The PSY supplement was better tolerated and participants did not report any adverse effects.

4. Discussion

Previous epidemiological and cohort studies have consistently revealed that higher fibre intakes are correlated with lower body weight, BMI, waist circumference [1,2], and improved plasma lipid profiles [3–12], glycaemia and insulinaemia [13], indicating the benefits and risk reduction for the metabolic syndrome, CVD and type 2 diabetes. Given that individuals find it difficult to eat the required amounts of fibre by increasing fruit and vegetable intake, it was hypothesised that fibre supplements can provide similar health benefits compared with increased dietary fibre intake. Therefore, this study investigated the effects of 15 g of PGX or psyllium compared to control (rice flour) supplementation for one year on lipids, insulin and glucose. Specifically, both the PGX and PSY groups demonstrated significant reductions at 3 months in fasting concentrations of total cholesterol by 8.2% and 7% respectively, LDL cholesterol by 13.9% and 8.1% respectively, insulin by 9% and 9.4% respectively and HOMA2-IR score by 11.9%, compared to control group. Only the PGX intervention improved fasting glucose and HDL cholesterol during the study.

Our results herein are supported by recent human and animal studies which suggest that psyllium fibre supplementation may provide cardiovascular benefits [22,31]. The effect of PGX on decreasing total and LDL cholesterol levels in this study concurs with similar reports in the literature describing the effects of viscous dietary fibre on lowering serum cholesterol levels. Carabin et al. [17] conducted a clinical trial with healthy subjects, 25 males and 29 females, mean age of 31.6 ± 10.5 years who consumed 2.5 g of PGX packaged with cereal and yoghurt twice a day as part of two main meals (breakfast and/or lunch, and/or dinner), for the first seven days, followed by 5 g PGX twice a day for the last 14 days of the study. The control product was a skimmed milk powder. Investigators observed significantly lower total and LDL cholesterol in the test group compared to the control group at day 8 (9.4% vs. 3.3% for total and 10.4% vs. 2.5% for LDL cholesterol, respectively) and at day 22 (14.1% vs. 8.3% for total and 16.6% vs. 8.2% for LDL cholesterol, respectively). The differences between groups was similar to the magnitude observed in our study. Reimer et al. [38] observed the effects of 14 weeks of short-term PGX supplementation in adults with abdominal obesity and also observed significant reductions in total and LDL cholesterol. In a pre-post study by Lyon & Reichert [18], 29 overweight and obese adults with a BMI between 25–36 kg/m^2, consumed 5 g of PGX in 500 mL of water 5–10 min before each meal, 2–3 times a day for 14 days and showed a significant reduction of total cholesterol and LDL cholesterol levels of 19% and 25% respectively, compared to baseline. As the supplement intervention in this latter study was combined with lifestyle changes, the decreases in cholesterol levels were greater than those observed in our current study. Although neither of the studies described above reported changes in HDL after PGX supplementation, we only observed this effect at 12 months, indicating a possible long term effect that has not been demonstrated previously. When looking at the effect of psyllium, another study [22] also found that simply adding a psyllium fibre supplement to a normal diet (10.2 g/day) was sufficient to see improvements in total cholesterol (−21%) and LDL cholesterol (−22%) at 12 weeks compared to control. Similar findings for psyllium have also been reported in various meta-analyses [39].

Animal studies have demonstrated a beneficial effect of PGX supplementation on glucose control and fasting insulin [40]. While many human studies have examined the short-term postprandial glucose response to PGX supplementation [20,41,42], few have looked at the long term effects. Lyon & Reichert [18] assessed changes to fasting insulin and glucose in their study. The PGX and lifestyle intervention caused a 6.96% reduction in fasting glucose and a 27.26% reduction in fasting insulin which is in agreement with our PGX intervention findings. Psyllium has been previously shown to improve glucose and insulin response [31,33]. In a study by Ziai et al. [23], psyllium was taken in combination with medication and a significant reduction in fasting glucose was observed. Gibb et al. [33] reported that psyllium improved glycaemic control proportional to loss of glycaemic control, which may explain why our non-diabetic psyllium group did not demonstrate any significant improvements to fasting blood glucose concentrations.

Due to its high viscosity, PGX swells in the stomach and increases feelings of fullness [23,42–45]. Psyllium has also been shown to increase fullness [29] but has a far lower viscosity than PGX [18]. This characteristic may have caused participants to decrease their food intake, which then lead to significant weight loss [46]. The changes to blood lipids and insulin observed are likely due to the changes in dietary intake and weight loss observed as well as the possible effect of PGX slowing gastric emptying and absorption of nutrients in the small intestine [47].

When comparing the PGX and PSY groups in the current study, there were no significant differences between them except for a lower concentration of TG at 3 months in the PSY group compared to the PGX group. However, when examining differences compared to control, HDL cholesterol was significantly higher in the PGX group at 12 months but not in the PSY group. LDL cholesterol was significantly lower in the PGX group at 3 and 6 months compared to control whereas LDL cholesterol was only significantly lower in the PSY group at 3 months compared to control. Glucose was significantly lower in the PGX group at 3 months but not in the PSY group. Intent-to-treat analysis was carried out but the outcome results were no different from the results presented. In this regard, the PGX group performed better overall than the PSY group and elicited more health benefits over the 12 months intervention period.

One of the strengths of this study was the duration, with a 12 months intervention period. Comparable studies have only been conducted for 14 weeks. This allowed us to investigate the long term effects of the fibre supplements, especially weight maintenance. This was a double-blinded study and supplements were packed in identical foil sachets. Investigators were not aware which participants were taking which supplement; however, due to the different characteristics of the supplements, participants may have been able to guess if they were taking a fibre supplement or the control, which is a limitation. The intervention was not combined with any other lifestyle modification advice, thus it would be simple for consumers to incorporate into their lifestyle or there could be added benefits if the supplements were combined with healthy lifestyle advice. Other study limitations include the use of a generally healthy population. We did not specifically recruit participants with elevated lipid, insulin or glucose concentrations which would have limited our ability to detect significant improvements. The majority of participants were women and hormonal changes over the 12 months may have impacted on lipids levels.

5. Conclusions

It is thought the high viscosity of PGX caused participants to decrease their food intake, which then lead to significant weight loss, lipid, insulin, and glucose reductions. Taking a fibre supplement before meals was a relatively easy task for people to incorporate into their daily routine and would be a simple intervention to implement. We observed similar results between PGX and PSY supplements when compared to the control group, however the PGX supplement was superior in terms of increased HDL cholesterol and decreased fasting blood glucose. Therefore, regular consumption of a PolyGlycopleX or a psyllium supplement is a simple and effective method to improve blood lipids, insulin and glucose control in overweight or obese people and may lead to risk reduction for metabolic syndrome, CVD and type 2 diabetes.

Supplementary Materials: The following are available online at http://www.mdpi.com/2072-6643/9/2/091/s1, Table S1: Lipids, Glucose and Insulin levels during 12 months of fibre supplementation (intention to treat analysis).

Acknowledgments: PGX®, PolyGlycopleX® and EnviroSimplex® are registered trademarks of InovoBiologic Inc., Calgary, AB, Canada. The proprietary Psyllium product (PgxSyl™) (PSY) was formulated by InovoBiologic Inc. We thank Michael Lyon, MD for helping with the design of this study. We thank all the participants for their time and contributions to this study.

Author Contributions: S.P., S.W. and R.J.G. designed research; S.H. (and Jenny McKay) conducted research; S.H. analysed data; S.P., S.H., S.W. and R.J.G. wrote the paper; S.P. and S.H. had primary responsibility for final content. All authors read and approved the final manuscript.

Conflicts of Interest: R.J.G. owns the Factors Group of Companies, which retains an interest in PGX®. S.W. receives consulting fees from InovoBiologic Inc. Funding: Financial support for the submitted work from Factors Group Australia Pty Ltd., which had no role in data collection, analysis and interpretation.

References

1. Du, H.; van der, A.D.L.; Boshuizen, H.C.; Forouhi, N.G.; Wareham, N.J.; Halkjaer, J.; Tjonneland, A.; Overvad, K.; Jakobsen, M.U.; Boeing, H.; et al. Dietary fiber and subsequent changes in body weight and waist circumference in European men and women. *Am. J. Clin. Nutr.* **2010**, *91*, 329–336. [CrossRef] [PubMed]
2. Newby, P.K.; Maras, J.; Bakun, P.; Muller, D.; Ferrucci, L.; Tucker, K.L. Intake of whole grains, refined grains, and cereal fiber measured with 7-D diet records and associations with risk factors for chronic disease. *Am. J. Clin. Nutr.* **2007**, *86*, 1745–1753. [PubMed]
3. National Health and Medical Research Council. *Australian Dietary Guidelines*; National Health and Medical Research Council: Canberra, Australia, 2013.
4. Wu, H.; Dwyer, K.M.; Fan, Z.; Shircore, A.; Fan, J.; Dwyer, J.H. Dietary fiber and progression of atherosclerosis: The Los Angeles Atherosclerosis Study. *Am. J. Clin. Nutr.* **2003**, *78*, 1085–1091. [PubMed]
5. Lairon, D. Macronutrient intake and modulation on chylomicron production and clearance. *Atheroscler. Suppl.* **2008**, *9*, 45–48. [CrossRef] [PubMed]
6. Kan, H.; Stevens, J.; Heiss, G.; Klein, R.; Rose, K.M.; London, S.J. Dietary fiber intake and retinal vascular caliber in the atherosclerosis risk in communities study. *Am. J. Clin. Nutr.* **2007**, *86*, 1626–1632. [PubMed]
7. Lairon, D.; Arnault, N.; Bertrais, S.; Planells, R.; Clero, E.; Hercberg, S.; Boutron-Ruault, M.C. Dietary fiber intake and risk factors for cardiovascular disease in French adults. *Am. J. Clin. Nutr.* **2005**, *82*, 1185–1194. [PubMed]
8. Venn, B.J.; Mann, J.I. Cereal grains, legumes and diabetes. *Eur. J. Clin. Nutr.* **2004**, *58*, 1443–1461. [CrossRef] [PubMed]
9. Weickert, M.O.; Pfeiffer, A.F. Metabolic effects of dietary fiber consumption and prevention of diabetes. *J. Nutr.* **2008**, *138*, 439–442. [PubMed]
10. McKeown, N.M.; Meigs, J.B.; Liu, S.; Wilson, P.W.; Jacques, P.F. Whole-grain intake is favorably associated with metabolic risk factors for type 2 diabetes and cardiovascular disease in the Framingham Offspring Study. *Am. J. Clin. Nutr.* **2002**, *76*, 390–398. [PubMed]
11. Pittler, M.H.; Ernst, E. Guar gum for body weight reduction: Meta-analysis of randomized trials. *Am. J. Med.* **2001**, *110*, 724–730. [CrossRef]
12. Brown, L.; Rosner, B.; Willett, W.W.; Sacks, F.M. Cholesterol-lowering effects of dietary fiber: A meta-analysis. *Am. J. Clin. Nutr.* **1999**, *69*, 30–42. [PubMed]
13. Ludwig, D.S.; Pereira, M.A.; Kroenke, C.H.; Hilner, J.E.; Van Horn, L.; Slattery, M.L.; Jacobs, D.R., Jr. Dietary fiber, weight gain, and cardiovascular disease risk factors in young adults. *JAMA* **1999**, *282*, 1539–1546. [CrossRef] [PubMed]

14. Clemens, R.; Kranz, S.; Mobley, A.; Nicklas, R.; Raimondi, M.; Rodriguez, J.; Slavin, J.; Jacobs, D.J. Filling America's Fiber Intake Gap: Summary of a Roundtable to Probe Realistic Solutions with a Focus on Grain-Based Foods. *J. Nutr.* **2012**, *142*, 1390S–1401S. [CrossRef] [PubMed]
15. US Department of Agriculture; US Department of Health and Human Services. *Dietary Guidelines for Americans*; US Government Printing Office: Washington, DC, USA, 2005.
16. Marlett, J.A.; McBurney, M.I.; Slavin, J.L. Position of the American Dietetic Association: Health implications of dietary fiber. *J. Am. Diet. Assoc.* **2002**, *102*, 993–1000. [CrossRef]
17. Carabin, I.G.; Lyon, M.R.; Wood, S.; Pelletier, X.; Donazzolo, Y.; Burdock, G.A. Supplementation of the diet with the functional fiber PolyGlycoplex is well tolerated by healthy subjects in a clinical trial. *Nutr. J.* **2009**, *8*, 9. [CrossRef] [PubMed]
18. Lyon, M.R.; Reichert, R.G. The effect of a novel viscous polysaccharide along with lifestyle changes on short-term weight loss and associated risk factors in overweight and obese adults: an observational retrospective clinical program analysis. *Altern. Med. Rev.* **2010**, *15*, 68–75. [PubMed]
19. Food and Nutrition Board of the Institute of Medicine of the National Academies. Dietary, functional, and total fiber. In *Dietary Reference Intakes for Energy, Carbohydrate, Fiber, Fat, Fatty Acids, Cholesterol, Protein, and Amino Acids*; Spears, G.E., Ed.; The National Academies Press: Washington, DC, USA, 2005; pp. 339–421.
20. Jenkins, A.L.; Kacinik, V.; Lyon, M.; Wolever, T.M. Effect of adding the novel fiber, PGX®, to commonly consumed foods on glycemic response, glycemic index and GRIP: A simple and effective strategy for reducing post prandial blood glucose levels—A randomized, controlled trial. *Nutr. J.* **2010**, *9*, 58. [CrossRef] [PubMed]
21. Reimer, R.A.; Pelletier, X.; Carabin, I.G.; Lyon, M.; Gahler, R.; Parnell, J.A.; Wood, S. Increased plasma PYY levels following supplementation with the functional fiber PolyGlycopleX in healthy adults. *Eur. J. Clin. Nutr.* **2010**, *64*, 1186–1191. [CrossRef] [PubMed]
22. Pal, S.; Khossousi, A.; Binns, C.; Dhaliwal, S.; Ellis, V. The effect of a fibre supplement compared to a healthy diet on body composition, lipids, glucose, insulin and other metabolic syndrome risk factors in overweight and obese individuals. *Br. J. Nutr.* **2011**, *105*, 90–100. [CrossRef] [PubMed]
23. Ziai, S.; Larijani, B.; Akhoondzadeh, S.; Fakhrzadeh, H.; Dastpak, A.; Bandarian, F.; Rezai, A.; Badi, H.; Emami, T. Psyllium decreased serum glucose and glycosylated hemoglobin significantly in diabetic outpatients. *J. Ethnopharmacol.* **2005**, *102*, 202–207. [CrossRef] [PubMed]
24. Karhunen, L.; Juvonen, K.; Flander, S.; Liukkonen, K.; Lahteenmaki, L.; Siloaho, M.; Laaksonen, D.; Herzig, K.; Uusitupa, M.; Poutanen, K. A psyllium fiber-enriched meal strongly attenuates postprandial gastrointestinal peptide release in healthy young adults. *J. Nutr.* **2010**, *140*, 737–744. [CrossRef] [PubMed]
25. Anderson, J.; Allgood, L.; Lawrence, A.; Altringer, L.; Jerdack, G.; Hengehold, D.; Morel, J. Cholesterol-lowering effects of psyllium intake adjunctive to diet therapy in men and women with hypercholesterolemia: Meta-analysis of 8 controlled trials. *Am. J. Clin. Nutr.* **2000**, *71*, 472–479. [PubMed]
26. Rodriguez-Moran, M.; Guerrero-Romero, F.; Lazcano-Burciaga, G. Lipid- and glucose-lowering efficacy of *Plantago*. Psyllium in type II diabetes. *J. Diabetes Complic.* **1998**, *12*, 273–278. [CrossRef]
27. Vuksan, V.; Jenkins, A.L.; Rogovik, A.L.; Fairgrieve, C.; Jovanovski, E.; Leiter, L. Viscosity rather than quantity of dietary fibre predicts cholesterol-lowering effect in healthy individuals. *Br. J. Nutr.* **2011**, *106*, 1349–1352. [CrossRef] [PubMed]
28. Tai, E.; Fok, A.; Chu, R.; Tan, C. A study to assess the effect of dietary supplementation with soluble fibre (Minolest) on lipid levels in normal subjects with hypercholesterolaemia. *Ann. Acad. Med. Singapore* **1999**, *28*, 209–213. [PubMed]
29. Turnbull, W.; Thomas, H. The effect of a *Plantago ovata* seed containing preparation on appetite variables, nutrient and energy intake. *Int. J. Obes. Relat. Metab. Disord.* **1995**, *19*, 338–342. [PubMed]
30. Delargy, H.; O'Sullivan, K.; Fletcher, R.; Blundell, J. Effects of amount and type of dietary fibre (soluble and insoluble) on short-term control of appetite. *Int. J. Food Sci. Nutr.* **1997**, *48*, 67–77. [CrossRef] [PubMed]
31. Pal, S.; Radavelli-Bagatini, S. Effects of psyllium on metabolic syndrome risk factors. *Obes. Rev.* **2012**, *13*, 1034–1047. [CrossRef] [PubMed]
32. Khossousi, A.; Binns, C.W.; Dhaliwal, S.S.; Pal, S. The acute effects of psyllium on postprandial lipaemia and thermogenesis in overweight and obese men. *Br. J. Nutr.* **2008**, *99*, 1068–1075. [CrossRef] [PubMed]

33. Gibb, R.; McRorie, J.; Russel, D.; Hasselblad, V.; D'Alessio, D. Psyllium fiber improves glycemic control proportional to loss of glycemic control: A meta-analysis of data in euglycemic subjects, patients at risk of type 2 diabetes mellitus, and patients being treated for type 2 diabetes mellitus. *Am. J. Clin. Nutr.* **2015**, *102*, 1604–1614. [CrossRef] [PubMed]
34. US Pharmacopeia. *Food Chemicals Codex (FCC)*, 9th ed.; US Pharmacopeia: Rockville, MD, USA, 2015.
35. Pal, S.; Ellis, V.; Dhaliwal, S. Effects of whey protein isolate on body composition, lipids, insulin and glucose in overweight and obese individuals. *Br. J. Nutr.* **2010**, *104*, 716–723. [CrossRef] [PubMed]
36. Bairaktari, E.; Hatzidimou, K.; Tzallas, C.; Vini, M.; Katsaraki, A.; Tselepis, A.; Elisaf, M.; Tsolas, O. Estimation of LDL cholesterol based on the Friedewald formula and on apo B levels. *Clin. Biochem.* **2000**, *33*, 549–555. [CrossRef]
37. Wallace, T.M.; Levy, J.C.; Matthews, D.R. Use and abuse of HOMA modeling. *Diabetes Care* **2004**, *27*, 1487–1495. [CrossRef] [PubMed]
38. Reimer, R.A.; Yamaguchi, H.; Eller, L.K.; Lyon, M.R.; Gahler, R.J.; Kacinik, V.; Juneja, P.; Wood, S. Changes in visceral adiposity and serum cholesterol with a novel viscous polysaccharide in Japanese adults with abdominal obesity. *Obesity* **2013**, *21*, E379–E387. [PubMed]
39. Bernstein, A.; Titgemeier, B.; Kirkpatrick, K.; Golubic, M.; Roizen, M. Major cereal grain fibers and psyllium in relation to cardiovascular health. *Nutrients* **2013**, *5*, 1471–1487. [CrossRef] [PubMed]
40. Grover, G.J.; Koetzner, L.; Wicks, J.; Gahler, R.J.; Lyon, M.R.; Reimer, R.A.; Wood, S. Effects of the soluble fiber complex PolyGlycopleX® on glucose homeostasis and body weight in young Zucker diabetic rats. *Front. Pharmacol.* **2011**, *2*, 47. [CrossRef] [PubMed]
41. Brand-Miller, J.C.; Atkinson, F.S.; Gahler, R.J.; Kacinik, V.; Lyon, M.R.; Wood, S. Effects of PGX, a novel functional fibre, on acute and delayed postprandial glycaemia. *Eur. J. Clin. Nutr.* **2010**, *64*, 1488–1493. [CrossRef] [PubMed]
42. Solah, V.A.; Brand-Miller, J.C.; Atkinson, F.S.; Gahler, R.J.; Kacinik, V.; Lyon, M.R.; Wood, S. Dose-response effect of a novel functional fibre, PolyGlycopleX®, PGX®, on satiety. *Appetite* **2014**, *77C*, 72–76. [CrossRef] [PubMed]
43. Vuksan, V.; Panahi, S.; Lyon, M.; Rogovik, A.L.; Jenkins, A.L.; Leiter, L.A. Viscosity of fiber preloads affects food intake in adolescents. *Nutr. Metab. Cardiovasc. Dis.* **2009**, *19*, 498–503. [CrossRef] [PubMed]
44. Yong, M.; Solah, V.; Johnson, S.; Meng, X.; Kerr, D.; James, A.; Fenton, H.; Gahler, R.J.; Wood, S. Effects of a viscous-fibre supplemented evening meal and the following un-supplemented breakfast on post-prandial satiety responses in healthy women. *Physiol. Behav.* **2016**, *154*, 34–39. [CrossRef] [PubMed]
45. Kacinik, V.; Lyon, M.R.; Purnama, M.; Reimer, R.A.; Gahler, R.J.; Green, T.J.; Wood, S. Effect of PGX, a novel functional fibre supplement, on subjective ratings of appetite in overweight and obese women consuming a 3-day structured, low-calorie diet. *Nutr. Diab.* **2011**, *1*, e22. [CrossRef] [PubMed]
46. Pal, S.; Ho, S.; Gahler, R.; Wood, S. Effect on body weight and composition in overweight/obese Australian adults over 12 months consumption of two different types of fiber supplementation in a randomized trial. *Nutr. Metab.* **2016**, *13*, 82. [CrossRef] [PubMed]
47. Matulka, R.A.; Lyon, M.R.; Wood, S.; Ann Marone, P.; Merkel, D.J.; Burdock, G.A. The safety of PolyGlycopleX (PGX) as shown in a 90-day rodent feeding study. *Nutr. J.* **2009**, *8*, 1. [CrossRef] [PubMed]

nutrients

MDPI

Article

A High Fiber Cookie Made with Resistant Starch Type 4 Reduces Post-Prandial Glucose and Insulin Responses in Healthy Adults

Maria L. Stewart * and J. Paul Zimmer

Global Nutrition R & D, Ingredion Incorporated, 10 Finderne Ave, Bridgewater, NJ 08807, USA; paul.zimmer@ingredion.com

* Correspondence: maria.stewart@ingredion.com; Tel.: +1-908-685-5470

Received: 6 January 2017; Accepted: 28 February 2017; Published: 5 March 2017

Abstract: Distarch phosphate is a resistant starch type 4 (RS4) containing phosphodiester cross-links within and between starch molecules. This study examined the glycemic effects of VERSAFIBE 1490™ resistant starch, a distarch phosphate derived from potato, containing 90% total dietary fiber (TDF, AOAC 991.43 method). In this double-blind, randomized, placebo-controlled, cross-over study, 28 healthy adults consumed a cookie containing 24 g fiber from distarch phosphate (fiber cookie) or a control cookie containing 0.5 g fiber that was matched for fat, protein, and total carbohydrate content. Intravenous blood glucose, intravenous blood insulin, and capillary glucose were measured for two hours after cookie consumption. The fiber cookie reduced the post-prandial blood glucose incremental area under the curve from 0 to 120 minutes ($iAUC_{0\text{-}120min}$) by 44% (p = 0.004) and reduced the maximum glucose concentration ($C_{max0\text{-}120min}$) by 8% (p = 0.001) versus the control cookie. Consumption of the fiber cookie resulted in a significant 46% reduction of the post-prandial serum insulin $iAUC_{0\text{-}120min}$ (p < 0.001) and a 23% reduction in $Cmax_{0\text{-}120min}$ (p = 0.007) versus the control cookie. This study shows that distarch phosphate RS4 can be incorporated into a cookie and significantly reduce post-prandial glucose and insulin responses in healthy adults.

Keywords: resistant starch type 4; dietary fiber; post-prandial; blood glucose; insulin; capillary glucose; glycemic response

1. Introduction

Resistant starch (RS) is a complex carbohydrate (glucose polymer) that resists digestion and absorption in the small intestine. Resistant starches are classified into five types: RS1 (physically inaccessible starches), RS2 (granular starches with B- or C-polymorph), RS3 (retrograded starches), RS4 (chemically modified starches), and RS5 (amylose-lipid complexes) [1]. Resistant starch type 4 is a unique class of resistant starch due to the diversity of chemical modifications that decrease digestibility. Common chemical modifications include cross-linking, substitution, and pyrodextrinization [2].

Resistant starch, in general, is known for improving physiological endpoints such as improving bowel function [3] and controlling glycemia [4]. In these reviews, all sources of RS are combined. However, it has been documented that different RSs exert different physiological effects. In a study using a porcine model, RS3 increased fecal nitrogen excretion compared to RS2 [5]. The composition of the human gut microbiota was affected in different manners, depending on the type of RS consumed (RS2 vs. RS4) [6]. Given these differences, clinical trials on specific resistant starch preparations are necessary to confirm the beneficial physiological effects.

As noted previously, RS4 includes starches that have a variety of chemical modifications to reduce digestibility. VERSAFIBE™ 1490 resistant starch is a distarch phosphate derived from potato that has been modified using phosphorus oxychloride [7]. Distarch phosphate is resistant to digestion due to the presence of diester phosphate crosslinks within and between starch molecules. Phosphated distarch phosphate is a similar type of RS4 with additional monophosphate esters, although the monophosphate esters do not substantially affect digestibility [8,9].

Resistant starch type 4, specifically distarch phosphate and phosphate distarch phosphate, is a relatively new form of resistant starch, with the earliest clinical trials on phosphated distarch phosphate published in 2010. The evidence on phosphated distarch phosphate RS4, albeit limited, supports improvement of metabolic endpoints such as reduced post-prandial glucose response and reduced serum lipids, after the ingredient is consumed [10–13]. To date, only one study examined post-prandial blood glucose response to distarch phosphate (consumed in a beverage) [14]. The aforementioned study demonstrated that distarch phosphate did not contribute to the post-prandial glycemic response, and this effect needed to be confirmed when the ingredient is incorporated into a solid, baked food with mixed nutrients. The present study assessed the acute, post-prandial glycemic and insulinemic response to a cookie containing RS4 in the form of distarch phosphate (VERSAFIBE 1490 resistant starch) in healthy adults. This is the first clinical study to examine these outcomes in a solid food containing distarch phosphate RS4.

2. Materials and Methods

2.1. Study Subjects

This study was conducted in accordance with the ethical principles outlined in the Declaration of Helsinki and approved by the Institutional Review Board (IRB Services, Aurora, ON, Canada). Clinical study visits were held at a clinical research facility (KGK Synergize, London, Ontario, Canada). Healthy subjects were recruited to participate in this study. Subjects that met the inclusion criteria (18 years of age or older, body mass index (BMI) 18.0–29.9 kg/m^2, fasting glucose $\leq$6.0 mmol/L; if female, not of childbearing potential (e.g., taking oral contraceptives, past hysterectomy)) and exclusion criteria (diagnosed metabolic or chronic diseases (e.g., type-2 diabetes); cancer diagnosis or treatment within 5 years; gastrointestinal problems; bowel cleansing during prior week; current medications to control blood glucose; blood cholesterol and/or blood pressure; smoker; use of medical marijuana; alcohol or drug abuse treatment in past 12 months; allergy or sensitivity to study products; blood donation in prior 2 months; if female, currently pregnant, currently breastfeeding, or planning to become pregnant) were qualified to participate in the study. Subjects provided informed consent and were randomly assigned to a treatment order at the time of enrollment: "control cookie-fiber cookie" or "fiber cookie-control cookie". A senior staff member not involved in the study procedures generated two randomization lists—one list for males and one list for females—by www.randomization.com. Fourteen male participants were randomized into seven blocks by utilizing a randomization seed 10,087 and fourteen female participants were randomized into seven blocks by utilizing a randomization seed 11,065. A total of twenty-eight subjects were enrolled in the study. Subject flow through the study is described in Figure 1.

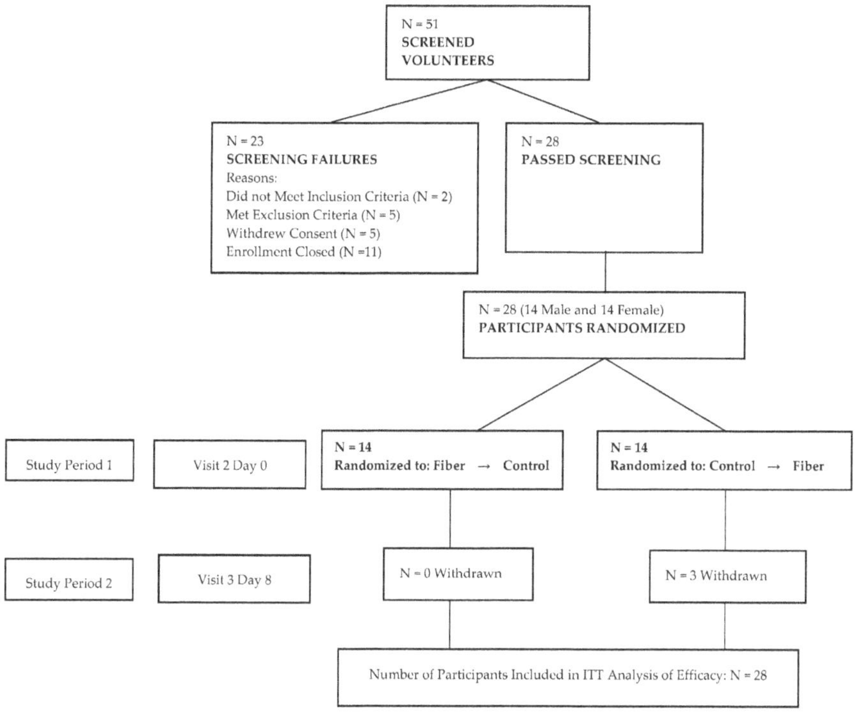

Figure 1. Subject flow through study.

2.2. Study Design

This study was a double-blind, randomized, controlled, cross-over intervention study. Fifty-one subjects were screened, and 28 subjects were enrolled in the study (Figure 1). The subjects participated in two 24-h study periods that began the evening before the clinical study visit. Prior to each clinical study visit, the subjects consumed a standard dinner meal. Subjects arrived at the study center the following morning, after fasting for 12 h. Fasting blood samples (intravenous and capillary) were taken prior to study product consumption. Both intravenous and capillary blood samples were taken because previous reports indicated differences in blood glucose measures, depending on the sampling technique [15]. The study product (cookie) was consumed with 250 mL water. Intravenous and capillary blood samples were taken at 15, 30, 45, 60, 90, and 120 min after cookie consumption. Biochemical analyses were conducted by Life Labs (Hamilton, ON, Canada). Subjects completed a seven-day washout period between study visits.

2.3. Study Foods

The fiber cookie contained 25 g of VERSAFIBE™ 1490 resistant starch (Ingredion Incorporated, Bridgewater, NJ, USA), which was the primary source of fiber in the cookie. VERSAFIBE™ 1490 resistant starch is a resistant starch type 4 with 90% dietary fiber (AOAC 991.43). VERSAFIBE™ 1490 resistant starch is produced from food grade potato starch. The raw food starch is slurried in water and maintained at a temperature not exceeding 100° F. The pH of the slurry is raised not to exceed pH 12 in the presence of salt. To phosphorylate the starch, phosphorus oxychloride is added to the slurry while maintaining the reaction pH. After the phosphorylation step is complete, the pH is neutralized with acid. The starch is washed, dewatered, and dried to a moisture content not to exceed 18%.

The fiber cookie and control cookie were matched for fat, protein, and total carbohydrate (Table 1). Nutrient composition of the cookies was calculated using Genesis R&D Food Labeling Software (ESHA Research, Salem, OR, USA). The cookies were identical in appearance. The cookies were packaged in an opaque enveloped with an alpha-numeric code for identification. Neither the study subjects nor the investigators knew the identity of the cookies. The subjects rated the cookies on appearance, texture, flavor and acceptance using modified visual analog scale with demarcations at whole numbers 1–10. The subjects were not trained sensory panelists.

Table 1. Nutrient composition of cookies.

Per Serving, As-Eaten	Control Cookie	Fiber Cookie
Weight (g)	47.02	48.00
Calories (kcal)	214.7	129.7
Fat (g)	3.99	3.92
Saturated fat (g)	0.56	0.54
Protein (g)	5.36	4.92
Total Carbohydrates (g)	36.84	36.84
Available Carbohydrates (g)	36.28	12.71
Dietary Fiber (g) *	0.55	24.13
Sugars (g)	11.51	11.72

* Fiber cookie contained VERSAFIBE 1490 resistant starch.

2.4. Sample Size Calculation

The sample size of 28 subjects was determined based on the primary outcome of detecting a difference in incremental area under the curve from 0 to 120 minutes ($iAUC_{0\text{-}120min}$) intravenous blood glucose at 80% power, 0.05 alpha, and expected subject dropout rate of 12.5%.

2.5. Statistical Analysis

Incremental area under the curve (iAUC) was calculated using the trapezoidal approximation but only included the positive area components above the baseline value [16]. The maximum concentration (Cmax) was taken to be the highest concentration within the respective time interval. The iAUC calculations as well as the Cmax values were reported and compared for each product group.

Each numeric outcome was assessed for normality using visual representations (histogram, quantile-quantile plot, etc.) and the Shapiro–Wilk normality test. Outcomes that were log-normally or square root normally distributed were analyzed in the logarithmic or square root domain respectively. Non-normal variables were analyzed by appropriate non-parametric tests (see below). All summary statistics were reported non-transformed, arithmetic means.

Numerical efficacy endpoints were formally tested for significance between groups by a linear mixed model with a fixed effect for study product group and a random effect for each participant [17]. The concentrations of the analytes at each time point included a covariate for the baseline value. Numerical endpoints that are intractably non-normal were assessed by the Wilcoxon sign-rank test. All statistical analysis was completed using the R Statistical Software Package Version 3.2.2 (R Core Team, 2015) for Microsoft Windows. Linear mixed models were run using the "nlme" package [18]. Statistical significance was achieved at $p < 0.05$.

3. Results

3.1. Demographics

Subject demographics are shown in Table 2. All of the subjects were healthy. The demographic characteristics are consistent with the typical North American adult population.

Table 2. Subject demographics.

Mean ± SD	All Participants (n = 28)
Age (y)	42.8 ± 18.5
Sex (male/female)	14/14
Race (white/nonwhite)	23/5
Weight (kg)	71.3 ± 12.0
Body Mass Index (kg/m^2)	24.7 ± 3.3
Fasting blood glucose (mmol/L)	5.03 ± 0.34

3.2. *Post-Prandial Blood Glucose and Insulin Response*

Three subjects who were randomized to the "control cookie-fiber cookie" sequence did not complete the second treatment. Blood samples obtained for up to two subjects in each treatment group could not be analyzed for the metabolite of interest. The sample size for each group and each outcome is noted in the footnote of Table 3.

Table 3. Post-prandial glucose and insulin iAUC and Cmax §.

Mean ± SD	Control Cookie	Fiber Cookie	p-Value §
Intravenous blood glucose *			
$iAUC_{0\text{-}120min}$ (mmol/L *·h)	1.31 ± 0.75	0.73 ± 0.90	0.004
$Cmax_{0\text{-}120min}$ (mmol/L *·h)	6.83 ± 0.90	6.29 ± 0.82	0.001
Capillary blood glucose †			
$iAUC_{0\text{-}120min}$ (mmol/L *·h)	2.35 ± 0.94	1.22 ± 1.18	<0.001
$Cmax_{0\text{-}120min}$ (mmol/L *·h)	7.22 ± 1.00	6.60 ± 1.00	0.005
Intravenous serum insulin ‡			
$iAUC_{0\text{-}120min}$ (pmol/L *·h)	229 ± 124	124 ± 94	<0.001
$Cmax_{0\text{-}120min}$ (pmol/L *·h)	280 ± 129	215 ± 94	0.007

§ iAUC = incremental area under the curve, Cmax = maximum concentration * n = 27 control cookie, n = 25 fiber cookie; † n = 26 control cookie, n = 23 fiber cookie; ‡ n = 27 control cookie, n = 25 fiber cookie; § iAUC intravenous blood glucose and iAUC intravenous serum insulin datasets were square root transformed prior to statistical analysis; Cmax intravenous blood glucose and Cmax intravenous serum insulin datasets were log transformed prior to statistical analysis.

Mean post-prandial intravenous blood glucose, capillary glucose, and intravenous serum insulin concentration over the two-hour study period are shown in the time-course graphs (Figure 2A–C). Intravenous blood glucose was significantly lower at 45 min after the fiber cookie was consumed, compared to the control cookie. Capillary blood glucose concentrations were significantly lower at 15, 30, 45, 60, 90, and 120 min after the fiber cookie was consumed, compared to the control cookie. At 45, 60, 90, and 120 min, intravenous blood insulin concentrations were significantly lower after subjects consumed the fiber cookie compared to the control cookie.

The significant reductions at individual time points for glucose and insulin values reflected significant reductions in iAUC and Cmax. After consuming the fiber cookie, the subjects experienced a 44% reduction in intravenous blood glucose $iAUC_{0\text{-}120min}$ compared to the control cookie (p = 0.004, Table 3). This was largely driven by a significant, 8% reduction in intravenous blood glucose $Cmax_{0\text{-}120min}$ after consuming the fiber cookie compared to the control cookie (p = 0.001). A similar response was noted for capillary blood glucose measures, with a significant, 48% reduction in $iAUC_{0\text{-}120min}$ and a significant 9% reduction in $Cmax_{0\text{-}120min}$. Intravenous blood insulin was significantly lower for $iAUC_{0\text{-}120min}$ (46% lower), and $Cmax_{0\text{-}120min}$ (23% lower), after subjects consumed the fiber cookie, compared to the control. The decrease in insulin concentrations after consuming the fiber cookie reflect the decreased intravenous and capillary blood glucose concentrations.

The subject ratings were favorable and did not differ between groups (Table 4).

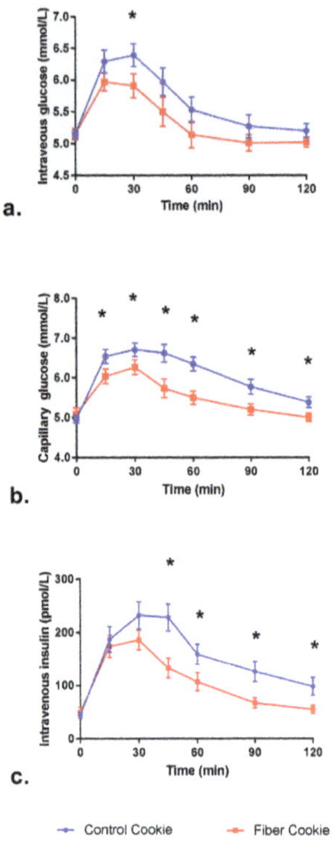

Figure 2. Post-prandial blood measurements over 120 min (**a**) intravenous blood glucose; (**b**) capillary blood glucose; (**c**) intravenous insulin concentrations. Data are presented as means ± SEM. * = Fiber cookie and control cookie were significantly different ($p < 0.05$).

Table 4. Sensory ratings of the fiber cookie and control cookie.

Question	Fiber Cookie	Control Cookie	Between Group p Value §
	Mean ± SD (n)	Mean ± SD (n)	
Rate the appearance of the cookie	5.69 ± 2.02 (26)	5.61 ± 1.89 (28)	0.811
Rate the texture of the cookie	6.23 ± 2.07 (26)	5.93 ± 2.07 (28)	0.525
Rate the flavor of the cookie	6.46 ± 2.14 (26)	6.79 ± 1.62 (28)	0.355
What is your overall acceptance of the cookie?	6.54 ± 2.21 (26)	6.50 ± 1.58 (28)	0.970

§ Between group comparisons were made using RM-ANOVA not adjusted for baseline. Probability values $p \leq 0.05$ are statistically significant.

4. Discussion

Dietary fiber has been long acknowledged for reducing post-prandial blood glucose and insulin concentrations through mechanisms of delayed nutrient absorption or replacement of digestible carbohydrates [19]. The RS4 used in this trial, VERSAFIBE 1490 resistant starch, replaced digestible carbohydrates from refined flour when formulated into processed foods such as bakery items. This fiber maintains sensory attributes of the final food while increasing dietary fiber and decreasing available carbohydrate content. Resistant starch type 4 is a broad class of resistant starches that have been chemically modified to reduce digestibility. The particular ingredient used in this study contains phosphodiester cross-links in the distarch phosphate molecules that reduce swelling and enzyme accessibility [8,9,20]. Previous work demonstrated the low glycemic response to distarch phosphate when mixed with water alone [14]. When the resistant starch type 4 was added to a dextrose beverage, the glycemic response was the same as the dextrose beverage alone. This demonstrates that the RS4 does not affect bioavailability of other carbohydrates, and the changes in post-prandial glycemic response are due to the nondigestible nature of the carbohydrate. The dietary fiber content is consistent when analyzed with both AOAC method 991.43 and AOAC method 2009.01, which indicates that the RS4 is heat-stable and resistant to prolong enzymatic digestion (unpublished data). We expect the RS4 content and dietary fiber content to be similar in the ingredient as well as the final food product (cookie).

Resistant starch type 4 may exert additional mechanisms to reduce post-prandial glycemic response, in addition to strictly replacing available carbohydrate. In a study where the treatments were matched for available carbohydrate, the RS4 treatment, phosphated distarch phosphate, resulted in significantly lower blood glucose $iAUC_{0\text{-}120min}$, peak blood glucose, blood insulin $iAUC_{0\text{-}120min}$ and peak insulin in healthy adults [10]. Additional research is needed to further define the mechanisms by which RS4 lowers post-prandial blood glucose response when treatments are matched for available carbohydrate.

The $iAUC_{0\text{-}120min}$ and $Cmax_{0\text{-}120min}$ for blood glucose were significantly lower after subjects consumed the fiber cookie compared to the control cookie, regardless of the sampling method. As noted by previous researchers, the absolute blood glucose values differ when measured intravenously or through capillary sampling [15]. When individual time points were compared, the capillary sampling method yielded significantly lower values after the fiber cookie was consumed at 45, 60, 90, and 120 min, whereas the intravenous sampling method yielded significantly different blood glucose values at 45 min, only. This can be attributed to the larger variability in blood glucose values when intravenous sampling was used. Previous researchers also noted this phenomenon [15]. Intravenous insulin $iAUC_{0\text{-}120min}$ and Cmax were lower after the subjects consumed the fiber cookie compared to the control cookie, which corresponds to the observed changes in blood glucose.

Resistant starch type 4, such as distarch phosphate, has functional properties that allow it to replace refined grain flour in product formulations. As a result, the available carbohydrates in a food can be reduced while maintaining the same sensory properties [2]. This provides the opportunity to formulate desirable foods with added health benefits such as improved post-prandial blood glucose management.

Reduced post-prandial glycemic response is a beneficial health effect for healthy individuals as well as individuals with compromised carbohydrate metabolism (e.g., pre-diabetes, Type-2 diabetes). The results from this study demonstrate how replacing refined flour with RS4 in a baked good (cookie) reduces post-prandial glucose and insulin response in healthy adults. Further research is warranted in individuals with compromised carbohydrate metabolism.

Acknowledgments: This study was funded by Ingredion Incorporated.

Author Contributions: J.P.Z. conceived and designed the experiments; M.L.S. and J.P.Z. wrote the paper.

Conflicts of Interest: M.L.S. and J.P.Z. are employees of Ingredion Incorporated.

References

1. Birt, D.F.; Boylston, T.; Hendrich, S.; Jane, J.L.; Hollis, J.; Li, L.; McClelland, J.; Moore, S.; Phillips, G.J.; Rowling, M.; et al. Resistant starch: Promise for improving human health. *Adv. Nutr.* **2013**, *4*, 587–601. [CrossRef] [PubMed]
2. Maningat, C.C.; Seib, P.A. Rs4-Type Resistant Starch: Chemistry, Functionality and Health Benefits. In *Resistant Starch: Sources, Applications and Health Benefits;* Shi, Y.C., Maningat, C.C., Eds.; John Wiley & Sons: Hoboken, NJ, USA, 2013; pp. 43–77.
3. Shen, D.; Bai, H.; Li, Z.; Yu, Y.; Zhang, H.; Chen, L. Positive effects of resistant starch supplementation on bowel function in healthy adults: A systematic review and meta-analysis of randomized controlled trials. *Int. J. Food Sci. Nutr.* **2017**, *68*, 149–157. [CrossRef] [PubMed]

4. Bindels, L.B.; Walter, J.; Ramer-Tait, A.E. Resistant starches for the management of metabolic diseases. *Curr. Opin. Clin. Nutr. Metab. Care* **2015**, *18*, 559–565. [CrossRef] [PubMed]
5. Heijnen, M.-L.A.; Beynen, A.C. Consumption of retrograded (rs3) but not uncooked (rs2) resistant starch shifts nitrogen excretion from urine to feces in cannulated piglets. *J. Nutr.* **1997**, *127*, 1828–1832. [PubMed]
6. Martínez, I.; Kim, J.H.; Duffy, P.R.; Schlegel, V.L.; Walter, J. Resistant starches types 2 and 4 have differential effects on the composition of the fecal microbiota in human subjects. *PLoS ONE* **2010**, *5*, e15046. [CrossRef] [PubMed]
7. IngredionIncorporated. Technical Specifications: Versafibe 1490 tm Resistant Starch. Available online: http://www.ingredion.us/content/dam/ingredion/technical-documents/na/VERSAFIBE%201490%20%20%2006400400%20%20%20Technical%20Specification.pdf (accessed on 15 December 2016).
8. Woo, K.S.; Seib, P.A. Cross-linked resistant starch: Preparation and properties. *Cereal Chem.* **2002**, *79*, 819–825. [CrossRef]
9. Sang, Y.J.; Seib, P.A.; Herrera, A.I.; Prakash, O.; Shi, Y.-C. Effects of alkaline treatment on the structure of phosphorylated wheat starch and its digestibility. *Food Chem.* **2010**, *118*, 323–327. [CrossRef]
10. Al-Tamimi, E.K.; Seib, P.A.; Snyder, B.S.; Haub, M.D. Consumption of cross-linked resistant starch (rs4(xl)) on glucose and insulin responses in humans. *J. Nutr. Metab.* **2010**. [CrossRef] [PubMed]
11. Haub, M.D.; Hubach, K.L.; Al-Tamimi, E.K.; Ornelas, S.; Seib, P.A. Different types of resistant starch elicit different glucose reponses in humans. *J. Nutr. Metab.* **2010**. [CrossRef] [PubMed]
12. Nichenametla, S.N.; Weidauer, L.A.; Wey, H.E.; Beare, T.M.; Specker, B.L.; Dey, M. Resistant starch type 4-enriched diet lowered blood cholesterols and improved body composition in a double blind controlled cross-over intervention. *Mol. Nutr. Food Res.* **2014**, *58*, 1365–1369. [CrossRef] [PubMed]
13. Upadhyaya, B.; McCormack, L.; Fardin-Kia, A.R.; Juenemann, R.; Nichenametla, S.; Clapper, J.; Specker, B.; Dey, M. Impact of dietary resistant starch type 4 on human gut microbiota and immunometabolic functions. *Sci. Rep.* **2016**, *6*, 28797. [CrossRef] [PubMed]
14. Haub, M.D.; Louk, J.A.; Lopez, T.C. Novel resistant potato starches on glycemia and satiety in humans. *J. Nutr. Metab.* **2012**, *2012*, 478043. [CrossRef] [PubMed]
15. Wolever, T.M.; Vorster, H.H.; Bjorck, I.; Brand-Miller, J.; Brighenti, F.; Mann, J.I.; Ramdath, D.D.; Granfeldt, Y.; Holt, S.; Perry, T.L.; et al. Determination of the glycaemic index of foods: Interlaboratory study. *Eur. J. Clin. Nutr.* **2003**, *57*, 475–482. [CrossRef] [PubMed]
16. Wolever, T.M. Effect of blood sampling schedule and method of calculating the area under the curve on validity and precision of glycaemic index values. *Br. J. Nutr.* **2004**, *91*, 295–301. [CrossRef] [PubMed]
17. Cnaan, A.; Laird, N.M.; Slasor, P. Using the general linear mixed model to analyse unbalanced repeated measures and longitudinal data. *Stat. Med.* **1997**, *16*, 2349–2380. [CrossRef]
18. Pinheiro, J.; Bates, D.; DebRoy, S.; Sarkar, D.; R Core Team. *Nlme: Linear and Nonlinear Mixed Effects Models*; R Foundation: Vienna, Austria, 2015.
19. Medicine, I.O. Dietary, Functional, and Total Fiber. In *Dietary Reference Intakes for Energy, Carbohydrate, Fiber, Fat, Fatty Acids, Cholesterol, Protein, and Amino Acids*; National Academies Press: Washington, DC, USA, 2005; pp. 339–421.
20. Janzen, J.G. Digestibility of starch and phosphate starches by pancreatin. *Starke* **1969**, *21*, 231–235. [CrossRef]

nutrients

MDPI

Article

Effects of Higher Dietary Protein and Fiber Intakes at Breakfast on Postprandial Glucose, Insulin, and 24-h Interstitial Glucose in Overweight Adults

Akua F. Amankwaah [1,2], R. Drew Sayer [3], Amy J. Wright [1], Ningning Chen [4], Megan A. McCrory [5] and Wayne W. Campbell [1,*]

1. Department of Nutrition Science, Purdue University, West Lafayette, IN 47907, USA; aamankwaah@calbaptist.edu (A.F.A.); amyjwright2@purdue.edu (A.J.W.)
2. Department of Public Health Sciences, College of Health Science, California Baptist University, Riverside, CA 92504, USA
3. Anschutz Health and Wellness Center, University of Colorado—Denver | Anschutz Medical Campus, Aurora, CO 80045, USA; drew.sayer@ucdenver.edu
4. Department of Statistics, Purdue University, West Lafayette, IN 47907, USA; chen929@purdue.edu
5. Department of Health Sciences, College of Health & Rehabilitation Sciences: Sargent College, Boston University, Boston, MA 02215, USA; mamccr@bu.edu

* Correspondence: campbellw@purdue.edu; Tel.: +1-765-494-8236; Fax: +1-765-494-0674

Received: 11 February 2017; Accepted: 30 March 2017; Published: 2 April 2017

Abstract: Dietary protein and fiber independently influence insulin-mediated glucose control. However, potential additive effects are not well-known. Men and women (n = 20; age: 26 ± 5 years; body mass index: 26.1 ± 0.2 kg/m^2; mean ± standard deviation) consumed normal protein and fiber (NPNF; NP = 12.5 g, NF = 2 g), normal protein and high fiber (NPHF; NP = 12.5 g, HF = 8 g), high protein and normal fiber (HPNF; HP = 25 g, NF = 2 g), or high protein and fiber (HPHF; HP = 25 g, HF = 8 g) breakfast treatments during four 2-week interventions in a randomized crossover fashion. On the last day of each intervention, meal tolerance tests were completed to assess postprandial (every 60 min for 240 min) serum glucose and insulin concentrations. Continuous glucose monitoring was used to measure 24-h interstitial glucose during five days of the second week of each intervention. Repeated-measures ANOVA was applied for data analyses. The HPHF treatment did not affect postprandial glucose and insulin responses or 24-h glucose total area under the curve (AUC). Higher fiber intake reduced 240-min insulin AUC. Doubling the amount of protein from 12.5 g to 25 g/meal and quadrupling fiber from 2 to 8 g/meal at breakfast was not an effective strategy for modulating insulin-mediated glucose responses in these young, overweight adults.

Keywords: dietary protein; dietary fiber; breakfast; overweight; continuous glucose monitoring; meal tolerance test

1. Introduction

Type 2 diabetes (T2D) is a chronic metabolic disease that is impacted by insulin resistance, glucose intolerance, and dyslipidemia [1–3]. Dietary factors that influence blood glucose control may modify these metabolic abnormalities [3–6]. Total dietary energy intake and macronutrient composition are well-known to modulate glycemia [4,7]. Restricting energy intake and the resultant reductions in body weight improves these modifiable risk factors for T2D [8–10]. Nevertheless, maintaining energy restriction and weight loss over the long-term is challenging [11]. Manipulating dietary macronutrient composition without restricting energy has also been shown to be an effective dietary strategy for prevention of T2D [12,13].

The quantity and quality of carbohydrate and protein in a mixed meal modulate postprandial glucose and insulin concentrations, with the total amount and the type of carbohydrate consumed being the major contributors to postprandial glucose concentration [14–16]. An increased amount of digestible/metabolizable carbohydrate consumed is associated with higher postprandial glycemia [17–19], which increases the risk of developing T2D [20,21]. On the other hand, a higher amount of complex/indigestible carbohydrates, such as soluble, viscous, and gel-forming fibers [22–24] may attenuate postprandial glucose concentrations [25–29]. Among different forms of soluble fibers, psyllium fiber is known to consistently attenuate fasting and postprandial glucose and insulin [30,31] and distinctly exert a laxation effect when consumed with meals [32]. Dietary protein appears to stimulate insulin secretion in people with normal glucose tolerance and T2D [33–35] and this insulinotropic effect of protein is related to secretagogue amino acids, such as arginine and leucine [33]. Eggs are a complete protein source with a relatively high leucine content [36]. Evidence supporting a glucose lowering effect of eggs is inconclusive [37–39]. Experimental evidence supports metabolic effects of protein and fiber in blunting postprandial and long-term glucose responses independently [7,12,13,35,40]. However, the extent to which the effects of protein and fiber intakes on postprandial glucose when co-consumed may be additive are uncertain, particularly in overweight individuals, who may be at risk of developing T2D.

While traditional meal tolerance tests adequately assess the impact of meals/diets on postprandial glucose and insulin responses, this method does not support the assessment of daylong glucose control. Continuous glucose monitoring (CGM) is an emerging technique that is used to determine the 24-h pattern of interstitial glucose concentrations in community-dwelling individuals [41,42]. The CGM technique may be preferred to inpatient meal tolerance tests to track the impact of dietary intake on daylong glucose responses, particularly when the impact of self-selected dietary intake on glycemia is of interest. By using this approach, the suggested extended favorable effects of protein and fiber intakes on daylong glucose control can be assessed.

We conducted a randomized controlled crossover trial to assess the independent and combined effects of normal versus higher egg-based protein and fiber intakes at breakfast on postprandial glycemic and insulinemic responses as well as 24-h glucose patterns with CGM. The study focused on breakfast because the typical intakes of protein and fiber at this meal are lower than at lunch and dinner [43]. In addition, some previous studies suggest that higher protein [13,44,45] or fiber [46,47] intake at breakfast, particularly protein, may have favorable metabolic benefits by enhancing insulin-mediated glucose disposal due to increased insulin secretion. We hypothesized that co-consumption of higher quantities of egg-based protein and fiber at breakfast would lower postprandial glucose and 24-h glucose responses.

2. Materials and Methods

2.1. Participants

Overweight male and female adults were recruited from the Greater Lafayette, Indiana, USA, area through advertisement to participate in the study. The inclusion criteria for selection of participants were: age 21–45 years; body mass index (BMI) 25–29.9 kg/m^2; females with regular menstrual cycles; non-smoking; not taking medications or dietary/herbal supplements known to affect energy regulation or appetite; not pregnant or lactating within the past 1 year or planning a pregnancy; weight stable ($\pm$3 kg) for the past 3 months; not following a vigorous exercise regimen or weight loss program within the past 6 months; no acute illness; not diabetic (fasting blood glucose $\leq$126 mg/dL (7 mmol/L); not severely claustrophobic; willing to eat study foods; and not skipping breakfast >2 day/week. Eligible individuals were approved by the study physician to participate based on routine blood chemistry assessments. All participants gave written informed consent and the study had approval from the Purdue University Biomedical Institutional Review Board. Figure 1 shows participants' flow through the study. Baseline participant characteristics were not statistically different ($p > 0.05$)

between groups of participants who did versus did not complete the study. Two male participants were withdrawn from the study after randomization by the investigators due to an inability to fully comply with study procedures. These participants did not find the CGM comfortable to wear (one after three days of wearing the device and the other at the end of first intervention period). Four participants had scheduling conflicts. One of these individuals was not able to show up for the first test day appointment. The other three withdrew from the study after completing one or two testing periods. Data for these three participants were not included in the analysis. We obtained and included data from the 20 study completers in the postprandial glucose and insulin analysis. However, one of these 20 participants was unable to wear the CGM because it interfered with his farming occupation. This trial was registered on ClinicalTrials.gov (NCT02169245).

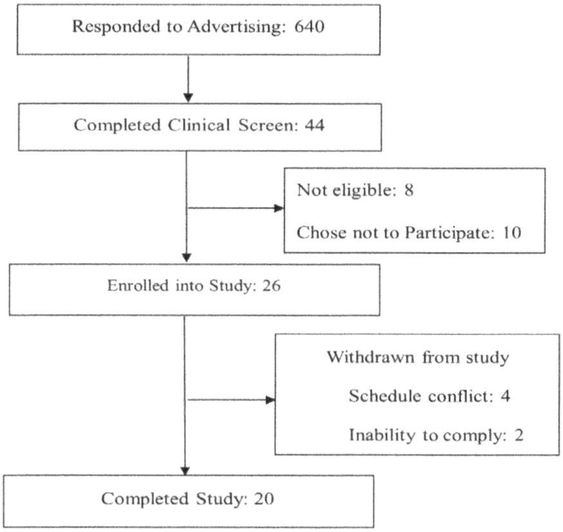

Figure 1. Consort diagram of the study.

2.2. Experimental Design

Participants completed this randomized crossover trial in approximately 15 weeks. Participants consumed four breakfast meals that varied in protein and fiber amounts daily for 2 weeks in random order. The breakfast types were normal protein and fiber (NPNF), normal protein and high fiber (NPHF), high protein and normal fiber (HPNF), and high protein and fiber (HPHF). During each 2-week intervention period, participants consumed the designated breakfast type every morning, but foods and beverages outside of breakfast were otherwise uncontrolled and self-chosen. Testing days were scheduled to occur on the last day of each 2-week intervention period. Twenty-four-hour interstitial glucose patterns were assessed by CGM during the second week of each 2-week intervention period. On the last day of each intervention period, a meal tolerance test was performed. Participants arrived at our clinical research facility after a 10-h overnight fast. Upon arrival, a fasting blood draw was obtained. Participants next consumed the same breakfast type (NPNF, NPHF, HPNF, and HPHF) that they had eaten for the preceding 2-week dietary intervention period. Participants were asked to consume the entire breakfast in no more than 15 min. Postprandial blood draws were obtained hourly for 4 h after the completion of breakfast. Fasting and postprandial serum samples were analyzed for glucose and insulin concentrations. Each 2-week period of dietary intervention was separated by $\geq$15 days (mean: 17 days, range: 15–36 days) during which time the participants were asked to consume their habitual diets. Study investigators (with the exception of the research dietitian, AJW) and participants were blinded to the protein and fiber content of the breakfast treatments during the study data collection period.

2.3. Breakfast Characteristics

All breakfast recipes (Tables S1–S16 were designed by a research dietitian (AJW) using ProNutra (Release 3.2, Viocare Technologies, Inc., Princeton, NJ, USA) and were prepared by metabolic research kitchen staff in conjunction with the NIH-supported bionutrition center at Purdue University. Breakfasts were provided to the participants to consume either on-site or at a self-chosen location. Four varieties (egg and potato casserole, quiche, breakfast sandwich, and breakfast burrito) of each breakfast type were provided within each 2-week intervention period to provide variety. Within each breakfast variety, pilot testing was completed to ensure comparable palatability and textural characteristics across NPNF, NPHF, HPNF, and HPHF breakfasts. While all breakfast varieties were designed to achieve the similar energy, macronutrient, and fiber amounts, the breakfast burrito was consumed on all testing days to provide additional consistency (Table 1).

Table 1. Energy and macronutrient distribution of provided breakfast treatments.

Dietary Variables	Breakfast Treatments			
	NPNF	HPNF	NPHF	HPHF
* Energy (kcal)	396	397	387	386
Available Carbohydrate (g)	51	50	51	48
Sugar (g)	18	22	11	14
Total Fiber (g)	2	2	8	8
Soluble Fiber (g)	0	1	6	7
Insoluble Fiber (g)	2	1	2	1
Total Protein (g)	12.5	25	12.5	25
Total Fat (g)	16	10	14	10
Saturated Fat (g)	4	3	4	3
Monounsaturated Fat (g)	6	3	6	3
Polyunsaturated Fat (g)	3	1	2	1
Trans Fat (g)	0	0	0	0
Cholesterol (mg)	114	325	114	325
Sodium (mg)	767	723	765	720

* Metabolizable energy. Data are based on information from ProNutra, Release 3.2, Viocare Technologies, Inc., Princeton, NJ, USA. NPNF: Normal Protein + Normal Fiber; HPNF: High Protein + Normal Fiber; NPHF: Normal Protein + High Fiber; HPHF: High Protein + High Fiber.

All four breakfast types (NPNF, NPHF, HPNF, and HPHF) provided ~400 kcals of metabolizable energy and contained ~50 g of available carbohydrate. High and normal protein were defined as 25 g and 12.5 g of protein, respectively. The increases in breakfast protein content for HPNF and HPHF were achieved by the addition of whole eggs and/or egg products such as egg white powder; and fat content was reduced to maintain similar total energy content among breakfast types. The high and normal fiber intakes were defined as 8 g, and 2 g, respectively. The additional fiber in NPHF and HPHF was achieved by adding powdered psyllium husk to the meals, which was shown to reduce postprandial glucose responses [30,31] and can easily be incorporated into meals for participant and investigator blinding. The energy, protein, and fiber content of the NPNF breakfasts were designed to resemble reported breakfast characteristics for adult males and females as described in the 2013–2014 What We Eat in America data tables [43]. The protein contents of HPNF and HPHF were doubled to 25 g (25% of energy at breakfast), which is consistent with published definitions of HP diets [48,49].

2.4. Dietary Intake

Self-selected food and beverage intakes during each intervention period were determined using the multiple-pass approach on three unscheduled days (one weekend day and two non-consecutive weekdays) and analyzed by the research dietitian using Nutrition Data System for Research

(NDSR) software, version 2013 (Nutrition Coordinating Center, Univ. MN, Minneapolis, MN, USA). Two-dimensional food portion visuals (Nutrition Coordinating Center, Univ. MN, Minneapolis, MN, USA) were used to assist subjects in estimating portion sizes.

2.5. Body Composition

Standing height without shoes was measured during baseline with a wall-mounted stadiometer. Whole body mass, fat mass, and lean mass were also determined at baseline using air displacement plethysmography (BOD POD, COSMED USA, Concord, CA, USA). Body mass index was calculated as body mass divided by height squared (kg/m^2).

2.6. 24-h Glucose (CGM)

A Medtronic iPro2 Professional CGM device (Northridge, CA, USA) was used to obtain 24-h continuous interstitial glucose concentration data from study participants during the last 7 days of each dietary intervention period. The glucose oxidase-based sensor inserted into the abdominal area at least 5 cm away from the umbilicus obtain an interstitial glucose measurement every 10 s and a recorder stored a smoothed and filtered average of these values every 5 min. Data obtained on the first and last day while participants wore the CGM device were excluded to obtain 24-h glucose data within periods where CGM sensor functional life was ideal. We considered 24-h glucose data valid when three or more self-monitoring glucose reading (finger sticks) were documented for calibration of CGM sensor glucose data [50]. CGM data were used to calculate 24-h interstitial glucose peak, mean, coefficient of variation (CV) and total area under the curve (AUC). The group mean and peak glucose were calculated from the individual participants' means of 2–5 days of useable CGM data. Similarly, group CV was calculated as mean of the ratio of the individual participants' standard deviation to mean. Also, in a subset of participants, the CGM data were used to document the postprandial glucose responses for 75 min after participants consumed the same trial-specific breakfast test treatment (breakfast burrito) as consumed during the corresponding meal tolerance test and also consumed their next meal or beverage by 75 min after consuming the test-specific breakfast treatment. Only participants who provided these data (obtained on different days) were used to graphically show the postprandial glucose responses in more detail (interstitial fluid samples every 5 min) to complement blood sampling (serum samples every hour) during the meal tolerance tests.

2.7. Biochemical Analyses and Calculation

Each blood sample was collected into vials containing serum separator and silica clot activator that were inverted several times and maintained at room temperature for 45 min to allow clotting and then centrifuged at 4 °C for 10 min at 4400 rpm. The resulting serum aliquots were stored at −80 °C until thawed for measurements of glucose by enzymatic colorimetry using an oxidase method on a COBAS Integra 400 analyzer (Roche Diagnostic Systems USA, Indianapolis, Indiana) and insulin by an electrochemiluminescence immunoassay method on the Elecsys 2010 analyzer (Roche Diagnostic USA, Indianapolis, Indiana). The trapezoidal method [51] was used to calculate total AUC for glucose and insulin at 0–120 min, 120–240 min, and 0–240 min time periods. The homeostatic model assessment (HOMA) insulin resistance (HOMA-IR), HOMA β-cell function (HOMA-%β) and whole-body (composite) insulin sensitivity index (ISI) were calculated as previously described [52,53].

2.8. Statistical Analysis

Independent *t*-test was used to assess baseline metabolic health indices between the individuals who completed vs. those who did not complete the study. Doubly repeated-measures ANOVA (PROC MIXED) was used to assess the effects of protein intake (normal vs. high), fiber intake (normal vs. high), and time (fasting-state (0) vs. 60 vs. 120 vs. 180 vs. 240 min), protein × time, fiber × time, and protein × fiber × time interactions on serum fasting and postprandial glucose and insulin. The 2 repeated factors in our model were time and intervention period. Repeated-measures

ANOVA (PROC MIXED) was used to assess the effects of breakfast meal treatments on 0–120, 120–240, and 0–240 min AUCs; 24-h interstitial glucose peak, mean, and CV, and predictive indices of glucose control measures HOMA-IR, HOMA-%β, and ISI. Data are presented as unadjusted mean ± standard deviation (SD) for participant characteristics and mean ± standard error of the mean (SEM) for all other results. We adjusted for fasting-dependent variable values (only when the outcome variable was expressed as AUC), sex, breakfast treatment order (chronological testing order: Period 1 vs. Period 2 vs. Period 3 vs. Period 4), and intervention carryover effect, as previously described [54]. Post hoc analyses were performed using Tukey–Kramer adjustment for multiple comparisons. Statistical significance was set using $\alpha = 0.05$, two-tailed. Statistical Analysis Systems software, version 9.3 (SAS Institute Inc., Cary, NC, USA) was used to perform all statistical analyses.

3. Results

3.1. *Participant Characteristics*

Participants were apparently healthy young overweight adults (seven females, 13 males). Baseline fasting glucose, lipid and lipoprotein concentrations were within the clinically normal reference ranges (Table 2).

Table 2. Baseline participant characteristics.

Variable	Mean ± SD
Age (years)	26 ± 5
Height (cm)	175 ± 10
Body Mass (kg)	83.4 ± 10.2
BMI (kg/m^2)	27.0 ± 1.3
% Body Fat	26.4 ± 9.5
Serum glucose (mmol/L)	5.2 ± 0.3
Total cholesterol (mmol/L)	4.3 ± 0.5
Low-density lipoprotein cholesterol (mmol/L)	2.6 ± 0.5
High-density lipoprotein cholesterol (mmol/L)	1.2 ± 0.2
Triglycerides (mmol/L)	1.1 ± 0.4

Values are means ± standard deviation (SD) for $n = 20$ participants. BMI: body mass index.

3.2. *Breakfast Treatments Effect on Outcome Measures*

3.2.1. The Effect of Breakfast Treatment on Fasting Glucose and Insulin Variables

Fasting serum glucose, insulin, and predictive indices of glucose control including HOMA-IR, ISI, and HOMA-β (%) measured on the last day of each two-week breakfast treatment were not different among treatments (Table 3).

Table 3. Fasting serum glucose, insulin, and indices of glucose control after two weeks of breakfast meals consumption.

Fasting Variables	Breakfast Treatments				
	NPNF	HPNF	NPHF	HPHF	*p*
Glucose (mmol/L)	5.3 ± 0.2	5.3 ± 0.2	5.2 ±0.1	5.2 ± 0.2	0.924
Insulin (pmol/L)	36 ± 6	36 ± 6	42 ± 6	42 ± 6	0.695
HOMA-IR	1.39 ± 0.1	1.51 ± 0.2	1.55 ± 0.2	1.54 ± 0.2	0.713
ISI	33 ± 5.2	32 ± 4.7	30 ± 5.6	31 ± 4.3	0.803
HOMA-β (%)	79 ± 10.2	79 ± 9.5	115 ± 36.9	88 ± 18.2	0.740

$n = 20$. Estimates are mean ± SEM. Homeostatic model assessment (HOMA) insulin resistance (HOMA-IR), HOMA β-cell function (HOMA-%β); whole-body (composite) insulin sensitivity index (ISI). The main effects of protein (high vs. low) and fiber (high vs. low) and their interaction on these fasting variables were assessed using a repeated-measures PROC mixed effects model, adjusting for sex, dietary treatment order, and carryover effect. NPNF: Normal Protein + Normal Fiber; HPNF: High Protein + Normal Fiber; NPHF: Normal Protein + High Fiber; HPHF: High Protein + High Fiber.

3.2.2. Time Course of Postprandial Glucose and Insulin Responses (AUC)

Results from meal tolerance testing showed that over time, postprandial glucose (p = 0.005) and insulin (p < 0.0001) responses occurred. Compared to fasting (time 0), insulin was higher at 60 and 120 min and glucose was lower at 60 min. The protein and/or fiber contents of the breakfast treatments did not affect 240-min glucose AUC. Protein intake did not affect 240-min insulin AUC, while higher fiber intake lowered 240-min insulin AUC (p = 0.030). Further analysis of the insulin AUCs indicated that higher fiber intake reduced insulin AUC at 120–240 min (p = 0.002), but not at 0–120 min (p = 0.245) (Figures 2 and 3). The apparent lack of a postprandial rise in glucose prompted an assessment of CGM-based interstitial glucose data from days that participants consumed the same treatment-specific breakfast burritos. Indeed, interstitial glucose increased after consumption of each breakfast meal treatment, peaking after about 30 min, and decreasing to baseline concentrations by 60–75 min (Figure 4). An effect was observed for fiber (p = 0.017) but not protein (p = 0.631) or their interaction (p = 0.795).

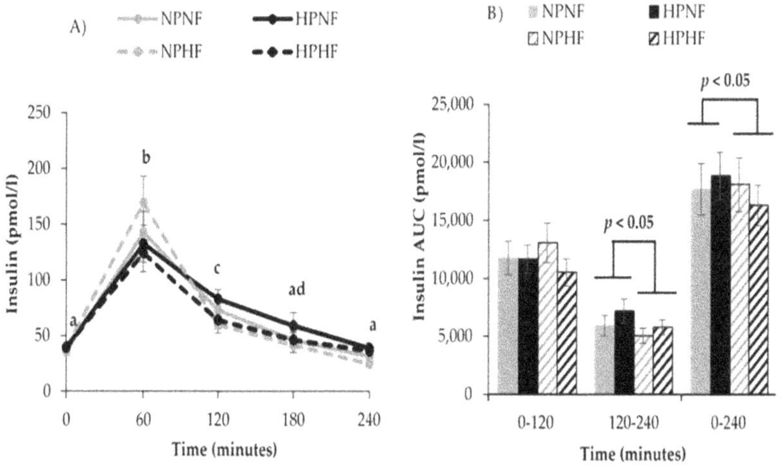

Figure 2. Postprandial time course (**A**) and total area under the curve (AUC) (**B**) for insulin response to breakfast treatments. Postprandial time points with different letters are statistically different (main effect of time, $p < 0.05$). $n = 20$, Estimates are unadjusted mean ± SEM. The main effects of protein (high vs. low) and fiber (high vs. low) and their interaction on postprandial insulin were assessed using a repeated-measures PROC mixed effects model, adjusting with fasting glucose (AUC only), for sex, dietary treatment order, and carryover effect. An effect was observed for fiber at 120–240 min (p = 0.002) and 0–240 min (p = 0.030) but not protein at 120–240 min (p = 0.113) or 0–240 min (p = 0.569) or their interaction (p = 0.944). NPNF: Normal Protein + Normal Fiber; HPNF: High Protein + Normal Fiber; NPHF: Normal Protein + High Fiber; HPHF: High Protein + High Fiber.

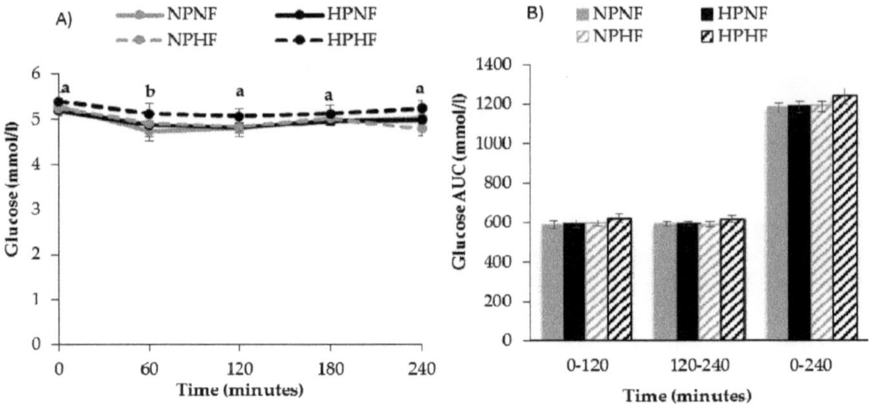

Figure 3. Postprandial time course (**A**) and total area under the curve (AUC) (**B**) for glucose response to breakfast treatments. n = 20, Estimates are unadjusted mean ± SEM. Values without a common letter are different, $p < 0.05$. The main effects of protein (high vs. low) and fiber (high vs. low) and their interaction on glucose were assessed using a repeated-measures PROC mixed effects model, adjusting for fasting glucose (AUC only), sex, dietary treatment order, and carryover effects. No effect or interaction effect was observed. NPNF: Normal Protein + Normal Fiber; HPNF: High Protein + Normal Fiber; NPHF: Normal Protein + High Fiber; HPHF: High Protein + High Fiber.

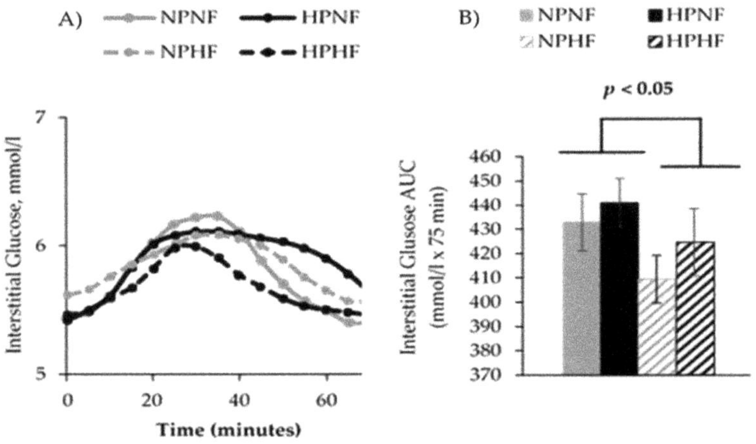

Figure 4. Postprandial time course (**A**) and total area under the curve (AUC) (**B**) for continuous glucose monitoring (CGM)-measured interstitial glucose after treatment-specific breakfast test meals (breakfast burrito) were consumed. Estimates are unadjusted mean ± SEM. The main effects of protein (high vs. low) and fiber (high vs. low) and their interaction on postprandial interstitial glucose were assessed using a repeated-measures PROC mixed effects model, adjusting with fasting glucose (AUC only), for sex, dietary treatment order, and carryover effect. An effect was observed for fiber (p = 0.017) but not protein (p = 0.631) or their interaction (p = 0.795). NPNF: Normal Protein + Normal Fiber; HPNF: High Protein + Normal Fiber; NPHF: Normal Protein + High Fiber; HPHF: High Protein + High Fiber. NPNF: n = 11, HPNF: n = 15, NPHF: n = 14, HPHF: n = 14.

3.3. 24-h Interstitial Glucose Variables

Among the four breakfast treatments, we did not observe differential responses in the interstitial glucose 24-h peak (p = 0.768), mean (p = 0.255), and CV (p = 0.534) and AUC (p = 0.179) (Table 4). Comparable 24-h interstitial glucose profiles were observed for all breakfast treatments (Supplementary Figure S1).

Table 4. Breakfast treatment effects on 24-h interstitial glucose variables.

Glucose Variables	Breakfast Treatments				
	NPNF	HPNF	NPHF	HPHF	p
Peak (mmol/L)	7.4 ± 0.2	7.1 ± 0.2	7.2 ± 0.1	7.2 ± 0.2	0.768
Mean (mmol/L)	5.5 ± 0.1	5.5 ± 0.1	5.5 ± 0.1	5.2 ± 0.1	0.255
Variability (CV)	0.99 ± 0.54	0.33 ± 0.23	0.30 ± 0.24	0.60 ± 0.38	0.534
AUC (mmol/L × 1440 min)	7982 ± 109	7977 ± 123	7755 ± 109	7860 ± 104	0.179

n = 19. Estimates are mean ± SEM. CV, coefficient of variation. AUC: total area under the curve. The main effects of protein (high vs. low) and fiber (high vs. low) and their interaction on 24-h interstitial glucose variables were assessed using a repeated-measures PROC mixed effects model, adjusting for sex, dietary treatment order, and carryover effect. No effect was observed for fiber and protein or their interaction. NPNF: Normal Protein + Normal Fiber; HPNF: High Protein + Normal Fiber; NPHF: Normal Protein + High Fiber; HPHF: High Protein + High Fiber.

3.4. Daily Energy and Macronutrients Intake

Among the four breakfast treatments, we did not observe differential responses in either the non-breakfast energy intake (self-chosen energy intake) (p = 0.421) or daily energy intakes (breakfast energy + self-chosen energy intakes after breakfast meals) (p = 0.394) (Supplementary Table S17 and S18), respectively. While we did not observe differences with the non-breakfast macronutrients intakes (Supplementary Table S17), we did observe differences in the daily total dietary fiber (p = 0.021), soluble fiber (p < 0.0001), and polyunsaturated fatty acids (p = 0.015) intakes but not the other macronutrients assessed (Supplementary Table S18).

4. Discussion

We conducted this study with the primary aim to assess the combined effect of higher intakes of protein and fiber consumed daily at breakfast over a 2-week period on postprandial glucose and insulin responses. We hypothesized that increasing protein and fiber amounts at breakfast would blunt postprandial serum glucose responses compared to increasing either protein or fiber alone. Contrary to our hypotheses, we observed that increasing protein and fiber amounts at breakfast did not influence postprandial glucose responses in overweight young adults. However, we observed an effect of fiber on insulin response (AUC). Increasing fiber lowered both the last two hours (120–240 min) and the composite 240-min insulin AUCs. Also, we did not observe protein and/or fiber breakfast meal effects on 24-h interstitial glucose or indices of glucose control.

Results from the meal tolerance tests suggested the lack of a postprandial glucose response that may be explained by the timing of blood sampling in the current study. Specifically, it is likely that postprandial glucose concentrations peaked and began returning to baseline levels before the first postprandial sample 60 min after breakfast. This is supported by interstitial glucose data obtained via CGM that showed peak glucose concentrations approximately 30 min after breakfast and declining to baseline concentration by 60–75 min. Generally, the expected postprandial glucose peak occurs one hour postprandial in overweight and obese adults [46]. This supported our choice of hourly blood sampling for the meal tolerance testing because our study participants were overweight adults. Other studies that included varying amounts of fiber [55] and protein [44,56] to meals also reported shorter postprandial glucose peaks occurring within 30–45 min but declining to either baseline or below baseline glucose concentration by 60 min. However, a modestly elevated postprandial insulin at 60 min was concurrently reported by those studies with meal tolerance testing. Our results are consistent with such studies. We observed that glucose concentration 60 min after breakfast was slightly, but statistically, lower than the fasting serum glucose concentration. Our results, together with others, suggest that future studies must always use frequent blood sampling (15-min interval within the first hour of feeding), particularly when both fiber and protein amounts are varied in test meals, to possibly avoid missing important data points within the first hour after feeding.

Studies assessing whether the consumption of higher amounts of protein and fiber simultaneously would better attenuate postprandial glucose response compared to when either protein or fiber is increased and consumed separately are lacking. To our knowledge, only one study assessed the effects of a moderate protein (from egg source) and high fiber (whole grains) breakfast treatment (protein = 20 g, fiber = 7 g, carbohydrates = 45 g) compared with a refined rice cereal breakfast (protein = 10 g, fiber = 1 g, carbohydrate = 55 g) [57]. Bonnema et al. [57] reported an attenuation of 3.5-h AUC glucose with the moderate protein and high fiber breakfast. Results of insulin AUC were not reported. Of note, the difference in carbohydrate content of those breakfasts may explain the glucose results as opposed to the combined effect of protein and fiber. In contrast, one previous study [58] systematically assessed the individual and combined effects of low vs. high glycemic index (GI) and protein breakfast treatments on postprandial insulin and glucose responses. Makris et al. [58] found that combining higher amounts of protein and low GI simultaneously did not have an effect on postprandial insulin and glucose responses. However, intake of higher amounts of the low GI breakfast meal attenuated postprandial insulin and glucose responses. We also did not observe an additive effect with intake of higher amounts of protein and fiber on postprandial insulin and glucose. Collectively, the expected favorable additive effect with increasing the amount of protein and either low GI carbohydrates or fiber from whole grains sources and fiber per se on postprandial insulin and glucose responses is inconclusive.

Our results partially supported the favorable metabolic effects established for soluble viscous fibers. The 6-g difference between the normal fiber (2 g) and high fiber (8 g) breakfast treatments was achieved by adding psyllium husk powder, which is known as a soluble fiber. We observed that increasing soluble fiber intake attenuated the postprandial insulin response. Other studies noted that increasing soluble fiber when a meal had greater amounts of high glycemic index foods/metabolizable carbohydrate content attenuated postprandial glucose [55,59] and insulin [55] responses. The lowering of insulin with increasing dietary fiber intake that was observed in our study is consistent with previous findings [27,55,60]. Reducing postprandial insulin with higher fiber intakes has beneficial metabolic effects in healthy overweight individuals who are at risk of developing hyperinsulinemia, an early abnormality preceding the development of type 2 diabetes. Insulin resistance with concurrent compensatory hyperinsulinemia is a major feature that underlies the development of metabolic morbidities, particularly, type 2 diabetes [61]. This compensatory elevation of insulin secretion is usually needed to achieve a normal postprandial glucose response in overweight and obese individuals [62] after a meal. Intervention strategies that alleviate the need for elevated insulin secretion for glucose clearance are beneficial. While dietary interventions that vary dietary macronutrient composition without inducing weight lost do not consistently improve insulin resistance, manipulating the dietary macronutrient content has been documented to impact the insulin resistance-induced hyperinsulinemia [46]. Therefore, increasing dietary fiber supported improvement in insulin sensitivity (lower insulin concentration to normalize blood glucose) as previously established [24,47].

In addition to assessing postprandial glucose and insulin responses by meal tolerance testing, our study design allowed us to evaluate potential "second meal effects" with CGM. Jenkins et al. [63] defined second meal effects as an effect of a first meal on the postprandial glucose response after eating the second meal. Consuming higher amounts of fiber and protein were previously shown to elicit "second meal effects" by reducing postprandial glucose responses following a second meal [64–67]. Other studies also reported an attenuation of daylong glucose (lunch and dinner meals) with intake of low GI foods [68]. Assessing such a prolonged effect of consuming a breakfast with controlled protein and fiber amounts on subsequent and uncontrolled meals was an important and novel aim of the current study. However, 24-h interstitial glucose variables, including AUC, were not influenced by the 4 breakfast treatments used in the current study, which suggests a lack of a "second meal effect". Our results may be due to the observed large variability between participants' self-selected intake after the breakfast meal (Tables S17 and S18). Our findings could also suggest that the inclusion of fiber in multiple meals across the day may be needed with the intake of a typical Western diet to improve daily glycemic control.

One limitation of the study was that the lack of provision of a standard meal the night before the acute measurement to metabolically stabilize our study participants may have confounded our study outcomes. Previous studies suggest a residual effect from dinner meals may impact the next morning glucose profile [68] particularly with high fiber intake. Another limitation was the fact that we could not match sugar, MUFA, PUFA, and total fat, across normal vs. the high breakfast treatment meals although these nutrients may influence our results. However, the magnitude of the differences in the amounts of the afore-mentioned nutrients between the normal vs. high protein and fiber breakfast treatments where not numerically substantial. Lastly, our study findings are only generalizable to overweight young adults. A strength of this study is that both researchers and study participants were blinded to the study dietary treatment. This potentially eliminates any biases with our dietary manipulation that may influence our study outcomes. Another strength is that the 2-week dietary acclimation period before our postprandial responses were assessed allowed us to determine the prolonged effects of consumption of protein and fiber breakfasts beyond a single meal.

5. Conclusions

In conclusion, consumption of a breakfast meal with both higher protein and fiber content did not differentially influence postprandial glucose response and 24-h glucose peak and AUC compared to the other three breakfast treatments. However, increasing fiber had an attenuation effect on the postprandial insulin response. Therefore, doubling the amount of protein from 12.5 g to 25 g/meal and quadrupling fiber from 2 to 8 g/meal simultaneously at breakfast may not be an effective therapeutic strategy to improve insulin and glucose responses acutely; however, higher fiber intake at breakfast may be effective for lowering the postprandial insulin response in healthy overweight, young adults.

Supplementary Materials: The following are available online at www.mdpi.com/2072-6643/9/4/352/s1, Figure S1: 24-hour time course interstitial glucose from CGM to breakfast treatments and self-selected intakes after provided breakfast. $n = 19$, Estimates are unadjusted means. NPNF: Normal Protein + Normal Fiber; HPNF: High Protein + Normal Fiber; NPHF: Normal Protein + High Fiber; HPHF: High Protein + High Fiber, Table S1: NPNF breakfast burrito recipe, Table S2: HPNF breakfast burrito recipe, Table S3: NPHF breakfast burrito recipe, Table S4: HPHF breakfast burrito recipe, Table S5: NPNF breakfast sandwich recipe, Table S6: NPHP breakfast sandwich recipe, Table S7: NPHF breakfast sandwich recipe, Table S8: HPHF breakfast sandwich recipe, Table S9: NPNF breakfast casserole recipe, Table S10: HPNF breakfast casserole recipe, Table S11: NPHF breakfast casserole recipe, Table S12: HPHF breakfast casserole recipe, Table S13: NPNF breakfast quiche recipe, Table S14: HPNF breakfast quiche recipe, Table S15: NPHF breakfast quiche recipe, Table S16: HPHF breakfast quiche recipe: Table S17: Non-breakfast energy and macronutrient distribution, Table S18: Daily energy and macronutrient distribution.

Acknowledgments: Funding: American Egg Board/Egg Nutrition Center; NIH Indiana Clinical and Translational Sciences Institute, Clinical Research Center (Grant #UL1TR001108); USDA 2011-38420-20038. Financial supporters had no role in the design and conduct of the study or collection, analysis, and interpretation of the data. We are also grateful for Doug Maish EMS-P, CCRC for his assistance with clinical testing and Gerald W. Wehr (MD), IU School of Medicine-West Lafayette, our study physician.

Author Contributions: M.A.M., W.W.C., and R.D.S. designed the research project; A.F.A. and R.D.S. conducted the research; A.J.W. designed the intervention diets; N.C. conducted statistical analysis; A.F.A. and W.W.C. wrote the manuscript; A.F.A., W.W.W., M.A.M. have primary responsibility for the final content. All authors take responsibility for the final content of the manuscript.

Conflicts of Interest: The authors declare no conflict of interest. The funding sponsors had no role in the design of the study; in the collection, analyses, or interpretation of data; in the writing of the manuscript, and in the decision to publish the results.

References

1. Geiss, L.S.; Pan, L.; Cadwell, B.; Gregg, E.W.; Benjamin, S.M.; Engelgau, M.M. Changes in Incidence of Diabetes in U.S. Adults, 1997–2003. *Am. J. Prev. Med.* **2006**, *30*, 371–377. [CrossRef] [PubMed]
2. Cowie, C.C.; Rust, K.F.; Byrd-Holt, D.D.; Eberhardt, M.S.; Flegal, K.M.; Engelgau, M.M.; Saydah, S.H.; Williams, D.E.; Geiss, L.S.; Gregg, E.W. Prevalence of diabetes and impaired fasting glucose in adults in the U.S. population: National Health And Nutrition Examination Survey 1999–2002. *Diabetes Care* **2006**, *29*, 1263–1268. [CrossRef] [PubMed]
3. Eckel, R.H.; Kahn, R.; Robertson, R.M.; Rizza, R.A. Preventing Cardiovascular Disease and Diabetes: A Call to Action From the American Diabetes Association and the American Heart Association. *Circulation* **2006**, *113*, 2943–2946. [CrossRef] [PubMed]
4. Thomas, T.; Pfeiffer, A.F. Foods for the prevention of diabetes: How do they work? *Diabetes Metab. Res. Rev.* **2012**, *28*, 25–49. [CrossRef] [PubMed]
5. Salas-Salvado, J.; Martinez-Gonzalez, M.A.; Bullo, M.; Ros, E. The role of diet in the prevention of type 2 diabetes. *Nutr. Metab. Cardiovasc. Dis.* **2011**, *21*, B32–B48. [CrossRef] [PubMed]
6. Wyness, L. Understanding the role of diet in type 2 diabetes prevention. *Br. J. Community Nurs.* **2009**, *14*, 374–379. [CrossRef] [PubMed]
7. Wheeler, M.L.; Dunbar, S.A.; Jaacks, L.M.; Karmally, W.; Mayer-Davis, E.J.; Wylie-Rosett, J.; Yancy, W.S., Jr. Macronutrients, food groups, and eating patterns in the management of diabetes: A systematic review of the literature, 2010. *Diabetes Care* **2012**, *35*, 434–445. [CrossRef] [PubMed]
8. Most, J.; Tosti, V.; Redman, L.M.; Fontana, L. Calorie restriction in humans: An update. *Ageing Res. Rev.* **2016**. [CrossRef] [PubMed]
9. Omodei, D.; Fontana, L. Calorie restriction and prevention of age-associated chronic disease. *FEBS Lett.* **2011**, *585*, 1537–1542. [CrossRef] [PubMed]
10. Cox, K.L.; Burke, V.; Morton, A.R.; Beilin, L.J.; Puddey, I.B. Independent and additive effects of energy restriction and exercise on glucose and insulin concentrations in sedentary overweight men. *Am. J. Clin. Nutr.* **2004**, *80*, 308–316. [PubMed]
11. Heymsfield, S.B.; Harp, J.B.; Reitman, M.L.; Beetsch, J.W.; Schoeller, D.A.; Erondu, N.; Pietrobelli, A. Why do obese patients not lose more weight when treated with low-calorie diets? A mechanistic perspective. *Am. J. Clin. Nutr.* **2007**, *85*, 346–354. [PubMed]
12. Blom, W.A.; Lluch, A.; Stafleu, A.; Vinoy, S.; Holst, J.J.; Schaafsma, G. Effect of a high-protein breakfast on the postprandial ghrelin response. *Am. J. Clin. Nutr.* **2006**, *83*, 211–220. [PubMed]
13. Erdmann, J.; Topsch, R.; Lippl, F.; Gussmann, P.; Schusdziarra, V. Postprandial response of plasma ghrelin levels to various test meals in relation to food intake, plasma insulin, and glucose. *J. Clin. Endocr. Metab.* **2004**, *89*, 3048–3054. [CrossRef] [PubMed]
14. Sheard, N.F.; Clark, N.G.; Brand-Miller, J.C.; Franz, M.J.; Pi-Sunyer, F.X.; Mayer-Davis, E.; Kulkarni, K.; Geil, P. Dietary carbohydrate (amount and type) in the prevention and management of diabetes: A statement by the american diabetes association. *Diabetes Care* **2004**, *27*, 2266–2271. [CrossRef] [PubMed]
15. Franc, S.; Dardari, D.; Peschard, C.; Riveline, J.-P.; Biedzinski, M.; Boucherie, B.; Petit, C.; Requeda, E.; Mistretta, F.; Varroud-Vial, M.; Charpentier, G. Can Postprandial Blood Glucose Excursion Be Predicted in Type 2 Diabetes? *Diabetes Care* **2010**, *33*, 1913–1918. [CrossRef] [PubMed]
16. AlEssa, H.B.; Bhupathiraju, S.N.; Malik, V.S.; Wedick, N.M.; Campos, H.; Rosner, B.; Willett, W.C.; Hu, F.B. Carbohydrate quality and quantity and risk of type 2 diabetes in US women. *Am. J. Clin. Nutr.* **2015**, *102*, 1543–1553. [CrossRef] [PubMed]
17. Gross, L.S.; Li, L.; Ford, E.S.; Liu, S. Increased consumption of refined carbohydrates and the epidemic of type 2 diabetes in the United States: An ecologic assessment. *Am. J. Clin. Nutr.* **2004**, *79*, 774–779. [PubMed]
18. Hu, F.B. Are refined carbohydrates worse than saturated fat? *Am. J. Clin. Nutr.* **2010**, *91*, 1541–1542. [CrossRef] [PubMed]
19. Liu, S. Intake of Refined Carbohydrates and Whole Grain Foods in Relation to Risk of Type 2 Diabetes Mellitus and Coronary Heart Disease. *J. Am. Coll. Nutr.* **2002**, *21*, 298–306. [CrossRef] [PubMed]

20. Lichtenstein, A.H.; Appel, L.J.; Brands, M.; Carnethon, M.; Daniels, S.; Franch, H.A.; Franklin, B.; Kris-Etherton, P.; Harris, W.S.; Howard, B.; et al. Diet and Lifestyle Recommendations Revision 2006: A Scientific Statement From the American Heart Association Nutrition Committee. *Circulation* **2006**, *114*, 82–96. [CrossRef] [PubMed]
21. Beulens, J.W.J.; de Bruijne, L.M.; Stolk, R.P.; Peeters, P.H.M.; Bots, M.L.; Grobbee, D.E.; van der Schouw, Y.T. High Dietary Glycemic Load and Glycemic Index Increase Risk of Cardiovascular Disease Among Middle-Aged Women: A Population-Based Follow-Up Study. *J. Am. Coll. Cardiol.* **2007**, *50*, 14–21. [CrossRef] [PubMed]
22. McRorie, J.W. Evidence-Based Approach to Fiber Supplements and Clinically Meaningful Health Benefits, Part 1: What to Look for and How to Recommend an Effective Fiber Therapy. *Nutr. Today* **2015**, *50*, 82–89. [CrossRef] [PubMed]
23. Chutkan, R.; Fahey, G.; Wright, W.L.; McRorie, J. Viscous versus nonviscous soluble fiber supplements: Mechanisms and evidence for fiber-specific health benefits. *J. Am. Acad. Nurse Pract.* **2012**, *24*, 476–487. [CrossRef] [PubMed]
24. Jenkins, D.J.; Wolever, T.M.; Leeds, A.R.; Gassull, M.A.; Haisman, P.; Dilawari, J.; Goff, D.V.; Metz, G.L.; Alberti, K.G. Dietary fibres, fibre analogues, and glucose tolerance: Importance of viscosity. *Br. Med. J.* **1978**, *1*, 1392–1394. [CrossRef] [PubMed]
25. Jenkins, D.J.A.; Kendall, C.W.C.; Vuksan, V.; Vidgen, E.; Parker, T.; Faulkner, D.; Mehling, C.C.; Garsetti, M.; Testolin, G.; Cunnane, S.C.; et al. Soluble fiber intake at a dose approved by the US Food and Drug Administration for a claim of health benefits: Serum lipid risk factors for cardiovascular disease assessed in a randomized controlled crossover trial. *Am. J. Clin. Nutr.* **2002**, *75*, 834–839. [PubMed]
26. Dall'Alba, V.; Silva, F.M.; Antonio, J.P.; Steemburgo, T.; Royer, C.P.; Almeida, J.C.; Gross, J.L.; Azevedo, M.J. Improvement of the metabolic syndrome profile by soluble fibre–guar gum–in patients with type 2 diabetes: A randomised clinical trial. *Br. J. Nutr.* **2013**, *110*, 1601–1610. [CrossRef] [PubMed]
27. Cicero, A.G.; Derosa, G.; Bove, M.; Imola, F.; Borghi, C.; Gaddi, A. Psyllium improves dyslipidaemia, hyperglycaemia and hypertension, while guar gum reduces body weight more rapidly in patients affected by metabolic syndrome following an AHA Step 2 diet. *Mediterr. J. Nutr. Metab.* **2010**, *3*, 47–54. [CrossRef]
28. Gunness, P.; Gidley, M.J. Mechanisms underlying the cholesterol-lowering properties of soluble dietary fibre polysaccharides. *Food Funct.* **2010**, *1*, 149–155. [CrossRef] [PubMed]
29. Wolever, T.M.; Tosh, S.M.; Gibbs, A.L.; Brand-Miller, J.; Duncan, A.M.; Hart, V.; Lamarche, B.; Thomson, B.A.; Duss, R.; Wood, P.J. Physicochemical properties of oat beta-glucan influence its ability to reduce serum LDL cholesterol in humans: A randomized clinical trial. *Am. J. Clin. Nutr.* **2010**, *92*, 723–732. [CrossRef] [PubMed]
30. Gibb, R.D.; McRorie, J.W.; Russell, D.A.; Hasselblad, V.; D'Alessio, D.A. Psyllium fiber improves glycemic control proportional to loss of glycemic control: A meta-analysis of data in euglycemic subjects, patients at risk of type 2 diabetes mellitus, and patients being treated for type 2 diabetes mellitus. *Am. J. Clin. Nutr.* **2015**, *102*, 1604–1614. [CrossRef] [PubMed]
31. Pal, S.; Radavelli-Bagatini, S. Effects of psyllium on metabolic syndrome risk factors. *Obes. Rev.* **2012**, *13*, 1034–1047. [CrossRef] [PubMed]
32. McRorie, J.W. Evidence-Based Approach to Fiber Supplements and Clinically Meaningful Health Benefits, Part 2: What to Look for and How to Recommend an Effective Fiber Therapy. *Nutr. Today* **2015**, *50*, 90–97. [CrossRef] [PubMed]
33. Layman, D.K.; Baum, J.I. Dietary Protein Impact on Glycemic Control during Weight Loss. *J. Nutr.* **2004**, *134*, 968S–973S. [PubMed]
34. Salehi, A.; Gunnerud, U.; Muhammed, S.J.; Östman, E.; Holst, J.J.; Björck, I.; Rorsman, P. The insulinogenic effect of whey protein is partially mediated by a direct effect of amino acids and GIP on β-cells. *Nutr. Metab.* **2012**, *9*, 48. [CrossRef] [PubMed]
35. Nuttall, F.Q.; Gannon, M.C. Metabolic response of people with type 2 diabetes to a high protein diet. *Nutr. Metab. (Lond.)* **2004**, *1*, 6. [CrossRef] [PubMed]
36. Norton, L.E.; Wilson, G.J.; Layman, D.K.; Moulton, C.J.; Garlick, P.J. Leucine content of dietary proteins is a determinant of postprandial skeletal muscle protein synthesis in adult rats. *Nutr. Metab.* **2012**, *9*, 67. [CrossRef] [PubMed]
37. Djoussé, L.; Gaziano, J.M.; Buring, J.E.; Lee, I.M. Egg Consumption and Risk of Type 2 Diabetes in Men and Women. *Diabetes Care* **2009**, *32*, 295–300. [CrossRef] [PubMed]

38. Virtanen, J.K.; Mursu, J.; Tuomainen, T.-P.; Virtanen, H.E.K.; Voutilainen, S. Egg consumption and risk of incident type 2 diabetes in men: The Kuopio Ischaemic Heart Disease Risk Factor Study. *Am. J. Clin. Nutr.* **2015**, *101*, 1088–1096. [CrossRef] [PubMed]
39. Blesso, C.N.; Andersen, C.J.; Barona, J.; Volek, J.S.; Fernandez, M.L. Whole egg consumption improves lipoprotein profiles and insulin sensitivity to a greater extent than yolk-free egg substitute in individuals with metabolic syndrome. *Metabolism* **2013**, *62*, 400–410. [CrossRef] [PubMed]
40. Livesey, G.; Tagami, H. Interventions to lower the glycemic response to carbohydrate foods with a low-viscosity fiber (resistant maltodextrin): Meta-analysis of randomized controlled trials. *Am. J. Clin. Nutr.* **2009**, *89*, 114–125. [CrossRef] [PubMed]
41. Bell, K.J.; Smart, C.E.; Steil, G.M.; Brand-Miller, J.C.; King, B.; Wolpert, H.A. Impact of Fat, Protein, and Glycemic Index on Postprandial Glucose Control in Type 1 Diabetes: Implications for Intensive Diabetes Management in the Continuous Glucose Monitoring Era. *Diabetes Care* **2015**, *38*, 1008–1015. [CrossRef] [PubMed]
42. Baek, Y.H.; Jin, H.Y.; Lee, K.A.; Kang, S.M.; Kim, W.J.; Kim, M.G.; Park, J.H.; Chae, S.W.; Baek, H.S.; Park, T.S. The Correlation and Accuracy of Glucose Levels between Interstitial Fluid and Venous Plasma by Continuous Glucose Monitoring System. *Korean Diabetes J.* **2010**, *34*, 350–358. [CrossRef] [PubMed]
43. United States Department of Agriculture Agricultural Research Service. *What We Eat in America, NHANES Service*; United States Department of Agriculture Agricultural Research Service: Washington, DC, USA, 2011–2012. Available online: https://www.ars.usda.gov/northeast-area/beltsville-md/beltsville-human-nutrition-research-center/food-surveys-research-group/docs/wweia-data-tables/ (accessed on 31 March 2017).
44. Rains, T.M.; Leidy, H.J.; Sanoshy, K.D.; Lawless, A.L.; Maki, K.C. A randomized, controlled, crossover trial to assess the acute appetitive and metabolic effects of sausage and egg-based convenience breakfast meals in overweight premenopausal women. *J. Nutr.* **2015**, *14*, 17. [CrossRef] [PubMed]
45. Park, Y.-M.; Heden, T.D.; Liu, Y.; Nyhoff, L.M.; Thyfault, J.P.; Leidy, H.J.; Kanaley, J.A. A High-Protein Breakfast Induces Greater Insulin and Glucose-Dependent Insulinotropic Peptide Responses to a Subsequent Lunch Meal in Individuals with Type 2 Diabetes. *J. Nutr.* **2015**, *145*, 452–458. [CrossRef] [PubMed]
46. Jenkins, A.L.; Jenkins, D.J.A.; Wolever, T.M.S.; Rogovik, A.L.; Jovanovski, E.; Božikov, V.; Rahelić, D.; Vuksan, V. Comparable Postprandial Glucose Reductions with Viscous Fiber Blend Enriched Biscuits in Healthy Subjects and Patients with Diabetes Mellitus: Acute Randomized Controlled Clinical Trial. *Croat. Med. J.* **2008**, *49*, 772–782. [CrossRef] [PubMed]
47. Wolever, T.M.S.; Campbell, J.E.; Geleva, D.; Anderson, G.H. High-Fiber Cereal Reduces Postprandial Insulin Responses in Hyperinsulinemic but not Normoinsulinemic Subjects. *Diabetes Care* **2004**, *27*, 1281–1285. [CrossRef] [PubMed]
48. Halton, T.L.; Hu, F.B. The effects of high protein diets on thermogenesis, satiety and weight loss: A critical review. *J. Am. Coll. Nutr.* **2004**, *23*, 373–385. [CrossRef] [PubMed]
49. Kim, J.E.; O'Connor, L.E.; Sands, L.P.; Slebodnik, M.B.; Campbell, W.W. Effects of dietary protein intake on body composition changes after weight loss in older adults: A systematic review and meta-analysis. *Nutr. Rev.* **2016**, *74*, 210–224. [CrossRef] [PubMed]
50. Medtronic. *A Practical Guide to Continuous Glucose Monitoring*; Medtronic: North Ryde, Australia, 2011.
51. Potteiger, J.A.; Jacobsen, D.J.; Donnelly, J.E. A comparison of methods for analyzing glucose and insulin areas under the curve following nine months of exercise in overweight adults. *Int. J. Obes. Relat. Metab. Disord.* **2002**, *26*, 87–89. [CrossRef] [PubMed]
52. Matthews, D.R.; Hosker, J.P.; Rudenski, A.S.; Naylor, B.A.; Treacher, D.F.; Turner, R.C. Homeostasis model assessment: Insulin resistance and beta-cell function from fasting plasma glucose and insulin concentrations in man. *Diabetologia* **1985**, *28*, 412–419. [CrossRef] [PubMed]
53. Matsuda, M.; DeFronzo, R.A. Insulin sensitivity indices obtained from oral glucose tolerance testing: Comparison with the euglycemic insulin clamp. *Diabetes Care* **1999**, *22*, 1462–1470. [CrossRef] [PubMed]
54. Sayer, R.D.; Amankwaah, A.F.; Tamer, G.G.; Chen, N.; Wright, A.J.; Tregellas, J.R.; Cornier, M.-A.; Kareken, D.A.; Talavage, T.M.; McCrory, M.A.; et al. Effects of Dietary Protein and Fiber at Breakfast on Appetite, ad Libitum Energy Intake at Lunch, and Neural Responses to Visual Food Stimuli in Overweight Adults. *Nutrients* **2016**, *8*, 21. [CrossRef] [PubMed]

55. Potter, J.G.; Coffman, K.P.; Reid, R.L.; Krall, J.M.; Albrink, M.J. Effect of Test Meals of Varying Dietary Fiber Content on Plasma-Insulin and Glucose Response. *Am. J. Clin. Nutr.* **1981**, *34*, 328–334. [PubMed]
56. Acheson, K.J.; Blondel-Lubrano, A.; Oguey-Araymon, S.; Beaumont, M.; Emady-Azar, S.; Ammon-Zufferey, C.; Monnard, I.; Pinaud, S.; Nielsen-Moennoz, C.; Bovetto, L. Protein choices targeting thermogenesis and metabolism. *Am. J. Clin. Nutr.* **2011**, *93*, 525–534. [CrossRef] [PubMed]
57. Bonnema, A.L.; Altschwager, D.K.; Thomas, W.; Slavin, J.L. The effects of the combination of egg and fiber on appetite, glycemic response and food intake in normal weight adults—A randomized, controlled, crossover trial. *Int. J. Food Sci. Nutr.* **2016**, *67*, 723–731. [CrossRef] [PubMed]
58. Makris, A.P.; Borradaile, K.E.; Oliver, T.L.; Cassim, N.G.; Rosenbaum, D.L.; Boden, G.H.; Homko, C.J.; Foster, G.D. The Individual and Combined Effects of Glycemic Index and Protein on Glycemic Response, Hunger, and Energy Intake. *Obesity* **2011**, *19*, 2365–2373. [CrossRef] [PubMed]
59. Aller, R.; de Luis, D.A.; Izaola, O.; La Calle, F.; del Olmo, L.; Fernandez, L.; Arranz, T.; Hernandez, J.M.G. Effect of soluble fiber intake in lipid and glucose leves in healthy subjects: A randomized clinical trial. *Diabetes Res. Clin. Pract.* **2004**, *65*, 7–11. [CrossRef] [PubMed]
60. Karhunen, L.J.; Juvonen, K.R.; Flander, S.M.; Liukkonen, K.H.; Lahteenmaki, L.; Siloaho, M.; Laaksonen, D.E.; Herzig, K.H.; Uusitupa, M.I.; Poutanen, K.S. A Psyllium Fiber-Enriched Meal Strongly Attenuates Postprandial Gastrointestinal Peptide Release in Healthy Young Adults. *J. Nutr.* **2010**, *140*, 737–744. [CrossRef] [PubMed]
61. Reaven, G.M. The insulin resistance syndrome: Definition and dietary approaches to treatment. *Annu. Rev. Nutr.* **2005**, *25*, 391–406. [CrossRef] [PubMed]
62. Kn, F. *Metabolic Regulation*, 3rd ed.; Blackwell Publishing: Hoboken, NJ, USA, 2010.
63. Jenkins, D.J.A.; Wolever, T.M.S.; Nineham, R.; Sarson, D.L.; Bloom, S.R.; Ahern, J.; Alberti, K.G.M.M.; Hockaday, T.D.R. Improved glucose tolerance four hours after taking guar with glucose. *Diabetologia* **1980**, *19*, 21–24. [CrossRef] [PubMed]
64. O'Connor, L.E.; Campbell, W.W. A novel fiber composite ingredient incorporated into a beverage and bar blunts postprandial serum glucose and insulin responses: A randomized controlled trial. *Nutr. Res.* **2016**, *36*, 253–261. [CrossRef] [PubMed]
65. Chen, M.J.; Jovanovic, A.; Taylor, R. Utilizing the Second-Meal Effect in Type 2 Diabetes: Practical Use of a Soya-Yogurt Snack. *Diabetes Care* **2010**, *33*, 2552–2554. [CrossRef] [PubMed]
66. Clark, C.A.; Gardiner, J.; McBurney, M.I.; Anderson, S.; Weatherspoon, L.J.; Henry, D.N.; Hord, N.G. Effects of breakfast meal composition on second meal metabolic responses in adults with type 2 diabetes mellitus. *Eur. J. Clin. Nutr.* **2006**, *60*, 1122–1129. [CrossRef] [PubMed]
67. Jovanovic, A.; Gerrard, J.; Taylor, R. The Second-Meal Phenomenon in Type 2 Diabetes. *Diabetes Care* **2009**, *32*, 1199–1201. [CrossRef] [PubMed]
68. Nilsson, A.C.; Östman, E.M.; Granfeldt, Y.; Björck, I.M.E. Effect of cereal test breakfasts differing in glycemic index and content of indigestible carbohydrates on daylong glucose tolerance in healthy subjects. *Am. J. Clin. Nutr.* **2008**, *87*, 645–654. [PubMed]

nutrients

MDPI

Article

Associations between Dietary Fiber Intake in Infancy and Cardiometabolic Health at School Age: The Generation R Study

Rafaëlle M. A. van Gijssel [1,2,†], Kim V. E. Braun [1,†], Jessica C. Kiefte-de Jong [1,3], Vincent W. V. Jaddoe [1,2,4], Oscar H. Franco [1] and Trudy Voortman [1,*]

1 The Department of Epidemiology, Erasmus MC, University Medical Center, Office Na-2909, P.O. Box 2040, Rotterdam 3000 CA, The Netherlands; rmavgijssel@gmail.com (R.M.A.v.G.); k.braun@erasmusmc.nl (K.V.E.B.); j.c.kiefte-dejong@erasmusmc.nl (J.C.K.-d.J.); v.jaddoe@erasmusmc.nl (V.W.V.J.); o.franco@erasmusmc.nl (O.H.F.)

2 The Generation R Study Group, Erasmus MC, University Medical Center, Rotterdam 3000 CA, The Netherlands

3 Department of Global Public Health, Leiden University, The Hague 3595 DG, The Netherlands

4 The Department of Pediatrics, Erasmus MC, University Medical Center, Rotterdam 3000 CA, The Netherlands

* Correspondence: trudy.voortman@erasmusmc.nl; Tel.: +31-10-704-3536; Fax: +31-10-704-4657

† These authors contributed equally to this work.

Received: 17 June 2016; Accepted: 23 August 2016; Published: 30 August 2016

Abstract: Dietary fiber (DF) intake may be beneficial for cardiometabolic health. However, whether this already occurs in early childhood is unclear. We investigated associations between DF intake in infancy and cardiometabolic health in childhood among 2032 children participating in a population-based cohort in The Netherlands. Information on DF intake at a median age of 12.9 months was collected using a food-frequency questionnaire. DF was adjusted for energy intake using the residual method. At age 6 years, body fat percentage, high-density lipoprotein (HDL)-cholesterol, insulin, triglycerides, and blood pressure were assessed and expressed in age- and sex-specific standard deviation scores (SDS). These five factors were combined into a cardiometabolic risk factor score. In models adjusted for several parental and child covariates, a higher DF intake was associated with a lower cardiometabolic risk factor score. When we examined individual cardiometabolic factors, we observed that a 1 g/day higher energy-adjusted DF intake was associated with 0.026 SDS higher HDL-cholesterol (95% CI 0.009, 0.042), and 0.020 SDS lower triglycerides (95% CI −0.037, −0.003), but not with body fat, insulin, or blood pressure. Results were similar for DF with and without adjustment for energy intake. Our findings suggest that higher DF intake in infancy may be associated with better cardiometabolic health in later childhood.

Keywords: body fat; blood pressure; cohort; dietary fiber; early childhood; HDL-C; insulin; triglyceride

1. Introduction

Several studies suggest that dietary fiber (DF) is beneficial for various aspects of cardiometabolic health in adults, such as lower insulin and cholesterol concentrations, and a lower blood pressure [1,2]. High DF intake has been proposed to lower cardiometabolic risk through lower absorption of cholesterol and fat, improved glucose and insulin metabolism after meals, or via increased satiety and a subsequent lower energy intake [3]. However, many of the cardiometabolic health consequences in adulthood are preceded by abnormalities that might begin in childhood [4]. For example, overweight often already occurs in early childhood and is associated with a higher risk of overweight, type 2 diabetes, hypertension, dyslipidemia, and atherosclerosis in later life [4,5]. Small changes in other cardiometabolic risk factors can also already start during childhood and predict later cardiometabolic disease risk [6,7]. Therefore, it is important to focus on cardiometabolic health and its determinants already in childhood. A few previous studies in children suggested that the beneficial effect of DF on cardiometabolic health may already be present in childhood: a higher DF intake was, for example, associated with a lower body fat percentage in children around the age of 9 years [8], and with lower serum total cholesterol in children at ages of 13 months to 9 years [9].

However, these previous studies on DF intake in children in relation to body composition and metabolic risk factors focused on school-age children and adolescents [8–16], whereas diet might be important for cardiometabolic health already earlier in childhood [17]. Whether DF intake in early childhood is associated with cardiometabolic risk remains unknown and there is a lack of well-founded guidelines for adequate DF intake in young children [18–20]. Potential effects of DF intake might also differ by type of DF, such as soluble versus insoluble DF [3,21–24]. An observational study in adolescents showed that a higher intake of specifically soluble DF was associated with a reduction of visceral body fat over a period of 2 years [13]. However, data about the effects of different sources of DF is scarce [3].

Therefore, we investigated the association between DF intake in infancy and cardiometabolic health at the age of 6 years in a large prospective cohort. Additionally, we examined whether associations were explained by differences in energy intake and we explored whether associations differ for DF from different food sources.

2. Subjects and Methods

2.1. Study Design and Subjects

In this study we examined data from The Generation R Study, a population-based prospective cohort study from fetal life onward in Rotterdam, The Netherlands [25]. Pregnant women were enrolled between April 2002 and January 2006, and 7893 live-born children were available for postnatal follow-up, of whom 4215 had a Dutch ethnic background [25].

Because the food-frequency questionnaire (FFQ) was designed for dietary assessment of a Dutch population and was validated in Dutch children, we restricted our analyses to Dutch children. Children without information on diet (n = 1778) or any of the cardiometabolic health measurements (n = 405) were excluded, resulting in a study population of 2032 children (Figure 1). Because not all of these children had information available on all outcomes, the population for analysis ranged from 1314 to 1995 per cardiometabolic outcome. The study was approved by the local Medical Ethics Committee of Erasmus Medical Center, Rotterdam (MEC 198.782/2001/31, 2001), and written consent was given by parents.

2.2. Dietary Intake Assessment

Dietary data were collected using a 211-item semiquantitative FFQ, as described in detail elsewhere [26,27]. This FFQ was validated against three 24 h-recalls and the intraclass correlation coefficient was 0.7 for DF intake [27]. The median age of the children was 12.9 (interquartile range (IQR) 12.6–13.9) months. Total DF intake was calculated using the Dutch Food Composition Table (NEVO), where DF is defined as plant cell wall components that are not digestible by human digestive enzymes, including for example, lignin, cellulose, hemicellulose, and pectin [28]. Thereafter, we divided DF intake in DF from four different food groups, based on the different types of DF that are mainly present in these food groups [3,22]: (1) DF from cereals, as proxy for insoluble DF, defined as fiber from bread, cereals, pasta, rice, cookies, cakes, pastries, crackers, and ready-to-eat meals; (2) DF from potatoes and potato products, containing resistant starch; (3) DF from fruits and vegetables; and (4) DF from legumes, containing different types of soluble DF, insoluble DF, and resistant starch [29].

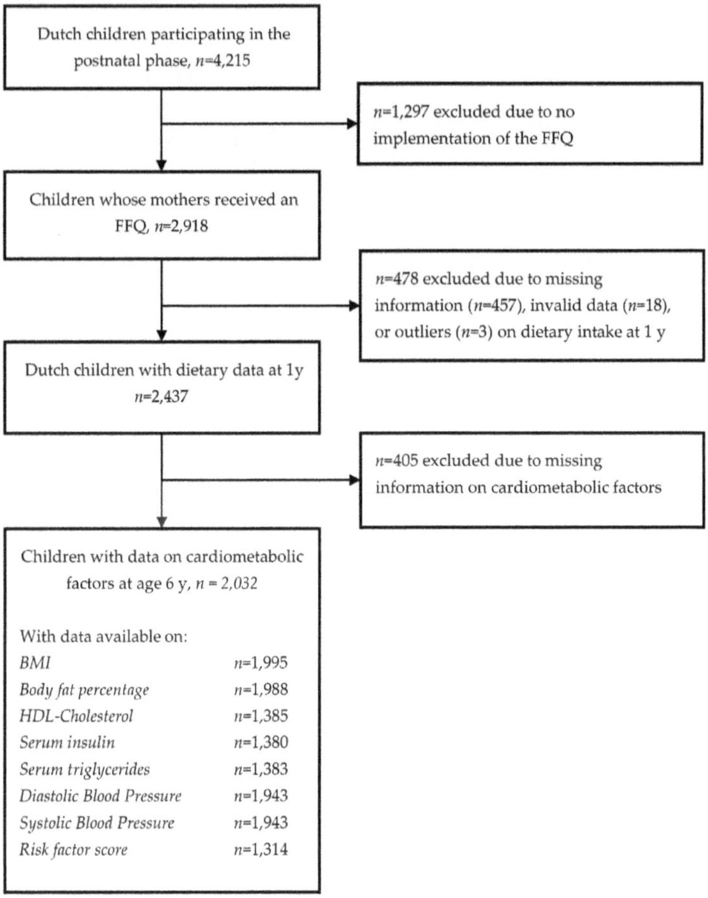

Figure 1. Flow chart of study participants included in the analysis.

2.3. Cardiometabolic Health Assessment

Children's height and weight up to the age of 4 years were repeatedly measured during routine visits to Child Health Centers [30]. At a median age of 5.9 (IQR 5.8–6.1) years, children visited our dedicated research center in the Sophia Children's Hospital in Rotterdam where they were examined in detail. As a primary outcome we used a cardiometabolic risk factor score including the components body fat percentage (BF%), high-density lipoprotein cholesterol (HDL-C), insulin, and triglyceride concentrations, and diastolic blood pressure (DBP) and systolic blood pressure (SBP). Body weight, measured with a mechanical personal scale (SECA), and body height, without shoes and heavy clothes, were measured to the nearest 0.1 kg or 0.1 cm, respectively, and BMI was calculated (kg/m^2). Body fat was determined using a dual-energy X-ray absorptiometry scanner (iDXA; General Electrics-Lunar, 2008, Madison, WI, USA) and enCORE software v.13.6 (GE Healthcare, Little Chalfont, UK) [31]. Total body fat was expressed as percentage of total body weight to define BF%. Additionally, we calculated fat mass index (FMI) as fat mass (kg)/m^2.

Non-fasting blood samples were drawn for measurements of HDL-C, insulin, and triglyceride concentrations, using enzymatic methods (using a Cobas 8000 analyzer, Roche, Almere, The Netherlands) [32]. Quality control samples demonstrated intra-assay and inter-assay coefficients of variation ranging from 0.77% to 1.69%. DBP and SBP were measured, while the children were lying down, at the right brachial artery, using the validated automatic sphygmomanometer Datascope

Accutorr Plus™ (Paramus, NJ, USA) [33]. Measurements were repeated four times with 1 min intervals and we used the mean of DBP and the mean of SBP of the last three measurements.

For all outcomes we calculated age- and sex-specific standard deviation scores (SDS) on the basis of our study population. Outliers, defined as the SDS $\geq |3.29|$ [34], were excluded (n = 0–7 per outcome). Individual cardiometabolic outcomes were combined into a continuous cardiometabolic risk factor score as described elsewhere [17,35]. This score included the sum of age- and sex-specific SD scores of BF%, the inverse of HDL-C, insulin, triglycerides, SBP, and DBP and was transformed into an SD score. A higher score is indicative of a less favorable cardiometabolic profile.

2.4. Covariates

Maternal age, household income, educational levels of both parents, and proxies for mother's pre-pregnancy cardiometabolic health (i.e., hypercholesterolemia, diabetes mellitus, or hypertension) were obtained with a questionnaire at enrolment in the study. Educational level of both parents was assessed with the same questionnaire and highest finished education was categorized into: no higher education; one parent with higher education; or both parents finished higher education, with higher education defined as higher vocational training, a Bachelor's degree, or university degree [36].

Maternal height and weight were measured at the research center at enrollment in the study, and BMI was calculated. Information about smoking, alcohol intake, and folic acid supplementation during pregnancy, as markers of health-conscious behavior of the mother, was obtained with questionnaires during pregnancy [27]. Information about pregnancy complications (i.e., gestational hypertension, preeclampsia, or gestational diabetes mellitus) was retrieved from medical records.

Medical records and hospital registries were used to collect information about child's sex, birth weight and gestational age. Sex- and gestational age-specific z-scores for birth weight were calculated using reference data [37]. Information about receiving breastfeeding at 4 months and timing of introduction of fruit and vegetables was collected with postnatal questionnaires [27].

A food-based diet score for preschool children was used to assess overall diet quality [27] and macronutrient intakes and glycemic load of the diet were calculated [38] from data obtained with the FFQ. Information about receiving dietary supplements (e.g., vitamins and mineral supplements) as a proxy of health-conscious behavior, was retrieved using the FFQ. Information about average screen time as proxy for sedentary behavior and about time spent walking or bicycling to school and playing outside as proxies for physical activity, and smoking in the household (categorized into never; less than once per week; or once per week or more) was obtained with a questionnaire at the child's age of 6 years.

2.5. Statistical Analysis

To explore whether potential associations of DF intake with cardiometabolic health were explained by energy intake, we examined both absolute DF (i.e., not adjusted for energy intake) and energy-adjusted DF intake. DF was adjusted for energy intake using the residual method [39]. Insulin was root-transformed, to obtain a normal distribution. Potential nonlinearity of the associations was assessed using natural cubic spline models with two to four degrees of freedom [40]. Because there were no indications for nonlinear associations for any of the outcomes (all $p > 0.05$), we assessed all associations using linear regression analyses only. In these models, we analyzed total DF intake and DF intake from different sources (per 1 g/day) and the cardiometabolic risk factor score and individual cardiometabolic health components at the age of 6 years.

In the crude model, we included child's age at FFQ and sex. To identify potential dietary confounders, we first examined correlations of DF intake with intake of total protein, vegetable protein, animal protein, fat, polyunsaturated fatty acids, monounsaturated fatty acids, saturated fatty acids, carbohydrates, glycemic load, and the diet quality score. We observed a strong correlation for energy intake, glycemic load, and the diet score with DF intakes, and therefore included these variables in the analyses. To avoid overadjustment, the diet quality score and glycemic load were adjusted for DF intake using the residual method. All other covariates described in the Covariates section were included as potential confounders using the manual forward stepwise method starting with the crude model. Variables were retained in the covariate-adjusted model when they resulted in a ≥5% change of the effect estimates of absolute or energy-adjusted DF intake on at least one of the outcomes. Following this procedure, all variables were retained, so covariate-adjusted models were adjusted for: maternal age, maternal BMI, household income, educational level of the parents, smoking, alcohol intake and folic acid supplementation during pregnancy, pregnancy complications, child's birth weight, sex, receiving breastfeeding at 4 months, timing of introduction of fruit and vegetables, age at FFQ, receiving dietary supplements, glycemic load, diet quality score, physical activity, screen time, and smoking in the household.

We tested for potential effect modification by child's sex, age at FFQ, and overweight status at the age of 6 years in the crude and covariate-adjusted models. We additionally explored whether DF intake was associated with repeatedly measured height, weight, and BMI using multivariable linear mixed models including the same covariates as in the main models. For the cardiometabolic risk factor score, we performed sensitivity analyses in which we excluded individual components from the score one at a time. Furthermore, we repeated the analyses in a selection of the children with complete data on all cardiometabolic outcomes (n = 1314).

Missing values of covariates were multiply imputed (n = 10 imputations) according to the Fully Conditional Specification method (predictive mean matching), with the assumption of no monotone missing pattern [41]. Effect estimates and population characteristics (Supplementary Materials Table S1) were similar before and after imputation and we report the pooled results after the multiple imputation procedure. Statistical analyses were performed using SPSS 21.0 (IBM Corp., version 21.0, Armonk, NY, USA) and R (The R Foundation for Statistical Computing, version 3.2.0, Aalborg, Denmark) and results were considered statistically significant at a p-value < 0.05.

3. Results

3.1. Population Characteristics

The population characteristics are shown in Table 1. At the age of 1 year, mean ± SD intake of total DF was 15.0 ± 4.3 g/day, with a range of 3.0–38.6 g/day, with 46.4% of the children having a DF intake above the Dutch recommended intake of 15 g/day for 1–3 year old children [42]. Most of the DF in the diet of our study population came from cereal products (median (IQR) 8.0 (6.2–10.0) g/day) and from fruits and vegetables (4.7 (3.2–6.2) g/day). Overall, parents of most of the children had a high educational level and a high income.

Table 1. Population characteristics (n = 2032).

	Mean ± SD, Median (IQR), or *n* (%)
Infancy Characteristics	
Gestational age at birth (weeks)	40.1 (39.3–41.1)
Birth weight (g)	3499 ± 563
Girls (n)	1031 (50.7%)
Receiving breastfeeding	
• Never	272 (13.3%)
• Partial in the first 4 months	1154 (56.8%)
• Exclusively in the first 4 months	606 (29.9%)
Timing of introduction of fruits and vegetables	
• <4 months	162 (7.9%)
• 4–6 months	1716 (84.4%)
• ≥6 months	154 (7.7%)
Characteristics at Dietary Assessment	
Age (months)	12.9 (12.6–13.9)

Table 1. Population characteristics (n = 2032).

	Mean ± SD, Median (IQR), or n (%)
Dietary fiber (DF) intake (g/day)	15.0 ± 4.3
• DF from cereals	8.0 (6.2–10.0)
• DF from potatoes	1.1 (0.4–1.9)
• DF from fruit and vegetables	4.7 (3.2–6.2)
• DF from legumes	0.2 (0.0–0.6)
Energy intake (kcal/day)	1267 (1070–1491)
Receiving any dietary supplements	973 (47.9%)
Characteristics at Cardiometabolic Health Assessment	
Age (year)	5.9 (5.8–6.1)
Height (cm)	118 (115–122)
Weight (kg)	21.8 (20.2–23.8)
BMI (kg/m^2) (n = 1995)	15.6 (15.0–16.5)
Body fat percentage (n = 1988)	23.1 (20.4–26.4)
Serum HDL-cholesterol (mmol/L) (n = 1385)	1.33 ± 0.30
Serum insulin (pmol/L) (n = 1380)	114 (63.8–183.6)
Serum triglycerides (mmol/L) (n = 1383)	0.98 (0.72–1.29)
Diastolic blood pressure (mmHg) (n = 1943)	60 ± 6
Systolic blood pressure (mmHg) (n = 1943)	102 ± 8
Physical activity (h/day)	1.60 (1.00–2.43)
Screen time (h/day)	1.14 (0.75–1.71)
Seldom or no smoking in household	1829 (90.0%)
Parental Characteristics	
Maternal age at enrolment (year)	32.3 (29.7–34.6)
Maternal BMI at enrolment (kg/m^2)	23.3 (21.7–25.8)
Household income ≥ €2,200 per month	1586 (78.0%)
Educational level parents	
• No higher education	421 (20.7%)
• One parent higher education	495 (24.4%)
• Both parents higher education	1116 (54.9%)
Maternal hypercholesterolemia, diabetes mellitus, or hypertension	93 (4.6%)
Smoking during pregnancy	
• Never	1606 (79.0%)
• Until pregnancy was known	213 (10.5%)
• Continued	213 (10.5%)
Alcohol consumption during pregnancy	
• Never	627 (30.9%)
• Until pregnancy was known	364 (17.9%)
• Continued	1041 (51.2%)
Use of folic acid supplements during pregnancy	
• Start periconceptional	1245 (61.3%)
• Start in first 10 weeks of pregnancy	599 (29.4%)
• No	188 (9.3%)
Gestational hypertension, preeclampsia, or gestational diabetes mellitus	183 (9.1%)

Abbreviations: DF, dietary fiber; HDL, high density lipoprotein; IQR, interquartile range.

3.2. Associations between DF Intake and Cardiometabolic Health

Table 2 presents the crude and covariate-adjusted associations between DF intake and energy-adjusted DF intake and age- and sex-adjusted outcomes of cardiometabolic health. In covariate-adjusted models, a 1 g/day higher energy-adjusted DF intake was associated with a 0.022 (95% CI −0.038, −0.006) SD lower cardiometabolic risk factor score. The effect estimate for DF without adjustment for energy was similar (−0.022 SDS; 95% CI −0.037, −0.006).

Table 2. Crude and covariate-adjusted associations between DF intake and energy-adjusted DF intake and cardiometabolic outcomes.

	DF Intake (per 1 g/day)		Energy-Adjusted DF Intake (per 1 g/day) [1]	
	Crude Model [2]	Covariate-Adjusted Model [3]	Crude Model [2]	Covariate-Adjusted Model [3]
Cardiometabolic risk factor score n = 1314	−0.014 * (−0.024, −0.003)	−0.022 * (−0.037, −0.006)	−0.023 * (−0.038, −0.007)	−0.022 * (−0.038, −0.006)
BF% (SDS) n = 1988	−0.005 (−0.014, 0.004)	−0.005 (−0.017, 0.007)	−0.004 (−0.016, 0.008)	−0.003 (−0.015, 0.010)
HDL-C (SDS) n = 1385	0.018 * (0.012, 0.024)	0.027 * (0.011, 0.044)	0.023 * (0.007, 0.039)	0.026 *,[4] (0.009, 0.043)
Insulin (SDS) n = 1380	0.001 (−0.005, 0.007)	0.002 (−0.014, 0.019)	−0.005 (−0.013, 0.003)	−0.003 (−0.020, 0.015)
Triglycerides (SDS) n = 1383	−0.008 (−0.020, 0.004)	−0.019 * (−0.035, −0.003)	−0.015 (−0.031, 0.001)	−0.018 *,[4] (−0.036, −0.002)
DBP (SDS) n = 1943	−0.006 (−0.015, 0.004)	−0.006 (−0.019, 0.008)	−0.004 (−0.017, 0.009)	−0.003 (−0.017, 0.011)
SBP (SDS) n = 1943	−0.001 (−0.006, 0.004)	−0.007 (−0.020, 0.007)	−0.009 (−0.022, 0.005)	−0.009 (−0.023, 0.005)

Values are based on multivariable linear regression models and reflect differences (95% confidence interval) in individual cardiometabolic outcomes and in cardiometabolic risk factor score (age- and sex-adjusted SDS) per 1 g/day increase in DF intake. [1] DF was analyzed as energy-adjusted DF using the residual method and models were additionally adjusted for energy intake; [2] Crude model is adjusted for child's sex and age at FFQ; [3] Covariate-adjusted model additionally includes maternal cardiometabolic health, age, BMI, smoking, alcohol intake and folic acid supplementation during pregnancy, pregnancy complications, household income, parental education, child's birth weight, breastfeeding, timing of introduction of fruit and vegetables, receiving dietary supplements, glycemic load, diet quality score, physical activity, screen time, and smoking in the household; [4] In our study population, a 0.026 SDS higher HDL-C corresponds to approximately 0.008 mmol/L or 0.31 mg/dL; and a 0.020 SDS lower triglyceride concentrations to approximately 0.010 mmol/L or 0.89 mg/dL; * p-value < 0.05. Abbreviations: BF%, body fat percentage; DBP, diastolic blood pressure; DF, dietary fiber; HDL-C, high-density lipoprotein cholesterol; SBP, systolic blood pressure; SDS, standard deviation score.

Thereafter, we analyzed the components of the cardiometabolic risk factor score separately (Table 2). A 1 g/day higher energy-adjusted DF intake was associated with 0.026 SDS (95% CI 0.089, 0.042) higher HDL-C concentrations. In addition, a higher energy-adjusted DF intake were associated with 0.020 SDS lower triglyceride concentrations (95% CI −0.037, −0.003). DF intake was not associated with BF%, insulin, DBP, or SBP. Intake of DF was also not associated with repeatedly measured height (−0.004 (95% CI −0.012, 0.005)), weight (−0.007 (95% CI −0.017, 0.003)), or BMI (−0.001 (95% CI −0.010, 0.008)), or with FMI at 6 years (−0.003 (95% CI −0.009, 0.009)). Also for the individual cardiometabolic outcomes, effect estimates with and without energy adjustment were similar (Table 2).

3.3. Associations between DF Intake from Different Sources and Cardiometabolic Health

Table 3 presents the covariate-adjusted associations between intake of DF from different sources and cardiometabolic health. A 1 g/day higher energy-adjusted DF intake from potatoes was associated with a 0.051 SDS (95% CI −0.094, −0.009) lower cardiometabolic risk factor score, and a 0.076 SDS lower triglyceride concentration (95% CI −0.121, −0.031). Effect estimates without energy adjustment were similar and in addition, there was a positive association between DF intake from potatoes and HDL-C (0.028 SDS; 95% CI 0.016, 0.072).

We observed that a 1 g/day higher energy-adjusted DF intake from fruit and vegetables was associated with a 0.028 SDS (95% CI 0.001, 0.054) higher HDL-C (similar without energy adjustment). Effect estimates for DF from legumes were similar to those obtained for total DF, however, the confidence intervals were wide and none of the associations for DF from legumes was statistically significant. For DF intake from cereals, we observed no associations with any of the outcomes.

Table 3. Covariate-adjusted associations between DF intake and energy-adjusted DF intake from cereals, from potatoes, from fruits and vegetables, and from legumes (per 1 g/day) and cardiometabolic outcomes.

	Cereals (per 1 g/day)		Potatoes (per 1 g/day)		Fruit & Vegetables (per 1 g/day)		Legumes (per 1 g/day)	
	DF Intake	Energy-Adjusted DF Intake [1]	DF Intake	Energy-Adjusted DF Intake [1]	DF Intake [1]	Energy-Adjusted DF Intake [1]	DF Intake	Energy-Adjusted DF Intake [1]
Cardiometabolic risk factor score (SDS) $n = 1311$	−0.006 (−0.026, 0.014)	−0.004 (−0.026, 0.019)	−0.050 * (−0.093, −0.008)	−0.051 * (−0.096, −0.009)	−0.009 (−0.034, 0.017)	−0.009 (−0.034, 0.016)	−0.032 (−0.111, 0.048)	−0.03 (−0.110, 0.049)
BF% (SDS) $n = 1984$	−0.009 (−0.024, 0.005)	−0.005 (−0.022, 0.011)	0 (−0.032, 0.032)	−0.001 (−0.033, 0.032)	0.006 (−0.012, 0.025)	0.006 (−0.013, 0.025)	−0.001 (−0.061, 0.059)	0 (−0.059, 0.060)
HDL-C (SDS) $n = 1383$	0.008 (−0.013, 0.029)	0.002 (−0.021, 0.024)	0.028 * (0.016, 0.072)	0.033 (−0.012, 0.077)	0.027 * (0.000, 0.054)	0.028 * (0.002, 0.054)	0.035 (−0.047, 0.117)	0.033 (−0.048, 0.115)
Insulin (SDS) $n = 1378$	0.001 (−0.019, 0.022)	−0.008 (−0.030, 0.015)	−0.018 (−0.055, 0.033)	−0.01 (−0.053, 0.034)	0.012 (−0.015, 0.039)	0.013 (−0.014, 0.040)	−0.015 (−0.097, 0.067)	−0.016 (−0.098, 0.066)
Triglycerides (SDS) $n = 1381$	0.011 (−0.010, 0.032)	−0.007 (−0.015, 0.000)	−0.075 * (−0.120, −0.030)	−0.076 * (−0.121, −0.032)	−0.02 (−0.048, 0.007)	−0.021 (−0.050, 0.006)	−0.015 (−0.098, 0.068)	−0.014 (−0.098, 0.069)
DBP (SDS) $n = 1939$	−0.007 (−0.024, 0.009)	−0.003 (−0.021, 0.016)	−0.001 (−0.038, 0.035)	−0.0034 (−0.040, 0.033)	−0.004 (−0.025, 0.017)	−0.005 (−0.026, 0.016)	−0.016 (−0.052, 0.084)	0.017 (−0.051, 0.085)
SBP (SDS) $n = 1939$	−0.009 (−0.026, 0.009)	−0.012 (−0.032, 0.008)	0.004 (−0.034, 0.041)	0.004 (−0.033, 0.042)	0.001 (−0.021, 0.023)	0.002 (−0.021, 0.024)	−0.008 (−0.028, 0.012)	−0.008 (−0.028, 0.012)

Values are based on multivariable linear regression models and reflect differences (95% confidence intervals) in individual cardiometabolic outcomes and in cardiometabolic risk factor score (age- and sex-adjusted SD scores) per 1 g/day increase in DF intake from different sources. All models are adjusted for maternal cardiometabolic health, age, BMI, smoking, alcohol intake and folic acid supplementation during pregnancy, pregnancy complications, household income, parental education, child's birth weight, sex, breastfeeding, timing of introduction of fruit and vegetables, age at food-frequency questionnaire (FFQ), receiving dietary supplements, glycemic load, diet quality score, physical activity, screen time, and smoking in the household. [1] DF was analyzed as energy-adjusted DF using the residual method and models were additionally adjusted for energy intake. * p-value < 0.05. Abbreviations: BF%, body fat percentage; DBP, diastolic blood pressure; DF, dietary fiber; HDL-C, high-density lipoprotein cholesterol; SBP, systolic blood pressure; SDS, standard deviation score.

3.4. Additional Analyses

We observed no significant interaction of DF intake with child's sex or age at FFQ on any of the outcomes. Crude associations were comparable with those after adjustment for confounders (Supplementary Materials Table S2). When we restricted our analyses to children with complete data on all cardiometabolic factors, we observed similar results as obtained for the full sample (Supplementary Materials Table S3). When we analyzed the cardiometabolic risk factor score without triglycerides (TG) or without HDL-C in sensitivity analyses, effect estimates only slightly attenuated (Supplementary Materials Table S4). Finally, we observed no significant differences in DF intake, BF%, or blood pressure between children with or without blood samples (Supplementary Materials Table S5).

4. Discussion

This is the first study that investigated the association between DF intake, including DF from different sources, and cardiometabolic health in a large cohort of young children. Overall, a higher DF intake was associated with a lower cardiometabolic risk factor score. This was mainly determined by a better blood lipid profile. Furthermore, we observed that the association between DF intake and better cardiometabolic health was not explained by differences in energy intake and seemed to be primarily driven by intake of DF from potatoes, fruits, and vegetables. Although effect sizes were modest and without clinical implications on the individual level, small variations in cardiometabolic risk factors in childhood have been shown to predict health in later life [6,7], and a high DF intake already in early childhood may thereby contribute to a reduction in the cardiometabolic disease burden of a population.

Our observation that a higher DF intake was associated with better combined cardiometabolic health is in line with previous studies in adolescents and adults that showed that a higher DF intake was associated with a lower risk of metabolic syndrome [1,43]. Although associations with all individual cardiometabolic outcomes were in the expected direction, we observed that the association with overall cardiometabolic health in our population was mainly driven by higher HDL-C and lower triglyceride concentrations. In line with our results, Ludwig et al. [2] showed that a higher DF intake was associated with higher HDL-C and with lower triglyceride concentrations in adults. In contrast, two previous studies that examined these associations in children found no associations between DF intake and HDL-C or triglycerides [9,16]. However, these studies were small (n = 543 and n = 147) and may have been underpowered to detect such associations. A potential beneficial effect of DF intake on blood lipid levels could be explained by two mechanisms. First, DF decreases gastric emptying, which reduces the acute postprandial responses, and thereby controls glucose and lipid concentrations after a meal [24,44]. In the long-term, lower fluctuations of glucose and lipids can reduce the risk of cardiometabolic disorders. Second, absorption of lipid is affected by dietary fiber intake, which leads to a reduction in hepatic cholesterol. [45].

Although associations were all in the expected direction (i.e., improved cardiometabolic health), DF intake was not significantly associated with the individual cardiometabolic components BF%, insulin, DBP, or SBP in our population. Results from previous studies in children and adolescents are mixed, with studies reporting either null or beneficial associations for higher DF intake. Jenner et al. [15] reported associations between a higher DF intake and energy-adjusted DF intake with a lower DBP in boys, but not in girls, at the age of 9 years. Two studies observed no associations of DF with BF% in young children [11] or with BF% and insulin dynamics in adolescents [12], whereas three other studies reported that higher energy-adjusted DF intake was associated with lower BMI [8,10], lower visceral adiposity [13], and improved insulin-related outcomes [10] in children and adolescents. Since most of these studies were performed in older children [8,10,13] or in higher risk populations, such as obese teenagers [10,13], there may have been insufficient variability in our young and generally healthy population to observe a potential beneficial effect of DF intake on these individual cardiometabolic factors. Although very high DF intake has been hypothesized to have harmful effects on growth, studies do not support that high DF intake compromises growth of children in developed countries [18,20]. In line with this, we observed no associations of DF intake with repeatedly measured height or weight and we observed no indications for nonlinear associations of DF intake with any of the growth or cardiometabolic factors, suggesting that associations did not differ for low or high DF intakes in our study population with a generally high DF intake.

Considering that DF intake may result in satiation that could lead to a lower energy intake [24], associations between DF intake and cardiometabolic health were hypothesized to be explained by differences in energy intake. However, we observed no clear differences in associations for DF with or without energy adjustment. If any, the effect estimates became stronger after adjustment for energy intake, which is in line with results from two previous studies among children that showed larger effect estimates of DF on cardiometabolic outcomes after adjustment for energy [9,15]. This suggests that the effects of satiation may not play a major role among young children. In other words, a high DF intake does not necessarily displace energy intake [9] and a higher DF intake might be beneficial for cardiometabolic health via other mechanisms.

These other mechanisms may differ for different types and food sources of DF. In our study, we observed that associations of DF intake with blood lipids were mainly explained by intake of DF from fruits, vegetables, and potatoes, but not from cereals. Fruits and vegetables contain hemicellulose A, pectin, gums, and mucilage; and these types of DF may increase the viscosity that result in distension of the stomach [22]. Potatoes contain resistant starch, and in line with our results on blood lipids, Higgins et al. [23] reported that a replacement of 5.4% of dietary carbohydrates with resistant starch increased postprandial lipid oxidation. Resistant starch has also been associated with an increase in satiety in adults [46], and the mechanism behind lowering triglyceride concentrations probably involves increased intestinal viscosity [47]. Other studies showed that the solubility of DF could influence the associations [13,14]. Unfortunately, we were only able to make a division of DF by food sources, and not by type of DF. Therefore, there is still an overlap between intake of soluble and insoluble DF in our analyses. Finally, because of the low legume intake in our population, we might not have been able to detect associations for DF intake from legumes.

Our study was performed in a large population-based cohort with information available on many potential confounders. Although not all information on confounders was complete for all participants, we used multiple imputation of covariates to reduce attrition bias. Another strength is the availability of blood samples to measure detailed markers of cardiometabolic health. Blood samples were available in only 68.3% of the children, which may have led to selection bias. However, we observed no significant differences in DF intake, BF%, and blood pressure between children with or without blood samples [17] and results were similar when we restricted our analyses to the subjects with complete data on cardiometabolic health available, suggesting that bias due to missing blood samples may not be a large issue in the current analyses. A limitation is that blood lipids and insulin concentrations were measured in blood samples that were collected in non-fasting state. According to studies in adults, fasting time has little influence on cholesterol levels [48], but concentrations of triacylglycerol [48] and insulin [49] vary more substantially with differences in fasting time. Assuming that fasting time of the children when visiting our research center is randomly distributed, this measurement error would have led to non-differential misclassification of the outcomes and may therefore have resulted in an underestimation of our effect estimates for associations with insulin and blood lipids.

Regarding the nutritional assessment, an FFQ is an appropriate method because it reflects habitual diet. Furthermore, although FFQs are prone to measurement error, our validation study showed an intra-class correlation coefficient of 0.7 for DF intake [26,27], indicating a reasonably good validity. Unfortunately, we had no information available on intake of specific subtypes of DF, such as soluble and insoluble DF. A limitation is that this is an observational study, therefore, we cannot establish a causal relation. Although we had information available on many potential confounders, residual confounding from, for example, physical activity may still be an issue. Finally, we did not have cardiometabolic health data at the age of 1 year or dietary data at the age of 6 years, consequently, we were not able to perform longitudinal analyses for the cardiometabolic factors.

5. Conclusions

Results of this prospective cohort study suggest that a higher DF intake in infancy is associated with better combined cardiometabolic health, especially with a healthier blood lipid profile. These associations were not explained by differences in energy intake. Intake of DF from potatoes, fruits, and vegetables rather than cereals seemed to drive this association. Future studies should investigate the longitudinal association of DF intake, including different subtypes of DF, in early childhood with long-term cardiometabolic health.

Supplementary Materials: The following are available online at http://www.mdpi.com/2072-6643/8/9/531/s1, Table S1: Population characteristics based on unimputed and imputed data; Table S2: Crude associations between DF intake and cardiometabolic outcomes; Table S3: Crude and covariate-adjusted associations between DF intake and cardiometabolic outcomes among children with complete data on cardiometabolic health (n = 1314); Table S4: Sensitivity analyses: associations between DF intake and the cardiometabolic risk factor score without TG or HDL-C; Table S5: Descriptives of children with and without blood samples available.

Acknowledgments: The Generation R Study was conducted by the Erasmus Medical Center in close collaboration with the School of Law and Faculty of Social Sciences of the Erasmus University Rotterdam, the Municipal Health Service-Rotterdam Metropolitan Area, the Rotterdam Homecare Foundation, and the Stichting Trombosedienst & Artsenlaboratorium Rijnmond, Rotterdam. The general design of the Generation R Study was made possible by financial support from the Erasmus Medical Center, Rotterdam; the Erasmus University, Rotterdam; the Dutch Ministry of Health, Welfare and Sport; and The Netherlands Organization for Health Research and Development (ZonMw). The authors Kim V. E. Braun, Jessica C. Kiefte-de Jong, Oscar H. Franco, and Trudy Voortman work in ErasmusAGE, a center for aging research across the life course funded by Nestle Nutrition (Nestec Ltd.), Metagenics Inc. and AXA. The funders had no role in design and conduct of the study; collection, management, analysis, and interpretation of the data; and preparation, review or approval of the manuscript.

Author Contributions: R.M.A.v.G., and K.V.E.B. designed the research project, conducted the analyses, and drafted the initial manuscript. J.C.K.-d.J., V.W.V.J., and O.H.F. were involved in the data collection and provided input regarding the interpretation of the results and writing of the manuscript. T.V. designed the research project and provided consultation regarding the data analysis, interpretation of results, and writing of the manuscript. All authors critically reviewed and approved the final manuscript as submitted and agree to be accountable for all aspects of the work.

Conflicts of Interest: The authors declare no conflict of interest. The funding sponsors had no role in the design of the study; in the collection, analyses, or interpretation of data; in the writing of the manuscript, or in the decision to publish the results.

Abbreviations

The following abbreviations have been used in the text:

BF%	Body Fat Percentage
BMI	Body Mass Index
DBP	Diastolic Blood Pressure
DF	Dietary Fiber
FFQ	Food Frequency Questionnaire
HDL-C	High Density Lipoprotein Cholesterol
LDL-C	Low Density Lipoprotein Cholesterol
SBP	Systolic Blood Pressure
SDS	Standard Deviation Score

References

1. Grooms, K.N.; Ommerborn, M.J.; Pham, D.Q.; Djousse, L.; Clark, C.R. Dietary fiber intake and cardiometabolic risks among us adults, nhanes 1999–2010. *Am. J. Med.* **2013**, *126*, 1059–1067. [CrossRef] [PubMed]
2. Ludwig, D.S.; Pereira, M.A.; Kroenke, C.H.; Hilner, J.E.; Van Horn, L.; Slattery, M.L.; Jacobs, D.R., Jr. Dietary fiber, weight gain, and cardiovascular disease risk factors in young adults. *JAMA* **1999**, *282*, 1539–1546. [CrossRef] [PubMed]
3. Satija, A.; Hu, F.B. Cardiovascular benefits of dietary fiber. *Curr. Atheroscler. Rep.* **2012**, *14*, 505–514. [CrossRef] [PubMed]

4. Dietz, W.H. Health consequences of obesity in youth: Childhood predictors of adult disease. *Pediatrics* **1998**, *101*, 518–525. [PubMed]
5. Juonala, M.; Magnussen, C.G.; Berenson, G.S.; Venn, A.; Burns, T.L.; Sabin, M.A.; Srinivasan, S.R.; Daniels, S.R.; Davis, P.H.; Chen, W.; et al. Childhood adiposity, adult adiposity, and cardiovascular risk factors. *N. Engl. J. Med.* **2011**, *365*, 1876–1885. [CrossRef] [PubMed]
6. Morrison, J.A.; Glueck, C.J.; Wang, P. Childhood risk factors predict cardiovascular disease, impaired fasting glucose plus type 2 diabetes mellitus, and high blood pressure 26 years later at a mean age of 38 years: The princeton-lipid research clinics follow-up study. *Metabolism* **2012**, *61*, 531–541. [CrossRef] [PubMed]
7. Morrison, J.A.; Glueck, C.J.; Woo, J.G.; Wang, P. Risk factors for cardiovascular disease and type 2 diabetes retained from childhood to adulthood predict adult outcomes: The princeton lrc follow-up study. *Int. J. Pediatr. Endocrinol.* **2012**. [CrossRef] [PubMed]
8. Cheng, G.; Karaolis-Danckert, N.; Libuda, L.; Bolzenius, K.; Remer, T.; Buyken, A.E. Relation of dietary glycemic index, glycemic load, and fiber and whole-grain intakes during puberty to the concurrent development of percent body fat and body mass index. *Am. J. Epidemiol.* **2009**, *169*, 667–677. [CrossRef] [PubMed]
9. Ruottinen, S.; Lagstrom, H.K.; Niinikoski, H.; Ronnemaa, T.; Saarinen, M.; Pahkala, K.A.; Hakanen, M.; Viikari, J.S.; Simell, O. Dietary fiber does not displace energy but is associated with decreased serum cholesterol concentrations in healthy children. *Am. J. Clin. Nutr.* **2010**, *91*, 651–661. [CrossRef] [PubMed]
10. Brauchla, M.; Juan, W.; Story, J.; Kranz, S. Sources of dietary fiber and the association of fiber intake with childhood obesity risk (in 2–18 year olds) and diabetes risk of adolescents 12–18 year olds: Nhanes 2003–2006. *J. Nutr. Metab.* **2012**. [CrossRef] [PubMed]
11. Buyken, A.E.; Cheng, G.; Gunther, A.L.; Liese, A.D.; Remer, T.; Karaolis-Danckert, N. Relation of dietary glycemic index, glycemic load, added sugar intake, or fiber intake to the development of body composition between ages 2 and 7 y. *Am. J. Clin. Nutr.* **2008**, *88*, 755–762. [PubMed]
12. Davis, J.N.; Alexander, K.E.; Ventura, E.E.; Kelly, L.A.; Lane, C.J.; Byrd-Williams, C.E.; Toledo-Corral, C.M.; Roberts, C.K.; Spruijt-Metz, D.; Weigensberg, M.J.; et al. Associations of dietary sugar and glycemic index with adiposity and insulin dynamics in overweight latino youth. *Am. J. Clin. Nutr.* **2007**, *86*, 1331–1338. [PubMed]
13. Davis, J.N.; Alexander, K.E.; Ventura, E.E.; Toledo-Corral, C.M.; Goran, M.I. Inverse relation between dietary fiber intake and visceral adiposity in overweight latino youth. *Am. J. Clin. Nutr.* **2009**, *90*, 1160–1166. [CrossRef] [PubMed]
14. Lin, Y.; Huybrechts, I.; Vereecken, C.; Mouratidou, T.; Valtuena, J.; Kersting, M.; Gonzalez-Gross, M.; Bolca, S.; Warnberg, J.; Cuenca-Garcia, M.; et al. Dietary fiber intake and its association with indicators of adiposity and serum biomarkers in european adolescents: The helena study. *Eur. J. Nutr.* **2015**, *54*, 771–782. [CrossRef] [PubMed]
15. Jenner, D.A.; English, D.R.; Vandongen, R.; Beilin, L.J.; Armstrong, B.K.; Miller, M.R.; Dunbar, D. Diet and blood pressure in 9-year-old australian children. *Am. J. Clin. Nutr.* **1988**, *47*, 1052–1059.
16. Rinaldi, A.E.; de Oliveira, E.P.; Moreto, F.; Gabriel, G.F.; Corrente, J.E.; Burini, R.C. Dietary intake and blood lipid profile in overweight and obese schoolchildren. *BMC Res. Notes* **2012**, *5*. [CrossRef] [PubMed]
17. Voortman, T.; van den Hooven, E.H.; Tielemans, M.J.; Hofman, A.; Kiefte-de Jong, J.C.; Jaddoe, V.W.; Franco, O.H. Protein intake in early childhood and cardiometabolic health at school age: The generation R study. *Eur. J. Nutr.* **2015**. [CrossRef] [PubMed]
18. Edwards, C.A.; Parrett, A.M. Dietary fibre in infancy and childhood. *Proc. Nutr. Soc.* **2003**, *62*, 17–23. [CrossRef] [PubMed]
19. Kranz, S.; Brauchla, M.; Slavin, J.L.; Miller, K.B. What do we know about dietary fiber intake in children and health? The effects of fiber intake on constipation, obesity, and diabetes in children. *Adv. Nutr.* **2012**, *3*, 47–53. [CrossRef] [PubMed]
20. Edwards, C.A.; Xie, C.; Garcia, A.L. Dietary fibre and health in children and adolescents. *Proc. Nutr. Soc.* **2015**, *74*, 292–302. [CrossRef] [PubMed]
21. Pereira, M.A.; O'Reilly, E.; Augustsson, K.; Fraser, G.E.; Goldbourt, U.; Heitmann, B.L.; Hallmans, G.; Knekt, P.; Liu, S.; Pietinen, P.; et al. Dietary fiber and risk of coronary heart disease: A pooled analysis of cohort studies. *Arch. Intern. Med.* **2004**, *164*, 370–376. [CrossRef] [PubMed]
22. Aggett, P.J.; Agostoni, C.; Axelsson, I.; Edwards, C.A.; Goulet, O.; Hernell, O.; Koletzko, B.; Lafeber, H.N.; Micheli, J.L.; Michaelsen, K.F.; et al. Nondigestible carbohydrates in the diets of infants and young children:

A commentary by the espghan committee on nutrition. *J. Pediatr. Gastroenterol. Nutr.* **2003**, *36*, 329–337. [CrossRef] [PubMed]
23. Higgins, J.A.; Higbee, D.R.; Donahoo, W.T.; Brown, I.L.; Bell, M.L.; Bessesen, D.H. Resistant starch consumption promotes lipid oxidation. *Nutr. Metab.* **2004**, *1*. [CrossRef] [PubMed]
24. Slavin, J.L. Dietary fiber and body weight. *Nutrition* **2005**, *21*, 411–418. [CrossRef] [PubMed]
25. Jaddoe, V.W.; van Duijn, C.M.; Franco, O.H.; van der Heijden, A.J.; van Iizendoorn, M.H.; de Jongste, J.C.; van der Lugt, A.; Mackenbach, J.P.; Moll, H.A.; Raat, H.; et al. The generation r study: Design and cohort update 2012. *Eur. J. Epidemiol.* **2012**, *27*, 739–756. [CrossRef] [PubMed]
26. Kiefte-de Jong, J.C.; de Vries, J.H.; Bleeker, S.E.; Jaddoe, V.W.; Hofman, A.; Raat, H.; Moll, H.A. Socio-demographic and lifestyle determinants of 'western-like' and 'health conscious' dietary patterns in toddlers. *Br. J. Nutr.* **2013**, *109*, 137–147. [CrossRef] [PubMed]
27. Voortman, T.; Kiefte-de Jong, J.C.; Geelen, A.; Villamor, E.; Moll, H.A.; de Jongste, J.C.; Raat, H.; Hofman, A.; Jaddoe, V.W.; Franco, O.H.; et al. The development of a diet quality score for preschool children and its validation and determinants in the generation R study. *J. Nutr.* **2015**, *145*, 306–314. [CrossRef] [PubMed]
28. Westenbrink, S.; Jansen-van der Vliet, M.; Brants, H.A.M.; van der Heijden, L.J.M.; Hulshof, K.F.A.M.; Langius, J.A.E.; van Oosten, H.M.; Pruissen-Boskaljon, J.C. *Nevo-Table 2006. Dutch Food Composition Table 2006*; The NEVO Foundation and the Dutch Nutrition Centre: The Hague, The Netherlands, 2006.
29. Bouchenak, M.; Lamri-Senhadji, M. Nutritional quality of legumes, and their role in cardiometabolic risk prevention: A review. *J. Med. Food* **2013**, *16*, 185–198. [CrossRef] [PubMed]
30. Braun, K.V.; Erler, N.S.; Kiefte-de Jong, J.C.; Jaddoe, V.W.; van den Hooven, E.H.; Franco, O.H.; Voortman, T. Dietary intake of protein in early childhood is associated with growth. *J. Nutr.* **2016**. in press.
31. Voortman, T.; Braun, K.V.; Kiefte-de Jong, J.C.; Jaddoe, V.W.; Franco, O.H.; van den Hooven, E.H. Protein intake in early childhood and body composition at the age of 6 years: The generation r study. *Int. J. Obes.* **2016**, *40*, 1018–1025. [CrossRef] [PubMed]
32. Kruithof, C.J.; Kooijman, M.N.; van Duijn, C.M.; Franco, O.H.; de Jongste, J.C.; Klaver, C.C.; Mackenbach, J.P.; Moll, H.A.; Raat, H.; Rings, E.H.; et al. The generation R study: Biobank update 2015. *Eur. J. Epidemiol.* **2014**, *29*, 911–927. [CrossRef] [PubMed]
33. Wong, S.N.; Tz Sung, R.Y.; Leung, L.C. Validation of three oscillometric blood pressure devices against auscultatory mercury sphygmomanometer in children. *Blood Press. Monit.* **2006**, *11*, 281–291. [CrossRef] [PubMed]
34. Field, A. *Discovering Statistics Using IBM SPSS Statistics*; SAGE Publications Ltd.: London, UK, 2013; pp. 176–180.
35. Eisenmann, J.C. On the use of a continuous metabolic syndrome score in pediatric research. *Cardiovasc. Diabetol.* **2008**, *7*. [CrossRef] [PubMed]
36. Statistics Netherlands. *Dutch Standard Classification of Education 2003 (Standaard Onderwijsindeling 2003)*; Statistics Netherlands (Centraal Bureau voor de Statistiek): Den Haag/Heerlen, The Netherlands, 2003.
37. Niklasson, A.; Ericson, A.; Fryer, J.G.; Karlberg, J.; Lawrence, C.; Karlberg, P. An update of the swedish reference standards for weight, length and head circumference at birth for given gestational age (1977–1981). *Acta Paediatr. Scand.* **1991**, *80*, 756–762. [CrossRef] [PubMed]
38. Kocevska, D.; Voortman, T.; Dashti, H.S.; van den Hooven, E.H.; Ghassabian, A.; Rijlaarsdam, J.; Schneider, N.; Feskens, E.J.; Jaddoe, V.W.; Tiemeier, H.; et al. Macronutrient intakes in infancy are associated with sleep duration in toddlerhood. *J. Nutr.* **2016**, *146*, 1250–1256. [CrossRef] [PubMed]
39. Willett, W.C.; Howe, G.R.; Kushi, L.H. Adjustment for total energy intake in epidemiologic studies. *Am. J. Clin. Nutr.* **1997**, *65*, 1220S–1228S. [PubMed]
40. Hastie, T.J. *Generalized Additive Models. Chapter 7 of Statistical Models in S*; Wadsworth & Brooks/Cole: Pacific Grove, CA, USA, 1992.
41. Sterne, J.A.; White, I.R.; Carlin, J.B.; Spratt, M.; Royston, P.; Kenward, M.G.; Wood, A.M.; Carpenter, J.R. Multiple imputation for missing data in epidemiological and clinical research: Potential and pitfalls. *BMJ* **2009**, *338*. [CrossRef] [PubMed]
42. Health Council of The Netherlands. *Guideline for Dietary Fiber Intake*; Health Council of The Netherlands: The Hague, The Netherlands, 2006; pp. 1–90.

43. Carlson, J.J.; Eisenmann, J.C.; Norman, G.J.; Ortiz, K.A.; Young, P.C. Dietary fiber and nutrient density are inversely associated with the metabolic syndrome in us adolescents. *J. Am. Diet. Assoc.* **2011**, *111*, 1688–1695. [CrossRef] [PubMed]
44. Heaton, K.W. Food fibre as an obstacle to energy intake. *Lancet* **1973**, *2*, 1418–1421. [CrossRef]
45. Fernandez, M.L. Soluble fiber and nondigestible carbohydrate effects on plasma lipids and cardiovascular risk. *Curr. Opin. Lipidol.* **2001**, *12*, 35–40. [CrossRef] [PubMed]
46. Willis, H.J.; Eldridge, A.L.; Beiseigel, J.; Thomas, W.; Slavin, J.L. Greater satiety response with resistant starch and corn bran in human subjects. *Nutr. Res.* **2009**, *29*, 100–105. [CrossRef] [PubMed]
47. Lattimer, J.M.; Haub, M.D. Effect of dietary fiber and its components on metabolic health. *Nutrients* **2010**, *2*, 1266–1289. [CrossRef] [PubMed]
48. Sidhu, D.; Naugler, C. Fasting time and lipid levels in a community-based population: A cross-sectional study. *Arch. Intern. Med.* **2012**, *172*, 1707–1710. [CrossRef] [PubMed]
49. Hancox, R.J.; Landhuis, C.E. Correlation between measures of insulin resistance in fasting and non-fasting blood. *Diabetol. Metab. Syndr.* **2011**, *3*, 23. [CrossRef] [PubMed]

nutrients

MDPI

Article

A Prospective Study of Different Types of Dietary Fiber and Risk of Cardiovascular Disease: Tehran Lipid and Glucose Study

Parvin Mirmiran [1], Zahra Bahadoran [1,*], Sajad Khalili Moghadam [1], Azita Zadeh Vakili [2] and Fereidoun Azizi [3,*]

1 Nutrition and Endocrine Research Center, Student Research Committee, Research Institute for Endocrine Sciences, Shahid Beheshti University of Medical Sciences, No. 24, Shahid-Erabi St., Yeman St., Velenjak, Tehran 19395-4763, Iran; mirmiran@endocrine.ac.ir (P.M.); sajadkhalili69@gmail.com (S.K.M.)

2 Cellular and Molecular Endocrine Research Center, Obesity Research Center, Research Institute for Endocrine Sciences, Shahid Beheshti University of Medical Sciences, No. 24, Shahid-Erabi St., Yeman St., Velenjak, Tehran 19395-4763, Iran; azitavakili@endocrine.ac.ir

3 Endocrine Research Center, Research Institute for Endocrine Sciences, Shahid Beheshti University of Medical Sciences, No. 24, Shahid-Erabi St., Yeman St., Velenjak, Tehran 19395-4763, Iran

* Correspondence: z.bahadoran@endocrine.ac.ir (Z.B.); azizi@endocrine.ac.ir (F.A.); Tel.: +98-21-224-32-500 (Z.B. & F.A.); Fax: +98-21-224-16-264 (Z.B. & F.A.) or +98-21-224-02-463 (Z.B. & F.A.)

Received: 2 August 2016; Accepted: 12 October 2016; Published: 7 November 2016

Abstract: Background and aim: This study was designed to examine the hypothesis that dietary of intake different types of fiber could modify the risk of cardiovascular disease (CVD) in a large prospective cohort among Iranian adults. Methods: In 2006–2008, we used a validated food frequency questionnaire to assess dietary fiber intake among 2295 health professionals with no previous history of heart disease. Subjects were subsequently followed until 2012 for incidence of CVD events. Multivariate Cox proportional hazard regression models, adjusted for potential confounders were used to estimate the risk of CVD across tertiles of total dietary fiber and different types of fiber. Linear regression models were also used to indicate the association of dietary fiber intakes with changes of cardiovascular risk factors during the follow-up. Results: Mean age of participants (42.8% men) was 38.2 ± 13.4, at baseline. Mean (SD) dietary intake of total fiber was 23.4 (8.9) g/day. After adjustment for cardiovascular risk score and dietary confounders, a significant inverse association was observed between intakes of total, soluble and insoluble dietary fiber and CVD risk, in the highest compared to the lowest tertiles (HR = 0.39, 95% CI = 0.18–0.83, HR = 0.19, 95% CI = 0.09–0.41, and HR = 0.31, 95% CI = 0.14–0.69, respectively). Inverse relations were observed between risk of CVD and dietary fiber from legumes, fruits and vegetables; however, dietary fiber intake from grain and nut sources was not related to risk of CVD. Conclusion: Our findings confirmed that higher intakes of dietary fiber from different sources is associated with CVD events and modify its major risk-related factors.

Keywords: coronary heart disease; dietary fiber; soluble fiber; insoluble fiber

1. Introduction

Dietary fiber, by its impact on the glycemic response and other aspects of metabolism, may also have important effects on cardiometabolic pathways [1]. An increasing number of studies have reported a reduced risk of cardiovascular disease (CVD) following regular diets high in fiber. Based on findings from epidemiologic studies regarding the protective effects of fiber intakes, the Dietary Reference Intakes (DRI) recommended consumption of dietary fiber is 14 g/1000 kcal, or 25 and 38 g/day for adult women and men, respectively [2]. Consuming a diet rich in high-fiber foods is also a critical component of the American Heart Association's strategy and other dietary recommendations for cardiovascular disease risk reduction in the general population [3,4].

It has been proposed that dietary fiber could modify underlying CVD risk factors including lipid and lipoprotein metabolism, insulin homeostasis, inflammatory markers and coagulation, and also improve insulin sensitivity, thereby reducing the risk of CVD mortality [5–7]. Although studies showed beneficial effects of soluble, gel-forming fiber on cardiometabolic risk factors, food sources of mainly insoluble fibers, primarily contributed by cereal products, have been the fiber most consistently associated with lower risk of CVD [5]. Findings of some investigations also suggest that the role of dietary fiber is more dependent on its types and sources, rather than the amount of intake [8,9]. Different types or sources of dietary fiber may induce different physiological effects; soluble fiber is responsible for the cholesterol-lowering effect of dietary fiber whereas insoluble fiber interacts with intestinal absorption of foods and contributes to reduction in clotting factors [10,11].

To examine the hypothesis that a greater intake of dietary fiber reduces risk of CVD, and different dietary fiber may lead to different CVD outcomes, we used prospective data from the Tehran Lipid and Glucose Study over a 6-year period to assess the relationship between total dietary fiber, soluble and insoluble fiber, and different fiber sources on the risk of CVD among Iranian adults.

2. Methods

2.1. Study Population

This study was conducted within the framework of the Tehran Lipid and Glucose Study (TLGS), an ongoing community-based prospective study being conducted to investigate and prevent non-communicable diseases in a representative sample in the district 13 of Tehran, the capital city of Iran [12]. During the third phase of the TLGS (2006–2008), of a total of 12,523 subjects who completed the examinations, 4920 were randomly selected for completing the dietary assessment based on their age and sex. The randomization was performed because of cost and complexity of dietary data collection in large populations and also the fact that this process is time-consuming. Finally, the dietary data for 3462 subjects who agreed to participate and completed the food frequency questionnaire (FFQ) were available. The characteristics of participants who completed the validated FFQ were similar to those of the total population in the third phase of TLGS [13]. For the purpose of the current study, among subjects aged $\geq$19 years, we recruited 2927 adult men and women, with complete data (demographics, anthropometrics, biochemicals). Participants were excluded from the final analysis if they had under- or over-reported energy intakes (<800 kcal/day or >4200 kcal/day, respectively), or were on specific diets (n = 563). Participants were also excluded if they had history of CVD at baseline examination (n = 88). The remaining participants (n = 2276) were followed until March 2012, for a mean duration of 4.7 years from the baseline examination. Participants who had left the study (n = 17) were also excluded and final analyses was conducted on data of 2259 adults (Figure 1).

Written informed consents were obtained from all participants. The study protocol, based on the ethical guidelines of the 1975 Declaration of Helsinki, was approved (ethics committee number: 57ECRIES94/02/15) by the Ethics Research Council of the Research Institute for Endocrine Sciences, Shahid Beheshti University of Medical Sciences.

2.2. Demographic and Anthropometric Measures

Demographics, anthropometrics and biochemical measures were assessed both at baseline (2006–2008) and again at the follow-up examination (2010–2012). Trained interviewers collected information including demographic data, medical history, medication use and smoking habits, using pretested questionnaires. Weight was measured to the nearest 100 g using digital scales, while the subjects were minimally clothed, without shoes. Height was measured to the nearest 0.5 cm, in a standing position without shoes, using a tape meter. Body mass index was calculated as weight (kg) divided by square of the height (m^2). Waist circumference was measured to the nearest 0.1 cm, midway between the lower border of the ribs and the iliac crest at the widest portion, over light clothing, using a soft measuring tape, without any pressure to the body. For blood pressure (BP) measurements, after a 15-min rest in the sitting position, two measurements of BP were taken on the right arm, during a standardized mercury sphygmomanometer; the mean of the two measurements was considered as the participant's BP.

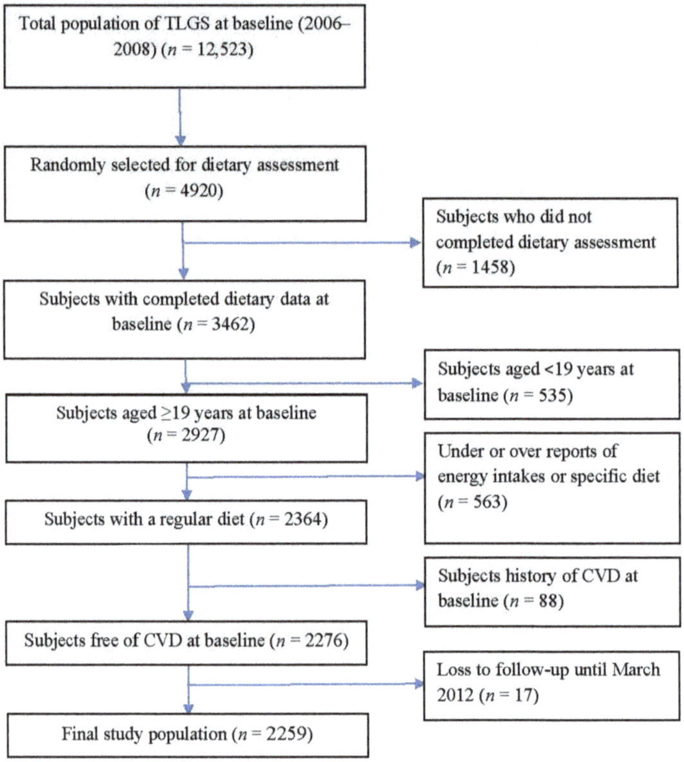

Figure 1. The flowchart of the study population.

2.3. *Biochemical Measures*

Fasting blood samples were taken after 12–14 h from all study participants, both at baseline and follow-up phase. Serum creatinine levels were assayed using kinetic colorimetric Jaffe method. Fasting serum glucose (FSG) was determined by the enzymatic colorimetric method using glucose oxidase. The standard 2 h serum glucose 2-h SG test was performed for all individuals who were not on anti-diabetic drugs. In a subsample of the population ($n = 904$), fasting serum insulin (FSI) was measured, by the electrochemiluminescence immunoasaay (ECLIA), using Roche Diagnostics kits and the Roche/Hitachi Cobas e-411 analyzer (GmbH, Mannheim, Germany). Intra- and inter-assay coefficients of variation for insulin were 1.2% and 3.5%, respectively.

Triglyceride (TG) levels were assessed by enzymatic colorimetric analysis with glycerol phosphate oxidase. High-density lipoprotein cholesterol (HDL-C) was measured after precipitation of the apolipoprotein B containing lipoproteins with phosphotungstic acid. Analyses were performed using Pars Azmoon kits (Pars Azmoon Inc., Tehran, Iran) and a Selectra 2 auto-analyzer (Vital Scientific, Spankeren, The Netherlands). Both inter- and intra-assay coefficients of variation of all assays were <5%.

2.4. Dietary Assessment

A 168-item food frequency questionnaire (FFQ) was used at the first examination to assess typical food intakes over the previous year. The validity and reliability of the FFQ had previously been assessed in a random sample, by comparing the data from two FFQs, completed 1 year apart and comparing the data from the FFQs and 12 dietary recalls, respectively; the validity and reliability of the FFQ for total dietary fat were acceptable; correlation coefficients between the FFQ and multiple 24 recalls were 0.59 and 0.38 and those between the two FFQs were 0.43 and 0.42 in male and female subjects, respectively [14]. Study of the reliability, comparative validity and stability of dietary patterns derived from the FFQ also showed that there was a reasonable reliability and validity of the dietary patterns among the population over time [15]. Trained dietitians asked participants to designate their intake frequency for each food item consumed during the past year on a daily, weekly, or monthly basis. Portion sizes of consumed foods reported in household measures were then converted to grams. Energy and nutrient content of foods and beverages were analyzed using the US Department of Agriculture Food Composition Table (FCT) because the Iranian FCT is incomplete, and has limited data on nutrient content of raw foods and beverages [13]. Finally, dietary intakes of participants, including dietary energy and energy density, macronutrients, and micronutrients were determined. In addition to calculating total dietary fiber from all foods, soluble and insoluble dietary fiber intakes were separately calculated. Additionally, we computed dietary fiber from different sources including cereal (traditional breads including barbari, taftoon, sangak, lavash, baguette breads, white rice, and barley), legumes (soya, cowpea, chickpea, broad bean, red bean, white bean, lentil, and split pea), nuts (almond, pistachio, walnut, hazelnut, and peanut), vegetables (green leafy vegetables, roots, starchy vegetables, and other vegetables including cucumber, tomato, scallion, zucchini, eggplant, cauliflower, onion, and garlic) and fruits (cantaloupe, melon watermelon, pear, apricot, cherries, apple, peach, nectarines, figs, grapes, kiwi, grapefruit, tangerine, pomegranate, strawberry, banana, lemons) as well.

2.5. Definition of Terms

History of cardiovascular disease was defined as previous ischemic heart disease and/or cerebrovascular accidents. Family history of premature cardiovascular disease reflected any prior diagnosis of cardiovascular disease in first-degree female relatives, aged <65 years, or first-degree male relatives, aged <55 years. Diabetes was defined as fasting serum glucose $\geq$126, 2 h serum glucose $\geq$200 or anti-diabetic medications [16]. Hypertension (HTN) was considered as systolic BP $\geq$140 mmHg or systolic BP $\geq$90 mmHg or current use of antihypertensive medications [17]. Homeostatic model assessment of insulin resistance was defined as follows: HOMA-IR = fasting insulin (μU/mL) $\times$ fasting glucose (mmol/L)/22.5; this index has been developed as a simple, inexpensive, and validated alternative tool for assessment of insulin resistance in epidemiological studies [18,19]. Insulin resistance was defined as HOMA-IR $\geq$3.2 [20].

2.6. Definition of Outcome in Our Study

Details of the collection of cardiovascular outcome data have been described elsewhere [21]. Briefly, each participant was followed up for any medical event annually by phone calls. Information of any medical condition or event was collected by a trained nurse, a trained physician and by utilization of data from medical files. The collected data were evaluated and confirmed by an outcome committee consisting of an internist, an endocrinologist, a cardiologist, an epidemiologist and other experts. CHD were included cases of definite myocardial infarction (MI) (diagnostic ECG and biomarkers), probable MI (positive ECG findings plus cardiac symptoms or signs plus missing biomarkers or positive ECG findings plus equivocal biomarkers), and angiographic proven CHD. Cardiovascular disease was defined as any CHD events, stroke (a new neurological deficit that lasted $\geq$24 h), or CVD death (definite fatal MI, definite fatal CHD, and definite fatal stroke) [22]. The CVD risk score was calculated according to the sex-specific "general CVD" algorithms were derived that incorporated age, total cholesterol, HDL-C, SBP, treatment for HTN, smoking, and diabetes status [23].

2.7. Statistical Methods

Dietary intakes of fiber and other nutrients were adjusted for total energy intake, according to residuals methods [24]. Mean (SD) values and the frequencies (%) of baseline characteristics of the participants, with and without CVD event were compared using independent t test or chi square test, respectively.

Linear associations of baseline intakes of total and different types of dietary fiber with changes of serum lipids, blood pressure and insulin levels during the follow-up period were estimated using linear regression models with adjustment of age, sex, and BMI.

A univariate analysis was performed for potential confounding variables including CVD risk score, dietary intake of total fats (% of energy), sodium (mg/1000 kcal), and vitamin C (mg/1000 kcal); variables with $P_E < 0.2$ in the univariate analyses were selected for the final multivariable models. Adjustment of CVD risk score, as a continuous potential risk factor of CVD, improve the stability of our models in the case of a limited number of events during the study follow-up.

To determine whether the associations of soluble and insoluble fiber intake are independent of each other, we adjusted the models in the presence of each type of the fiber. Similarly, the analyses of fiber from each different source were adjusted for fiber from all of the other sources.

Cox proportional hazard regression was used to assess the hazard ratios (HRs) of dietary fiber intakes for CVD. Time to event was defined by time of censoring or having event, whichever came first. The proportional hazards assumption was tested. We censored participants at the time of other causes of death, leaving the district or being in the study until March 2012 without event. The energy-adjusted amount of dietary fiber and its different types was categorized into tertiles, and the first tertile was given as a reference. Two Cox proportional hazard regression models were defined; model 1 was adjusted for CVD risk score and model 2 was further adjusted for dietary intakes of total fats, sodium and vitamin C. To assess the overall trends of HRs across tertiles of dietary fiber intakes, the median of each tertile was used as a continuous variable in Cox proportional hazard regression models.

All analyses were performed using IBM SPSS for Windows version 19 and STATA version 12 SE (StataCorp LP, College Station, TX, USA), with a two-tailed p value < 0.05 being considered significant.

3. Results

Mean age of participants (42.8% men) was 38.2 ± 13.4, at baseline. Mean (SD) dietary intake of total fiber was 23.4 (8.9) g/day. Legumes (35.8%), fruits (30.4%), vegetables (27.8%), and grains (24.0%) had greater contributions to total intakes of dietary fiber, respectively. During the average 4.7 ± 1.4 year of follow-up, 57 participants experienced CVD events; of which the more common events were angiographic proven CVD (40.4%), definite MI (24.6%), unstable angina (12.2%) and stroke (8.8%).

The distributions of the major known CVD risk factors and some biochemical values for the participants who had a CVD event and for those who did not are shown in Table 1. Higher prevalence of diabetes (14.3 vs. 3.9, p = 0.002) and HTN (43.9 vs. 8.3, p = 0.001), as well as higher rate of medications, including lipid-lowering drugs, anti-hypertensive drugs and aspirin, was observed in subjects with CVD events, compared to the rest of the cohort. Compared with non-CVD subjects, CVD patients were more likely to be older, and had higher BMI, waist circumference, blood pressure, serum creatinine, FPG, TG, TG/HDL-C ratio and CVD risk score at baseline (p for all < 0.05). Compared to non-CVD subjects, CVD patients had also higher intakes of dietary carbohydrate and lower intake of mono-unsaturated fatty acids and fiber (p for all < 0.05).

Results of linear regression showed a significant association between grain fiber intake and baseline CVD risk score (β = 0.05, 95% CI = 0.02–0.08) as well as changes of HOMA-IR (β = 0.04, 95% CI = 0.01–0.08) during the study follow-up. Legume fiber was associated with baseline CVD risk score (β = −0.14, 95% CI = −0.23, −0.04) and changes of HDL-C (β = 0.64, 95% CI = 0.19–1.08). Furthermore, dietary fiber from vegetables (β = −0.24, 95% CI = −0.34, −0.15), nuts (β = −0.23, 95% CI = −0.33, −0.13), fruits (β = −0.18, 95% CI = −0.28, −0.08) was inversely related to CVD risk score at baseline. Higher intake of dietary fiber from vegetables was related to lower levels of TG (β = −7.4, 95% CI = −12.7, −2.1) and TG/HDL-C ratio (β = −0.18, 95% CI = −0.29, −0.03), whereas dietary fiber intake from fruits was inversely related to changes of insulin levels (β = −7.80, 95% CI = −12.8, −2.7) and DBP (β = −0.50, 95% CI = −1.08, −0.03); compared to baseline values, higher intake of fruit-based fiber was also related to higher HDL-C levels (β = 0.54, 95% CI = 0.09–0.98).

Table 1. Baseline characteristics of the participants.

	Participants with CVD Outcome (*n* = 57)	Participants without CVD Outcome (*n* = 2202)	*p* Value
Age (years)	58.6 ± 9.7	37.3 ± 13.0	0.001
Male (%)	59.6	42.5	0.001
Smoking (%)	26.3	22.7	0.31
Body mass index (m^2/kg)	28.4 ± 4.4	26.5 ± 4.8	0.005
Lipid-lowering drugs (%)	10.5	1.5	0.001
Anti-hypertensive drugs (%)	14.3	1.5	0.001
Aspirin (%)	8.9	2.3	0.001
Waist circumference (cm)	97.2 ± 10.1	88.0 ± 13.2	0.001
Serum creatinine (μmol/L)	1.13 ± 0.18	1.03 ± 0.15	0.001
Systolic blood pressure (mmHg)	130 ± 17.4	109 ± 14.9	0.001
Diastolic blood pressure (mmHg)	80.2 ± 10.6	72.5 ± 10.3	0.001
Fasting blood glucose (mg/dL)	106 ± 39.9	88.5 ± 16.7	0.001
Serum triglycerides (mg/dL)	190 ± 107	132 ± 78.0	0.001
HDL-C (mg/dL)	40.2 ± 8.0	43.3 ± 10.4	0.03
TG/HDL-ratio	5.0 ± 3.2	3.4 ± 2.7	0.001
Serum insulin	7.4 ± 3.4	8.8 ± 4.9	0.13
HOMA-IR	1.5 ± 0.8	1.9 ± 0.8	0.28
Hyperinsulinemia (%)	12.5	17.6	0.57
Diabetes (%)	14.3	3.9	0.002
Hypertension (%)	43.9	8.3	0.001
Cardiovascular disease risk score	22.1	21.2	0.001
Dietary intakes			
Total fats (g/day)	74.1 ± 2.5	79.5 ± 0.4	0.03
Saturated fats (g/day)	24.8 ± 1.8	27.1 ± 0.3	0.22
Mono-unsaturated fat (g/day)	21.9 ± 1.0	27.6 ± 0.2	0.01
Sodium (mg/day)	4883 ± 410	4421 ± 66	0.26
Total carbohydrate (g/day)	337 ± 5.8	323 ± 0.9	0.02
Total fiber (g/day)	25.3 ± 1.1	29.0 ± 0.2	0.003

Data are mean ± SD unless stated otherwise (independent *t*-test for continuous variables and chi-square test for dichotomous variables was used.

There was also a significant negative association between fiber from nuts with body weight changes during the study period (β = −2.01, $p < 0.05$); no significant association was observed between other sources of dietary fiber or total fiber with changes of body weight.

The hazard ratios (95% CIs) of CVD across tertiles of dietary fiber and its categories are shown in Table 2. After adjustment of all potential confounding variables, a lower risk of CVD was observed in the highest compared to the lowest tertile of total dietary fiber intakes (HR = 0.39, 95% CI = 0.18–0.83, *p* for trend = 0.05). Soluble and insoluble dietary fiber was also negatively related to risk of CVD (HR = 0.19, 95% CI = 0.09–0.41, and HR = 0.31, 95% CI = 0.14–0.69) with a significant decreasing trend across increasing intakes (*p* for trend < 0.01).

Table 3 shows HRs (95% CIs) across tertile categories of different dietary sources of fiber. Dietary intake of grain and nut fiber had no significant association with the risk of CVD, whereas legume fiber intake was inversely related to risk of CVD (HR = 0.31, 95% CI = 0.15–0.65, in the third compared to the first tertile, *p* for trend = 0.003); similar associations were also observed for dietary intakes of fiber from fruit and vegetable sources. A combination of dietary fiber intake from vegetables, fruits and legumes also had similar impact on the risk of CVD (HR = 0.65, 95% CI = 0.34–1.24, and HR = 0.46, 95% CI = 0.22–0.96, in the second and third tertiles, respectively, p for trend = 0.11).

Table 2. The hazard ratio (95% CI) of coronary heart disease across tertiles of dietary fiber and its categories.

Dietary Fiber Intakes	T1	T2	T3	p for Trend
Total fiber				
Crude	Ref.	0.83 (0.45–1.54)	0.69 (0.36–1.33)	0.56
Model 1	Ref.	0.87 (0.46–1.62)	0.75 (0.38–1.46)	0.69
Model 2	Ref.	0.67 (0.35–1.26)	0.39 (0.18–0.83)	0.05
Soluble fiber				
Crude	Ref.	0.49 (0.26–0.91)	0.39 (0.20–0.76)	0.01
Model 1	Ref.	0.54 (0.29–1.03)	0.41 (0.20–0.82)	0.04
Model 2 [a]	Ref.	0.39 (0.21–0.75)	0.19 (0.09–0.41)	0.001
Insoluble fiber				
Crude	Ref.	0.64 (0.34–1.18)	0.53 (0.28–1.02)	0.15
Model 1	Ref.	0.72 (0.39–1.33)	0.58 (0.29–1.14)	0.25
Model 2 [b]	Ref.	0.54 (0.28–1.03)	0.31 (0.14–0.69)	0.014

Cox proportional hazard regression models were used. Model 1 was adjusted for cardiovascular disease risk score. Model 2 was additionally adjusted for dietary intake of total fats (% of energy), sodium (mg/1000 kcal), and vitamin C (mg/1000 kcal); [a] additionally adjusted for insoluble fiber; and [b] additionally adjusted for soluble fiber.

Table 3. The hazard ratio (95% CI) of coronary heart disease across tertiles of dietary fiber and its categories.

Dietary Fibers	T1	T2	T3	p for Trend
Grain fiber				
Crude	Ref.	0.89 (0.46–1.72)	1.11 (0.59–1.07)	0.79
Model 1	Ref.	0.83 (0.42–1.62)	0.98 (0.52–1.84)	0.84
Model 2	Ref.	0.79 (0.39–1.61)	0.90 (0.44–1.86)	0.82
Legume fiber				
Crude	Ref.	0.61 (0.34–1.11)	0.36 (0.18–0.73)	0.01
Model 1	Ref.	0.59 (0.32–1.09)	0.38 (0.18–0.77)	0.02
Model 2	Ref.	0.47 (0.25–0.89)	0.31 (0.15–0.65)	0.003
Nut fiber				
Crude	Ref.	0.78 (0.43–1.41)	0.47 (0.24–0.94)	0.10
Model 1	Ref.	0.77 (0.43–1.42)	0.54 (0.27–1.07)	0.21
Model 2	Ref.	0.65 (0.33–1.27)	0.49 (0.24–1.02)	0.14
Fruit fiber				
Crude	Ref.	0.74 (0.39–1.39)	0.81 (0.43–1.50)	0.61
Model 1	Ref.	0.74 (0.38–1.41)	0.83 (0.44–1.58)	0.65
Model 2	Ref.	0.56 (0.29–1.09)	0.44 (0.22–0.89)	0.05
Vegetable fiber				
Crude	Ref.	0.83 (0.45–1.52)	0.59 (0.31–1.16)	0.32
Model 1	Ref.	0.82 (0.45–1.51)	0.61 (0.31–1.21)	0.37
Model 2	Ref.	0.64 (0.34–1.20)	0.34 (0.16–0.72)	0.02

Cox proportional hazard regression models were used. Model 1 was adjusted for cardiovascular disease risk score. Model 2 was additionally adjusted for dietary intake of total fats (% of energy), sodium (mg/1000 kcal), and vitamin C (mg/1000 kcal), and other types of dietary fiber (g/day).

4. Discussion

In this prospective cohort study, conducted on a representative Iranian population, a mean 4.7-year follow-up showed that dietary fiber intake especially from legume, fruit, vegetable and nut sources had protective effect against the development of CVD events. Following adjustment of multiple CVD risk factors and dietary variables, most negative trends in the current study remained statistically significant.

Beneficial effects of vegetable fiber in reduced risk of CVD, in our study, could be related to decreased TG and TG to HDL-C ratio during the study follow-up. Lower risk of CVD across increasing intakes of dietary fiber from fruit sources could also be attributed to its inverse association with insulin levels and DBP as well as positive association with HDL-C. Lack of the beneficial effects of grain fiber on the risk of CVD may be explained by its positive relation with CVD risk score at baseline and its association with increased insulin resistance index during the study follow-up. It should be noted that in our study, high intakes of refined grains such as white rice and white breads had major contributions to dietary intakes of grain fiber, whereas the protective effects of grain fiber, reported in some previous studies, were mainly related to whole grains intake [11]. Aside from chance and biases, another explanation is that other characteristics of refined grains such as high-glycemic index nature, rather than fiber per se, may be responsible for the associations observed.

In a 6-year follow-up study among adult men, higher fiber intake (28.9 vs. 12.4 g/day) was inversely related to risk of total myocardial infarction by 0.41 (RR = 0.59, 95% CI = 0.46–0.76); the inverse association was strongest for fatal myocardial infarction (RR = 0.45, 95% CI = 0.28–0.72) [25]. Each 10-g increase in total dietary fiber corresponded to an RR for total myocardial infarction of 0.81 (95% CI, 0.70–0.93); among the three main food contributors to total fiber intake, cereal fiber had a stronger effect on the reduced risk of total myocardial infarction (RR = 0.71, 95% CI = 0.55–0.91 for each 10-g increase in cereal fiber/day) [25]. In another prospective cohort of elderly men, only cereal fiber consumption was associated with lower incident total stroke and ischemic stroke, whereas neither fruit fiber intake nor vegetable fiber intake were associated with incident CVD; compared to cereal fiber from other sources, fiber from dark breads including wheat, rye, and pumpernickel were associated with a lower risk of CVD (HR = 0.76, 95% CI = 0.64–0.90) [26].

Findings of a recent meta-analysis of 22 prospective cohorts showed that total dietary fiber intake was inversely associated with risk of CVD (Risk ratio = 0.91 per 7 g/day, 95% CI = 0.88 to 0.94) and CVD (Risk ratio = 0.91, 95% CI = 0.87–0.94); insoluble fiber and fiber from cereal and vegetable sources were inversely associated with the incident CVD and CVD, whereas fruit fiber intake was only inversely associated with risk of CVD [27]. No clear differences in the effect of dietary fiber intake from various food groups on CVD mortality have been observed in a cohort of adult men, although every additional 10 g/day intake of dietary total fiber reduced CVD mortality by 17% (95% CI = 2%–30%) and all-cause mortality by 9% (95% CI = 0%–18%) [28] (Table 4). The cardioprotective effect of dietary fiber has been found to be stronger for cereal fiber than for fruit or vegetable fiber [29]. In a cross-sectional study conducted on adult men and women, higher intakes of total fiber and insoluble fiber were inversely related to systolic blood pressure [30].

In our previous study, we showed that higher intake of total dietary fiber reduced the risk of metabolic syndrome by 47% (OR = 0.53, 95% CI = 0.39–0.74, p for trend < 0.05); soluble and insoluble fiber intakes were also related to lower risk of metabolic syndrome (OR = 0.60, 95% CI = 0.43–0.84, and OR = 0.51, 95% CI = 0.35–0.72). Similar findings were also observed for dietary fiber from fruits, cereals and legumes sources but not for vegetable and nut fiber [9]. In the National Health and Nutrition Examination Survey, dietary fiber intake was related to a low and intermediate lifetime CVD risk and there was a significant inverse linear association between dietary fiber intake and log-transformed C-reactive protein [31].

Some differences between our findings and those of other cohorts may be related to different dietary habits and dietary patterns; previous studies among Iranians demonstrated some major dietary patterns including traditional dietary pattern with higher load of white rice, traditional breads, vegetables, full-fat dairy products, hydrogenated fats, legumes, dried fruits and nuts; the healthy dietary pattern was related to a higher load of vegetables and fruits, whereas the Western pattern had higher load of fast foods, salty snacks, sweets, mayonnaise, and soft drinks [32,33]. Lack of significant associations between fiber from grains and nuts may be related to types of these food groups consumed among our population. Main grains consumed among the population were refined grains including white rice, and breads with a relatively low-fiber wheat flour; moreover, in our population, nuts were mainly consumed in the form of salty and roasted; these factors may reduce the expected protective effects of fiber from grains and nut sources.

Table 4. The association of dietary fiber intakes and the risk of cardiovascular disease.

Author	Study Population	Findings
Rimm et al. [25]	6-year follow-up study among adult men	Dietary intake of fiber 28.9 vs. 12.4 g/day decreased risk of total myocardial infarction (RR = 0.59, 95% CI = 0.46–0.76) and fatal myocardial infarction RR = 0.45, 95% CI = 0.28–0.72. Cereal fiber reduced risk of total MI (RR = 0.71, 95% CI = 0.55–0.91 for each 10 g/day increase in cereal fiber)
Mozaffarian et al. [26]	8.6-year follow-up of elderly men and women	Highest compared to the lowest quintile of cereal fiber consumption, decreased incident CVD (HR = 0.79; 95% CI = 0.62–0.99) Fruit fiber and vegetable fiber intake were not associated with incident CVD. Higher intake of cereal fiber was associated with lower risk of total stroke, ischemic stroke and ischemic heart disease death.
Streppel et al. [28]	40-year follow-up of adult men	Every additional 10 g/day of dietary fiber intake decreased CVD mortality by 17% (95% CI: 2%, 30%) and all-cause mortality by 9% (0%, 18%).
Threapleton et al. [27]	Meta-analysis of 22 prospective cohorts	Total fiber intake was inversely associated with risk of CVD (RR = 0.91 per 7 g/day, 95% CI = 0.88–0.94) and CVD (RR = 0.91, 95% CI = 0.87–0.94). Each 7 g/day increase in insoluble fiber (RR = 0.82, 95% CI = 0.70–0.96), fiber from cereal (RR = 0.84, 95% CI = 0.76 0.94), and each 4 g/day increase in fiber from vegetable sources (RR = 0.94, 95% CI = 0.89–1.00) decreased risk of CVD and CVD.

MI: Myocardial infarction; CVD: Coronary heart disease; CVD: Cardiovascular disease; HR + Hazard ratio; RR = Relative risk.

Several mechanisms have been proposed to explain beneficial effects of dietary fiber on metabolic pathways; Figure 2 displays some important mechanisms of cardioprotective effects of dietary fiber intakes. Colonic fermentation and subsequent production of short chain fatty acids is another metabolic effect of most types of dietary fiber especially soluble fibers; dietary fiber intake can also regulate gut hormonal responses that may act as satiety factors [34]. The lowering effect of dietary fiber on plasminogen activator inhibitor type 1 and factor VII coagulation activity is also another proposed mechanism for the biological actions of dietary fiber against cardiovascular outcomes [35,36]. Interplay between dietary fiber intakes and the intestinal microbiome has been found to modify the inflammatory responses in the body [37]. Considering the contributory role of gut microbiota in the development of cardiometabolic disorders, such as atherosclerosis, obesity, and type 2 diabetes, and the favorable effects of dietary fiber in modulation of gut microbiota, some cardioprotective properties of dietary fibers may be attributed to this mechanism [38–40].

Some strengths and limitations in the current study should be considered. Among the strength, its prospective population-based design, high participation rate and completeness of the follow-up, and use of a validated comprehensive FFQ to assess regular dietary intakes of the participants provided us an opportunity to investigate the associations of total intakes and different types of dietary fiber with 5-year incidence of CVD, relationship that have not been previously examined among Iranian population. Use of CVD risk score, based on age, total cholesterol, HDL-C, SBP, use of antihypertensive drugs, diabetes, and smoking status, in multivariate models allowed us to account for major CVD confounders without adding many variables that would lead to instability of our models. Of the study limitation, due to potential changes in CVD risk factors during the study follow-up, some degree of misclassification might have occurred which could lead to biased estimated hazard ratios towards the null, as inherent in any prospective study. Furthermore, both the participants' diets and the composition of food may have changed over the follow-up time, leading to errors in assessing dietary exposure of interest. Moreover, the young age of the participants resulted in low incidence of CVD during the study follow-up.

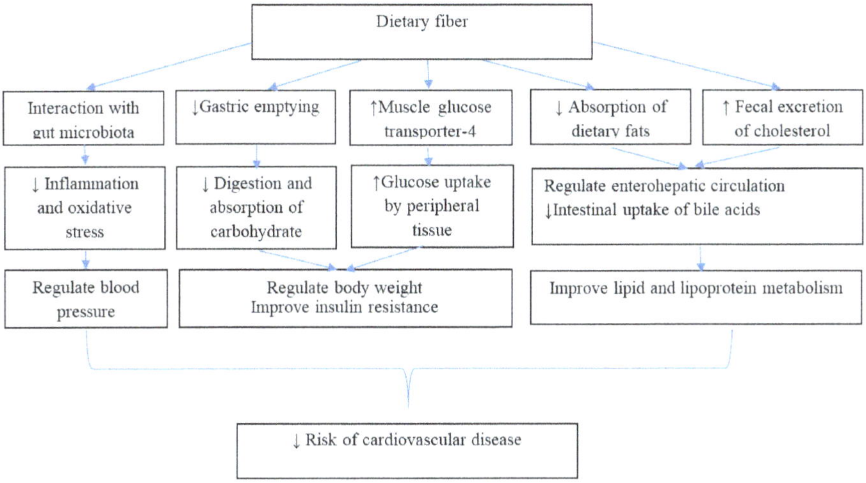

Figure 2. Mechanisms of protective effects of dietary fiber against development of cardiovascular disease. Dietary fiber improved insulin resistance by delaying gastric emptying, reduced absorption and digestion of carbohydrate and increased glucose uptake by peripheral tissue [34]. Dietary fiber also improved lipid and lipoprotein metabolism by decreased absorption of dietary fats, increased fecal excretion of cholesterol and decreased hepatic cholesterol synthesis; dietary fiber especially from cereal sources improved CVD health through multiple mechanisms including lipid reduction, body weight regulation, improved glucose metabolism, blood pressure control, and attenuation of oxidative stress and sub-clinical chronic inflammation [29]. Dietary fiber also modulated gut microbiota and modified cardiometabolic disorders [38–40].

5. Conclusions

In conclusion, our findings provided more evidence to confirm that increased intakes of fiber in a regular diet is an important cardioprotective dietary factor. Both soluble and insoluble dietary fibers have similar beneficial effects against the development of CVD. Dietary fiber intakes from legumes, vegetables and fruits may have stronger impact on cardiovascular outcomes.

Acknowledgments: We thank the TLGS participants and the field investigators of the TLGS for their cooperation and assistance in physical examinations, biochemical and nutritional evaluation and database management. We would like to acknowledge N. Shiva for critical editing of English grammar and syntax of the manuscript. This study was supported by grant No. 121 from the National Research Council of the Islamic Republic of Iran and the Research Institute for Endocrine Sciences of Shahid Beheshti University of Medical Sciences. This study was also supported by the Student Research Committee, Shahid Beheshti University of Medical Sciences (1395/S/47808).

Author Contributions: P.M., Z.B. and F.A. carried out the study design and analysis. P.M., Z.B., S.K.M., A.Z.V. and F.A. prepared the manuscript. All authors read and approved the final manuscript.

Conflicts of Interest: The authors declare no conflict of interest.

References

1. Pereira, M.A.; Liu, S. Types of carbohydrates and risk of cardiovascular disease. *J. Womens Health* **2003**, *12*, 115–122. [CrossRef] [PubMed]

2. Slavin, J.L. Position of the American Dietetic Association: Health implications of dietary fiber. *J. Am. Diet. Assoc.* **2008**, *108*, 1716–1731. [PubMed]
3. Lichtenstein, A.H.; Appel, L.J.; Brands, M.; Carnethon, M.; Daniels, S.; Franch, H.A.; Appel, L.J.; Brands, M.; Carnethon, M.; Daniels, S.; et al. Diet and lifestyle recommendations revision 2006: A scientific statement from the American Heart Association Nutrition Committee. *Circulation* **2006**, *114*, 82–96. [CrossRef] [PubMed]
4. Eilat-Adar, S.; Sinai, T.; Yosefy, C.; Henkin, Y. Nutritional recommendations for cardiovascular disease prevention. *Nutrients* **2013**, *5*, 3646–3683. [CrossRef] [PubMed]
5. Erkkila, A.T.; Lichtenstein, A.H. Fiber and cardiovascular disease risk: How strong is the evidence? *J. Cardiovasc. Nurs.* **2006**, *21*, 3–8. [CrossRef] [PubMed]
6. Eshak, E.S.; Iso, H.; Date, C.; Kikuchi, S.; Watanabe, Y.; Wada, Y.; Wakai, K.; Tamakoshi, A.; JACC Study Group. Dietary fiber intake is associated with reduced risk of mortality from cardiovascular disease among Japanese men and women. *J. Nutr.* **2010**, *140*, 1445–1453. [CrossRef] [PubMed]
7. Kokubo, Y.; Iso, H.; Saito, I.; Yamagishi, K.; Ishihara, J.; Inoue, M.; Tsugane, S.; JPHC Study Group. Dietary fiber intake and risk of cardiovascular disease in the Japanese population: The Japan Public Health Center-based study cohort. *Eur. J. Clin. Nutr.* **2011**, *65*, 1233–1241. [CrossRef] [PubMed]
8. McKeown, N.M.; Meigs, J.B.; Liu, S.; Saltzman, E.; Wilson, P.W.; Jacques, P.F. Carbohydrate nutrition, insulin resistance, and the prevalence of the metabolic syndrome in the Framingham Offspring Cohort. *Diabetes Care* **2004**, *27*, 538–546. [CrossRef] [PubMed]
9. Hosseinpour, S.M.P.; Sohrab, G.; Hosseini-Esfahani, F.; Azizi, F. Inverse association between fruit, legume, and cereal fiber and the risk of metabolic syndrome: Tehran Lipid and Glucose Study. *Diabetes Res. Clin. Pract.* **2011**, *94*, 276–283. [CrossRef] [PubMed]
10. Brown, L.; Rosner, B.; Willett, W.W.; Sacks, F.M. Cholesterol-lowering effects of dietary fiber: A meta-analysis. *Am. J. Clin. Nutr.* **1999**, *69*, 30–42. [PubMed]
11. Liu, S.; Buring, J.E.; Sesso, H.D.; Rimm, E.B.; Willett, W.C.; Manson, J.E. A prospective study of dietary fiber intake and risk of cardiovascular disease among women. *J. Am. Coll. Cardiol.* **2002**, *39*, 49–56. [CrossRef]
12. Azizi, F.; Rahmani, M.; Emami, H.; Mirmiran, P.; Hajipour, R.; Madjid, M.; Ghanbili, J.; Ghanbarian, A.; Mehrabi, Y.; Saadat, N.; et al. Cardiovascular risk factors in an Iranian urban population: Tehran lipid and glucose study (phase 1). *Soz. Praventivmed.* **2002**, *47*, 408–426. [CrossRef] [PubMed]
13. Hosseini-Esfahani, F.; Jessri, M.; Mirmiran, P.; Bastan, S.; Azizi, F. Adherence to dietary recommendations and risk of metabolic syndrome: Tehran Lipid and Glucose Study. *Metab. Clin. Exp.* **2010**, *59*, 1833–1842. [CrossRef] [PubMed]
14. Mirmiran, P.; Esfahani, F.H.; Mehrabi, Y.; Hedayati, M.; Azizi, F. Reliability and relative validity of an FFQ for nutrients in the Tehran lipid and glucose study. *Public Health Nutr.* **2010**, *13*, 654–662. [CrossRef] [PubMed]
15. Panagiotakos, D.B.; Pitsavos, C.; Skoumas, Y.; Stefanadis, C. The Association between Food Patterns and the Metabolic Syndrome Using Principal Components Analysis: The ATTICA Study. *J. Am. Diet. Assoc.* **2007**, *107*, 979–987. [CrossRef] [PubMed]
16. American Diabetes Association. Standards of medical care in diabetes—2014. *Diabetes Care* **2014**, *37*, S14–S80.
17. Chobanian, A.V.; Bakris, G.L.; Black, H.R.; Cushman, W.C.; Green, L.A.; Izzo, J.L., Jr.; Jones, D.W.; Materson, B.J.; Oparil, S.; Wright, J.T., Jr.; et al. The Seventh Report of the Joint National Committee on Prevention, Detection, Evaluation, and Treatment of High Blood Pressure: The JNC 7 report. *JAMA* **2003**, *289*, 2560–2572. [CrossRef] [PubMed]
18. Borai, A.; Livingstone, C.; Kaddam, I.; Ferns, G. Selection of the appropriate method for the assessment of insulin resistance. *BMC Med. Res. Methodol.* **2011**, *11*, 158. [CrossRef] [PubMed]
19. Muniyappa, R.; Lee, S.; Chen, H.; Quon, M.J. Current approaches for assessing insulin sensitivity and resistance in vivo: Advantages, limitations, and appropriate usage. *Am. J. Physiol. Endocrinol. Metab.* **2008**, *94*, E15–E26. [CrossRef] [PubMed]
20. Enzevaei, A.; Salehpour, S.; Tohidi, M.; Saharkhiz, N. Subclinical hypothyroidism and insulin resistance in polycystic ovary syndrome: Is there a relationship? *Iran. J. Reprod. Med.* **2014**, *12*, 481–486. [PubMed]
21. Hadaegh, F.; Harati, H.; Ghanbarian, A.; Azizi, F. Association of total cholesterol versus other serum lipid parameters with the short-term prediction of cardiovascular outcomes: Tehran Lipid and Glucose Study. *Eur. J. Cardiovasc. Prev. Rehabil.* **2006**, *13*, 571–577. [CrossRef] [PubMed]

22. Nejat, A.; Mirbolouk, M.; Mohebi, R.; Hasheminia, M.; Tohidi, M.; Saadat, N.; Azizi, F.; Hadaegh, F. Changes in lipid measures and incident coronary heart disease: Tehran Lipid & Glucose Study. *Clin. Biochem.* **2014**, *47*, 1239–1244. [PubMed]
23. D'Agostino, R.B., Sr.; Vasan, R.S.; Pencina, M.J.; Wolf, P.A.; Cobain, M.; Massaro, J.M.; Kannel, W.B. General cardiovascular risk profile for use in primary care: The Framingham Heart Study. *Circulation* **2008**, *117*, 743–753. [CrossRef] [PubMed]
24. Yilmaz, B.; Sahin, K.; Bilen, H.; Bahcecioglu, I.H.; Bilir, B.; Ashraf, S.; Halazun, K.J.; Kucuk, O. Carotenoids and non-alcoholic fatty liver disease. *Hepatobiliary Surg. Nutr.* **2015**, *4*, 161–171. [PubMed]
25. Rimm, E.B.; Ascherio, A.; Giovannucci, E.; Spiegelman, D.; Stampfer, M.J.; Willett, W.C. Vegetable, fruit, and cereal fiber intake and risk of coronary heart disease among men. *JAMA* **1996**, *275*, 447–451. [CrossRef] [PubMed]
26. Mozaffarian, D.; Kumanyika, S.K.; Lemaitre, R.N.; Olson, J.L.; Burke, G.L.; Siscovick, D.S. Cereal, fruit, and vegetable fiber intake and the risk of cardiovascular disease in elderly individuals. *JAMA* **2003**, *289*, 1659–1666. [CrossRef] [PubMed]
27. Threapleton, D.E.; Greenwood, D.C.; Evans, C.E.; Cleghorn, C.L.; Nykjaer, C.; Woodhead, C.; Cade, J.E.; Gale, C.P.; Burley, V.J. Dietary fibre intake and risk of cardiovascular disease: Systematic review and meta-analysis. *BMJ* **2013**, *347*, f6879. [CrossRef] [PubMed]
28. Streppel, M.T.; Ocké, M.C.; Boshuizen, H.C.; Kok, F.J.; Kromhout, D. Dietary fiber intake in relation to coronary heart disease and all-cause mortality over 40 years: The Zutphen Study. *Am. J. Clin. Nutr.* **2008**, *88*, 1119–1125. [PubMed]
29. Satija, A.; Hu, F.B. Cardiovascular benefits of dietary fiber. *Curr. Atheroscler. Rep.* **2012**, *14*, 505–514. [CrossRef] [PubMed]
30. Aljuraiban, G.S.; Griep, L.M.; Chan, Q.; Daviglus, M.L.; Stamler, J.; Van Horn, L.; Elliott, P.; Frost, G.S. Total, insoluble and soluble dietary fibre intake in relation to blood pressure: The INTERMAP Study. *Br. J. Nutr.* **2015**, *114*, 1480–1486. [CrossRef] [PubMed]
31. Ning, H.; Van Horn, L.; Shay, C.M.; Lloyd-Jones, D.M. Associations of Dietary Fiber Intake with Long-Term Predicted Cardiovascular Disease Risk and C-Reactive Protein Levels (from the National Health and Nutrition Examination Survey Data. *Am. J. Cardiol.* **2014**, *113*, 287–291. [CrossRef] [PubMed]
32. Doostvandi, T.; Bahadoran, Z.; Mozaffari-Khosravi, H.; Mirmiran, P.; Azizi, F. Food intake patterns are associated with the risk of impaired glucose and insulin homeostasis: A prospective approach in the Tehran Lipid and Glucose Study. *Public Health Nutr.* **2016**, *19*, 2467–2474. [CrossRef] [PubMed]
33. Moslehi, N.; Hosseini-Esfahani, F.; Hosseinpanah, F.; Mirmiran, P.; Azizi, F. Patterns of food consumption and risk of type 2 diabetes in an Iranian population: A nested case–control study. *Nutr. Diet.* **2016**, *73*, 169–176. [CrossRef]
34. Weickert, M.O.; Pfeiffer, A.F.H. Metabolic Effects of Dietary Fiber Consumption and Prevention of Diabetes. *J. Nutr.* **2008**, *138*, 439–442. [PubMed]
35. Anderson, J.W.; Tietyen-Clark, J. Dietary fiber: Hyperlipidemia, hypertension, and coronary heart disease. *Am. J. Gastroenterol.* **1986**, *81*, 907–919. [PubMed]
36. Anderson, J.W.; Chen, W.J. Plant fiber. Carbohydrate and lipid metabolism. *Am. J. Clin. Nutr.* **1979**, *32*, 346–363. [PubMed]
37. Kuo, S.M. The interplay between fiber and the intestinal microbiome in the inflammatory response. *Adv. Nutr.* **2013**, *4*, 16–28. [CrossRef] [PubMed]
38. Miele, L.; Giorgio, V.; Alberelli, M.A.; De Candia, E.; Gasbarrini, A.; Grieco, A. Impact of Gut Microbiota on Obesity, Diabetes, and Cardiovascular Disease Risk. *Curr. Cardiol. Rep.* **2015**, *17*, 120. [CrossRef] [PubMed]
39. Hamaker, B.R.; Tuncil, Y.E. A perspective on the complexity of dietary fiber structures and their potential effect on the gut microbiota. *J. Mol. Biol.* **2014**, *426*, 3838–3850. [CrossRef] [PubMed]
40. Parnell, J.A.; Reimer, R.A. Prebiotic fiber modulation of the gut microbiota improves risk factors for obesity and the metabolic syndrome. *Gut Microbes* **2012**, *3*, 29–34. [CrossRef] [PubMed]

nutrients

MDPI

Article

Exercise and Beta-Glucan Consumption (*Saccharomyces cerevisiae*) Improve the Metabolic Profile and Reduce the Atherogenic Index in Type 2 Diabetic Rats (HFD/STZ)

Eric Francelino Andrade [1,*], Andressa Ribeiro Veiga Lima [2], Ingrid Edwiges Nunes [3], Débora Ribeiro Orlando [4], Paula Novato Gondim [1], Márcio Gilberto Zangeronimo [1], Fernando Henrique Ferrari Alves [2] and Luciano José Pereira [2]

1 Department of Veterinary Medicine, Federal University of Lavras, Mail Box 3037, Lavras 37200-000, Brazil; pngondim@hotmail.com (P.N.G.); zangeronimo@prpg.ufla.br (M.G.Z.)

2 Department of Health Sciences, Federal University of Lavras, Mail Box 3037, Lavras 37200-000, Brazil; andressaveigalima@outlook.com (A.R.V.L.); fernando.ferrari@dsa.ufla.br (F.H.F.A.); lucianojosepereira@dsa.ufla.br (L.J.P.)

3 Department of Animal Sciences, Federal University of Lavras, Mail Box 3037, Lavras 37200-000, Brazil; inunes2611@gmail.com

4 Department of Agricultural Sciences, Federal University of Jequitinhonha and Mucuri Valleys, Rua Vereador João Narciso, 1380—Bairro Cachoeira, Unaí 3861-000, Brazil; debora.ribeiro@ufvjm.edu.br

* Correspondence: ericfrancelinoandrade@gmail.com; Tel.: +55-35-99187-2385

Received: 22 September 2016; Accepted: 29 November 2016; Published: 17 December 2016

Abstract: Physical activity and the ingestion of dietary fiber are non-drug alternatives commonly used as adjuvants to glycemic control in diabetic individuals. Among these fibers, we can highlight beta-glucans. However, few studies have compared isolated and synergic effects of physical exercise and beta-glucan ingestion, especially in type 2 diabetic rats. Therefore, we evaluated the effects beta-glucan (*Saccharomyces cerevisiae*) consumption, associated or not to exercise, on metabolic parameters of diabetic Wistar rats. The diabetes *mellitus* (DM) was induced by high-fat diet (HFD) associated with a low dose of streptozotocin (STZ—35 mg/kg). Trained groups were submitted to eight weeks of exercise in aquatic environment. In the last 28 days of experiment, animals received 30 mg/kg/day of beta-glucan by gavage. Isolated use of beta-glucan decreased glucose levels in fasting, Glycated hemoglobin (HbA1c), triglycerides (TAG), total cholesterol (TC), low-density lipoprotein (LDL-C), the atherogenic index of plasma. Exercise alone also decreased blood glucose levels, HbA1c, and renal lesions. An additive effect for reducing the atherogenic index of plasma and renal lesions was observed when both treatments were combined. It was concluded that both beta-glucan and exercise improved metabolic parameters in type 2 (HFD/STZ) diabetic rats.

Keywords: dietary fibers; glycemic control; metabolic profile

1. Introduction

Diabetes *mellitus* (DM) is a metabolic disorder characterized by chronic hyperglycemia, caused by the absence or reduction in insulin production (type 1 DM) as well as the resistance to the action of this hormone, featuring type 2 DM [1]. About 90% of DM cases are of type 2, and this fact is associated with increased incidence of obesity and obesity in the general population, especially in developing nations [2,3]. In addition, DM may predispose to diseases, such as retinopathy, nephropathy, neuropathy and heart disease, further aggravating the health condition of patients [2,4].

Glycemic control in diabetic patients can be achieved through the use of exogenous insulin and/oral hypoglycemic drugs [5]. However, the interaction between medications could cause side effects, and does not prevent the diseases associated with DM, making necessary the search for non-pharmacological alternatives to assist in the maintenance of blood sugar levels [4,6]. In this sense, the practice of physical exercise and diet therapy has been recommended as a treatment or therapeutic adjuvant [7]. Physical exercise increases the uptake and utilization of circulating glucose and improves insulin sensitivity [8]. The ingestion of some dietary fibers has also been reported to show antihyperglycemic action—mainly by reducing the absorption of carbohydrates and lipids in the intestine. Among these fibers, we can highlight beta-glucans that are polysaccharides found in the composition of cereal, fungi, bacteria and some grass cell walls [9].

The chemical structure of beta-glucan varies according to its origin [10]. Beta-glucans found in plants and cereals are linear and have branchings with β-1,3/1,4-type glycosidic linkages (soluble with low molecular weight), while those found in yeasts and fungi have β-1,3/1,6-type glycosidic linkages (insoluble with high molecular weight) [11]. These conformations make beta-glucans exhibit distinct physicochemical characteristics, such as molecular mass and solubility [12,13]. Cereal beta-glucans are reported to show metabolic potential, while those from fungi and yeast increase immune response [10,14,15]. Although fungi beta-glucans are recognized to modulate the immune response [16], recent studies from our group have also demonstrated interesting metabolic effects of yeast beta-glucans (*Saccharomyces cereviseae*) [10,17,18].

Considering the previously known effects of both exercise and the beta-glucan on glycemic control and metabolism, it is necessary to investigate the concomitant action of these agents in the treatment of type DM. In addition, there is a shortage of studies evaluating such effects in type 2 diabetes model. Thus, the present study aimed to evaluate the effects of beta-glucan (*Saccharomyces cerevisiae*), associated or not to physical exercise, on the metabolic parameters of type 2 diabetic rats (HFD/STZ).

2. Materials and Methods

2.1. Animals

This study was approved by the Ethics Committee on Animal Use of Federal University of Lavras (CEUA protocol 002/2015). The animals were kept in accordance with the Guide to the Care and Use of Experimental Animals (1993). The number of animals per group was kept at a minimum for ethical reasons but still enough to reach statistical significance. Thus, a power calculation test was performed to determine the sample size. The sample size was determined to provide 80% power to recognize a significant difference of 20% among groups and a standard deviation of 15% with a 95% confidence interval ($\alpha = 0.05$).

We used adult male Wistar rats (*Rattus norvegicus albinos*)—from the Animal Laboratory of the Federal University of Lavras (UFLA). Animals weighed 195.0 ± 15.7 g at the beginning of the study. Initially, rats were submitted to seven days of acclimatization in polypropylene boxes (dimensions 41 cm × 34 cm × 17.5 cm), containing wood shavings (for absorbing urine and water). Six animals were placed in each box. Throughout the experimental period, the rodents remained under controlled temperature (22 ± 2 °C), humidity (45% ± 15%) and luminosity (12–12 h light-dark cycle) conditions. High-fat diet and water were provided ad libitum throughout the experiment.

2.2. Induction of Diabetes Mellitus

At the end of the acclimatization period, all animals were submitted to type 2 diabetes induction protocol as described by Wang et al. [19]. The animals received high-fat diet (HFD—25% fat, 48% carbohydrates and 20% protein) for 28 days. Then, a low dose of streptozotocin (dissolved in citrate buffer—pH = 4.5) was injected intraperitoneally (STZ—35 mg/kg). Blood glucose levels were measured 48 h after STZ injection. Rats with blood glucose levels above 200 mg/dL [19] were considered diabetic. This model mimic advanced stages of type 2 diabetes in humans [19,20]. Rats that did not reach these glucose values were excluded from the experiment. Glycemia was checked weekly to ensure that diabetes was not reversed.

After diabetes induction, animals were randomly divided into four groups containing six animals each. A completely randomized experimental design in a 2 × 2 factorial scheme was used: with or without exercise and with or without beta-glucan.

2.3. Physical Training

After an acclimatization period, an adaptation to the aquatic environment was performed. Animals undergoing physical training remained for two hours daily, during seven days, in a polyethylene tank with a total capacity of 300 L, containing five centimeters of water at a temperature of approximately 32 ± 2 °C. The purpose of this acclimatization was to reduce stress against the aquatic environment, without causing, however, changes arising from the physical training [21].

In the following week, animals were submitted to progressive swimming sessions with time increments. This phase consisted of swimming without load, in 50 cm of water (in order to avoid animal tail contact with the bottom of the tank), where the animals swam 10 min in the first day, increasing 10 min daily until the end of six days, when each animal was swimming for 60 uninterrupted minutes without load [22].

In the subsequent eight weeks, the animals swam for 60 min daily, five times a week with a load of 5% of their body weight. This load causes improvement in the animals' endurance capacity, characterizing moderate intensity aerobic exercise [22]. After training sessions, we dried the animals with absorbent towels, before returning them to their cages [21].

2.4. Administration of Beta-Glucans

Simultaneously with training, in the last 28 days of the experiment, the animals in beta-glucan groups received a experimental solution and controls received saline—both by gavage. Beta-glucan solutions that contained 30 mg/kg of powder diluted in 0.3 mL saline solution prepared daily.

Beta-glucan used in the present study were derived from yeast *Saccharomyces cerevisiae*, with structural β-1,3/1,6 conformation. The beta-glucan powder presented the following composition: β-glucans—Min. 60.0%; Crude Protein—Max. 8.0%; pH (solution 2%) 4.0–7.0; Ash—Max. 10.0 g/100 g. Distribution of particle size: mean—41 μm; <20 μm 19%; 20–50 μm 43%; 50–100 μm 28%; 100–200 μm 10%; >200 μm 0%; Fluidity (seconds)—70.2; Angle of repose (degrees) 31.2; Compressibility 37%; Water retention capacity (mean) 7.4; and Solubility rate in water 7.9. The solutions were always administered daily in the morning. In animals under physical training, gavage was always performed with a minimum of 45 min before exercise, as described in previous studies [21,23].

2.5. Collection of Biological Material and Assessment of the Atherogenic Index of Plasma

At the end of the experimental period (eight weeks), the animals fasted for eight hours. Euthanasia was conducted by cardiac puncture under anesthesia (sodium thiopental 50 mg/kg ip). Glycated hemoglobin (HbA1c) and other blood biochemical parameters such as glucose, triacylglycerols (TAG), high density lipoprotein (HDL-C) and total cholesterol (TC) were determined using commercial kits (Labtest Diagnostica®, Belo Horizonte, Brazil and Gold analyzes diagnoses®, Belo Horizonte, Brazil) as described by Amr and Abeer [24]. The low-density lipoprotein (LDL) + very-low-density lipoprotein cholesterol (VLDL-C) levels of each animal were obtained by using the following equation: total cholesterol − HDL-C = LDL + VLDL-C [25]. Additionally, the animals' atherogenic index of plasma was calculated using the equation: log (TG)/(HDL-C), which is used as a significant predictor of atherosclerosis [26]. This index was used because type 2 diabetes increases one's chances of developing atherosclerosis [27].

2.6. Lee Index Assessment and Chemical Composition of the Body

The Lee index was calculated dividing the cubic root of body weight (grams) by the naso-anal length (cm) [18,28]. Internal organs, skin, head, feet and tail were removed from the animals and the clean carcasses were weighed and processed. Percentages of water, protein, fat and mineral matter present in the carcasses were evaluated by the meat FoodScan™ NIR analyzer (near-infra-red) (Foss, Warrington, UK) as performed by Vickers et al. [29]. This evaluation method of carcass composition has been considered as the gold standard [29].

2.7. Histological Analysis

Fragments of the right kidney and liver were fixed in 10% buffered formalin for 48 h, and then processed routinely for preparation of histological slices, which were then colored with hematoxylin-eosin [30]. An experienced veterinary pathologist conducted all histopathologic analysis (blind about experimental treatments). Tissue integrity, as well as the presence of alterations, were considered in the evaluations. Liver tissue ratings were assigned according to the presence and/or degree of steatosis as follows: no change—1; discreet—2; light—3; moderate—4; and severe—5. Steatosis was classified according to the presence of vacuoles in hepatocytes. Staining was performed with Periodic acid-Schiff (PAS) indicating accumulation of lipids or glycogen.

Similarly, the presence of renal lesions was scored as: no change—1; mild degeneration—2; low degeneration—3; moderate degeneration—4; marked degeneration 5. We observed the presence of alterations in the proximal and distal convoluted tubules, and the presence of calcifications in the glomerulus.

2.8. Statistical Analysis

Data were subjected to analysis of variance (two-way ANOVA) and means were compared by Tukey test ($p < 0.05$). Nonparametric data of liver and kidney damage scores were analyzed by the Kruskal–Wallis test ($p < 0.05$). We performed all analyses using statistical program Sisvar (version 5.3, Universidade Federal de Lavras, Lavras, Minas Gerais, Brazil) [31].

3. Results

Animals submitted to physical training, or consuming beta-glucan isolated and in association, presented lower fast blood glucose and HbA1c levels than diabetic animals (Table 1). Serum levels of TAG, TC and LDL-C were significantly reduced in animals consuming beta-glucan, independently of physical training. In addition, HDL-C levels were higher in animals treated with beta-glucan. Exercise did not significantly alter this parameter (Table 1). The atherogenic index of plasma in animals treated with beta-glucan was lower in comparison to without treatment. An additive effect of beta-glucan and physical exercise was observed for the atherogenic index of plasma. Blood parameters and atherogenic index of plasma means and standard deviations are presented in Table 1.

All treatments promoted similar results in the percentage of protein, fat and water in animals' carcasses. An increase in the percentage of mineral matter was observed in groups under physical training and beta-glucan consumption, with an extra increase when both treatments were associated. Exercise promoted a decrease in the Lee index compared to controls, with similar results among the other groups (Figure 1).

Liver histopathology slices revealed similar signs of steatosis in all groups (Table 2). Likewise, hydropic degeneration was found in the renal tissue from all groups. The degree of these lesions was attenuated by both physical exercise and beta-glucan ingestion (Table 3). Figures 2 and 3 represent, respectively, hepatic steatosis and renal degeneration in the different experimental groups.

Table 1. Biochemical parameters and atherogenic index of plasma in type 2 diabetic rats (high-fat diet/streptozotocin) submitted to physical training and treated beta-glucan (30 mg/kg/day).

	Beta-Glucan	Physical Training	
		Without	With
Glucose (mg/dL)	Without	371.0 (±21.4) [A,a]	335.0 (±10.4) [b]
	With	311.0 (±25.0) [b]	327.5 (±42.6)
HbA1c (mg/dL)	Without	9.4 (±0.4) [A,a]	8.8 (±0.3) [B]
	With	8.33 (±0.1) [b]	8.8 (±0.4)
Triacylglycerols (mg/dL)	Without	105.8 (±11.1) [a]	99.7 (±2.2) [a]
	With	71.5 (±7.2) [b]	57.5 (±12.8) [b]
Total cholesterol (mg/dL)	Without	88.8 (±22.9) [a]	85.4 (±9.4) [a]
	With	65.1 (±3.3) [b]	63.8 (±7.2) [b]
HDL-C (mg/dL)	Without	34.33 (±3.8) [a]	37.7 (±6.9)
	With	42.66 (±5.2) [b]	44.26 (±4.0)
LDL-C (mg/dL)	Without	34.6 (±20.1) [a]	33.4 (±5.8) [a]
	With	10.95 (±3.4) [b]	19.6 (±4.9) [b]
Atherogenic index of plasma	Without	1.6 (±0.6) [a]	1.3 (±0.2) [a]
	With	0.6 (±0.1) [A,b]	0.4 (±0.1) [B,b]

[a,b] Means followed by different letters in columns indicate significant differences between groups with and without beta-glucan treatment ($p < 0.05$); [A,B] Means followed by different letters in lines indicate significant difference between groups with and without physical training ($p < 0.05$).

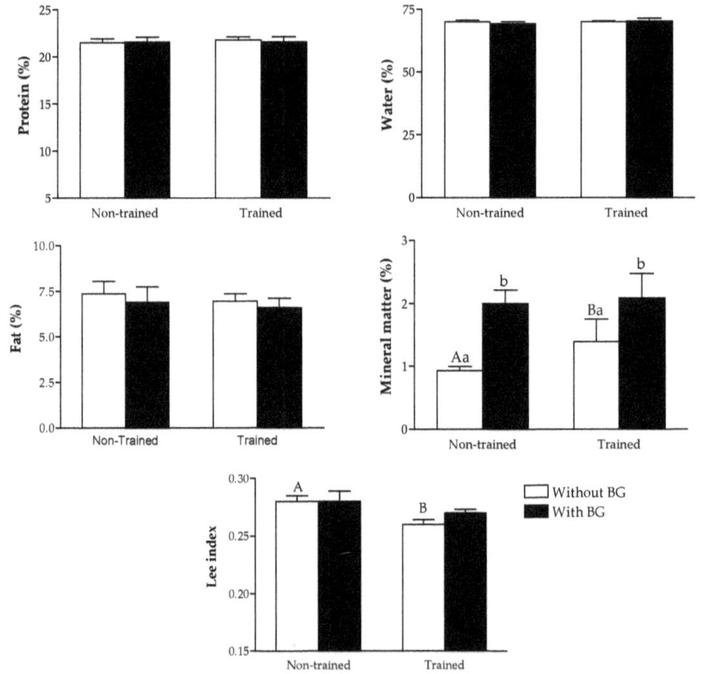

Figure 1. Chemical body composition (water, protein, fat and mineral matter) and Lee index of type 2 diabetic rats (high-fat diet/streptozotocin) submitted to physical training and treated with beta-glucan (30 mg/kg/day). [A,B] Significant difference between trained and non-trained groups; [a,b] Significant difference between groups with and without beta-glucans.

Table 2. Degree of hepatic steatosis in type 2 diabetic rats (HFD/STZ) submitted to physical training and/or treated with beta-glucans (30 mg/kg/day).

Group	Score of Steatosis				
	*	**	***	****	*****
A	0	3	0	3	0
B	1	3	2	0	0
C	2	3	0	1	0
D	1	5	0	0	0

* No change. ** Discreet Degeneration; *** Mild degeneration; **** Moderate degeneration; ***** Marked degeneration; A: diabetes *mellitus*; B: diabetes *mellitus* + beta-glucan; C: diabetes *mellitus* + exercise; D: diabetes *mellitus* + beta-glucan + exercise.

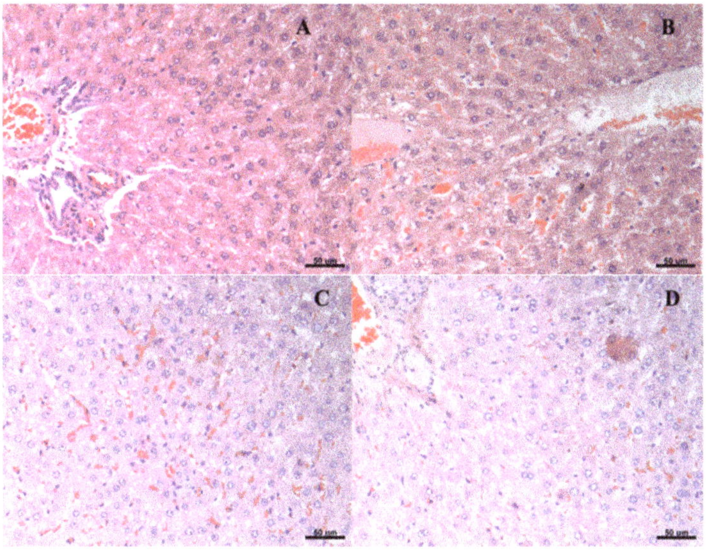

Figure 2. Histological representation (hematoxylin and eosin—20×) of degrees of hepatic steatosis in type 2 diabetic rats (HFD/STZ) submitted to physical training and/or treated with beta-glucans (30 mg/kg/day). (**A**) diabetes *mellitus*; (**B**) diabetes *mellitus* + beta-glucan; (**C**) diabetes *mellitus* + exercise; (**D**) diabetes *mellitus* + beta-glucan + exercise.

Table 3. Degree of renal degeneration in type 2 diabetic rats (HFD/STZ) submitted to physical training and/or treated with beta-glucans (30 mg/kg/day).

	Score of Renal Degeneration				
Group	*	**	***	****	*****
A	0	0	0	2	4
B	0	0	0	6	0
C	0	0	1	5	0
D #	0	0	1	5	0

* No change; ** Discreet Degeneration; *** Mild degeneration; **** Moderate degeneration; ***** Marked degeneration; # Difference compared to the DM group; A: diabetes *mellitus*; B: diabetes *mellitus* + beta-glucan; C: diabetes *mellitus* + exercise; D: diabetes *mellitus* + beta-glucan + exercise.

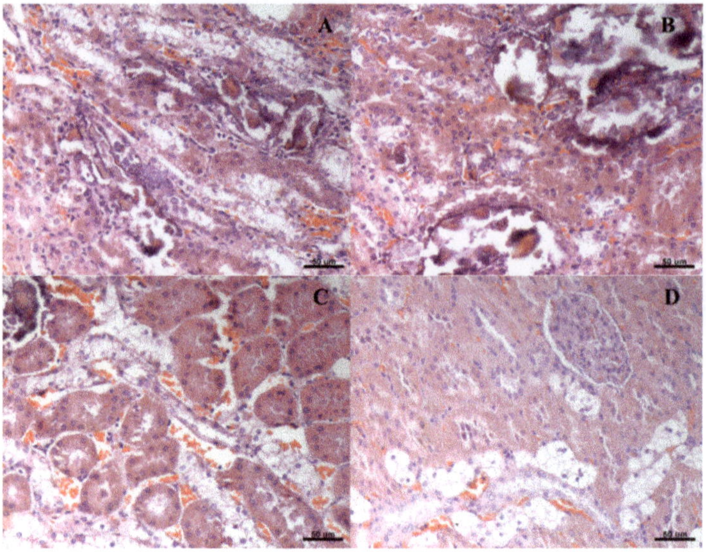

Figure 3. Histological representation (hematoxylin and eosin—20×) of degrees of renal degeneration in type 2 diabetic rats (HFD/STZ) submitted to physical training and/or treated with beta-glucans (30 mg/kg/day). (**A**) diabetes *mellitus*; (**B**) diabetes *mellitus* + beta-glucan; (**C**) diabetes *mellitus* + exercise; (**D**) diabetes *mellitus* + beta-glucan + exercise.

4. Discussion

The main findings of this study were related to improved glycemic control and reduced predisposition to atherosclerosis in animals subjected to both exercise beta-glucan consumption. Moreover, circulating lipoproteins levels, such as total cholesterol, LDL-C, and HDL-C, were improved in animals consuming beta-glucan, independently of physical exercise.

The effects of physical exercise on the improvement of glycemic control in diabetic patients (decrease in HbA1c and fasting glucose) are frequently reported [32–34]. Generally, this effect is due to the increased glucose uptake by skeletal muscle during exercise and increased insulin sensitivity for some hours after physical activity [35]. A beneficial effect in the glycemic control, in our study, was also observed after beta-glucan ingestion, as reported elsewhere in both animal [10] and in human studies [36]. Blood glucose control by beta-glucan consumption is probably due to the fact that these fibers form a gelatinous barrier in the intestinal lumen, hindering the absorption of carbohydrates and lipids by enterocytes [10,37,38]. In this sense, the same mechanism can be used to justify a reduction in circulating levels of total cholesterol, LDL-C and TAG found in groups treated with beta-glucan, with and without exercise. The improvement of the lipid profile, despite the consumption of beta-glucan, was a feature also observed in previous studies from our group [10,17]. The lower lipid absorption in the intestine favors the use of excessive cholesterol to the formation of bile salts in the liver, causing decreased blood concentrations of total cholesterol and LDL-C [39]. This mechanism is generally used to explain the anti-hypercholesterolemic effect of dietary fibers [39].

Among the possible beta-glucan's action, we can highlight the stimulation of intestinal motility, as well as changes in the microbiota and modulation of hormones secretion in the intestine [27,40,41]. Intestinal motility can be stimulated by the increase in the viscosity of the digesta in the lumen, due to the formation of a gelatinous layer [42,43]. In addition, beta-glucan decreases carbohydrates and lipid absorption [42], and consequently decreasing constipation problems [11]. High molecular weight beta-glucans (1,3/1,6) can also serve as a substrate for symbiotic microorganisms present in the intestine, increasing IgA and lysozyme secretion, and, as a consequence, immune resistance [40]. Another mechanism related to the functional effect of beta-glucans is satiety, mediated by gastrointestinal hormones [41]. Beta-glucans modulate the secretion of ghrelin and peptide YY, in order to inhibit hunger, acting indirectly in glycemic and lipidemic control [44].

In this study, we did not observe reduction of circulating lipids in trained animals. This may be related to the training time or duration of exercise sessions. Moura et al. [45] also found similar levels of HDL-C, LDL-C and TAG in diabetic rats (induced by alloxan) and subjected to 44 days of training, compared to sedentary diabetic rats. Another study demonstrated that twelve weeks of aquatic training decreased cholesterol levels and TAG in diabetic Zucker rats [46]. However, in the present study, no significant differences were observed in circulating lipids in animals submitted to physical training, and the atherosclerotic plasma index was reduced when there was an association of exercise and beta-glucan consumption. This additive effect may be related to improvement of the lipid profile provided by the dietary fiber [47], and to the recognized cardiovascular benefits of exercise [48].

Liver and renal lesions observed in all groups are consistent with those observed in type 2 diabetes, where circulating lipid levels promote increased fat deposition both in the liver and kidney [49,50]. However, even with the benefits observed with beta-glucan consumption or exercise, no changes were found in the degree of steatosis in any treatment. Beta-glucan consumption did not significantly alter steatosis either in a recent study of our group that investigated the effects of these fibers in rats submitted to high-fat diet [18]. On the other hand, it was observed that, in Sprague–Dawley rats, hepatic steatosis was reversed after eight weeks of treadmill exercise associated with restrictive diet (low-fat) [51]. Thus, it is possible that, in this study, steatosis was not attenuated because the animals were consuming a high-fat diet throughout the experimental period.

Regarding the effects of exercise, with or without the beta-glucan on the attenuation of renal lesions, it can be considered two mechanisms. The first one involves the reduction in lipotoxicity against moderate exercise [52], since the oxidative stress observed in diabetic patients is one of the factors that predispose to kidney damage [53]. The second one, more likely to explain the results of the present study, is the fact that exercise in moderate intensity promotes improvement in glycemic control, which consequently reduces the generation of advanced glycation-end products (AGE) [54]. Thus, the higher the blood glucose levels, the higher the formation of AGE that attack the kidney tissue and cause diabetic nephropathy [55].

Results of the present research show very promising effects of beta-glucan ingestion for glucose control. Complimentary studies are encouraged, evaluating insulin/leptin levels and inflammatory and cardiovascular parameters as well. The improvement of metabolic parameters in animals that consumed beta-glucans may be related to a decrease in the absorption of nutrients that increase plasma levels of glucose and lipids [37,39]. These changes were not as evident in animals subjected to exercise, possibly due to high-fat diet maintenance for the entire period.

5. Conclusions

Both exercise and beta-glucan consumption alone improved glycemic control in diabetic rats. In the present study, the combination of exercise and beta-glucans improved the atherosclerotic index and decreased renal lesions when compared to the isolated use of the treatments.

Acknowledgments: The authors thank the Coordination of Improvement of Higher Education Personnel (CAPES), the Research Foundation of the State of Minas Gerais (FAPEMIG), the National Council for Research and Technological Development (CNPq), and the Federal University of Lavras (UFLA), Brazil.

Author Contributions: E.F.A., L.J.P. and M.G.Z. conceptualized the study. E.F.A., A.R.V.L., P.N.G. and I.E.N. conducted the experiments. D.R.O. performed histopathologic analysis. M.G.Z. contributed to statistical analysis. E.F.A., F.H.F.A., and L.J.P. were involved in writing and editing the manuscript. All authors participated in the design of the study, study supervision, data interpretation, and revision and approval of the final version of the manuscript.

Conflicts of Interest: The authors declare no conflict of interest.

References

1. Forbes, J.M.; Cooper, M.E. Mechanisms of diabetic complications. *Physiol. Rev.* **2013**, *93*, 137–188. [CrossRef] [PubMed]
2. Chen, L.; Magliano, D.J.; Zimmet, P.Z. The worldwide epidemiology of type 2 diabetes mellitus—Present and future perspectives. *Nat. Rev. Endocrinol.* **2012**, *8*, 228–236. [CrossRef] [PubMed]
3. Kahn, S.E.; Cooper, M.E.; del Prato, S. Pathophysiology and treatment of type 2 diabetes: Perspectives on the past, present, and future. *Lancet (Lond. Engl.)* **2014**, *383*, 1068–1083. [CrossRef]
4. Atkinson, M.A.; Eisenbarth, G.S.; Michels, A.W. Type 1 diabetes. *Lancet* **2014**, *383*, 69–82. [CrossRef]
5. American Diabetes Association. Standards of medical care in diabetes—2015 abridged for primary care providers. *Clin. Diabetes* **2015**, *33*, 97–111.
6. Teixeira-Lemos, E.; Nunes, S.; Teixeira, F.; Reis, F. Regular physical exercise training assists in preventing type 2 diabetes development: Focus on its antioxidant and anti-inflammatory properties. *Cardiovasc. Diabetol.* **2011**, *10*, 12. [CrossRef] [PubMed]
7. Stevens, J.W.; Khunti, K.; Harvey, R.; Johnson, M.; Preston, L.; Woods, H.B.; Davies, M.; Goyder, E. Preventing the progression to type 2 diabetes mellitus in adults at high risk: A systematic review and network meta-analysis of lifestyle, pharmacological and surgical interventions. *Diabetes Res. Clin. Pract.* **2015**, *107*, 320–331. [CrossRef] [PubMed]
8. Thompson, D.; Karpe, F.; Lafontan, M.; Frayn, K. Physical activity and exercise in the regulation of human adipose tissue physiology. *Physiol. Rev.* **2012**, *92*, 157–191. [CrossRef] [PubMed]
9. Samuelsen, A.B.C.; Schrezenmeir, J.; Knutsen, S.H. Effects of orally administered yeast-derived beta-glucans: A review. *Mol. Nutr. Food Res.* **2014**, *58*, 183–193. [CrossRef] [PubMed]
10. De Oliveira Silva, V.; Lobato, R.V.; Andrade, E.F.; de Macedo, C.G.; Napimoga, J.T.C.; Napimoga, M.H.; Messora, M.R.; Murata, R.M.; Pereira, L.J. β-Glucans (*Saccharomyces cereviseae*) Reduce Glucose Levels and Attenuate Alveolar Bone Loss in Diabetic Rats with Periodontal Disease. *PLoS ONE* **2015**, *10*, e0134742.
11. Rahar, S.; Swami, G.; Nagpal, N.; Nagpal, M.A.; Singh, G.S. Preparation, characterization, and biological properties of β-glucans. *J. Adv. Pharm. Technol. Res.* **2011**, *2*, 94–103. [CrossRef] [PubMed]
12. Sonck, E.; Stuyven, E.; Goddeeris, B.; Cox, E. The effect of beta-glucans on porcine leukocytes. *Vet. Immunol. Immunopathol.* **2010**, *135*, 199–207. [CrossRef] [PubMed]
13. Mantovani, M.S.; Bellini, M.F.; Angeli, J.P.F.; Oliveira, R.J.; Silva, A.F.; Ribeiro, L.R. Beta-Glucans in promoting health: Prevention against mutation and cancer. *Mutat. Res.* **2008**, *658*, 154–161. [CrossRef] [PubMed]
14. Andrade, E.F.; Lobato, R.V.; Araújo, T.V.; Zangerônimo, M.G.; Sousa, R.V.; Pereira, L.J. Effect of beta-glucans in the control of blood glucose levels of diabetic patients: A systematic review. *Nutr. Hosp.* **2014**, *31*, 170–177.
15. Akramiene, D.; Kondrotas, A.; Didziapetriene, J.; Kevelaitis, E. Effects of beta-glucans on the immune system. *Medicina (Kaunas)* **2007**, *43*, 597–606. [PubMed]
16. Stier, H.; Ebbeskotte, V.; Gruenwald, J. Immune-modulatory effects of dietary Yeast Beta-1,3/1,6-D-glucan. *Nutr. J.* **2014**, *13*, 38. [CrossRef] [PubMed]
17. Lobato, R.V.; de Silva, V.O.; Andrade, E.F.; Orlando, D.R.; Zangeronimo, M.G.; de Sousa, R.V.; Pereira, L.J. Metabolic effects of β-glucans (*Saccharomyces cerevisae*) per os administration in rats with streptozotocin-induced diabetes. *Nutr. Hosp.* **2015**, *32*, 256–264.
18. De Araújo, T.V.; Andrade, E.F.; Lobato, R.V.; Orlando, D.R.; Gomes, N.F.; de Sousa, R.V.; Zangeronimo, M.G.; Pereira, L.J. Effects of beta-glucans ingestion (*Saccharomyces cerevisiae*) on metabolism of rats receiving high-fat diet. *J. Anim. Physiol. Anim. Nutr. (Berl)* **2016**. [CrossRef] [PubMed]
19. Wang, L.; Duan, G.; Lu, Y.; Pang, S.; Huang, X.; Jiang, Q.; Dang, N. The effect of simvastatin on glucose homeostasis in streptozotocin induced type 2 diabetic rats. *J. Diabetes Res.* **2013**, *2013*, 274986. [CrossRef] [PubMed]
20. Skovsø, S. Modeling type 2 diabetes in rats using high-fat diet and streptozotocin. *J. Diabetes Investig.* **2014**, *5*, 349–358. [CrossRef] [PubMed]
21. Rambo, L.M.; Ribeiro, L.R.; Oliveira, M.S.; Furian, A.F.; Lima, F.D.; Souza, M.A.; Silva, L.F.A.; Retamoso, L.T.; Corte, C.L.D.; Puntel, G.O.; et al. Additive anticonvulsant effects of creatine supplementation and physical exercise against pentylenetetrazol-induced seizures. *Neurochem. Int.* **2009**, *55*, 333–340. [CrossRef] [PubMed]

22. Gobatto, C.A.; de Mello, M.A.; Sibuya, C.Y.; de Azevedo, J.R.; dos Santos, L.A.; Kokubun, E. Maximal lactate steady state in rats submitted to swimming exercise. *Comp. Biochem. Physiol. A Mol. Integr. Physiol.* **2001**, *130*, 21–27. [CrossRef]
23. Andrade, E.F.; Lobato, R.V.; de Araújo, T.V.; Orlando, D.R.; da Costa, D.V.; de Oliveira Silva, V.; Rogatto, G.P.; Zangeronimo, M.G.; Rosa, P.V.; Pereira, L.J. Adaptation to physical training in rats orally supplemented with glycerol. *Can. J. Physiol. Pharmacol.* **2015**, *93*, 63–69. [CrossRef] [PubMed]
24. Amr, A.R.; Abeer, E.E.-K. Hypolipideimic and Hypocholestermic Effect of Pine Nuts in Rats Fed High Fat, Cholesterol-Diet. *World Appl. Sci. J.* **2011**, *15*, 1667–1677.
25. Martinez-flores, H.E.; Kil, Y. Effect of high fiber products on blood lipids and lipoproteins in hamsters. *Nutr. Res.* **2004**, *24*, 85–93. [CrossRef]
26. Hemmati, M.; Zohoori, E.; Mehrpour, O.; Karamian, M.; Asghari, S.; Zarban, A.; Nasouti, R. Anti-atherogenic potential of jujube, saffron and barberry: Anti-diabetic and antioxidant actions. *EXCLI J.* **2015**, *14*, 908–915. [PubMed]
27. Gleissner, C.A.; Galkina, E.; Nadler, J.L.; Ley, K. Mechanisms by which diabetes increases cardiovascular disease. *Drug Discov. Today Dis. Mech.* **2007**, *4*, 131–140. [CrossRef] [PubMed]
28. Lee, M.O. Determination of the surface area of the white rat with its application to the expression of metabolic results. *Am. J. Physiol.* **1929**, *89*, 24–33.
29. Vickers, S.P.; Cheetham, S.; Headland, K.; Dickinson, K.; Grempler, R.; Mayoux, E.; Mark, M.; Klein, T. Combination of the sodium-glucose cotransporter-2 inhibitor empagliflozin with orlistat or sibutramine further improves the body-weight reduction and glucose homeostasis of obese rats fed a cafeteria diet. *Diabetes Metab. Syndr. Obes. Targets Ther.* **2014**, *7*, 265–275. [CrossRef] [PubMed]
30. Andrade, E.F.; Lobato, R.V.; Araújo, T.V.; Orlando, D.R.; Gomes, N.F.; Alvarenga, R.R.; Rogatto, G.P.; Zangeronimo, M.G.; Pereira, L.J. Metabolic effects of glycerol supplementation and aerobic physical training on Wistar rats. *Can. J. Physiol. Pharmacol.* **2014**, *92*, 744–751. [CrossRef] [PubMed]
31. Ferreira, D.F. Sisvar: A computer statistical analysis system. *Ciênc. Agrotec.* **2011**, *35*, 1039–1042.
32. Hall, K.E.; McDonald, M.W.; Grisé, K.N.; Campos, O.A.; Noble, E.G.; Melling, C.W.J. The role of resistance and aerobic exercise training on insulin sensitivity measures in STZ-induced Type 1 diabetic rodents. *Metabolism* **2013**, *62*, 1485–1494. [CrossRef] [PubMed]
33. Ghiasi, R.; Ghadiri Soufi, F.; Somi, M.H.; Mohaddes, G.; Mirzaie Bavil, F.; Naderi, R.; Alipour, M.R. Swim Training Improves HOMA-IR in Type 2 Diabetes Induced by High Fat Diet and Low Dose of Streptozotocin in Male Rats. *Adv. Pharm. Bull.* **2015**, *5*, 379–384. [CrossRef] [PubMed]
34. Silveira, A.P.S.; Bentes, C.M.; Costa, P.B.; Simão, R.; Silva, F.C.; Silva, R.P.; Novaes, J.S. Acute effects of different intensities of resistance training on glycemic fluctuations in patients with type 1 diabetes mellitus. *Res. Sports Med.* **2014**, *22*, 75–87. [CrossRef] [PubMed]
35. Borghouts, L.B.; Keizer, H.A. Exercise and insulin sensitivity: A review. *Int. J. Sports Med.* **2000**, *21*, 1–12. [CrossRef] [PubMed]
36. He, L.; Zhao, J.; Huang, Y.; Li, Y. The difference between oats and beta-glucan extract intake in the management of HbA1c, fasting glucose and insulin sensitivity: A meta-analysis of randomized controlled trials. *Food Funct.* **2016**, *7*, 1413–1428. [CrossRef] [PubMed]
37. Tappy, L.; Gügolz, E.; Würsch, P. Effects of breakfast cereals containing various amounts of beta-glucan fibers on plasma glucose and insulin responses in NIDDM subjects. *Diabetes Care* **1996**, *19*, 831–834. [CrossRef] [PubMed]
38. Choi, J.S.; Kim, H.; Jung, M.H.; Hong, S.; Song, J. Consumption of barley beta-glucan ameliorates fatty liver and insulin resistance in mice fed a high-fat diet. *Mol. Nutr. Food Res.* **2010**, *54*, 1004–1013. [CrossRef] [PubMed]
39. Rideout, T.C.; Harding, S.V.; Jones, P.J.; Fan, M.Z. Guar gum and similar soluble fibers in the regulation of cholesterol metabolism: Current understandings and future research priorities. *Vasc. Health Risk Manag.* **2008**, *4*, 1023–1033. [CrossRef] [PubMed]
40. Raa, J. Immune modulation by non-digestible and non-absorbable beta-1,3/1,6-glucan. *Microb. Ecol. Health Dis.* **2015**, *26*, 27824. [CrossRef] [PubMed]
41. Rebello, C.J.; Burton, J.; Heiman, M.; Greenway, F.L. Gastrointestinal microbiome modulator improves glucose tolerance in overweight and obese subjects: A randomized controlled pilot trial. *J. Diabetes Complicat.* **2015**, *29*, 1272–1276. [CrossRef] [PubMed]

42. Reyna, N.Y.; Cano, C.; Bermúdez, V.J.; Medina, M.T.; Souki, A.J.; Ambard, M.; Nuñez, M.; Ferrer, M.A.; Inglett, G.E. Sweeteners and beta-glucans improve metabolic and anthropometrics variables in well controlled type 2 diabetic patients. *Am. J. Ther.* **2003**, *10*, 438–443. [CrossRef] [PubMed]
43. Battilana, P.; Ornstein, K.; Minehira, K.; Schwarz, J.M.; Acheson, K.; Schneiter, P.; Burri, J.; Jéquier, E.; Tappy, L. Mechanisms of action of beta-glucan in postprandial glucose metabolism in healthy men. *Eur. J. Clin. Nutr.* **2001**, *55*, 327–333. [CrossRef] [PubMed]
44. Vitaglione, P.; Lumaga, R.B.; Stanzione, A.; Scalfi, L.; Fogliano, V. β-Glucan-enriched bread reduces energy intake and modifies plasma ghrelin and peptide YY concentrations in the short term. *Appetite* **2009**, *53*, 338–344. [CrossRef] [PubMed]
45. Moura, L.P.; Puga, G.M.; Beck, W.R.; Teixeira, I.P.; Ghezzi, A.C.; Silva, G.A.; Mello, M.A.R. Exercise and spirulina control non-alcoholic hepatic steatosis and lipid profile in diabetic Wistar rats. *Lipids Health Dis.* **2011**, *10*, 2–7. [CrossRef] [PubMed]
46. De Lemos, E.T.; Pinto, R.; Oliveira, J.; Garrido, P.; Sereno, J.; Mascarenhas-Melo, F.; Páscoa-Pinheiro, J.; Teixeira, F.; Reis, F. Differential effects of acute (extenuating) and chronic (training) exercise on inflammation and oxidative stress status in an animal model of type 2 diabetes mellitus. *Mediat. Inflamm.* **2011**, *2011*, 253061.
47. Bays, H.E.; Evans, J.L.; Maki, K.C.; Evans, M.; Maquet, V.; Cooper, R.; Anderson, J.W. Chitin-glucan fiber effects on oxidized low-density lipoprotein: A randomized controlled trial. *Eur. J. Clin. Nutr.* **2013**, *67*, 2–7. [CrossRef] [PubMed]
48. Roberts, C.K.; Chen, A.K.; Barnard, R.J. Effect of a short-term diet and exercise intervention in youth on atherosclerotic risk factors. *Atherosclerosis* **2007**, *191*, 98–106. [CrossRef] [PubMed]
49. Alsaad, K.O.; Herzenberg, A.M. Distinguishing diabetic nephropathy from other causes of glomerulosclerosis: An update. *J. Clin. Pathol.* **2007**, *60*, 18–26. [CrossRef] [PubMed]
50. Birkenfeld, A.L.; Shulman, G.I. Nonalcoholic fatty liver disease, hepatic insulin resistance, and type 2 Diabetes. *Hepatology* **2014**, *59*, 713–723. [CrossRef] [PubMed]
51. Gauthier, M.-S.; Couturier, K.; Latour, J.-G.; Lavoie, J.-M. Concurrent exercise prevents high-fat-diet-induced macrovesicular hepatic steatosis. *J. Appl. Physiol.* **2003**, *94*, 2127–2134. [CrossRef] [PubMed]
52. Ghosh, S.; Khazaei, M.; Moien-Afshari, F.; Ang, L.S.; Granville, D.J.; Verchere, C.B.; Dunn, S.R.; McCue, P.; Mizisin, A.; Sharma, K.; et al. Moderate exercise attenuates caspase-3 activity, oxidative stress, and inhibits progression of diabetic renal disease in db/db mice. *Am. J. Physiol. Renal Physiol.* **2009**, *296*, 700–708. [CrossRef] [PubMed]
53. Tanaka, Y.; Kume, S.; Araki, S.; Isshiki, K.; Chin-Kanasaki, M.; Sakaguchi, M.; Sugimoto, T.; Koya, D.; Haneda, M.; Kashiwagi, A.; et al. Fenofibrate, a PPARα agonist, has renoprotective effects in mice by enhancing renal lipolysis. *Kidney Int.* **2011**, *79*, 871–882. [CrossRef] [PubMed]
54. Boor, P.; Celec, P.; Behuliak, M.; Grančič, P.; Kebis, A.; Kukan, M.; Pronayová, N.; Liptaj, T.; Ostendorf, T.; Šebeková, K. Regular moderate exercise reduces advanced glycation and ameliorates early diabetic nephropathy in obese Zucker rats. *Metabolism* **2009**, *58*, 1669–1677. [CrossRef] [PubMed]
55. Yamagishi, S.-I.; Matsui, T. Advanced glycation end products, oxidative stress and diabetic nephropathy. *Oxid. Med. Cell. Longev.* **2010**, *3*, 101–108. [CrossRef] [PubMed]

nutrients

MDPI

Article

Consumption of Fruit or Fiber-Fruit Decreases the Risk of Cardiovascular Disease in a Mediterranean Young Cohort

Pilar Buil-Cosiales [1,2,3], Miguel Angel Martinez-Gonzalez [2,3,4,5], Miguel Ruiz-Canela [2,3,4], Javier Díez-Espino [1,2,3], Ana García-Arellano [6] and Estefania Toledo [2,3,4,*]

1. Atención Primaria, Servicio Navarro de Salud-Osasunbidea, 08010 Navarra, Spain; pilarbuil@ono.com (P.B.-C.); javierdiezesp@ono.com (J.D.-E.)
2. Centro de Investigación Biomédica en Red Fisiopatología de la Obesidad y Nutrición (CIBERobn), Instituto de Salud Carlos III, 28029 Madrid, Spain; mamartinez@unav.es (M.A.M.-G.); mcanela@unav.es (M.R.C.)
3. IdiSNA, Navarra Institute for Health Research, 31008 Pamplona, Navarra, Spain
4. Department of Preventive Medicine and Public Health, University of Navarra, 31008 Pamplona, Navarra, Spain
5. Department of Nutrition, Harvard School of Public Health, Boston, MA 02115, USA
6. Department of Emergency, Complejo Hospitalario de Navarra Servicio Navarro de Salud-Osasunbidea, 31008 Pamplona, Navarra, Spain; agarare@gmail.com

* Correspondence: etoledo@unav.es or etoledo@unav.com; Tel.: +34-948-425600 (ext. 806224)

Received: 3 January 2017; Accepted: 10 March 2017; Published: 17 March 2017

Abstract: Fiber and fiber-rich foods have been inversely associated with cardiovascular disease (CVD), but the evidence is scarce in young and Mediterranean cohorts. We used Cox regression models to assess the association between quintiles of total fiber and fiber from different sources, and the risk of CVD adjusted for the principal confounding factors in a Mediterranean cohort of young adults, the SUN (Seguimiento Universidad de Navarra, Follow-up) cohort. After a median follow-up of 10.3 years, we observed 112 cases of CVD among 17,007 participants (61% female, mean age 38 years). We observed an inverse association between fiber intake and CVD events (p for trend = 0.024) and also between the highest quintile of fruit consumption (hazard ratio (HR) 0.51, 95% confidence interval (CI) 0.27–0.95) or whole grains consumption (HR 0.43 95% CI 0.20–0.93) and CVD compared to the lowest quintile, and also a HR of 0.58 (95% CI 0.37–0.90) for the participants who ate at least 175 g/day of fruit. Only the participants in the highest quintile of fruit-derived fiber intake had a significantly lower risk of CVD (HR 0.52, 95% CI 0.28–0.97). The participants who ate at least one serving per week of cruciferous vegetables had a lower risk than those who did not (HR 0.52, 95% CI 0.30–0.89). In conclusion, high fruit consumption, whole grain consumption, or consumption of at least one serving/week of cruciferous vegetables may be protective against CVD in young Mediterranean populations.

Keywords: fiber; fruit; vegetables; cardiovascular disease; legumes; whole grains

1. Introduction

Cardiovascular disease (CVD) is the leading cause of morbidity and mortality in developed countries [1,2] and its prevalence is increasing in developing countries. Lifestyles are the most important determinants of CVD, among which nutritional habits play an important role.

Higher dietary fiber intake has been recognized to be inversely associated with coronary heart disease (CHD) [3] and stroke [4]. Nevertheless, studies that have assessed the association between fiber intake and CVD in Mediterranean countries are scarce. It is also noteworthy that the foods that mainly contribute to the high intake of fiber—namely fruits, vegetables, legumes, and whole grains—have other micronutrients that have been postulated to be even more important for the prevention of CVD [5,6].

Fruits and vegetables are a heterogeneous food group with different contents of vitamins, minerals, and other bioactive phytochemicals [7]. There are not many studies that have evaluated the association between specific fruits or vegetables or groups of them, and it is unclear which fruit or vegetable subgroup may be the most protective against CVD. Also, fruits and vegetables consumed in different regions differ, and this could explain the differences observed in their reported effects [8].

Epidemiologic studies that have analyzed the relationship between fruit and vegetable consumption, which represent the principal source of fiber in Mediterranean countries, and CHD found inconsistent results. A meta-analysis published in 2015 [8], that analyzed 23 studies assessing this relationship, found an inverse association but showed heterogeneity with geographical differences. Concretely, an inverse association between fruit and vegetable consumption and CHD was observed only in Western countries. In addition, only one of the included studies had been conducted in a Mediterranean country [9] and this latter study found no significant association of fruit and vegetable consumption with the risk of CHD. More recently, two studies [10,11] conducted within the PREDIMED trial (PREvención con DIeta MEDiterránea) that recruited older participants in the Mediterranean area found an inverse association between fruit consumption and cardiovascular mortality, but not with non-fatal CVD. Albeit there are cohort studies and even a meta-analysis [12] that have observed an inverse association between fruits and vegetables and stroke, none of the included studies had been conducted in Mediterranean countries.

On the other hand, legumes and whole grains are also good sources of dietary fiber, and both have been suggested to be protective against CVD [13–15]. There is a wide body of evidence regarding the inverse association between whole grains and the risk of cardiovascular risk factors, such as type 2 diabetes [16,17], dyslipidaemia [18,19], high blood pressure [20], and obesity [17], but the research on their association with CVD clinical hard end-points is not large. A meta-analysis [21] included only nine publications that assessed the relationship between whole grains and CVD and found an inverse association. Six out of the nine studies had been conducted in the US, and only one in a Mediterranean country, and this latter study only reported on cardiovascular mortality. Even less are the studies which have assessed the relationship between legume consumption and the risk of CVD events [19,22,23].

Additionally, most of the studies have been conducted in aged adults and older people, and none in young adults. Therefore, we analyzed the association between fiber-rich foods and CVD in a Mediterranean cohort of young adults in order to advance in the knowledge of this relationship.

2. Materials and Methods

The SUN (Seguimiento Universidad de Navarra, Follow-up) project is a prospective, multipurpose, dynamic cohort of university graduates conducted in Spain. As a dynamic cohort, the recruitment of the participants is permanently open. Methodological aspects of this cohort have been published in detail previously [24]. Briefly, the cohort began in December 1999 and the recruitment of participants is permanently open. Information is gathered biennially by mailed questionnaires. Several validation studies of this self-reported information have been conducted, including anthropometric data [25], physical activity [26], the diagnosis of hypertension [27] and the specific criteria used for metabolic syndrome definition [28], all of them supporting the quality of the collected information.

For the present study, we included 22,476 subjects recruited before March 2013, so that they could have at least one follow-up questionnaire by the time of the last update of the dataset (December 2015). For the current analysis, we excluded 2113 participants with an energy intake out of sex specific predefined limits (>4000 kcal/day and <800 kcal/day for men and >3500 kcal/day and <500 kcal/day for women) [29]. We also excluded 947 participants who had prevalent cardiovascular disease at baseline and 2409 subjects with no follow-up information. After exclusions, the final sample population included a total of 17,007 participants. The retention in the cohort was 88%.

The study was approved by the Institutional Review Board of the University of Navarra on 30 August 2001. Voluntary completion of the first questionnaire was considered to imply informed consent.

Dietary intake was assessed through a validated 136-item semi-quantitative food-frequency questionnaire [30,31], which showed an intra-class correlation coefficient of 0.71 for fruits and 0.82 for vegetables.

Each item in the questionnaire included a typical portion size. Daily food consumption was estimated by multiplying the portion size by the consumption frequency for each item (nine options ranging from never or almost never to six times per day). Nutrient intake was estimated using Spanish food composition tables. We defined moderate alcohol consumption between 5 and 25 g/day for women and between 10 and 50 g/day for men. Based on the dietary information collected with the food-frequency questionnaire we calculated a score of adherence to the traditional Mediterranean diet [13].

Incidence of cardiovascular events, defined as non-fatal myocardial infarction, non-fatal stroke reported by participants on a follow-up questionnaire, or deaths due to cardiovascular disease, was the primary endpoint. An expert panel of physicians, blinded to the information on diet, anthropometric indexes, and risk factors, reviewed medical records of participants and adjudicated events applying universal criteria for myocardial infarction and clinical criteria for the other outcomes. A non-fatal stroke was defined as a focal neurological deficit of sudden onset and vascular mechanism lasting >24 h. Cases of fatal stroke were documented if there was evidence of a cerebrovascular mechanism. Deaths were reported to our research team by the participants' next of kin, work associates, and postal authorities. For participants lost to follow-up, we consulted the National Death Index every six months to identify deceased cohort members and to obtain their cause of death. Cases of fatal CHD or stroke reported by families or postal authorities were confirmed by a review of medical records with permission of the next of kin.

Statistical Analysis

Participants were categorized in quintiles of fiber, fruits, vegetables, legumes, or whole grain consumption. We used the residuals method to adjust the assessed foods for total energy intake.

Baseline characteristics are presented according to quintiles of baseline consumption of fruit and vegetables, as mean (SD) for quantitative traits, and percentage for categorical variables.

We used Cox regression models to assess the relationship between quintiles of baseline fiber, fruit, vegetables, legumes, or whole grains consumption and the subsequent incidence of CVD during follow-up. Hazard ratios (HRs) and their 95% confidence intervals (95% CIs) were calculated using the first quintile as the reference category. We used age as the underlying time variable. Entry time was defined as the date of completion of the first questionnaire and exit time as the date of CVD, the date of the completion of the last questionnaire, or date of death, whichever occurred first.

In addition, we analyzed specific subgroups of fruit and vegetables. The definition of composite groups was based on a report by Joshipura et al. [32] which we adapted to our Food Frequency Questionnaire (FFQ) and to the usual habits of the Spanish population. The fruits and vegetables included in each subgroup are presented in Table 1.

Three multivariable models were constructed to adjust for the known or suspected predictors of CVD. First, we adjusted only for sex. In the second model, we adjusted additionally for marital status (married, single, widowed, separated, others), highest attained educational level (five categories), family history of CHD (dichotomous), type 2 diabetes (dichotomous), high blood pressure (dichotomous), dyslipidemia (dichotomous), smoking status (four categories), total energy intake (kcal/day), body mass index (kg/m^2), alcohol intake (three categories), and use of cholesterol-lowering drugs. We also fitted a third model with additional adjustments for nutritional variables: olive oil (g/day) for all the groups and vegetables (g/day), legumes (g/day), and whole grains (g/day) in the analysis of fruit consumption; fruits (g/day), legumes (g/day), and whole grains (g/day) in an analysis that assessed vegetable consumption; fruits (g/day), vegetables (g/day), and whole grains (g/day) consumption in the analysis of legumes and fruits (g/day), vegetables (g/day), and legumes (g/day) consumption in the analysis that assessed whole grains consumption. All the models were also stratified by age in decades.

Table 1. Definitions for various fruit and vegetable subgroups.

Subgroups	Individual Foods
Orange group	Orange, tangerine, grapefruit
Apple/pear group	Apple/pear
Green leafy vegetables	Spinach, lettuce, chard greens
Cruciferous vegetables	Broccoli, cabbage, cauliflower, Brussels sprouts
β-carotene-rich fruits and vegetables	Carrots, spinach, pumpkin, chard greens
Lutein-rich fruits and vegetables	Spinach, chard greens
Lycopene-rich fruits and vegetables	Tomatoes, tomato sauce, "gazpacho" *
Vitamin C-rich fruits and vegetables	Orange, tangerine, grapefruit, peppers

* Cold tomato-based soup with pepper, cucumber, garlic, and onion.

Tests for linear trend were conducted by assigning the quintile specific median value of consumption of each food item or nutrient and regressing the risk of CVD on the resulting variable, which was treated as a continuous variable.

For some foods for which the point estimates obtained with the quintiles suggested a threshold effect, we generated a new dichotomous variable and assessed the relationship between this new variable and CVD with the same multivariable models.

Statistical tests were two-sided, and p values of less than 0.05 were considered to indicate statistical significance.

3. Results

The final sample comprised 17,007 participants, of whom 61% were women and the mean age was 38 years. The median follow-up was 10.3 years (mean = 9.6 years). We observed 112 confirmed cases of CVD during this follow-up period (56 myocardial infarctions, 32 strokes, and 33 cardiovascular deaths). The mean consumption of fruits, vegetables, legumes, and whole grains was 343 g/day, 525 g/day, 23 g/day, and 12 g/day, respectively. The most consumed fruit was oranges and the most consumed vegetables were tomatoes and lettuce. The main sources of fiber were mostly vegetables (10.4 g/day) and fruits (6 g/day).

Table 2 presents the baseline characteristics of the study participants according to quintiles of baseline fiber consumption. Participants in the highest quintile were older, and more likely to be diagnosed with dyslipidemia, type 2 diabetes, and high blood pressure. As expected, participants in the higher quintiles consumed more fruits, vegetables, legumes, and whole grains, and of all the items of the fruits and vegetables groups. Also, participants with the highest fiber intake showed a higher adherence to the traditional Mediterranean diet.

When we compared the highest quintile of fruit or whole grains consumption with the lowest quintile, we observed an inverse association between them and CVD in the fully adjusted model, and also a significant inverse trend for fiber intake. Table 3 shows the association of fiber intake, fruits, vegetables, legumes, or whole grains consumption at baseline with the incidence of CVD. When we compared the participants who consumed at least 160 g/day of fruit (two servings) with those with a lower consumption we found a HR of CVD of 0.62 (95% CI 0.39–0.99, $p = 0.045$) and HR of 0.58 (95% CI 0.37–0.90; $p = 0.015$) for the participants who consumed at least 175 g/day compared with those with a lower consumption. We observed no threshold for vegetables consumption.

Table 2. Baseline characteristics * of the study participants according to baseline quintiles of fiber intake, SUN (Seguimiento Universidad de Navarra, Follow-up) Project 1999–2013.

	Quintiles of Fiber Intake				
	Q1	Q2	Q3	Q4	Q5
Age (years)	34 (10)	36 (11)	38 (12)	40 (12)	42 (13)
Sex (% women)	60.6	60.6	60.6	60.6	60.6
Marital Status, %					
Single	55.3	47.4	42.9	40.6	37.9
Married	41.8	48.9	52.6	53.8	55.6
Others	2.9	3.8	4.6	5.6	6.5
Highest attained educational level					
Degree or licenciate degree, %	56	53	53	52	53
Master's degree, %	7	8	8	8	8
Doctoral degree, %	7	9	11	11	11
Family history of CHD, %	11	12	14	14	16
Use of lipid-lowering drugs, %	1.2	1.5	3.0	3.1	4.0
Type 2 diabetes, %	0.7	0.9	1.7	2.2	3.0
Body mass index (Kg/m^2)	23 (11)	23 (3.3)	24 (3.5)	24 (3.5)	24 (3.5)
Hypertension, %	3.7	4.9	6.7	7.9	9.3
Dyslipidemia, %	11.7	14.9	16.9	16.2	20.1
Smoking status, %					
Current smoker	28.5	23.4	21.6	18.6	16.1
Former smoker	22.5	26.5	28.0	32.6	33.3
Carbohydrate intake (% of total energy)	40 (7)	42 (7)	43 (7)	44 (7)	48 (7)
Protein intake (% of total energy)	17 (4)	18 (3)	18 (3)	19 (3)	19 (3)
Fat intake (% of total energy)	40 (7)	38 (6)	37 (6)	36 (6)	32 (6)
Olive oil consumption (g/day) **	18 (14)	18 (14)	19 (13)	19 (13)	18 (13)
Fiber intake (g/day) **	16 (3.4)	22 (1.5)	26 (1.6)	31 (2.1)	44 (10.0)
Fruit consumption (g/day) **	144 (116)	246 (143)	312 (159)	407 (219)	604 (419)
Vegetable consumption (g/day) **	271 (138)	397 (151)	493 (176)	601 (218)	863 (458)
Legume consumption (g/day) **	16 (9)	20 (10)	22 (12)	24 (14)	31 (29)
Whole grains (g/day) **	2 (10)	6 (15)	10 (21)	16 (29)	32 (52)
Orange group (portions/week) **	1.8 (2.7)	3.3 (3.5)	4.5 (4.4)	5.7 (5.3)	8.2 (7.7)
Apples/pear (portions/week) **	1.1 (1.5)	1.9 (2.0)	2.5 (2.6)	3.3 (3.4)	5.2 (5.8)
Lutein-rich fruits and vegetables (portions/week) **	0.4 (0.4)	0.6 (0.6)	0.8 (0.7)	1.0 (1.0)	1.7 (1.9)
Cruciferous (portions/week) **	0.3 (0.4)	0.5 (0.5)	0.6 (0.6)	0.8 (0.9)	1.2 (1.6)
Green-leafy vegetables (portions/week) **	2.5 (1.9)	3.6 (2.3)	4.5 (2.5)	5.5 (3.1)	7.8 (5.6)
Lycopene-rich fruits and vegetables (portions/week) **	2.0 (2.1)	3.7 (2.3)	3.7 (2.8)	4.5 (3.1)	6.2 (5.5)
Carotene-rich fruits and vegetables (portions/week) **	1.0 (1.0)	1.7 (1.2)	2.3 (1.5)	3.0 (1.9)	5.1 (4.1)
Vitamin C-rich fruits and vegetables (portions/week) **	3.1 (3.0)	5.0 (3.8)	6.5 (4.6)	8.1 (5.6)	11.5 (8.7)
Alcohol consumption (g/day) **	6.1 (11.7)	5.0 (7.8)	4.3 (6.8)	4.2 (12.9)	3.5 (6.0)
Moderate alcohol consumption (%) **	24.6	22.38	19.43	18.32	15.08
Physical activity (METs-h/week) **	21.6 (19.0)	21.6 (19.0)	22.4 (19.4)	23.3 (20.0)	24.3 (20.0)
Total energy intake (Kcal/day) **	2525 (616)	2283 (591)	2223 (595)	2237 (610)	2420 (610)
MDS (0–9 items) ***	2.7 (1.4)	3.5 (1.5)	4.1 (1.4)	4.8 (1.4)	5.6 (1.4)

* Mean (SD) unless otherwise stated; ** Adjusted for total energy intake by the residual method; *** MDS, Mediterranean diet score [13]; CHD, coronary heart disease; METs, metabolic equivalent of task.

Table 3. Hazard ratios (HRs) (95% confidence intervals) of cardiovascular disease (CVD) according to baseline quintiles (Q) of fiber, fruit, vegetables, pulses, or whole-grain consumption.

	Quintiles of Fiber Intake					
	Q1	Q2	Q3	Q4	Q5	*p* for Trend
N	3402	3401	3402	3401	3401	
Time at risk	33,643	33,107	32,496	32,132	31,381	
# of cases	18	24	22	22	26	
Median g/day	16.76	22.06	26.09	31.12	40.88	
Sex adjusted	1 (ref)	1.24 (0.66–2.30)	0.77 (0.41–1.45)	0.67 (0.36–1.28)	0.57 (0.31–1.06)	0.015
Multivariable adjusted 1	1 (ref)	1.31 (0.70–2.49)	0.81 (0.42–1.57)	0.70 (0.37–1.35)	0.61 (0.32–1.16)	0.025
Multivariable adjusted 2	1 (ref)	1.32 (0.70–2.49)	0.81 (0.42–1.56)	0.70 (0.36–1.35)	0.60 (0.32–1.15)	0.024
	Quintiles of Fruit Consumption					
	Q1	Q2	Q3	Q4	Q5	*p* for Trend
N	3402	3401	3402	3401	3401	
Time at risk	33,824	32,929	32,684	31,714	31,608	
# of cases	23	19	17	25	28	
Median g/day	90	192	280	398	653	
Sex adjusted	1 (ref)	0.60 (0.32–1.11)	0.45 (0.24–0.85)	0.49 (0.28–0.88)	0.45 (0.25–0.81)	0.036
Multivariable adjusted 1	1 (ref)	0.61 (0.32–1.17)	0.48 (0.24–0.94)	0.51 (0.27–0.94)	0.48 (0.26–0.87)	0.057
Multivariable adjusted 3	1 (ref)	0.62 (0.32–1.18)	0.50 (0.26–0.98)	0.54 (0.29–1.00)	0.51 (0.27–0.95)	0.114
	Quintiles of Vegetable Consumption					
	Q1	Q2	Q3	Q4	Q5	*p* for Trend
N	3402	3401	3402	3401	3401	
Time at risk	33,695	32,816	32,870	32,100	31,278	
# of cases	20	24	25	18	25	
Median g/day	209	348	468	609	884	
Sex adjusted	1 (ref)	1.18 (0.65–2.15)	1.06 (0.58–1.92)	0.71 (0.37–1.35)	0.80 (0.44–1.47)	0.191
Multivariable adjusted 1	1 (ref)	1.29 (0.70–2.38)	1.07 (0.58–1.96)	0.77 (0.40–1.48)	0.81 (0.44–1.49)	0.180
Multivariable adjusted 4	1 (ref)	1.37 (0.74–2.54)	1.14 (0.62–2.11)	0.86 (0.44–1.67)	0.96 (0.51–1.82)	0.458

Table 3. *Cont.*

	Q1	Q2	Q3	Q4	Q5	*p* for Trend
			Quintiles of Legumes Consumption			
N	3402	3401	3402	3401	3401	
Time at risk	32,311	32,682	32,726	33,244	31,796	
# of cases	26	24	20	15	27	
Median g/day	8.4	15.2	20	25	36	
Sex adjusted	1 (ref)	0.91 (0.52–1.60)	0.78 (0.43–1.40)	0.58 (0.30–1.10)	0.96 (0.59–1.65)	0.674
Multivariable adjusted 1	1 (ref)	0.92 (0.52–1.62)	0.80 (0.44–1.45)	0.58 (0.30–1.11)	0.92 (0.53–1.59)	0.559
Multivariable adjusted 5	1 (ref)	0.95 (0.54–1.68)	0.83 (0.46–1.52)	0.59 (0.31–1.15)	0.95 (0.54–1.66)	0.622
			Quintiles of Whole Grains Consumption			
	Q1	Q2	Q3	Q4	Q5	*p* for Trend
N	3402	3401	3402	3401	3401	
Time at risk	34,089	34,090	33,207	32,620	31,255	
# of cases	26	17	25	28	16	
Median g/day	0	0	1.9	5.7	54.7	
Sex adjusted	1 (ref)	0.59 (0.31–1.10)	0.79 (0.45–1.37)	0.71 (0.41–1.22)	0.51 (0.27–0.95)	0.110
Multivariable adjusted 1	1 (ref)	0.49 (0.24–0.99)	0.62 (0.29–1.31)	0.48 (0.20–1.15)	0.40 (0.19–0.86)	0.102
Multivariable adjusted 6	1 (ref)	0.51 (0.25–1.02)	0.64 (0.30–1.36)	0.49 (0.20–1.18)	0.43 (0.20–0.93)	0.149

Note: Multivariable adjusted 1: sex, marital status (five categories), highest attained educational level (five categories), family history of CHD (yes/no), type 2 diabetes (yes/no), high blood pressure (yes/no), dyslipidaemia (yes/no), smoking status (four categories), total energy intake (kcal/day), body mass index, physical activity (METs-h/day), alcohol intake (three categories) and use of lipid-lowering drugs, and stratified by age in decades. Age as underlying time variable. Multivariable adjusted 2: additionally adjusted for and olive oil consumption (g/day). Multivariable adjusted 3: additionally adjusted for olive oil (g/day), vegetables, legumes (g/day), and whole-grains (g/day) consumption. Multivariable adjusted 4: additionally adjusted for olive oil (g/day), fruits (g/day), legumes (g/day), and whole-grains (g/day) consumption. Multivariable adjusted 5: additionally adjusted for olive oil (g/day), fruits (g/day), vegetables (g/day), and whole-grains (g/day) consumption. Multivariable adjusted 6: additionally adjusted for olive oil (g/day), fruits (g/day), vegetables (g/day), and legumes (g/day) consumption.

When we analyzed fiber intake according to its source as exposure, participants in the highest quintile of fruit fiber consumption had the lowest risk of CVD, which was significantly lower than the risk of those in the first quintile (HR 0.52, 95% CI 0.28–0.97). No statistically significant differences were found for other fiber sources.

We found no significant association between legume consumption and CVD.

When we analyzed specific groups of fruits and vegetables, only higher intakes of cruciferous vegetables were associated with CVD with a HR of 0.52 (95% CI 0.30–0.89, $p = 0.16$) for the participants who ate at least one serving/week in comparison with those who did not. We also observed an inverse significant trend in the association between cruciferous vegetable consumption and CVD (Table 4).

Table 4. Hazard ratios (HRs) of CVD according to baseline quintiles (Q) of specific groups of fruits and vegetables consumption. (HR and 95% confidence intervals).

	Q1	Q2	Q3	Q4	Q5	*p* for Trend
			Orange Group			
N	3402	3401	3402	3401	3401	
Time at risk	32,607	32,155	32,253	32,686	33,057	
# of cases	21	22	21	21	27	
Median (servings/week)	0.23	1.58	3.09	5.64	15.34	
Sex adjusted	1 (ref)	0.80 (0.43–1.46)	0.73 (0.40–1.34)	0.53 (0.29–0.98)	0.60 (0.34–1.08)	0.166
Multivariable adjusted 1	1 (ref)	0.81 (0.43–1.55)	0.79 (0.42–1.50)	0.56 (0.30–1.05)	0.65 (0.35–1.19)	0.234
Multivariable adjusted 2	1 (ref)	0.81 (0.43–1.56)	0.80 (0.42–1.52)	0.56 (0.30–1.07)	0.65 (0.35–1.20)	0.267
			Apple/Pear Group			
	Q1	Q2	Q3	Q4	Q5	*p* for Trend
N	3402	3401	3402	3401	3401	
Time at risk	33,274	32,993	32,058	31,793	32,641	
# of cases	24	16	17	25	30	
Median (servings/week)	0.16	0.79	1.55	3.12	6.68	
Sex adjusted	1 (ref)	0.51 (0.27–0.97)	0.47 (0.25–0.89)	0.75 (0.42–1.32)	0.61 (0.35–1.06)	0.715
Multivariable adjusted 1	1 (ref)	0.46 (0.23–0.92)	0.44 (0.22–0.88)	0.74 (0.41–1.35)	0.61 (0.34–1.08)	0.816
Multivariable adjusted 2	1 (ref)	0.47 (0.24–0.93)	0.45 (0.23–0.91)	0.79 (0.44–1.44)	0.65 (0.37–1.16)	0.997

Table 4. *Cont.*

	Q1	Q2	Q3	Q4	Q5	p for Trend
Green Leafy Group						
	Q1	Q2	Q3	Q4	Q5	p for Trend
N	3402	3401	3402	3401	3401	
Time at risk	32,830	32,494	32,226	32,498	32,711	
# of cases	19	23	25	22	23	
Median (servings/week)	1.14	2.81	3.99	6.16	8.21	
Sex adjusted	1 (ref)	1.47 (0.79–2.72)	1.42 (0.77–2.59)	0.90 (0.48–1.66)	0.92 (0.50–1.71)	0.268
Multivariable adjusted 1	1 (ref)	1.48 (0.79–2.77)	1.57 (0.85–2.91)	0.90 (0.48–1.68)	0.97 (0.52–1.80)	0.298
Multivariable adjusted 2	1 (ref)	1.54 (0.82–2.89)	1.61 (0.87–2.99)	0.93 (0.49–1.75)	1.05 (0.56–1.96)	0.431
Cruciferous Group						
	Q1	Q2	Q3	Q4	Q5	p for Trend
N	3402	3401	3402	3401	3401	
Time at risk	32,604	32,972	32,488	32,817	31,878	
# of cases	19	26	27	21	19	
Median (servings/week)	0	0.37	0.48	0.93	1.07	
Sex adjusted	1 (ref)	1.03 (0.56–1.88)	1.25 (0.69–2.27)	0.81 (0.43–1.51)	0.56 (0.30–1.08)	0.035
Multivariable adjusted 1	1 (ref)	0.97 (0.52–1.79)	1.35 (0.73–2.47)	0.82 (0.43–1.55)	0.54 (0.28–1.04)	0.033
Multivariable adjusted 2	1 (ref)	0.98 (0.53–1.81)	1.37 (0.75–2.52)	0.83 (0.44–1.58)	0.56 (0.29–1.09)	0.046
Carotene-Rich Fruits and Vegetables						
	Q1	Q2	Q3	Q4	Q5	p for Trend
N	3402	3401	3402	3401	3401	
Time at risk	33,385	33,226	32,328	32,002	31,817	
# of cases	25	19	24	20	24	
Median (servings/week)	0.44	1.16	1.78	3–28	5.92	
Sex adjusted	1 (ref)	0.69 (0.38–1.26)	0.82 (0.47–1.45)	0.62 (0.34–1.14)	0.60 (0.33–1.06)	0.111
Multivariable adjusted 1	1 (ref)	0.74 (0.40–1.38)	0.90 (0.50–1.62)	0.67 (0.36–1.24)	0.64 (0.35–1.14)	0.142
Multivariable adjusted 2	1 (ref)	0.77 (0.41–1.43)	0.92 (0.51–1.67)	0.71 (0.38–1.31)	0.68 (0.38–1.23)	0.218
Lutein-Rich Fruits and Vegetables						
	Q1	Q2	Q3	Q4	Q5	p for Trend
N	3402	3401	3402	3401	3401	
Time at risk	32,106	32,994	32,316	32,995	32,408	
# of cases	21	23	22	18	27	
Median (servings/week)	0	0.4	0.58	0.98	2.88	
Sex adjusted	1 (ref)	0.90 (0.49–1.65)	0.90 (0.49–1.65)	0.76 (0.40–1.43)	0.76 (0.43–1.36)	0.381
Multivariable adjusted 1	1 (ref)	1.07 (0.58–1.99)	1.0 (0.54–1.87)	0.82 (0.43–1.56)	0.81 (0.45–1.48)	0.354
Multivariable adjusted 2	1 (ref)	1.10 (0.59–2.05)	1.03 (0.56–1.93)	0.84 (0.44–1.60)	0.86 (0.47–1.55)	0.439
Lycopene-Rich Fruits and Vegetables						
	Q1	Q2	Q3	Q4	Q5	p for Trend
N	3402	3401	3402	3401	3401	
Time at risk	34,332	33,347	32,602	31,537	31,041	
# of cases	23	26	19	23	21	
Median (servings/week)	0.44	1.91	3.24	4.87	7.23	
Sex adjusted	1 (ref)	1.04 (0.59–1.84)	0.81 (0.44–1.50)	0.78 (0.43–1.39)	0.70 (0.38–1.27)	0.137
Multivariable adjusted 1	1 (ref)	0.98 (0.54–1.76)	0.80 (0.43–1.49)	0.81 (0.44–1.47)	0.69 (0.38–1.28)	0.181
Multivariable adjusted 2	1 (ref)	1.0 (0.55–1.79)	0.8 (0.43–1.49)	0.84 (0.46–1.53)	0.73 (0.40–1.35)	0.249
Vitamin C-rich fruits and vegetables						
	Q1	Q2	Q3	Q3	Q5	p for Trend
N	3402	3401	3402	3401	3401	
Time at risk	32,746	32,672	32,371	32,628	32,341	
# of cases	20	21	25	19	27	
Median (servings/week)	1.46	3.4	5.33	7.84	16.41	
Sex adjusted	1 (ref)	0.78 (0.42–1.46)	0.91 (0.50–1.65)	0.55 (0.29–1.03)	0.61 (0.33–1.11)	0.103
Multivariable adjusted 1	1 (ref)	0.79 (0.42–1.53)	0.99 (0.54–1.84)	0.56 (0.29–1.07)	0.66 (0.38–1.22)	0.171
Multivariable adjusted 2	1 (ref)	0.83 (0.43–1.61)	1.00 (0.54–1.86)	0.58 (0.30–1.11)	0.68 (0.37–1.27)	0.191

Note: Multivariable adjusted 1: sex, marital status (five categories), studies (five categories), family history of CHD (yes/no), type 2 diabetes (yes/no), high blood pressure (yes/no), dyslipidemia (yes/no), smoking status (four categories), total energy intake (kc/day), body mass index, physical activity (METs-h/day), alcohol intake (three categories), stratified by age in decades. Age as underlying time variable. Multivariable adjusted 2: additionally adjusted for legumes (g/day), whole-grains (g/day), and olive oil consumption (g/day).

4. Discussion

In this young, highly educated, Mediterranean cohort, we found an inverse association between fiber intake and CVD. This observed association was consistent with previous studies [3,33,34], but the results for fruit and vegetables subtypes, for the different fiber sources, or for rich-fiber foods remain unclear.

We also found an inverse association between fruit consumption and fruit fiber and CVD. Our findings are consistent with various meta-analyses [12,33–37], even though the individual studies seldom reached statistical significance. In a previous work with participants of an old Mediterranean cohort [11], our results suggested that higher fruit consumption was likely to be inversely associated with the future occurrence of CVD, but the results were no longer statistically significant in the multivariable analysis. The EPIC study (European Prospective Investigation into Cancer and Nutrition) that included participants from several Mediterranean countries did not find an association between fruit consumption and cardiovascular mortality either [38]. A meta-analysis [33] found a marginally significant inverse association for each 4 g/day greater intake of fiber fruit with CVD (HR 0.96 (95% CI 0.93–1.00)), but another meta-analysis that included one further publication [3] found a clearly decreased risk of 8% (95% CI 2%–14%) for CHD. None of these meta-analyses included studies with Mediterranean populations. In our work, we also found that consumptions of at least two portions a day of fruit (160 g/day) could be protective against CVD, and higher consumptions did not appear to provide additional protection.

We found no significant association with vegetable consumption nor with fiber from vegetables. Similarly, a recent meta-analysis [3] did not find a statistically significant association between vegetable fiber and CVD. It is also noteworthy that in our study vegetable consumption was very high (mean 525 g/day) and the median of the first quintile was already 209 g/day. Lack of variability in a lower range of vegetable consumption may have precluded us from finding significant associations. In addition, the number of observed cases was low, as expected in this educated, slim, and young Mediterranean cohort. The statistical power of our study would be sufficient only to detect relative risks between extreme quintiles in the range of 0.40–0.55, but not other relative risks closer to the null. However, we expected to find strong associations, on the basis of a previous case-control study conducted by our group [39].

Fruit and vegetables are rich sources of fiber, but they also provide antioxidants, vitamin K, folate, and other phytochemicals—some of them have other micronutrients, thus leading to heterogeneity between the different types. Therefore, some classifications have been suggested according these differences. Nevertheless, studies that have assessed the association between a food or group and CVD are scarce. Oude Griep et al. [40] found no significant association between different varieties of fruits and vegetables and CHD or stroke, but found a strong correlation between the different fruit varieties and total fruit intake (0.72), and a less strong correlation between the different vegetables varieties and total vegetable consumption (0.53). Their results suggest that the quantity of fruit and vegetable consumption may be more relevant than their variety for the prevention of CVD. In a different classification according to the color of vegetables, the same authors [41,42] found a significant protective association with stroke only for white fruits and vegetables; no significant association was observed for CHD. In our analysis, we found an inverse association between cruciferous vegetable consumption and CVD, where eating at least one serving of cruciferous vegetables per week could reduce the risk of CVD by 48%. Our results differ from other studies that found no association between cruciferous vegetables and stroke [12] or CHD [32,43], but are consistent with our results from a previous study on an old Mediterranean cohort [11]. Bendinelli [9] analyzed the association between fruit and vegetable consumption and CHD in a Mediterranean cohort of women, and found an inverse association with green leafy vegetables, which was consistent with other studies [32,44,45], but did not report the results for cruciferous vegetables alone. Cruciferous vegetables contain sulforaphane [7], the most widely studied and best characterized isothiocyanate [46] which is a long-acting antioxidant, but also has anti-inflammatory activity by inhibition of cytokine production. The relationship between sulforaphane and the atherosclerosis process seems to be clear [46]. In animal models, sulforaphane has shown an inverse association with hypertension, diabetes, and diabetes complications [47,48].

A higher consumption of legumes did not have any association with the risk of CVD in our cohort. Legumes are high in vegetable proteins and dietary fiber, and have a low glycemic index. To our knowledge, only Bazzano et al. [49] and Wang et al. [50] reported an inverse association between the consumption of legumes and CVD, with tangible benefits observed for the consumption of legumes at least four times per week. A recently published meta-analysis [51] found an inverse association between legume consumption and CHD (HR 0.90 CI 95% 0.84–0.97). Additionally, the authors of this latter meta-analysis also found a marginally significant association between legume consumption and CVD (HR 0.94 CI 95% 0.89–1.00). Our participants had a high legume consumption (median in the fifth quintile: 36 g/day) and a priori we expected to find a risk reduction. Legumes are an important food in the Mediterranean diet and Trichopoulou et al. [13] found that the observed inverse association between adherence to the Mediterranean diet and cardiovascular mortality was toned down when legumes were taken out from their score. Another meta-analysis [52] conducted with 20 studies that analyzed the association between adherence to the Mediterranean diet or its individual components and CVD also found an inverse association between legume consumption and CVD (HR 0.90 CI 95% 0.83–0.98). Our results are similar in the magnitude and the direction of the association, but we did not achieve statistical significance. Again, the low number of cases could explain this result. Moreover, there are important differences in composition across legumes in macronutrients [53] (specifically in their protein content), fiber content, micronutrients, and phytochemicals, which could also explain the differences across different cohorts. Additionally, there are differences in the way they are cooked in the different Mediterranean countries, which could also contribute to the diverse results in the different studies.

We found an inverse association between whole grain consumption and risk of CVD (HR for the fifth vs. first quintile of 0.43 (95% CI 0.20–0.93)). Our study is consistent with a meta-analysis of ten cohort studies [21] that found an inverse association between whole grain consumption and risk of CHD, stroke, and CVD, with no evidence of linearity and with a stronger risk reduction from no consumption up to 50 g/day than with higher intakes. Most of the studies included in the last meta-analysis were from USA, only one of the included cohorts originating from a Mediterranean setting, and even then, only cardiovascular mortality was assessed. We found no association between whole grain consumption and CVD in a cohort with older Mediterranean participants [11].

Different plant foods, including fruits, vegetables, and whole grains among others, have their distinctive phytochemical contents. These distinctive phytochemicals have different biochemical properties, such as molecular size and solubility [5]. All these properties will affect the interactions between the various biochemicals and thus their antioxidant or anti-inflammatory effect. Also, different plant-based foods contain different fiber types. Eating a wide variety of fruits, vegetables, whole grains, and other plant foods and following a health dietary pattern—like the Mediterranean diet—has been postulated as being more important for CVD prevention than eating isolated food items [54]. A recent meta-analysis has shed light on this association [52], finding that some of the individual components did not achieve significance, but that the overall diet decreased CVD disease rates.

We acknowledge that our study may have some limitations. First, our participants have a high educational level, and are young and predominantly females, potentially limiting the generalizability of our results. However, the high educational level of our participants enhances the quality of their self-reported information and increases the internal validity of our results. In addition, lack of representativeness does not preclude from finding associations valid for other populations [55]. In fact, there are no biological mechanisms that suggest that our observed associations may no longer hold for other populations. Finally, literature on the covered topic in middle-aged cohort was previously absent. Second, the use of a validated FFQ does not rule out the existence of an information bias, but it has good or reasonable correlation coefficients for the considered exposures. Since the possible measurement error in the assessment of diet is expected to be non-differential, it would presumably bias our results towards the null value. Third, the absence of repeated measurements may have also led to a misclassification bias, because our participants may have experienced changes in their consumption along the follow-up. Fourth, we might have missed some CVD events. Nevertheless, all of our participants are university graduates, who are highly educated and highly motivated, and more than half of them are health professionals, thereby reducing the risk of underreporting. Additionally, we regularly consulted the National Death Index. Fifth, the incidence of CVD was low in our cohort. Thus, we may have low statistical power to assess associations, especially in adjusted models. Nevertheless, it is noteworthy that the point estimates hardly changed with successive adjustment and that the point estimates point towards the a priori expected association based on the available literature. Finally, observing significant associations may have been hindered by a considerably high consumption of healthy foods in the lowest quintiles, compared to other available studies. High consumption of the considered food items may show protective effects when compared to really low consumptions, but may show no additional protection beyond moderate consumptions.

The major strengths of the current study include its prospective design, its relatively large sample and long-term follow-up, and its high retention rate. Another potential strength is the use of a validated FFQ, with good correlations with the analyzed foods. Moreover, we adjusted the models for a wide array of potential confounders, in an attempt to control for potential confounders.

In conclusion, consumptions of at least two servings/day of fruit, and one serving/week of cruciferous vegetables or whole grains may be protective against CVD in young Mediterranean populations.

Acknowledgments: The authors are indebted to the participants of the SUN study for their continued cooperation and participation. We are also grateful to the members of the Department of Nutrition of the Harvard School of Public Health (Willett WC, Hu FB, and Ascherio A) who helped us to design the SUN study. We also thank the other members of the SUN Group: Alonso A, Barrio López MT, Basterra-Gortari FJ, Benito Corchón S, Bes-Rastrollo M, Beunza JJ, Carlos Chillerón S, Carmona L, Cervantes S, de Irala Estévez J, de la Rosa PA, Delgado Rodríguez M, Donat Vargas CL, Donázar M, Fernández Montero A, Galbete Ciáurriz C, García López M, Gea A, Goñi Ochandorena E, Guillén Grima F, Hernández A, Lahortiga F, Llorca J, López del Burgo C, Marí Sanchís A, Martí del Moral A, Martín Calvo N, Martínez JA, Núñez-Córdoba JM, Pimenta AM, Ramallal R, Ruiz Zambrana A, Sánchez Adán D, Sayón Orea C, Toledo Atucha J, Vázquez Ruiz Z, and Zazpe García I. The SUN Project has received funding from the Spanish Government-Instituto de Salud Carlos III, and the European Regional Development Fund (FEDER) (RD 06/0045, CIBER-OBN, Grants PI10/02658, PI10/02293, PI13/00615, PI14/01668, PI14/01798, PI14/01764, and G03/140), the Navarra Regional Government (45/2011, 122/2014), and the University of Navarra.

Author Contributions: M.A.M.-G. and M.R.-C. conceived and designed the experiments; J.D.-E. and A.G.-A. contributed to data collection; P.B.-C. and E.T. analyzed the data and wrote the paper. All authors have revised the manuscript critically for important intellectual content and have given final approval of the version to be published.

Conflicts of Interest: The authors declare no conflict of interest.

References

1. Mozaffarian, D.; Benjamin, E.J.; Go, A.S.; Arnett, D.K.; Blaha, M.J.; Cushman, M.; Das, S.H.; De Ferranti, S.; Despres, J.D.; Fullerton, H.J.; et al. Heart Disease and Stroke Statistics—2016 Update. *Circulation* **2016**, *133*, e38–e360. [CrossRef] [PubMed]
2. World Health Organization. Global Health Observatory (GHO) data. *World Health Statistics 2016: Monitoring health for the SDGs*. Available online: http://www.who.int/gho/publications/world_health_statistics/2016/en/ (accessed on 16 March 2017).
3. Wu, Y.; Qian, Y.; Pan, Y.; Li, P.; Yang, J.; Ye, X.; Xu, G. Association between dietary fiber intake and risk of coronary heart disease: A meta-analysis. *Clin. Nutr.* **2015**, *34*, 603–611. [CrossRef] [PubMed]
4. Wang, S.; Moustaid-Moussa, N.; Chen, L.; Mo, H.; Shastri, A.; Su, R.; Bapak, P.; KWun, J.; Shen, C.L. Novel insights of dietary polyphenols and obesity. *J. Nutr. Biochem.* **2014**, *25*, 1–18. [CrossRef] [PubMed]
5. Liu, R.H. Health-promoting components of fruits and vegetables in the Diet. *Adv. Nutr.* **2013**, *4*, 384S–392S. [CrossRef] [PubMed]
6. Liu, R.H. Potential synergy of phytochemicals in cancer prevention: Mechanism of action. *J. Nutr.* **2004**, *134*, 3479S–3485S. [PubMed]
7. Rodriguez-Casado, A. The health potential of fruits and vegetables phytochemicals: Notable examples. *Crit. Rev. Food Sci. Nutr.* **2014**. [CrossRef] [PubMed]
8. Gan, Y.; Tong, X.; Li, L.; Cao, S.; Yin, X.; Gao, C.; Merath, C.; Li, W.; Jin, Z.; Chen, Y.; et al. Consumption of fruit and vegetable and risk of coronary heart disease: A meta-analysis of prospective cohort studies. *Int. J. Cardiol.* **2015**, *183*, 129–137. [CrossRef] [PubMed]

9. Bendinelli, B.; Masala, G.; Saieva, C.; Salvini, S.; Calonico, C.; Sacerdote, C.; Agnoli, C.; Grioni, S.; Frasca, G.; Mattiello, A.; et al. Fruit, vegetables, and olive oil and risk of coronary heart disease in Italian women: The EPICOR Study. *Am. J. Clin. Nutr.* **2011**, *93*, 275–283. [CrossRef] [PubMed]
10. Buil-Cosiales, P.; Zazpe, I.; Toledo, E.E.; Corella, D.; Salas-Salvadó, J.; Diez-Espino, J.; Ros, E.; Fernandez-Creuet Navajas, J.; Santos-Lozano, J.M.; Aros, F.; et al. Dietary Fiber intake and all-cause mortality in the Prevencio (PREDIMED) study Mediterra. *Am. J. Clin. Nutr.* **2014**, *100*, 1498–1507. [CrossRef] [PubMed]
11. Buil-Cosiales, P.; Toledo, E.; Salas-Salvadó, J.; Zazpe, I.; Farràs, M.; Basterra-Gortari, F.J.; Diez-Espino, J.; Estruch, R.; Corella, D.; Ros, E.; et al. Association between dietary fibre intake and fruit, vegetable or whole-grain consumption and the risk of CVD: Results from the PREvención con DIeta MEDiterránea (PREDIMED) trial. *Br. J. Nutr.* **2016**, *1*, 1–13. [CrossRef] [PubMed]
12. Hu, D.; Huang, J.; Wang, Y.; Zhang, D.; Qu, Y. Fruits and vegetables consumption and risk of stroke: A meta-analysis of prospective cohort studies. *Stroke* **2014**, *45*, 1613–1619. [CrossRef] [PubMed]
13. Trichopoulou, A.; Bamia, C.; Trichopoulos, D. Anatomy of health effects of Mediterranean diet: Greek EPIC prospective cohort study. *BMJ* **2009**, *338*, b2337. [CrossRef] [PubMed]
14. Nagura, J.; Iso, H.; Watanabe, Y.; Maruyama, K.; Date, C.; Toyoshima, H.; Yamamoto, A.; Kikuchi, S.; Koizumi, A.; Kondal, T.; et al. Fruit, vegetable and bean intake and mortality from cardiovascular disease among Japanese men and women: The JACC Study. *Br. J. Nutr.* **2009**, *102*, 285–292. [CrossRef] [PubMed]
15. Flight, I.; Clifton, P. Cereal grains and legumes in the prevention of coronary heart disease and stroke: A review of the literature. *Eur. J. Clin. Nutr.* **2006**, *60*, 1145–1159. [CrossRef] [PubMed]
16. De Munter, J.S.L.; Hu, F.B.; Spiegelman, D.; Franz, M.; Van Dam, R.M. Whole grain, bran, and germ intake and risk of type 2 diabetes: A prospective cohort study and systematic review. *PLoS Med.* **2007**, *4*, 1385–1395. [CrossRef] [PubMed]
17. Ye, E.; Chacko, S.; Chou, E.; Kugizaki, M.; Liu, S. Greater whole-grain intake is associated with lower risk of type 2 diabetes, cardiovascular disease, and weight gain. *J. Nutr.* **2012**, *142*, 1304–1313. [CrossRef] [PubMed]
18. Leinonen, K.S.; Poutanen, K.S.; Mykkänen, H.M. Rye bread decreases serum total and LDL cholesterol in men with moderately elevated serum cholesterol. *J. Nutr.* **2000**, *130*, 164–170. [PubMed]
19. Ha, V.; Sievenpiper, J.L.; de Souza, R.J.; Jayalath, V.H.; Mirrahimi, A.; Agarwal, A.; Chiavaroli, L.; Mejia, S.B.; Sacks, F.H.; Di Buono, M.; et al. Effect of dietary pulse intake on established therapeutic review and meta-analysis of randomized controlled trials. *Can. Med. Assoc. J.* **2014**, *186*, 252–262. [CrossRef] [PubMed]
20. Kirwan, J.P.; Malin, S.K.; Scelsi, A.R.; Kullman, E.L.; Navaneethan, S.D.; Haus, J.M.; Fillion, J.; Godin, J.P.; Kochher, S.; Ross, A.B. A whole grain diet reduces cardiovascular risk factors in overweight and obese adults: A randomized controlled trial. *J. Nutr.* **2016**, *146*, 2244–2251. [CrossRef] [PubMed]
21. Aune, D.; Keum, N.; Giovannucci, E.; Fadnes, L.T.; Boffetta, P.; Greenwood, D.C.; Tonstad, S.; Vatten, L.J.; Riboli, E.; Narat, T. Whole grain consumption and risk of cardiovascular disease, cancer, and all cause and cause specific mortality: Systematic review and dose-response meta-analysis of prospective studies. *BMJ* **2016**, *353*, i2716. [CrossRef] [PubMed]
22. Bouchenak, M.; Lamri-Senhadji, M. Nutritional quality of legumes, and their role in cardiometabolic risk prevention: A review. *J. Med. Food* **2013**, *16*, 1–14. [CrossRef] [PubMed]
23. Hosseinpour-Niazi, S.; Mirmiran, P.; Amiri, Z.; Hosseini-Esfahani, F.; Shakeri, N.; Azizi, F. Legume intake is inversely associated with metabolic syndrome in adults. *Arch. Iran. Med.* **2012**, *15*, 538–544. [PubMed]
24. Seguí-Gómez, M.; de la Fuente, C.; Vázquez, Z.; de Irala, J.; Martínez-González, M.A. Cohort profile: The "Seguimiento Universidad de Navarra" (SUN) study. *Int. J. Epidemiol.* **2006**, *35*, 1417–1422. [CrossRef] [PubMed]
25. The British Geriatrics Society. Fit for Frailty-Consensus Best Practice Guidance for the Care of Older People Living in Community and Outpatient Settings-a Report from the British Geriatrics Society 2014. Available online: http://www.bgs.org.uk/campaigns/fff/fff_full.pdf (accessed on 15 March 2017).
26. Eguaras, S.; Toledo, E.; Hernández-Hernández, A.; Cervantes, S.; Martínez-González, M.A. Better adherence to the mediterranean diet could mitigate the adverse consequences of obesity on cardiovascular disease: The SUN prospective cohort. *Nutrients* **2015**, *7*, 9154–9162. [CrossRef] [PubMed]
27. Alonso, A.; Beunza, J.J.; Delgado-Rodríguez, M.; Martínez-González, M.A. Validation of self reported diagnosis of hypertension in a cohort of university graduates in Spain. *BMC Public Health* **2005**, *5*, 94. [CrossRef] [PubMed]

28. Fernandez-Montero, A.; Beunza, J.J.; Bes-Rastrollo, M.; Barrio, M.T.; de la Fuente-Arrillaga, C.; Moreno-Galarraga, L.; Martinez-Gonzalez, M.A. Validacion de los componentes del sindrome metabolico autodeclarados en un estudio de cohortes. *Gac. Sanit.* **2011**, *25*, 303–307. (In Spanish) [CrossRef] [PubMed]
29. Willett, W.C. Implications of total energy intake for epidemiologic analyses. In *Nutritional Epidemiology*, 3rd ed.; Willett, W.C., Ed.; Oxford University Press: New York, NY, USA, 2013.
30. Martin-Moreno, J.M.; Boyle, P.; Gorgojo, L.; Maisonneuve, P.; Fernandez-Rodriguez, J.C.; Salvini, S.; Willet, W.C. Development and validation of a food frequency questionnaire in Spain. *Int. J. Epidemiol.* **1993**, *22*, 512–519. [CrossRef] [PubMed]
31. Fernández-Ballart, J.D.; Piñol, J.L.; Zazpe, I.; Corella, D.; Carrasco, P.; Toledo, E.; Perez-Bauer, M.; Fernandez-Gonzalez, M.A.; Salas-Salvado, J.; Martin-Moreno, J.M. Relative validity of a semi-quantitative food-frequency questionnaire in an elderly Mediterranean population of Spain. *Br. J. Nutr.* **2010**, *103*, 1808–1816. [CrossRef] [PubMed]
32. Joshipura, K.J.; Hu, F.B.; Manson, J.E.; Stampfer, M.J.; Rimm, E.B.; Speizer, F.E.; Colditz, G.; Ascherio, A.; Rossner, B.; Spiegelman, D.; et al. The effect of fruit and vegetable intake on risk for coronary heart disease. *Ann. Intern. Med.* **2001**, *134*, 1106–1114. [CrossRef] [PubMed]
33. Threapleton, D.E.; Greenwood, D.C.; Evans, C.E.L.; Cleghorn, C.L.; Nykjaer, C.; Woodhead, C.; Cade, J.E.; Gale, C.P.; Burley, V.J. Dietary fibre intake and risk of cardiovascular disease: Systematic review and meta-analysis. *BMJ* **2013**, *347*, f6879. [CrossRef] [PubMed]
34. Dauchet, L.; Amouyel, P.; Hercberg, S.; Dallongeville, J. Fruit and vegetable consumption and risk of coronary heart disease: A meta-analysis of cohort studies. *J. Nutr.* **2006**, *136*, 2588–2593. [PubMed]
35. Chen, G.-C.C.; Lv, D.-B.B.; Pang, Z.; Dong, J.-Y.Y.; Liu, Q.-F.F. Dietary fiber intake and stroke risk: A meta-analysis of prospective cohort studies. *Eur. J. Clin. Nutr.* **2013**, *67*, 96–100. [CrossRef] [PubMed]
36. He, F.J.; Nowson, C.A.; MacGregor, G.A. Fruit and vegetable consumption and stroke: Meta-analysis of cohort studies. *Lancet* **2006**, *367*, 320–326. [CrossRef]
37. Dauchet, L.; Amouyel, P.; Dallongeville, J. Fruit and vegetable consumption and risk of stroke: A meta-analysis of cohort studies. *Neurology* **2005**, *65*, 1193–1197. [CrossRef] [PubMed]
38. Leenders, M.; Sluijs, I.; Ros, M.M.; Boshuizen, H.C.; Siersema, P.D.; Ferrari, P.; Weikert, C.; Tjonneland, A.; Olsen, D.; Boutron-Ruault, M.C. Fruit and vegetable consumption and mortality European prospective investigation into cancer and nutrition. *Am. J. Epidemiol.* **2013**. [CrossRef] [PubMed]
39. Martínez-González, M.A.; Fernández-Jarne, E.; Martínez-Losa, E.; Prado-Santamaría, M.; Brugarolas-Brufau, C.; Serrano-Martinez, M. Role of fibre and fruit in the Mediterranean diet to protect against myocardial infarction: A case-control study in Spain. *Eur. J. Clin. Nutr.* **2002**, *56*, 715–722. [CrossRef] [PubMed]
40. Oude Griep, L.M.; Verschuren, W.M.; Kromhout, D.; Ocké, M.C.; Geleijnse, J.M. Variety in fruit and vegetable consumption and 10-year incidence of CHD and stroke. *Public Health Nutr.* **2012**, 1–7. [CrossRef] [PubMed]
41. Oude Griep, L.M.; Verschuren, W.M.M.; Kromhout, D.; Ocké, M.C.; Geleijnse, J.M. Colors of fruit and vegetables and 10-year incidence of stroke. *Stroke* **2011**, *42*, 3190–3195. [CrossRef] [PubMed]
42. Oude Griep, L.M.; Monique Verschuren, W.M.; Kromhout, D.; Ocké, M.C.; Geleijnse, J.M. Colours of fruit and vegetables and 10-year incidence of CHD. *Br. J. Nutr.* **2011**, *106*, 1562–1569. [CrossRef] [PubMed]
43. Bhupathiraju, S.N.; Wedick, N.M.; Pan, A.; Manson, J.E.; Rexrode, K.M.; Willett, W.C.; Rimm, E.B.; Hu, F.B. Quantity and variety in fruit and vegetable intake and risk of coronary heart disease. *Am. J. Clin. Nutr.* **2013**. [CrossRef] [PubMed]
44. Joshipura, K.J.; Ascherio, A.; Manson, J.E.; Stampfer, M.J.; Rimm, E.B.; Speizer, F.E.; Mennkens, C.H.; Spiegelmam, D.; Willet, W.C. Fruit and vegetable intake in relation to risk of ischemic stroke. *JAMA* **1999**, *282*, 1233–1239. [CrossRef] [PubMed]
45. Pollock, R.L. The effect of green leafy and cruciferous vegetable intake on the incidence of cardiovascular disease: A meta-analysis. *JRSM Cardiovasc. Dis.* **2016**, *5*, 1–9. [CrossRef] [PubMed]
46. Bai, Y.; Wang, X.; Zhao, S.; Ma, C.; Cui, J.; Zheng, Y. Sulforaphane Protects against Cardiovascular Disease via Nrf2 Activation. *Oxid. Med. Cell. Longev.* **2015**. [CrossRef] [PubMed]
47. Bahadoran, Z.; Mirmiran, P.; Hosseinpanah, F.; Rajab, A.; Asghari, G.; Azizi, F. Broccoli sprouts powder could improve serum triglyceride and oxidized LDL/LDL-cholesterol ratio in type 2 diabetic patients: A randomized double-blind placebo-controlled clinical trial. *Diabetes Res. Clin. Pract.* **2012**, *96*, 348–354. [CrossRef] [PubMed]

48. Bahadoran, Z.; Tohidi, M.; Nazeri, P.; Mehran, M.; Azizi, F.; Mirmiran, P. Effect of broccoli sprouts on insulin resistance in type 2 diabetic patients: A randomized double-blind clinical trial. *Int. J. Food Sci. Nutr.* **2012**, *63*, 767–771. [CrossRef] [PubMed]
49. Bazzano, L.A.; He, J.; Ogden, L.G.; Loria, C.; Vupputuri, S.; Myers, L.; Whelton, P.K. Legume Consumption and Risk of Coronary Heart Disease in US Men and Women. *Arch. Intern. Med.* **2001**, *161*, 2573. [CrossRef] [PubMed]
50. Wang, J.-B.; Fan, J.-H.; Dawsey, S.M.; Sinha, R.; Freedman, N.D.; Taylor, P.R.; Qiao, Y-L.; Abnet, C.C. Dietary components and risk of total, cancer and cardiovascular disease mortality in the Linxian Nutrition Intervention Trials cohort in China. *Sci. Rep.* **2016**, *6*, 22619. [CrossRef] [PubMed]
51. Marventano, S.; Izquierdo Pulido, M.; Sánchez-González, C.; Godos, J.; Speciani, A.; Galvano, F.; Grosso, G. Legume consumption and CVD risk: A systematic review and meta-analysis. *Public Health Nutr.* **2017**, *20*, 245–254. [CrossRef] [PubMed]
52. Grosso, G.; Marventano, S.; Yang, J.; Micek, A.; Pajak, A.; Scalfi, L.; Galvano, F.; Kales, S.N. A comprehensive meta-analysis on evidence of Mediterranean diet and cardiovascular disease: Are individual components equal? *Crit. Rev. Food Sci. Nutr.* **2015**. [CrossRef] [PubMed]
53. Ros, E.; Hu, F.B. Consumption of plant seeds and cardiovascular health: Epidemiological and clinical trial evidence. *Circulation* **2013**, *128*, 553–565. [CrossRef] [PubMed]
54. Martínez-González, M.A.; Gea, A. Mediterranean diet: The whole is more than the sum of its parts. *Br. J. Nutr.* **2012**, *108*, 577–578. [CrossRef] [PubMed]
55. Rothman, K.J. Six persistent research misconceptions. *J. Gen. Intern. Med.* **2014**, *29*, 1060–1064. [CrossRef] [PubMed]

Section 6:
Other Health Outcomes

nutrients

MDPI

Article

Soluble Fibre Meal Challenge Reduces Airway Inflammation and Expression of GPR43 and GPR41 in Asthma

Isabel Halnes [1], Katherine J. Baines [1], Bronwyn S. Berthon [1], Lesley K. MacDonald-Wicks [2], Peter G. Gibson [1] and Lisa G. Wood [1,*]

[1] Centre for Healthy Lungs, Hunter Medical Research Institute, University of Newcastle, Callaghan, NSW 2308, Australia; isabel_h90@hotmail.com (I.H.); Katherine.baines@newcastle.edu.au (K.J.B.); bronwyn.berthon@newcastle.edu.au (B.S.B.); peter.gibson@newcastle.edu.au (P.G.G.)

[2] School of Health Sciences, University of Newcastle, Callaghan, NSW 2305, Australia; lesley.wicks@newcastle.edu.au

* Correspondence: lisa.wood@newcastle.edu.au; Tel.: +61-240-420-147

Received: 16 November 2016; Accepted: 27 December 2016; Published: 10 January 2017

Abstract: Short chain fatty acids (SCFAs) are produced following the fermentation of soluble fibre by gut bacteria. In animal models, both dietary fibre and SCFAs have demonstrated anti-inflammatory effects via the activation of free fatty acid receptors, such as G protein-coupled receptor 41 and 43 (GPR41 and GPR43). This pilot study examined the acute effect of a single dose of soluble fibre on airway inflammation—including changes in gene expression of free fatty acid receptors—in asthma. Adults with stable asthma consumed a soluble fibre meal (n = 17) containing 3.5 g inulin and probiotics, or a control meal (n = 12) of simple carbohydrates. Exhaled nitric oxide (eNO) was measured and induced sputum was collected at 0 and 4 h for differential cell counts, measurement of interleukin-8 (IL-8) protein concentration, and GPR41 and GPR43 gene expression. At 4 h after meal consumption, airway inflammation biomarkers, including sputum total cell count, neutrophils, macrophages, lymphocytes, sputum IL-8, and eNO significantly decreased compared to baseline in the soluble fibre group only. This corresponded with upregulated GPR41 and GPR43 sputum gene expression and improved lung function in the soluble fibre group alone. Soluble fibre has acute anti-inflammatory effects in asthmatic airways. Long-term effects of soluble fibre as an anti-inflammatory therapy in asthma warrants further investigation.

Keywords: asthma; prebiotics; G-protein coupled receptor; inflammation; short chain fatty acids

1. Introduction

Asthma is a chronic inflammatory disease of the airways, affecting approximately 300 million people worldwide [1]. In Australia, over two million people are affected [2]. Glucocorticoids are the mainstay of asthma management [3]. However, treatment can predispose individuals to long-term side effects (e.g., osteoporosis, hypertension, insulin resistance, neuropsychiatric effects), and some patients respond poorly [3]. Thus, new ways to treat inflammation in asthma are urgently needed.

While asthma has a significant genetic component, environmental factors also play a role. Epidemiological studies report increased asthma risk with consumption of westernized diets [4–7], which are often high in fat and processed foods, and low in fibre. Dietary fibres are complex carbohydrates found in plant-based foods and are classified based on their solubility in water [8]. Insoluble fibres (e.g., cellulose) are biologically inert substances that assist in the alleviation of constipation by promoting bowel movements [8]. Soluble fibres such as oligosaccharides and fructans (e.g., inulin) act as substrates for fermentation by intestinal microbes [9]. Partial digestion of soluble fibre produces short chain fatty acids (SCFAs), primarily acetate, propionate and butyrate [9]. Butyrate is the preferred fuel source for colonocytes, propionate is mainly metabolized by the liver, while acetate is the main SCFA to enter the circulation where it can act on immune cells and peripheral tissues and potentially elicit anti-inflammatory effects [9,10].

Recently, we reported that fibre intake was inversely associated with lung function and eosinophilic airway inflammation [11,12]. One mechanism potentially linking dietary fibre intake and inflammatory responses, involves the activation of the free fatty acid receptors, G protein-coupled receptor 41 and 43 (GPR41 and GPR43). These are cell surface receptors that are activated by SCFAs on cells of the gastrointestinal tract, as well as immune cells (e.g., eosinophils and neutrophils) and adipocytes [13]. To date, there are no human intervention trials that have assessed how dietary fibre—in particular soluble fibre—can impact airway inflammation. Airway inflammation can be assessed in subjects with asthma by collecting induced sputum (which enables quantification of inflammatory cells) and the use of molecular techniques to measure gene expression to examine mechanistic pathways [14]. Furthermore, sputum can be induced serially, in a safe manner to assess changes in inflammation [15].

We hypothesised that increased intake of soluble fibre would reduce airway inflammation in asthma via activation of free fatty acid receptors. Therefore, in this pilot study, we aimed to investigate the effects of an acute soluble fibre challenge on airway inflammation and free fatty acid receptor activity in asthma.

2. Materials and Methods

2.1. Subjects

Twenty-nine subjects with stable asthma, aged $\geq$18 years and with a body mass index (BMI) between 18 and 30 kg/m^2 were recruited from the John Hunter Hospital Asthma Clinic, NSW, Australia, from existing study volunteer databases and by advertisement. A subset of data from these participants has previously been reported [16]. Asthma stability was confirmed, defined as no exacerbation, respiratory tract infection, or oral corticosteroids in the past four weeks. Asthma control was assessed using the seven-item Asthma Control Questionnaire (ACQ-7) [17]. Clinical asthma pattern (intermittent, mild, moderate, or severe persistent) was determined according to the Global Initiative for Asthma (GINA) guidelines [18]. Subjects were excluded from the study if they were current smokers or had any respiratory-related illness other than asthma on presentation. This trial was conducted at the Hunter Medical Research Institute, Newcastle, Australia according to the guidelines laid down in the Declaration of Helsinki, and all procedures involving human subjects were approved by the Hunter New England Human Research Ethics Committee (HREC) (06/10/25/5.03, 11/06/15/4.02) and registered with the University of Newcastle HREC. Written informed consent was obtained from all subjects. The trial was registered with the Australian and New Zealand Clinical Trials Registry (number ACTRN12607000236493) prior to the study commencing.

2.2. Study Design

All subjects fasted for 12 h, withheld short acting β_2-agonist medications (for 12 h) and long acting β_2-agonist medications (for 24 h), and underwent exhaled nitric oxide (eNO, Ecomedics CLD 88sp, Ecomedics, Duernten, Switzerland), spirometry, and hypertonic saline challenge with combined sputum induction, and then consumed the study meal (soluble fibre n = 17, control n = 12) within 15 min. Four hours after meal consumption, eNO, spirometry, and sputum induction were repeated. The soluble fibre meal consisted of commercial probiotic yoghurt (Vaalia, low fat, 175 g), containing 806 kJ, the soluble fibre inulin (3.5 g), and the probiotics *Lactobacillus acidophilus* strain LA5, *Bifidobacterium lactis* strain Bb12, and *Lactobacillus rhamnosus* strain GG, each at a concentration of $\geq 10^8$ colony forming units. The control meal consisted of an isocaloric meal of 200 g plain mashed potato.

2.3. *Hypertonic Saline Challenge*

Baseline spirometry (Minato Autospiro AS-600; Minato Medical Science, Osaka, Japan) was performed to measure lung function, and predicted values for forced expiratory volume in one second (FEV_1) and forced vital capacity (FVC) were calculated using NHANES (National Health and Nutrition Examination Survey) III data, which accounts for gender, age, and height [19]. Using predicted values for FEV_1 and FVC allows for interpretation of actual lung function values (L) as a percent of expected values developed from reference data in healthy populations [20]. Combined bronchial provocation and sputum induction with nebulized (ULTRA-NEBTM ultrasonic nebulizer, Model 2000; DeVilbiss, Tipton, West Midlands, United Kingdom) hypertonic saline (4.5%) were performed as previously described [21]. If FEV_1 dropped below 15% of baseline, subjects were considered to have airway hyperresponsiveness (AHR). The response of all subjects to hypertonic saline was also described by the dose response slope (DRS, the percent decline in FEV_1 per mL hypertonic saline).

2.4. *Sputum Processing*

Sputum was selected from saliva [21,22], dispersed with dithiothreitol, and a total cell count of leukocytes and viability were performed. Cytospins were prepared, stained (May-Grunwald Geimsa), and a differential cell count obtained from 400 non-squamous cells. The remaining solution was centrifuged (400× *g*, 10 min, 4 °C) and the cell-free supernatant was aspirated and stored at −80 °C. For GPR41 and GPR43 gene expression analysis, 100 μL of selected sputum was added to Buffer RLT (Qiagen, Hilden, Germany) and stored at −80 °C until RNA extraction.

2.5. *Sputum Supernatant Measurements*

The concentration of interleukin 8 (IL-8) was determined by Enzyme-linked Immunosorbent Assay (ELISA) using R&D Systems Human CXCL8/IL-8 DuoSet Ancillary Reagent ELISA kit (R&D Systems, Minneapolis, MN, USA). IL-8 has been previously validated for assessment in induced sputum [23,24].

2.6. *RNA Extraction and cDNA Synthesis*

Total RNA was extracted from sputum samples stored in Buffer RLT using the RNeasy Mini Kit (Qiagen) as per kit instructions. Sputum RNA was quantitated using the Quant-iT RiboGreen RNA Assay Kit (Invitrogen, Eugene, OR, USA), whereby fluorescence was measured by FLUOstar OPTIMA spectrometer (BMG LabTech, Ortenberg, Germany). Genomic DNA was removed via treatment with DNase I (Life Technologies, Scoresby, Australia) and cDNA was generated via reverse transcription from 200ng of RNA using the High Capacity cDNA Reverse Transcription Kit, as per kit instructions (Applied Biosystems, Forster City, CA, USA).

2.7. *mRNA Quantification by Real-Time qRT-PCR*

Taqman gene expression assays for GPR41 and GPR43 were purchased as proprietary pre-optimised reagents (Applied Biosystems) and combined with cDNA and Taqman master mix in duplicate singleplex quantitative real-time polymerase chain reactions (qRT-PCR) (ABI 7500 Real time PCR system). 18S ribosomal RNA was utilised as the housekeeping reference gene. Relative fold change in gene expression after the soluble fibre and control meal challenge was calculated using $2^{-\Delta\Delta Ct}$ relative to the housekeeping gene 18S rRNA (ΔCt) and the baseline (ΔΔCt).

2.8. *Statistical Analysis*

Data were analysed with STATA 11 (StataCorp, College Station, TX, USA) and reported as mean ± standard error of mean (SEM) for parametric and median (interquartile range, IQR) for nonparametric data. Data was tested for normality using the D'Agostino–Pearson omnibus normality test. To compare baseline characteristics between groups, normally distributed variables were analysed using Students t-tests, and non-parametric variables were analysed using the Wilcoxon rank sum test. Categorical variables were analysed by Fisher's exact test. Within-group changes were compared using Wilcoxon matched-pairs signed rank test, and between group changes were analysed using the Wilcoxon rank sum test. Significance was accepted if $p < 0.05$.

3. Results

3.1. Baseline Characteristics

Twenty-nine subjects with stable asthma were included in the study, allocated to the soluble fibre ($n = 17$) or control group ($n = 12$). The clinical characteristics at baseline were similar between the two groups (Table 1).

Table 1. Baseline clinical characteristics.

Clinical Characteristic	Soluble Fibre Group ($n = 17$)	Control Group ($n = 12$)	p *
Gender Male n (%)	7 (41)	6 (50)	0.716
Female n (%)	10 (59)	6 (50)	
Age (years)	42.1 ± 3.4	40.4 ±4.6	0.770
BMI (kg/m^2)	24.9 ± 0.7	26.6 ± 0.7	0.099
Ex-smokers n (%)	6 (35)	3 (25)	0.694
ACQ-7 (units)	0.7 ± 0.1	0.7 ± 0.2	0.941
Atopy n (%)	14 (82)	8 (67)	0.403
AHR n (%)	10 (59]	5 (41.7)	0.462
DRS (%ΔFEV$_1$/mL), med [IQR]	2.2 [0.4, 6.4]	0.6 [0.2, 2.4]	0.109
ICS dose † (μg/day), med [IQR]	1000 [400, 1000]	1000 [563, 1000]	0.679

Data are means ± SEM unless otherwise stated. BMI: body mass index; ACQ: 7-item asthma control questionnaire; AHR: airway hyperresponsiveness; DRS: dose–response slope (% fall in forced expiratory volume in one second (FEV$_1$)/mL saline); ICS: inhaled corticosteroids. * Difference between soluble fibre and control groups. † Beclomethasone equivalents.

3.2. Airway Inflammatory Markers

There was no difference in airway inflammation at baseline between groups; however, the response to the soluble fibre and control meals was different (Table 2, Figure 1). Following the control meal, there were no changes in airway inflammation. Within the soluble fibre group, there was a significant decrease in sputum total cell count which was significantly different to the control group (Figure 1a). Sputum neutrophils (Figure 1b), macrophages (Figure 1d), lymphocytes, sputum IL-8 (Figure 1c), and eNO (Figure 1f) also decreased significantly in the soluble fibre group at 4 h compared to baseline, though these changes were not significantly different between the control and intervention groups.

Table 2. Airway inflammation at baseline and change at 4 h following soluble fibre or control meal challenge ^.

Airway Inflammation	Soluble Fibre Group		$p^{\dagger}$	Control Group		$p^{\dagger}$	p^{*}
	0 h	Δ4 h		0 h	Δ4 h		
Sputum (*n*)	16	14		10	9		
TCC (×10^6/mL)	3.7 [2.2, 6.3]	−2.0 [−2.8, −1.1]	0.013	3.0 [1.4, 6.0]	0.2 [−0.8, 1.4]	0.833	0.037
Neutrophils (×10^4/mL)	76.2 [54.6, 249.4]	−67.5 [−158.0, −6.4]	0.033	92.4 [7.2, 342.7]	−1.1 [−94.9, 105.1]	1.000	0.148
Eosinophils (×10^4/mL)	3.3 [1.3, 16.0]	−1.2 [−5.8, 1.8]	0.490	2.4 [0.0, 4.5]	2.6 [−1.7, 6.7]	0.440	0.393
Macrophages (×10^4/mL)	144.0 [93.0, 386.3]	−99.1 [−244.6, −12.2]	0.030	124.5 [104.5, 211.5]	3.4 [−47.6, 85.1]	0.779	0.117
Lymphocytes (×10^4/mL)	1.6 [0.2, 7.1]	−1.4 [−3.9, −0.3]	0.002	4.1 [0.4, 6.7]	2.1 [−1.5, 3.9]	0.401	0.034
Sputum IL-8 (ng/mL)	5.7 [3.9, 9.7]	−1.9 [−7.6, −1.1]	0.005	3.7 [3.0, 22.6]	−1.3 [−10.1, 1.2]	0.208	0.539
Exhaled NO (ppb)	17.5 [14.5, 70.5]	−3.4 [−7.9, −0.6]	0.028	14.9 [11.0, 51.0]	−1.9 [−4.6, 1.0]	0.170	0.301

TCC: total cell count; NO: nitric oxide; ppb: parts per billion. ^ Data are nonparametric, presented as median [quartile 1, quartile 3], within-group changes analyzed by Wilcoxon matched pairs signed-rank test, and group comparison performed using Wilcoxon rank-sum test. † Difference in change from 0 to 4 h within group. * Difference in change from 0 to 4hrs between the soluble fibre and control group.

Table 3. Sputum mRNA gene expression at baseline, 4 h, and fold change at 4 h following soluble fibre or control meal challenge ^.

Gene	Soluble Fibre Group ($n = 8$)			$p^{\dagger}$	Control Group ($n = 4$)			$p^{\dagger}$	p^{*}
	0 h	4 h	FC		0 h	4 h	FC		
GPR43	0.07 [0.05, 0.29]	0.79 [0.26, 2.01]	6.26 [1.66, 13.5]	0.124	1.53 [0.29, 3.64]	0.24 [0.17, 0.27]	0.31 [0.07, 0.67]	0.068	0.007
GPR41	0.07 [0.04, 0.35]	1.70 [0.14, 5.18]	5.15 [3.96, 22.9]	0.161	1.27 [0.80, 1.42]	0.58 [0.41, 1.22]	0.41 [0.31, 2.37]	0.715	0.027

GPR: G protein-coupled receptor; FC: fold change. ^ Data are nonparametric, presented as median [quartile 1, quartile 3], within-group changes analyzed by Wilcoxon matched pairs signed-rank test and group comparison performed using Wilcoxon rank-sum test. † Difference in change from 0 to 4 h within group. * Difference in fold change between the soluble fibre and control group.

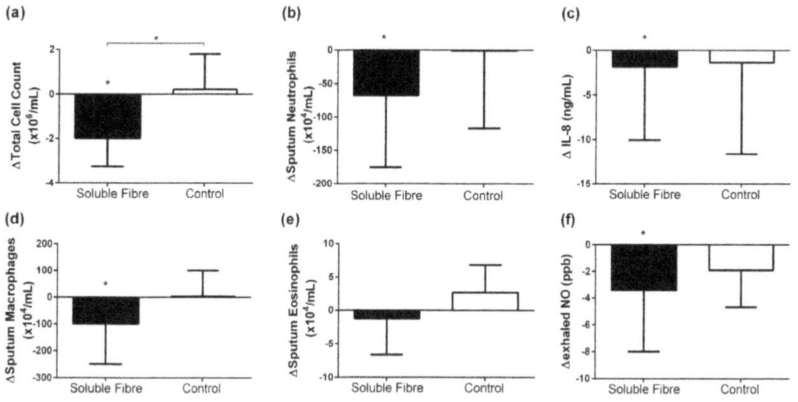

Figure 1. Change in airway inflammatory markers: (**a**) sputum total cell count; (**b**) sputum neutrophils; (**c**) sputum interleukin 8 (IL-8); (**d**) sputum macrophages; (**e**) sputum eosinophils; (**f**) exhaled nitric oxide 4 h following soluble fibre challenge (soluble fibre group) or control meal challenge (control group). Data expressed as median (IQR) and analyzed by Wilcoxon matched pairs signed-rank for within group and Wilcoxon rank-sum for between group comparisons. * $p < 0.05$.

3.3. GPR41 and GPR43 Sputum Gene Expression

GPR41 and GPR43 gene expression fold change in sputum was compared between the two groups after the soluble fibre and the control meals. Both GPR43 and GPR41 expression were significantly upregulated following the soluble fibre meal compared to the control meal (Table 3, Figure 2).

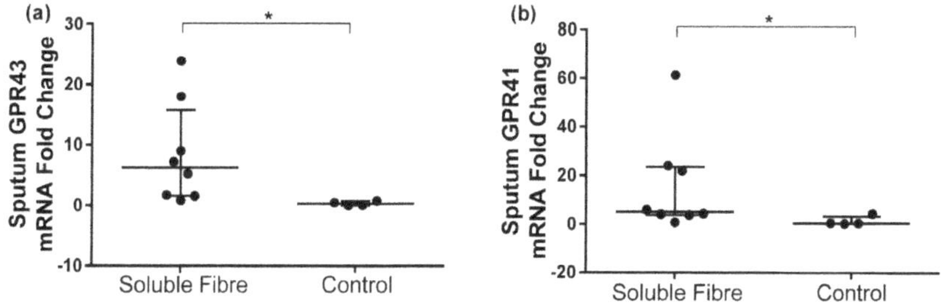

Figure 2. Change in sputum (**a**) GPR43 and (**b**) GPR41 gene expression 4 h following soluble fibre challenge (soluble fibre group $n = 8$) or control meal challenge (control group $n = 4$). Data expressed as median (IQR) and analyzed by Wilcoxon rank-sum test.* $p < 0.05$.

3.4. Lung Function

At baseline, forced vital capacity (FVC % predicted) was lower in the control group, but both groups were within normal range (80–120) of percentage predicted FVC [25]. FEV_1 and FEV_1/FVC improved 4 h following the soluble fibre meal, while no changes in lung function were seen following the control meal (Table 4, Figure 3). There were no significant differences in lung function changes between groups.

Table 4. Lung function at baseline and change at 4 h following soluble fibre or control meal challenge.

Lung Function	Soluble Fibre Group		$p^{\dagger}$	Control Group		$p^{\dagger}$	p^{*}
	0 h	Δ4 h		0 h	Δ4 h		
(n)	17	17		12	12		
FEV_1 (L) ^	2.7 [2.2, 3.6]	0.1 [0.0, 0.2]	0.022	2.9 [2.0, 3.5]	0.1 [−0.1, 0.2]	0.347	0.341
FEV_1 (% predicted) #	82.4 ± 4.4	4.0 ± 1.6	0.024	77.7 ± 6.8	1.0 ± 1.4	0.506	0.190
FVC (L) ^	4.1 [3.4, 4.7]	0.0 [−0.1, 0.1]	0.331	4.0 [3.5, 4.9]	0.01 [−0.04, 0.1]	0.503	0.595
FVC (% predicted) #	98.9 ± 3.4 §	1.6 ± 1.2	0.193	86.9 ± 4.5	−0.2 ± 1.0	0.859	0.285
FEV_1/FVC (%) #	69.2 ± 2.5	3.8 ± 1.1	0.002	71.9 ± 4.6	1.2 ± 0.7	0.101	0.070

FEV_1: forced expiratory volume in 1 s; FVC: forced vital capacity. ^ Data are nonparametric, presented as median [quartile 1, quartile 3], within-group changes analyzed by Wilcoxon matched pairs signed-rank test and group comparison performed using Wilcoxon rank-sum test. # Data are normally distributed and presented as means ± SEMs, within group changes analyzed by paired t-test and group comparison performed using two-sample t-test. § $p < 0.05$ versus control group at baseline. † Difference in change from 0 to 4 h within group. * Difference in change from 0 to 4 h between the soluble fibre and control group.

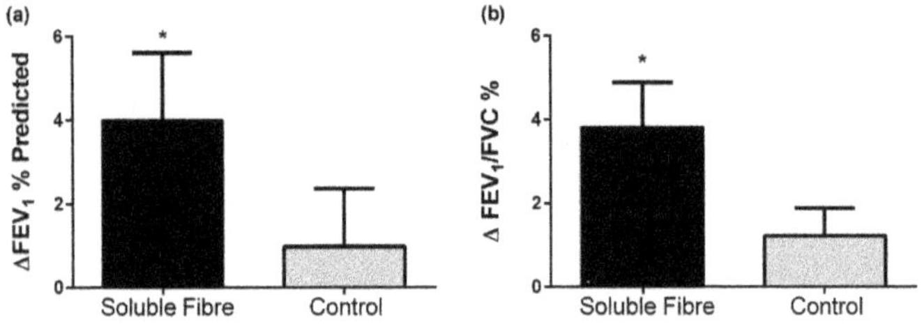

Figure 3. Change in lung function (**a**) FEV_1% predicted and (**b**) FEV_1/FVC % 4 h following soluble fibre challenge (soluble fibre group) or control meal challenge (control group). Data expressed as mean ± SEMs and analyzed by two-sample t-test. * $p < 0.05$.

4. Discussion

To gain a better understanding of the effects of soluble fibre on airway inflammation in people with asthma, this pilot study examined changes in airway inflammatory biomarkers at 4 h versus baseline (0 h), following a soluble fibre or control meal. We observed significant reductions in airway inflammation four hours after the consumption of a single dose of soluble fibre (3.5 g inulin). This was characterised by decreases in sputum total cell count, neutrophils, macrophages, lymphocytes, sputum IL-8 and eNO. When compared to the control subjects, we also found significantly upregulated GPR41 and GPR43 sputum cell gene expression in the soluble fibre group. We also observed an improvement in lung function (FEV_1 and FEV_1/FVC) in the soluble fibre group.

Several studies in the general population have reported an inverse relationship between dietary fibre intake and systemic inflammation [26,27]. We have previously extended these observations by demonstrating that dietary fibre is also inversely associated with eosinophilic airway inflammation in asthma [12]. The current study suggests that a key mechanism driving the anti-inflammatory actions of soluble fibre is the activation of free fatty acid receptors. The soluble fibre inulin is partially fermented by commensal bacteria in the colon, providing the substrate for production of physiologically active by-products, including the SCFAs: acetate, propionate, and butyrate. Our observations suggest that fermentation of inulin leads to activation of GPR41 and GPR43 in immune cells in the airways, which results in a reduction in airway inflammation. While we did not observe a reduction in airway eosinophils in the current study, we did observe a decrease in eNO, which is a marker of eosinophilic inflammation [28].

Our observations support findings from animal models, which have shown that GPR43/41 stimulation by SCFAs is necessary for the resolution of airway inflammation. In an allergic airways model, GPR43-deficient mice showed more severe inflammation, with increased inflammatory cell numbers in the lung lining fluid and higher levels of eosinophil peroxidase activity and inflammatory cells in lung tissue [29]. In another study in mice with allergic airways disease [30], a fibre-rich diet changed the composition of the gut microbiota by increasing proportions of the Bacteroidaceae and Bifidobacteriaceae families, which are potent fermenters of soluble fibre into SCFA. Increased circulating SCFA levels were observed and airway inflammation was attenuated, with dendritic cells having an impaired ability to activate Th2 effector cells in the lung [30]. Consequently, in mice fed either a high fibre diet or directly administered with acetate or propionate in their drinking water, airway inflammation could not be sustained; after an allergen challenge, cellular infiltration (eosinophils), IL-4, IL-5, IL-13, and IL-17A levels were reduced in the lungs and AHR improved. The effects were dependent on GPR41, but not GPR43. This highlights the importance of measuring both free fatty acid receptors in order to understand their anti-inflammatory actions.

This is the first study to examine the effects of SCFAs on inflammation in human airways. The majority of previous studies in humans that have looked at the role of SCFAs have examined gut inflammation, predominantly ulcerative colitis where sodium butyrate is administered either orally (using capsules with slow release coating to release butyrate into the colon), or through enemas [10]. We are interested in the effects of SCFAs on inflammation in peripheral tissues, in particular the lungs [31]. Certainly, it has previously been shown that soluble fibre can affect inflammation in the circulation. In a randomized, double-blind, placebo-controlled crossover study on inflammation and gut microbiota following soluble fibre supplementation, improvements in the composition and metabolic activity of gut microbiota—such as increased production of butyrate—was seen after two and four weeks [32]. In addition, significant reductions in circulating pro-inflammatory mediators such as tumour necrosis factor-alpha (TNF-α), IL-6, and IL-8 were observed [32]. We sought to extend our investigations to the airways, and have shown that a single dose of soluble fibre can modulate airway inflammation. This was associated with an improvement in lung function, and hence appears to be clinically important.

The single meal challenge design that we employed mimics many previous studies that have shown that a single meal high in carbohydrates and/or fat causes postprandial systemic inflammation [33]. We have also previously shown that a single high fat mixed meal increases airway inflammation within 4 h [16]. This is biologically plausible, as it is known that at 4 h after the consumption of inulin, the SCFAs acetate, propionate, and butyrate are all elevated compared to baseline in plasma [34]. Nonetheless, a clinical trial of longer duration is warranted to determine what clinical effects would occur with chronic supplementation.

As the importance of SCFAs in human health is being increasingly recognized, further research is required to assess changes that occur in circulating SCFA levels and inflammation following the intake of various types of soluble fibres. In addition, research is also needed to determine the optimal delivery form for increasing circulating SCFAs. In animal studies, SCFAs are often administered directly through the drinking water of animals, however oral delivery of SCFA is not optimal for humans, as the majority of acetate delivered orally is oxidized, with plasma levels only remaining elevated for 60 min [35]. Hence, supplementation with soluble fibre (as we have done in this study) is a useful strategy to increase circulating SCFA levels [34].

From our study, we are unable to determine whether SCFA reach the lungs, and this is an important area for future research. Previous animal studies have shown that SCFA are not detectable in lung tissue following soluble fibre supplementation [30]. Hence, it appears likely that effects of SCFA on immune function initially occur systemically. Supporting this hypothesis, it has been reported that mice treated with propionate have altered haematopoiesis in bone marrow, characterised by changes in the types of dendritic cell (DC) precursors generated, which have greater phagocytic ability but reduced ability to promote Th2 responses once in the lungs [30].

A limitation of this study is the small sample size; however, this was adequate for us to demonstrate, for the first time, that soluble fibre can reduce airway inflammation in people with asthma. Another potential limitation is the short duration of the study, as the soluble fibre was delivered as a single meal. Nonetheless, the chronic effects of soluble fibre on airway inflammation in asthma are likely to be even greater, as in addition to activation of free fatty acid receptors, gut microbial changes will also be induced, which further enhance SCFA production [36]. Hence, long-term studies of soluble fibre supplementation are warranted.

5. Conclusions

In summary, we have shown that a single dose of soluble fibre was able to significantly reduce airway inflammation in stable asthma. The long-term benefits of increasing soluble fibre intake are likely to have a greater impact on inflammation, as soluble fibre also enhances the growth of SCFA-producing gut bacteria, which will further enhance the production of beneficial SCFAs. Supplementing with a prebiotic such as inulin has the potential to be widely accepted and adopted, and could potentially reduce the amount of inhaled glucocorticoids required for treatment. As such, this approach provides a less costly strategy for managing asthma, as well as lowering the risk of asthma patients experiencing adverse side effects due to pharmacological treatment.

Acknowledgments: The authors would like to acknowledge the research participants and the HMRI Respiratory Research clinical team including Amber Smith, Joanne Smart, Hayley Scott and the laboratory team including Bridgette Donati, Michelle Gleeson, Kellie Fakes and Naomi Fibbens for assistance with collection, processing and analysis of samples. This trial was supported by a National Health and Medical Research Council of Australia Project Grant and a Hunter Medical Research Institute project grant sponsored by the Piggott family.

Author Contributions: I.H. conducted the laboratory work and statistical analysis and contributed to drafting the manuscript, K.J.B. contributed to the conception and design of the study, analysis, interpretation of data and revising the manuscript, B.S.B. contributed to the data acquisition, interpretation of data and revising the manuscript, P.G.G. contributed to the conception and design of the study, analysis, interpretation of data and revising the manuscript, L.K.M.-W. contributed to the study design, interpretation of data and revising the manuscript, L.G.W. had overall responsibility for the conception and design of the study, analysis, interpretation of data, revising the manuscript and obtaining funding for the work.

Conflicts of Interest: The authors declare no conflict of interest.

References

1. Masoli, M.; Fabian, D.; Holt, S.; Beasley, R. Global initiative for asthma (GINA) program. The global burden of asthma: Executive summary of the GINA dissemination committee report. *Allergy* **2004**, *59*, 469–478. [CrossRef] [PubMed]
2. Australian Centre for Asthma Monitoring. Asthma in Australia 2011. In *AIHW Asthma Series No. 4. Cat. No. ACM 22*; Australian Institute of Health and Welfare (AIHW): Canberra, Australia, 2011.
3. Barnes, P.J.; Adcock, I.M. Glucocorticoid resistance in inflammatory diseases. *Lancet* **2009**, *373*, 1905–1917. [CrossRef]
4. Wickens, K.; Barry, D.; Friezema, A.; Rhodius, R.; Bone, N.; Purdie, G.; Crane, J. Fast foods—Are they a risk factor for asthma? *Allergy* **2005**, *60*, 1537–1541. [CrossRef] [PubMed]
5. Hijazi, N.; Abalkhail, B.; Seaton, A. Diet and childhood asthma in a society in transition: A study in urban and rural Saudi Arabia. *Thorax* **2000**, *55*, 775–779. [CrossRef] [PubMed]
6. Carey, O.J.; Cookson, J.B.; Britton, J.; Tattersfield, A.E. The effect of lifestyle on wheeze, atopy, and bronchial hyperreactivity in Asian and white children. *Am. J. Respir. Crit. Care Med.* **1996**, *154*, 537–540. [CrossRef] [PubMed]
7. Huang, S.-L.; Pan, W.-H. Dietary fats and asthma in teenagers: Analyses of the first Nutrition and Health Survey in Taiwan (NAHSIT). *Clin. Exp. Allergy* **2001**, *31*, 1875–1880. [CrossRef] [PubMed]
8. Rolfes, S.R.; Pinna, K.; Whitney, E. *Understanding Normal and Clinical Nutrition*, 8th ed.; Wadsworth: Belmont, CA, USA, 2009.
9. Ganapathy, V.; Thangaraju, M.; Prasad, P.D.; Martin, P.M.; Singh, N. Transporters and receptors for short-chain fatty acids as the molecular link between colonic bacteria and the host. *Curr. Opin. Pharmacol.* **2013**, *13*, 869–874. [CrossRef] [PubMed]
10. Vinolo, M.A.R.; Rodrigues, H.G.; Nachbar, R.T.; Curi, R. Regulation of Inflammation by Short Chain Fatty Acids. *Nutrients* **2011**, *3*, 858–876. [CrossRef] [PubMed]

11. Root, M.M.; Houser, S.M.; Anderson, J.J.; Dawson, H.R. Healthy Eating Index 2005 and selected macronutrients are correlated with improved lung function in humans. *Nutr. Res.* **2014**, *34*, 277–284. [CrossRef] [PubMed]
12. Berthon, B.S.; Macdonald-Wicks, L.K.; Gibson, P.G.; Wood, L.G. Investigation of the association between dietary intake, disease severity and airway inflammation in asthma. *Respirology* **2013**, *18*, 447–454. [CrossRef] [PubMed]
13. Brown, A.J.; Goldsworthy, S.M.; Barnes, A.A.; Eilert, M.M.; Tcheang, L.; Daniels, D.; Muir, A.I.; Wigglesworth, M.J.; Kinghorn, I.; Fraser, N.J.; et al. The Orphan G protein-coupled receptors GPR41 and GPR43 are activated by propionate and other short chain carboxylic acids. *J. Biol. Chem.* **2003**, *278*, 11312–11319. [CrossRef] [PubMed]
14. Baines, K.J.; Simpson, J.L.; Wood, L.G.; Scott, R.J.; Gibson, P.G. Transcriptional phenotypes of asthma defined by gene expression profiling of induced sputum samples. *J. Allergy Clin. Immunol.* **2011**, *127*, 153–160. [CrossRef] [PubMed]
15. Fahy, J.V.; Liu, J.; Wong, H.; Boushey, H.A. Analysis of cellular and biochemical constituents of induced sputum after allergen challenge: A method for studying allergic airway inflammation. *J. Allergy Clin. Immunol.* **1994**, *93*, 1031–1039. [CrossRef]
16. Wood, L.G.; Garg, M.L.; Gibson, P.G. A high fat challenge increases airway inflammation and impairs bronchodilator recovery in asthma. *J. Allergy Clin. Immunol.* **2011**, *127*, 1133–1140. [CrossRef] [PubMed]
17. Juniper, E.F.; Bousquet, J.; Abetz, L.; Bateman, E.D. Identifying 'well-controlled' and 'not well-controlled' asthma using the Asthma Control Questionnaire. *Respir. Med.* **2006**, *100*, 616–621. [CrossRef] [PubMed]
18. Global Initiative for Asthma (GINA). Global Strategy for Asthma Management and Prevention 2012 (Update). Available online: http://wwwginasthmaorg (accessed on 30 July 2012).
19. Hankinson, J.; Odencrantz, J.; Fedan, K. Spirometric reference values from a sample of the general U.S. population. *Am. J. Respir. Crit. Care Med.* **1999**, *159*, 179–187. [CrossRef] [PubMed]
20. Stanojevic, S.; Wade, A.; Stocks, J. Reference values for lung function: Past, present and future. *Eur. Respir. J.* **2010**, *36*, 12–19. [CrossRef] [PubMed]
21. Gibson, P.G.; Wlodarczyk, J.W.; Hensley, M.J.; Gleeson, M.; Henry, R.L.; Cripps, A.W.; Clancy, R.L. Epidemiological Association of Airway Inflammation with Asthma Symptoms and Airway Hyperresponsiveness in Childhood. *Am. J. Respir. Crit. Care Med.* **1998**, *158*, 36–41. [CrossRef] [PubMed]
22. Gibson, P.G.; Henry, R.L.; Thomas, P. Noninvasive assessment of airway inflammation in children: Induced sputum, exhaled nitric oxide, and breath condensate. *Eur. Respir. J.* **2000**, *16*, 1008–1015. [PubMed]
23. Simpson, J.L.; Scott, R.J.; Boyle, M.J.; Gibson, P.G. Differential proteolytic enzyme activity in eosinophilic and neutrophilic asthma. *Am. J. Respir. Crit. Care Med.* **2005**, *172*, 559–565. [CrossRef] [PubMed]
24. Wood, L.G.; Garg, M.L.; Simpson, J.L.; Mori, T.A.; Croft, K.D.; Wark, P.A.B.; Gibson, P.G. Induced Sputum 8-Isoprostane Concentrations in Inflammatory Airway Diseases. *Am. J. Respir. Crit. Care Med.* **2005**, *171*, 426–430. [CrossRef] [PubMed]
25. Altalag, A.; Road, J.; Wilcox, P. *Pulmonary Function Tests in Clinical Practice*; Springer: London, UK, 2009.
26. Ma, Y.; Griffith, J.A.; Chasan-Taber, L.; Olendzki, B.C.; Jackson, E.; Stanek, E.J.; Li, W.; Pagoto, S.L.; Hafner, A.R.; Ockene, I.S. Association between dietary fiber and serum C-reactive protein. *Am. J. Clin. Nutr.* **2006**, *83*, 760–766. [PubMed]
27. Ajani, U.A.; Ford, E.S.; Mokdad, A.H. Dietary fiber and C-reactive protein: Findings from national health and nutrition examination survey data. *J. Nutr.* **2004**, *134*, 1181–1185. [PubMed]
28. Taylor, D.R.; Pijnenburg, M.W.; Smith, A.D.; Jongste, J.C.D. Exhaled nitric oxide measurements: Clinical application and interpretation. *Thorax* **2006**, *61*, 817–827. [CrossRef] [PubMed]
29. Maslowski, K.M.; Vieira, A.T.; Ng, A.; Kranich, J.; Sierro, F.; Yu, D.; Schilter, H.C.; Rolph, M.S.; Mackay, F.; Artis, D.; et al. Regulation of inflammatory responses by gut microbiota and chemoattractant receptor GPR43. *Nature* **2009**, *461*, 1282–1286. [CrossRef] [PubMed]
30. Trompette, A.; Gollwitzer, E.S.; Yadava, K.; Sichelstiel, A.K.; Sprenger, N.; Ngom-Bru, C.; Blanchard, C.; Junt, T.; Nicod, L.P.; Harris, N.L.; et al. Gut microbiota metabolism of dietary fiber influences allergic airway disease and hematopoiesis. *Nat. Med.* **2014**, *20*, 159–166. [CrossRef] [PubMed]
31. De Filippo, C.; Cavalieri, D.; Di Paola, M.; Ramazzotti, M.; Poullet, J.B.; Massart, S.; Collini, S.; Pieraccini, G.; Lionetti, P. Impact of diet in shaping gut microbiota revealed by a comparative study in children from Europe and rural Africa. *Proc. Natl. Acad. Sci. USA* **2010**, *107*, 14691–14696. [CrossRef] [PubMed]

32. Macfarlane, S.; Cleary, S.; Bahrami, B.; Reynolds, N.; Macfarlane, G.T. Synbiotic consumption changes the metabolism and composition of the gut microbiota in older people and modifies inflammatory processes: A randomised, double-blind, placebo-controlled crossover study. *Aliment. Pharmacol. Ther.* **2013**, *38*, 804–816. [CrossRef] [PubMed]
33. Nappo, F.; Esposito, K.; Cioffi, M.; Giugliano, G.; Molinari, A.M.; Paolisso, G.; Marfella, R.; Giugliano, D. Postprandial endothelial activation in healthy subjects and in Type 2 diabetic patients: Role of fat and carbohydrate meals. *J. Am. Coll. Cardiol.* **2002**, *39*, 1145–1150. [CrossRef]
34. Tarini, J.; Wolever, T.M. The fermentable fibre inulin increases postprandial serum short-chain fatty acids and reduces free-fatty acids and ghrelin in healthy subjects. *Appl. Physiol. Nutr. Metab.* **2010**, *35*, 9–16. [CrossRef] [PubMed]
35. Smith, G.I.; Jeukendrup, A.E.; Ball, D. Sodium acetate induces a metabolic alkalosis but not the increase in fatty acid oxidation observed following bicarbonate ingestion in humans. *J. Nutr.* **2007**, *137*, 1750–1756. [PubMed]
36. Roberfroid, M.B. Introducing inulin-type fructans. *Br. J. Nutr.* **2005**, *93*, S13–S25. [CrossRef] [PubMed]

nutrients

Communication

Validity and Reproducibility of a Habitual Dietary Fibre Intake Short Food Frequency Questionnaire

Genelle Healey [1,2,*], Louise Brough [1], Rinki Murphy [3], Duncan Hedderley [2], Chrissie Butts [2] and Jane Coad [1]

[1] Massey Institute of Food Science and Technology, School of Food and Nutrition, Massey University, Palmerston North 4442, New Zealand; l.brough@massey.ac.nz (L.B.); j.coad@massey.ac.nz (J.C.)

[2] Food, Nutrition and Health, The New Zealand Institute for Plant & Food Research Limited, Palmerston North 4442, New Zealand; duncan.hedderley@plantandfood.co.nz (D.H.); chrissie.butts@plantandfood.co.nz (C.B.)

[3] Faculty of Medical and Health Sciences, The University of Auckland, Auckland 1023, New Zealand; r.murphy@auckland.ac.nz

* Correspondence: genelle.healey@plantandfood.co.nz; Tel.: +64-6-355-6108

Received: 22 July 2016; Accepted: 5 September 2016; Published: 10 September 2016

Abstract: Low dietary fibre intake has been associated with poorer health outcomes, therefore having the ability to be able to quickly assess an individual's dietary fibre intake would prove useful in clinical practice and for research purposes. Current dietary assessment methods such as food records and food frequency questionnaires are time-consuming and burdensome, and there are presently no published short dietary fibre intake questionnaires that can quantify an individual's total habitual dietary fibre intake and classify individuals as low, moderate or high habitual dietary fibre consumers. Therefore, we aimed to develop and validate a habitual dietary fibre intake short food frequency questionnaire (DFI-FFQ) which can quickly and accurately classify individuals based on their habitual dietary fibre intake. In this study the DFI-FFQ was validated against the Monash University comprehensive nutrition assessment questionnaire (CNAQ). Fifty-two healthy, normal weight male (n = 17) and female (n = 35) participants, aged between 21 and 61 years, completed the DFI-FFQ twice and the CNAQ once. All eligible participants completed the study, however the data from 46% of the participants were excluded from analysis secondary to misreporting. The DFI-FFQ cannot accurately quantify total habitual dietary fibre intakes, however, it is a quick, valid and reproducible tool in classifying individuals based on their habitual dietary fibre intakes.

Keywords: dietary fibre; short food frequency questionnaire; validation

1. Introduction

Dietary fibre are non-digestible plant polysaccharides found in high amounts in fruits, vegetables, breads and cereals, legumes and nuts and seeds. Dietary fibre has been shown to have important implications on human health, including preventing and alleviating constipation, reducing gastrointestinal cancer incidence and blood glucose levels, lowering blood cholesterol levels and blood pressure, and beneficially modulating gut microbiota [1]. It is also possible that the efficacy of a dietary intervention is altered as a result of the influence habitual dietary fibre intake has on gut microbiota responsiveness and host outcomes. Therefore, being able to quickly assess an individual's habitual dietary fibre intake and classify individuals based on their dietary fibre intakes will prove useful in clinical practice and in nutrition and health research. Dietary assessment methods such as diet records and food frequency questionnaires have inherent limitations such as being difficult to complete accurately, time-consuming and may not accurately assess a person's habitual diet [2]. A small number of dietary fibre assessment questionnaires have been developed, however these questionnaires assess general dietary behaviours, do not estimate total dietary fibre amounts, and/or do not classify individuals based on habitual dietary fibre intakes [3–6]. Therefore, the primary aim of this study was to determine whether a newly developed dietary fibre intake short food frequency questionnaire (DFI-FFQ) can accurately classify individuals based on their habitual dietary fibre intake and the secondary aim of the study was to determine whether the DFI-FFQ can accurately quantify total habitual dietary fibre intakes.

2. Methods

2.1. Subjects

Participants were recruited via email and poster advertisement in multiple locations around Palmerston North, New Zealand. A diverse cross-section of the population was targeted to help ensure a good representation of the New Zealand population was recruited. Sixty-eight individuals provided informed consent to participate in this study, of which fifty-two healthy participants met the inclusion criteria (aged >19 and <65 years, healthy, BMI >18.5 and <30 kg/m^2, no significant weight loss or weight gain within the past year, no significant dietary change within the past year, not pregnant or breastfeeding, no food intolerances which cause gastrointestinal symptoms (i.e., lactose intolerance, gluten sensitivity), no adverse gastrointestinal symptoms, non-smoker and not high alcohol consumers). Participants completed the DFI-FFQ twice, at least 2 weeks apart, and the comprehensive nutrition assessment questionnaire (CNAQ) once. The DFI-FFQ was completed initially, followed by the CNAQ, and lastly the repeated DFI-FFQ was completed. The CNAQ and DFI-FFQ were both completed online. An energy intake: basal metabolic rate (EI:BMR) of <1.1 and >2.19 was used to exclude participants who appeared to have over- or under-reported using the CNAQ [7]. Ethical approval was obtained from the Massey University Human Ethics Committee (Southern A, Application 15/34).

2.2. Development of the DFI-FFQ

The DFI-FFQ (Figure S1) was designed to quickly and accurately classify individuals as low, moderate or high habitual dietary fibre consumers and quantify an individual's habitual dietary fibre intake (g/day). The DFI-FFQ consists of five high dietary fibre containing food groups (vegetables, fruits, breads and cereals, nuts and seeds and legumes) which account for 73.5% of the dietary fibre in a typical New Zealand diet [8]. Examples of what one serve is equivalent to, for each food group, is detailed within the DFI-FFQ. The frequency of consumption for the average number of serves consumed over the past year, was given as follows: Never, <1/month, 1–3/month, 1/week, 2–4/week, 5–6/week, 1/day, 2/day, 3/day, 4/day, 5/day and 6+/day.

2.3. DFI-FFQ Scoring Sheet

A scoring sheet was developed to quantify the amount of dietary fibre consumed and to classify individuals as low, moderate and high dietary fibre consumers. FoodWorks version 7.0.3016 (Xyris Software Pty Ltd., Brisbane, Queensland, Australia) was used to quantify the average amount of dietary fibre provided by the five food groups for each frequency of consumption. An individual's total dietary fibre intake was calculated by adding together the average amount of dietary fibre consumed from each food group in relation to the number of serves consumed.

2.4. Dietary Fibre Classification

The cut-offs used to classify individuals based on their dietary fibre intakes are outlined in Table 1. The high dietary fibre intake cut-offs were selected to reflect the New Zealand Ministry of Health recommended dietary fibre intake guidelines; >25 g/day for females and >30 g/day for males [9]. The low dietary fibre intake cut-offs were selected as the median dietary fibre intake in New Zealand was 17.5 g/day for females and 22.1 g/day for males, which are below recommended amounts [8].

Similar cut-offs have been used previously however the specific cut-offs used in this study were modified to be applicable to a New Zealand population [3].

Table 1. The dietary fibre intake cut-offs used to classify individuals as low, moderate and high dietary fibre consumers.

	Females	Males
Low	<18 g/day	<22 g/day
Moderate	18–24.9 g/day	22–29.9 g/day
High	≥25 g/day	≥30 g/day

2.5. *Dietary Assessment Method Used for Comparison*

The Monash University online CNAQ was used for comparison with the DFI-FFQ. The 297-item food frequency questionnaire has been shown to be valid in assessing habitual dietary intakes when compared to four 7-day food records, each completed three months apart [10].

2.6. *Statistical Analysis*

We aimed to recruit enough participants to ensure that correlations over 0.7 would be statistically significant and that the assumptions of *chi-squared* tests would not be over stretched. The relationship between results of the DFI-FFQ when compared to the CNAQ was determined using Spearman correlation, Pearson correlation, Bland-Altman plot, *chi-squared* test and linear weighted kappa score. Test-retest repeatability was assessed using Pearson correlation, Bland-Altman plot and Cronbach's alpha. *T*-tests were used to determine whether there were any differences in dietary fibre intakes between the DFI-FFQ and CNAQ and the repeated DFI-FFQ. A p value of < 0.05 is considered significant. Statistical analysis was carried out using GenStat 17th edition (VSNi Ltd., Hemel Hempstead, UK), Minitab 16th edition (Cronbach's alpha) (Minitab Inc., State College, PA, USA) and the calculator at http://vassarstats.net/kappa.html (kappa score) [11].

3. Results

All eligible participants (n = 52) completed the study. The data from 28 participants (54%) were used as the data from 24 participants (46%) were excluded from the analysis secondary to likely misreporting on the CNAQ; with 18 participants (34.5%) having over-reported and six participants (11.5%) having under-reported their energy intakes. The group mean EI:BMR was 2.8 (SD 4.7) prior to exclusion and reduced to 1.6 (SD 0.3) after exclusion. Participant characteristics, total dietary fibre intakes and classifications determined by the DFI-FFQ and CNAQ are summarised in Table 2. The median dietary fibre intake in New Zealand (20.3 g/day) [8] is similar to the average dietary fibre intake of the study cohort, with dietary fibre intakes from both groups being below the New Zealand recommended dietary fibre intake guidelines [9]. The DFI-FFQ took on average 3.5 min to complete in comparison to the estimated completion time of 20–40 min for the CNAQ.

When comparing the DFI-FFQ to the CNAQ for dietary fibre classification, exact agreement occurred 79% of the time and gross misclassification occurred 7% of the time (Table 3). There was a significant difference in dietary fibre intakes between the DFI-FFQ and CNAQ (CNAQ was on average 5 g/day higher than the DFI-FFQ). The two dietary assessment methods were however correlated (Pearson correlation 0.65, Spearman correlation 0.53). A *chi-squared* test indicated an association between the classifications based on the DFI-FFQ and CNAQ (p = 0.002) and the linear weighted kappa score showed good agreement [12] (Table 4). The Bland-Altman plot is available within the Supplementary information (Figure S2A).

Table 2. Characteristics, dietary fibre intakes and classifications for the study participants.

Mean (SD)	Male (n = 8)	Female (n = 20)	Total (n = 28)
Participant characteristics			
Age (years)	40 (11.02)	38 (9.37)	39 (9.91)
BMI (kg/m^2)	24 (1.9)	23 (3.1)	24 (2.82)
Ethnicity (No.)			
New Zealand European	4	14	18
Asian	3	0	3
Maori	0	2	2
Other	1	4	5
Dietary fibre intakes and classifications			
DFI-FFQ			
Dietary fibre intake (g/day)	27 (11.77)	23 (10.33)	24 (10.85)
Dietary fibre classification (No.)			
Low	2	5	7
Moderate	2	4	6
High	4	11	15
Monash CNAQ			
Dietary fibre intake (g/day)	31 (11.35)	29 (9.43)	29 (10.09)
Dietary fibre classification (No.)			
Low	1	4	5
Moderate	3	1	4
High	4	15	19

DFI-FFQ: dietary fibre intake short food frequency questionnaire; CNAQ: comprehensive nutrition assessment questionnaire; SD: standard deviation.

Table 3. Comparison in dietary fibre classification between the comprehensive nutrition assessment questionnaire (CNAQ) and the dietary fibre intake food frequency questionnaire (DFI-FFQ).

		CNAQ			Total
		Low	Moderate	High	
DFI-FFQ	Low	5 (18%)	0 (0%)	2 (7%)	7 (25%)
	Moderate	0 (0%)	3 (11%)	3 (11%)	6 (21%)
	High	0 (0%)	1 (3%)	14 (50%)	15 (54%)
Total		5 (18%)	4 (14%)	19 (68%)	28 (100%)

Table 4. Correlation and test-retest repeatability statistical analysis.

Correlation between DFI-FFQ and CNAQ		p Value
Pearson correlation	0.65	<0.001
Spearman correlation	0.53	0.001
Chi-square test	9.6	0.002
Linear weighted kappa *	0.68	
Standard error	0.14	
Magnitude of agreement	Good	
Bland-Altman plot		
Limits of agreement (g/day)	−12.5–22.6	
Standard error	1.7	
Mean difference (g/day)	5	0.007
Test-Retest Repeatability		**p value**
Pearson correlation	0.94	<0.001
Cronbach's alpha	0.97	
Bland-Altman plot		
Limits of agreement (g/day)	−6.0–9.6	
Standard error	0.72	
Mean difference (g/day)	1.8	0.019

CNAQ: comprehensive nutrition assessment questionnaire; DFI-FFQ: dietary fibre intake short food frequency questionnaire; * One category disagreement had a weight of 3/4.

Pearson correlation (0.94) and Cronbach's alpha (0.97) showed that the repeated DFI-FFQ correlated. The estimated dietary fibre intake from the second DFI-FFQ was significantly lower than the first DFI-FFQ by 1.8 g/day (Table 4). The Bland-Altman plot is available within the Supplementary information (Figure S2B).

4. Discussion

Presently, there are no known short dietary fibre intake questionnaires that are able to classify individuals based on their habitual dietary fibre intake. Having the ability to be able to quickly and accurately classify an individual based on their dietary fibre intake will prove useful as low dietary fibre intakes have been associated with poorer health outcomes [13]. This study has shown that the DFI-FFQ can accurately classifying individuals based on their habitual dietary fibre intakes.

There was however, a significant difference in habitual dietary fibre intakes between the repeated DFI-FFQs and the DFI-FFQ and CNAQ, which suggests the DFI-FFQ might not accurately quantify total habitual dietary fibre intakes. Research has shown that large food item FFQs overestimate fruit and vegetable consumption, which may help explain the higher dietary fibre intakes determined from the CNAQ [14]. The addition of other dietary fibre contributing food groups, such as cakes and muffins, pies and pastries and biscuits, to the DFI-FFQ may have helped to improve the questionnaire's accuracy in quantifying total habitual dietary fibre intakes as these food groups collectively contribute 6.3% of the dietary fibre in a typical New Zealand diet [8]. Another reason why the DFI-FFQ may not have been able to accurately quantify total habitual dietary fibre intakes may be related to the serving size examples provided. The examples provided did not include all possible foods within a particular food group and relied on participants to use their own judgement regarding the number of serves consumed for foods that were not specifically listed.

There are a handful of short questionnaires that have been developed to assess dietary fibre intakes however these questionnaires assess general dietary behaviours [4–6], do not estimate total dietary fibre amounts [4–6], and/or do not classify individuals based on habitual dietary fibre intakes [3–6]. The DFI-FFQ is novel as it can accurately classify individuals based on habitual dietary fibre intake. Unlike previously developed questionnaires, the DFI-FFQ was validated against an FFQ which assesses dietary intake over the past year, providing a more accurate account of long term rather than current dietary fibre intakes. Additionally, some of the questionnaires were validated using fairly homogenous populations, such as factory workers [3] and patients [5], making these questionnaires less useful in more diverse populations, such as in this study.

When comparing the study cohorts average dietary fibre intake to the Adult Nutrition Survey data [8] it appeared the study cohort has a similar dietary fibre intake to the New Zealand population. Therefore, the DFI-FFQ is a valid tool for classifying individuals based on their habitual dietary fibre intakes in New Zealand. In countries where dietary fibre intakes are distinctly different from New Zealand, the DFI-FFQ may need to be re-validated in these populations.

Forty-six percent of participants were excluded from the study secondary to misreporting on the CNAQ, which reduced the data available for analysis. A known limitation of FFQs is the high rate of misreporting, however the rate of misreporting in this study was much higher than previously reported [15]. It may therefore be useful to compare the DFI-FFQ to another dietary assessment method (i.e., 3- or 7-day diet records, or shorter validated FFQ) to confirm these results. The sample size for this study was small however a sufficient number of participants were recruited based on the sample size calculations, even after exclusion for misreporting. Additionally, other dietary questionnaire validation studies have similarly small participant numbers [16,17]. Despite the limitations discussed, we believe the DFI-FFQ will be a valuable tool in research and clinical practice as it is quick to complete (3.5 min on average), has low respondent burden and is a valid and reproducible method of classifying individuals based on their habitual dietary fibre intakes.

5. Conclusions

The DFI-FFQ has been shown to be a quick, valid and reproducible tool in classifying individuals based on their habitual dietary fibre intakes. The DFI-FFQ cannot however, accurately estimate total habitual dietary fibre intakes.

Author Contributions: G.H. was involved in the conception, study design, recruitment, conducting the study, and writing and editing the manuscript. J.C., C.B., R.M. and L.B. were involved in the conception, study design and editing of the manuscript. D.H. conducted the statistical analysis and was involved in editing the manuscript. All authors read and approved the manuscript.

Acknowledgments: The authors would like to take the opportunity to thank the individuals who participated in this study. The study was supported by the Foods for Health programme (C11X1312). The funds for the Foods for Health programme were provided to a number of collaborating New Zealand organisations, including The New Zealand Institute for Plant & Food Research Limited, by the Ministry of Business, Innovation and Employment, New Zealand Government.

Conflicts of Interest: The authors declare no conflict of interest.

References

1. Fuller, S.; Beck, E.; Salman, H.; Tapsell, L. New horizons for the study of dietary fiber and health: A review. *Plant Foods Hum. Nutr.* **2016**, *71*, 1–12. [CrossRef] [PubMed]
2. Thompson, F.E.; Subar, A.F. Dietary assessment methodology. In *Nutrition in the Prevention and Treatment of Disease*, 2nd ed.; Coulston, A.M., Boushey, C.J., Eds.; Elsevier: London, UK, 2008; pp. 3–39.
3. Roe, L.; Strong, C.; Whiteside, C.; Neil, A.; Mant, D. Dietary intervention in primary care: Validity of the DINE method for diet assessment. *Fam. Pract.* **1994**, *11*, 375–381. [CrossRef] [PubMed]
4. Wright, J.L.; Scott, J.A. The fat and fibre barometer, a short food behaviour questionnaire: Reliability, relative validity and utility. *Aust. J. Nutr. Diet.* **2000**, *57*, 33–39.
5. Shannon, J.; Kristal, A.R.; Curry, S.J.; Beresford, S.A. Application of a behavioral approach to measuring dietary change: The fat- and fiber-related diet behavior questionnaire. *Cancer Epidemiol. Biomark. Prev.* **1997**, *6*, 355–361.
6. Svilaas, A.; Strom, E.C.; Svilaas, T.; Borgejordet, A.; Thoresen, M.; Ose, L. Reproducibility and validity of a short food questionnaire for the assessment of dietary habits. *Nutr. Metab. Cardiovasc. Dis.* **2002**, *12*, 60–70. [PubMed]
7. Black, A.E. Critical evaluation of energy intake using the Goldberg cut-off for energy intake: Basal metabolic rate. A practical guide to its calculation, use and limitations. *Int. J. Obes.* **2000**, *24*, 1119–1130. [CrossRef]
8. Ministry of Health. A Focus on Nutrition Key Findings of the 2008/09 New Zealand Adult Nutrition Survey. Available online: https://www.health.govt.nz/system/files/documents/publications/a-focus-on-nutrition-v2.pdf (accessed on 15 July 2016).
9. Ministry of Health; Department of Health and Ageing. Nutrient Reference Values for Australia and New Zealand. Available online: http://www.health.govt.nz/publication/nutrient-reference-values-australia-and-new-zealand (accessed on 15 July 2016).
10. Barrett, J.S.; Gibson, P.R. Development and validation of a comprehensive semi-quantitative food frequency questionnaire that includes FODMAP intake and glycemic index. *J. Am. Diet. Assoc.* **2010**, *110*, 1469–1476. [CrossRef] [PubMed]
11. Kappa as a Measure of Concordance in Categorical Sorting. Available online: http://vassarstats.net/kappa.html (accessed on 15 July 2016).
12. Masson, L.F.; McNeill, G.; Tomany, J.O.; Simpson, J.A.; Peace, H.S.; Wei, L.; Grubb, D.A.; Bolton-Smith, C. Statistical approaches for assessing the relative validity of a food-frequency questionnaire: Use of correlation coefficients and the kappa statistic. *Public Health Nutr.* **2003**, *6*, 313–321. [CrossRef] [PubMed]
13. Buil-Cosiales, P.; Zazpe, I.; Toledo, E.; Corella, D.; Salas-Salvadó, J.; Diez-Espino, J.; Ros, E.; Navajas, J.F.C.; Santos-Lozano, J.M.; Arós, F.; et al. Fiber intake and all-cause mortality in the Prevención con Dieta Mediterránea (PREDIMED) study. *Am. J. Clin. Nutr.* **2014**, *100*, 1498–1507. [CrossRef] [PubMed]
14. Krebs-Smith, S.M.; Heimendinger, J.; Subar, A.F.; Patterson, B.H.; Pivonka, E. Using food frequency questionnaires to estimate fruit and vegetable intake: Association between the number of questions and total intakes. *J. Nutr. Educ.* **1995**, *27*, 80–85. [CrossRef]

15. Molag, M.L.; De Vries, J.H.; Ocke, M.C.; Dagnelie, P.C.; Van Den Brandt, P.A.; Jansen, M.C.; van Staveren, W.A.; van't Veer, P. Design characteristics of food frequency questionnaires in relation to their validity. *Am. J. Epidemiol.* **2007**, *166*, 1468–1478. [CrossRef] [PubMed]
16. O'Reilly, S.; McCann, L. Development and validation of the Diet Quality Tool for use in cardiovascular disease prevention settings. *Aust. J. Prim. Health* **2012**, *18*, 138–147. [CrossRef] [PubMed]
17. Spoon, M.; Devereux, P.; Benedict, J.; Leontos, C.; Constantino, N.; Christy, D.; Snow, G. Usefulness of the food habits questionnaire in a worksite setting. *J. Nutr. Educ. Behav.* **2002**, *34*, 268–272. [CrossRef]

nutrients

MDPI

Article

Wheat Bran Does Not Affect Postprandial Plasma Short-Chain Fatty Acids from ^{13}C-inulin Fermentation in Healthy Subjects

Lise Deroover [1], Joran Verspreet [2,3], Anja Luypaerts [1], Greet Vandermeulen [1], Christophe M. Courtin [2,3] and Kristin Verbeke [1,3,*]

1 Translational Research in Gastrointestinal Disorders, KU Leuven, Leuven 3000, Belgium; lise.deroover@kuleuven.be (L.D.); anja.luypaerts@kuleuven.be (A.L.); greet.vandermeulen@kuleuven.be (G.V.)
2 Centre for Food and Microbial Technology, KU Leuven, Leuven 3000, Belgium; joran.verspreet@kuleuven.be (J.V.); christophe.courtin@kuleuven.be (C.M.C.)
3 Leuven Food Science and Nutrition Research Centre, KU Leuven, Leuven 3000, Belgium
* Correspondence: kristin.verbeke@kuleuven.be; Tel.: +32-163-301-50; Fax: +32-163-307-23

Received: 14 December 2016; Accepted: 17 January 2017; Published: 20 January 2017

Abstract: Wheat bran (WB) is a constituent of whole grain products with beneficial effects for human health. Within the human colon, such insoluble particles may be colonized by specific microbial teams which can stimulate cross-feeding, leading to a more efficient carbohydrate fermentation and an increased butyrate production. We investigated the extent to which WB fractions with different properties affect the fermentation of other carbohydrates in the colon. Ten healthy subjects performed four test days, during which they consumed a standard breakfast supplemented with 10 g ^{13}C-inulin. A total of 20 g of a WB fraction (unmodified WB, wheat bran with a reduced particle size (WB RPS), or de-starched pericarp-enriched wheat bran (PE WB)) was also added to the breakfast, except for one test day, which served as a control. Blood samples were collected at regular time points for 14 h, in order to measure ^{13}C-labeled short-chain fatty acid (SCFA; acetate, propionate and butyrate) concentrations. Fermentation of ^{13}C-inulin resulted in increased plasma SCFA for about 8 h, suggesting that a sustained increase in plasma SCFA can be achieved by administering a moderate dose of carbohydrates, three times per day. However, the addition of a single dose of a WB fraction did not further increase the ^{13}C-SCFA concentrations in plasma, nor did it stimulate cross-feeding (Wilcoxon signed ranks test).

Keywords: colonic fermentation; short-chain fatty acids; wheat bran; inulin

1. Introduction

The short-chain fatty acids (SCFA) acetate, propionate, and butyrate, constitute a major class of bacterial metabolites that are derived from colonic carbohydrate fermentation. They are increasingly considered as signaling molecules with a beneficial impact on gut and systemic health [1,2]. Indeed, besides serving as energy substrates for the colonocytes, SCFA influence the expression of many genes by acting as inhibitors of histone deacetylases, and affect metabolic processes through the activation of G-protein coupled receptors (GPR41 and GPR43, later renamed as free fatty acid receptor (FFAR)-3 and (FFAR)-2). Several studies have indicated that SCFA, and in particular butyrate, improve the intestinal barrier function and reduce inflammation by inhibiting NFκB activation [3,4]. In addition, SCFA that enter the systemic circulation modulate energy homeostasis, and peripheral glucose and lipid metabolism [4–6]. Furthermore, SCFA regulate immune function by affecting T cell differentiation into effector and regulatory T cells (Treg) [7], and colonic Treg cell homeostasis [8].

As a consequence, strategies that target the microbiota to improve health often aim at increasing saccharolytic fermentation. The production of colonic SCFA may be stimulated by modulating the intestinal microbiota and increasing the numbers of acetate and butyrate producing bacteria via administration of probiotics. Many probiotics are selected strains of lactobacilli or bifidobacteria [9], which are known lactate and acetate producers. In addition, there is a growing interest in the use of butyrate producing bacteria, such as *Faecalibacterium prausnitzii* and *Butyrcicoccus pullicaecorum*, as probiotics [10–13].

An alternative strategy for increasing SCFA production is to stimulate the indigenous saccharolytic bacterial population by administration of prebiotics or fermentable dietary fibers [14]. The best studied prebiotic substrates are inulin-type fructans (comprising oligofructose), galacto-oligosaccharides, xylo-oligosaccharides, and arabinoxylanoligosaccharides. In vitro fermentation studies with fecal inocula indicate that the amount and proportion of SCFA produced, depends on the type of fermentable substrate [15]. For example, inulin-type fructans induce a relatively high proportion of acetate, whereas resistant starch favors butyrate production [16].

Here, we applied a third strategy for modulating the entire intestinal ecosystem, which involves the administration of disperse insoluble particles that act as platforms on which the bacteria can adhere, grow, and interact. We hypothesize that these particles facilitate the exchange of microbial nutrients and metabolites, resulting in a more complete carbohydrate fermentation and increased cross-feeding. For example, the production of butyrate requires collaboration between primary degraders, such as bifidobacteria, that produce acetate and lactate, and butyrate producing bacteria, such as *Faecalibacterium* and *Roseburia*, that convert acetate into butyrate [17,18]. This interaction may be facilitated if both species adhere to the dietary platforms. Wheat bran (WB) was selected as an interesting dietary component for this purpose, as bacterial communities attached to WB that was incubated in vitro with human fecal inocula, were found to be dominated by *Clostridium* cluster XIVa bacteria, known as butyrate producers [19]. In addition, WB can be easily technically modified to control its physical properties. In this study, we evaluated the impact of three WB fractions that differed in particle size and tissue composition, on the fermentation of a readily fermentable carbohydrate (^{13}C-inulin) in healthy subjects. Concentrations of ^{13}C-SCFA were measured in plasma as an indication of carbohydrate fermentation and the relative proportions of acetate, propionate, and butyrate, were considered as a marker of cross-feeding.

2. Materials and Methods

2.1. WB Fractions

2.1.1. Unmodified WB

Commercial WB with a particle size of 1690 μm was obtained from Dossche Mills (Deinze, Belgium) and was used without further modification. Its chemical composition (amounts of dietary fiber, starch, protein, lipid, and ash) was analysed as previously described [20–22].

2.1.2. Wheat Bran with Reduced Particle Size (WB RPS)

The unmodified commercial WB mentioned above was milled in a Cyclotec 1093 Sample mill (FOSS, Höganäs, Sweden), as described previously [22], in order to obtain WB particles with an average size of 150 μm.

2.1.3. Destarched Pericarp-Enriched Wheat Bran (PE WB)

PE WB was ascertained from Fugeia N.V. (Leuven, Belgium) and was obtained after an amylase and xylanase treatment of untreated WB, as described by Swennen et al. [23]. Subsequently, the PE WB was reduced in particle size to about 280 μm, using the same method as mentioned above.

2.2. Fermentable Substrate

Highly ^{13}C-enriched inulin with an atom percent (AP) beyond 97% was purchased from Isolife (Wageningen, The Netherlands) and was mixed with unlabeled native inulin (Fibruline instant, Cosucra Groupe Warcoing SA, Warcoing, Belgium; AP 0.98%), to form a homogeneous mixture with an AP of 1.93%.

2.3. Study Population

Ten healthy men and woman, aged between 18 and 65 years, were recruited to participate in the study. All subjects had a body mass index (BMI) between 18 and 27 kg/m^2 and a regular diet defined as three meals per day, on at least five days per week. Exclusion criteria were the use of antibiotics, prebiotics and probiotics, in the month preceding the study and during the study, consumption of a low calorie diet or another special diet in the month prior to the study, the use of medication that could affect the gastrointestinal tract in the two weeks before the start of the study and during the study, abdominal surgery in the past (except for appendectomy), chronic gastrointestinal diseases, blood donation in the three months prior to the study, hemoglobin (Hb) levels below reference values, and for woman, pregnancy or breast feeding. Subjects that had participated in a clinical trial involving radiation exposure in the year prior to the study were also excluded. The study protocol conformed to the Declaration of Helsinki and was approved by the Ethics Committee of the University of Leuven (Belgian Registration Number: B322201423101). All participants signed written informed consent. The study has been registered at ClinicalTrials.gov (clinical trial number: NCT02422537).

2.4. Study Design

Each subject performed four test days, with at least one week in between each test. During the three days prior to each test day, subjects were instructed to consume a low fiber diet, consisting of a maximum of one piece of fruit per day, white bread instead of wholegrain products, and no more than 100 g vegetables per day. They were also asked to avoid alcohol consumption. On the evening prior to the test day, the subjects consumed a completely digestible and non-fermentable meal (lasagna), eventually supplemented with white bread. After an overnight fast, the subjects presented themselves at the laboratory and provided two basal breath samples for the measurement of $^{13}CO_2$ and $^{14}CO_2$. A catheter (BD, Erembodegem, Belgium) was placed into an antecubital vein in the forearm to collect all blood samples during the test day. After collection of a basal blood sample, a standard breakfast was administered to the subjects. The breakfast consisted of 250 g low-fat yoghurt labeled with inulin-^{14}C-carboxylic acid (74 kBq, Perkin Elmer, Boston, MA, USA), a marker for oro-cecal transit time (OCTT), and 10 g of ^{13}C-labeled inulin, which served as a model fermentable substrate. The OCTT was defined as the time that elapses between the intake of the meal, and the arrival in the colon, which is reflected by the appearance of $^{14}CO_2$ in the breath. Depending on the test day, the breakfast was further supplemented with 20 g of one of the three WB fractions, or no supplement on the control test day. The participants were blind to the order of the different WB fractions and control tests, which were randomized using online software [24]. Breath samples were collected every 20 min, up to 14 h after consumption of the breakfast. Blood samples were collected every hour during the first 4 h, every 40 min from 4 h to 10 h, and again every hour from 10 h to 14 h. A light digestible meal was offered to the subjects 4 h and 8 h after consumption of the breakfast. Water was offered *ad libitum* during the whole test day. The course of a test day is represented in Figure 1.

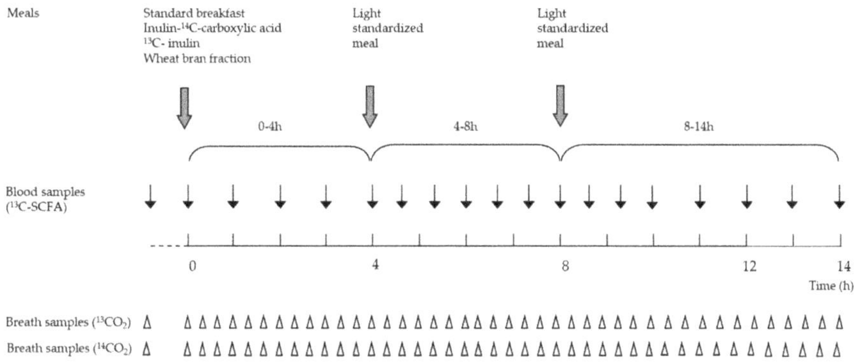

Figure 1. After a standard breakfast, labeled with ^{13}C-inulin, inulin-^{14}C-carboxylic acid and a WB fraction, breath samples were collected for the measurement of $^{13}CO_2$ and $^{14}CO_2$ and blood samples were collected for the analysis of ^{13}C-SCFA concentrations for 14 h. A light standardized meal was administered after 4 h and 8 h. The participants were blind to the order of the different WB fractions and control tests, which were randomized.

2.5. Collection and Analysis of Breath Samples

Subjects deposited breath samples for the analysis of $^{13}CO_2$ by blowing through a straw, into a 12-mL glass tube (Exetainer®, Labco Ltd., Ceredigion, UK), whereas samples for the measurement of $^{14}CO_2$ were collected by blowing through a pipet, into a plastic scintillation vial (Sarstedt, Nümbrecht, Germany) containing 4 mL of a 0.5 M hyamine hydroxide solution (Perkin Elmer, Boston MA, USA). Thymolphtaleine acted as a color indicator, which became discolored when 2 mmol CO_2 was exhaled.

The abundance of $^{13}CO_2$ was measured using isotope ratio mass spectrometry (ABCA, Sercon, Crewe, UK) and the results were expressed as delta over baseline (DOB). $^{14}CO_2$ was measured using β-scintillation counting (Packard Tricarb Liquid Scintillation Spectrometer, model 3375, Packard Instruments, Downers Grove, IL, USA), after addition of 10 mL hionic fluor (Perkin Elmer, Boston MA, USA), and was expressed as disintegrations per minute (DPM) [25]. The arrival time of the breakfast in the colon (OCTT) and the start of the fermentation, were defined as the time at which a significant increase in $^{14}CO_2$ and $^{13}CO_2$, respectively, from the background was observed in the breath. This increase was defined as 2.5 times the standard deviation of all previous points, above the running average of all previous points [26].

2.6. Analysis of Plasma ^{13}C-Abundance

Blood samples were centrifuged at 3000× *g* and 4 °C for 10 min to obtain plasma. The samples were immediately aliquoted and stored at −80 °C until analysis. Plasma samples were deproteinized using Amicon® Ultra-15 filters (Molecular weight cut-off: 30 kDa, Merck, Kenilworth, NJ, USA). Before application of the sample, the filters were rinsed twice using 0.2 N HCl to avoid SCFA contamination. Subsequently, 3 mL plasma was mixed with 3 mL MilliQ® water (Sartorius Arium® 611-VF, Sartorius, Göttingen, Germany) and 150 μL 0.15 N NaOH, and centrifuged at 2000× *g* and 4 °C for 20 min. Following this, the samples were transferred to the cleaned filters and deproteinized by centrifugation at 3000× *g* and 4 °C for 3 h. After addition of 120 μL 1 M NaOH, the filtrate was dried overnight in a vacuum concentrator (RVC 2-18, Christ, Germany) at 50 °C.

Prior to injection, the dried samples were acidified with 100 μL 4 M HCl with trypan blue (0.4%, Sigma, UK), and extracted in 400 μL diethyl ether (Sigma-Aldrich, Steinheim, Germany). The ether layer was pipetted into a crimp neck vial (1.5 mL) and evaporated with nitrogen gas (N_2) to about 50 μL, before injection in the gas chromatograph combustion isotope ratio mass spectrometer (GC-C-IRMS) (Delta plus-XP, Thermo Fisher, Bremen, Germany), equipped with a trace gas chromatograph (Interscience, Breda, The Netherlands) and a combustion interface type 3 (Thermo Fisher). Four μL of the SCFA solution was injected on an AT-Aquawax-DA column (30 m × 0.53 mm, i.d., 1.00 μm, Grace, Lokeren, Belgium), with the injector temperature at 240 °C. Helium 5.0 was used as a carrier gas at a constant flow of 2.5 mL/min. The initial oven temperature was held at 80 °C for 3 min and was increased by 4 °C/min to 140 °C, then further increased by 8 °C/min to 240 °C, and kept at this temperature for 10 min. The separated GC-effluents were combusted and oxidised to NO_x, CO_2, and H_2O in an oxidation furnace (CuO/NiO/Pt) at 940 °C [25]. All oxidised components were passed over the reduction column at 640 °C and the H_2O in the system was eliminated by a Nafion membrane (Thermo Fisher). The delta (δ^{13} Pee Dee Belemnite (PDB)) values were calculated by Isodat 2.0 software (Thermo Fisher) and converted to AP. The measured AP at any time point *t* was subtracted from the abundance measured in the baseline sample at time point 0, to obtain results in atom per cent excess (APE) [25]. The linearity of the system (slope < 0.06) was confirmed to be in the range between 0.8 and 11 volts, with CO_2 as the reference gas (5.0 quality, $\delta = -32.16‰$).

2.7. Analysis of Total SCFA Concentrations in Plasma

The total concentration of acetate, propionate, and butyrate in the plasma was measured using gas chromatography coupled with a flame ionization detector (GC-FID) after preconcentration of the SCFA, using a hollow fiber liquid membrane extraction. Plasma samples were thawed prior to analysis, and prepared and analyzed as described by Zhao et al. [27], with slight modifications. Plasma samples (100 μL) were rapidly spiked with internal standard (12.5 μg 2-ethyl butyric acid and 30 μg 3-methyl-valeric acid), acidified with 20 μL 0.2 N HCl, and diluted to 1.5 mL. A hollow fiber coated with tri-n-octylphoshphine oxide and filled with 10 μL 0.15 N NaOH, was immersed in the diluted plasma and shaken overnight. In this way, protonated SCFA diffuse into the fiber, where they become ionized and remain trapped. After acidification of the fiber content, 0.5 μL of the acidified SCFA solution was injected in a GC (HP 6890 series, Agilent, Wilmington, NC, USA) equipped with a FID and a DB-FAPP capillary column (30 m × 0.53 mm id, 1.00 μm film, Agilent, Wilmington, NC, USA). Helium was used as a carrier gas at a flow rate of 4.2 mL/min. The initial oven temperature was 100 °C for 3 min, raised by 4 °C/min to 140 °C, and held at this temperature for 5 min, before being further increased by 40 °C/min to 235 °C, and finally held at 235 °C for 5 min. The temperature of the FID heater and the injection port were set at 240 °C and 200 °C, respectively. The flow rates of hydrogen, air, and nitrogen as the make-up gas, were 30, 300, and 20 mL/min, respectively.

2.8. Calculations

At each time point, the concentration of ^{13}C-SCFA in plasma is the sum of the concentration that was already present at the baseline, and the concentration that originates from the colon (Equation (1)).

$$\left[^{13}\text{C-SCFA}\right] = \left[^{13}\text{C-SCFA}\right]_{t_0} + \left[^{13}\text{C-SCFA}\right]_{\text{colon}} \quad (1)$$

where $\left[^{13}\text{C-SCFA}\right]_{t_0}$ is the concentration of ^{13}C-SCFA present in plasma at time point 0 and $\left[^{13}\text{C-SCFA}\right]_{\text{colon}}$ is the concentration of ^{13}C-SCFA coming from the colon at time point t.

Substitution of the concentration of ^{13}C-SCFA by the product of its total concentration and abundance, results in Equation (2).

$$n_t \times AP_t = n_0 \times AP_{\text{plasma}_{t_0}} + n_{\text{colon}} \times AP_{\text{colon}} \quad (2)$$

In addition, the total concentration of SCFA at each time point t is the sum of the SCFA already present in the plasma, and the SCFA produced in the colon (Equation (3)).

$$n_t = n_0 + n_{\text{colon}} \quad (3)$$

Substitution of n_0 by n_t-n_{colon} in Equation (2), allows one to calculate the concentration of SCFA originating from the colon, thus produced from the ^{13}C-inulin at a time point t, according to Equation (4).

$$n_{colon} = n_t \times \frac{\left(AP_t - AP_{plasma_{t_0}}\right)}{\left(AP_{colon} - AP_{plasma_{t_0}}\right)} \quad (4)$$

where n_{colon} is the concentration of SCFA originating from the colon; n_t is the total concentration of SCFA at time point t; AP_t is the AP of ^{13}C-acetate, ^{13}C-propionate, or ^{13}C-butyrate at time point t; AP_{colon} is the AP of the administered inulin; $AP_{plasma_{t_0}}$ is the atom percent of ^{13}C-acetate, ^{13}C-propionate, or ^{13}C-butyrate in the plasma at time point t_0.

The concentrations of ^{13}C-acetate, ^{13}C-propionate, and ^{13}C-butyrate, originating from the colon at each time point, were used to draw concentration versus time curves for each test day. Subsequently, the cumulative concentrations of ^{13}C-acetate, ^{13}C-propionate, and ^{13}C-butyrate (area under the curve (AUC)) were calculated using the trapezoidal rule and were expressed in μmol·h/L.

The starting point of the fermentation was ascertained by calculating the mean time at which ^{13}C-acetate, ^{13}C-propionate, and ^{13}C-butyrate concentrations in plasma increased. The end of the fermentation was the mean time at which ^{13}C-acetate, ^{13}C-propionate, and ^{13}C-butyrate concentrations returned to the baseline. The duration of the fermentation was the difference between the end and start points of the fermentation.

2.9. Statistical Analysis

Statistical analysis was performed using SPSS software, version 23.0 (IBM, Brussels, Belgium). Because of the small sample size, non-parametric tests were used (Wilcoxon signed ranks test).

3. Results

3.1. Characterisation of the WB Fractions

Untreated WB had an average particle size of 1690 μm and was composed of 50% dietary fiber (arabinoxylan, cellulose, β-glucan, lignin and fructan), 17% starch, 20% protein, 6% lipids, and 7% ash (Figure 2a). WB RPS did not differ in tissue composition from the unmodified WB (Figure 2a). In contrast, PE WB was composed of 71% dietary fiber (mainly insoluble), 2% starch, 18% protein, 6% lipids, and 7% ash (Figure 2b).

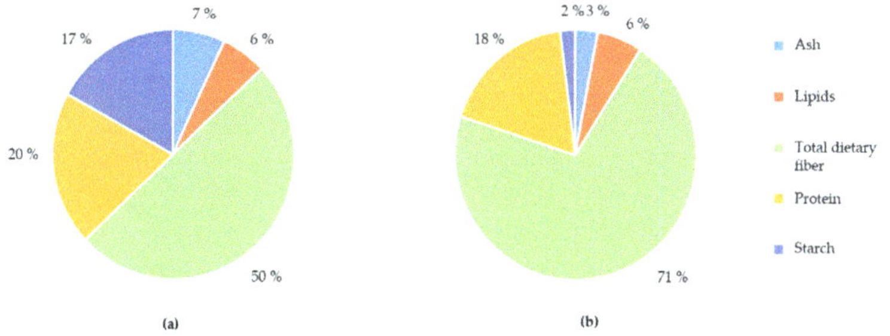

Figure 2. Unmodified wheat bran (WB) and wheat bran with reduced particle size (WB RPS) (**a**) contain less total dietary fiber and more starch compared to destarched pericarp-enriched wheat bran (PE WB) (**b**).

3.2. Study Population

From the 58 subjects that responded to the advertisement, 15 subjects underwent screening, which included an assessment of height and body weight, plasma Hb levels, medical history, and dietary habits (Figure 3). Five volunteers withdrew from the study before the start because of a lack of time (*n* = 3), pregnancy (*n* = 1), or because they did not meet the inclusion criteria (*n* = 1). Ten subjects (4M/6F, aged 25 ± 4 years, BMI 23.7 ± 2.0 kg/m^2) completed the four test days according to the study protocol.

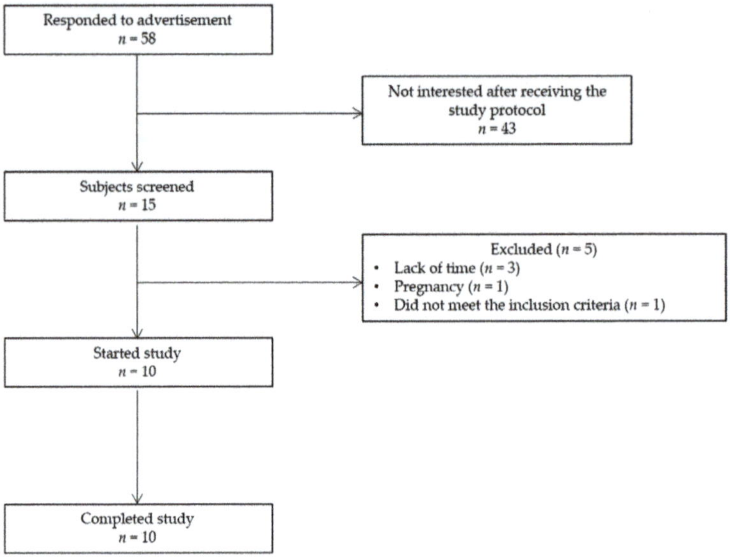

Figure 3. Flow chart depicting the passage of subjects through the study.

3.3. *Estimation of the OCTT and the Start of the Fermentation Using Breath and Plasma Samples*

The start of the fermentation was defined as the time point at which $^{13}CO_2$ started to increase in the breath, or as the mean time point at which the concentration of ^{13}C-acetate, ^{13}C-propionate, and ^{13}C-butyrate started to increase in the plasma. An increase in breath $^{14}CO_2$, which was generated from bacterial fermentation of ^{14}C-labeled inulin carboxylic acid, was used as a marker for the OCTT. Figure 4a,b compare the OCTT to the start of fermentation, based on breath $^{13}CO_2$ excretion and plasma ^{13}C-SCFA concentrations, respectively. The increase in breath $^{13}CO_2$ and in plasma ^{13}C-SCFA occurred slightly before the increase in breath $^{14}CO_2$, suggesting that fermentation of ^{13}C-inulin had already started in the terminal ileum.

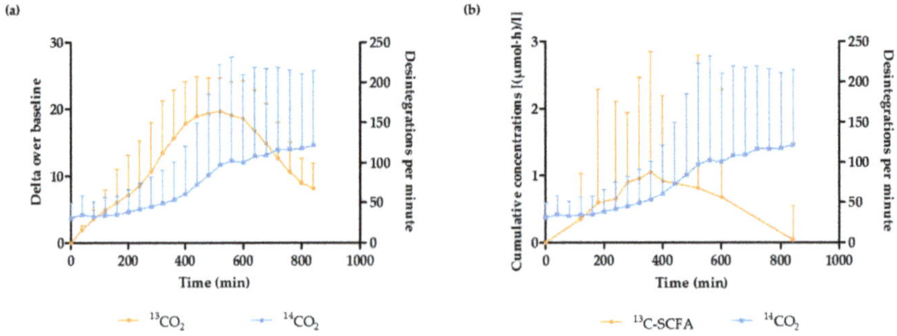

Figure 4. Both ^{13}C-excretion in breath (**a**) and plasma ^{13}C-SCFA concentrations (**b**) start to increase before the increase in breath $^{14}CO_2$ (*n* = 40).

On average, the fermentation started 208.5 ± 29 min and 219 ± 24.2 min after consumption of the breakfast, based on the breath samples and the plasma samples, respectively. The start of the fermentation was not affected by the addition of any of the WB fractions, when compared to the control (Wilcoxon signed ranks test; Breath samples: $p_{WB} = 0.073$, $p_{WBRPS} = 0.125$, $p_{PEWB} = 0.619$; Plasma samples: $p_{WB} = 0.123$, $p_{WBRPS} = 0.482$, $p_{PEWB} = 0.066$) (Figure 5a,b).

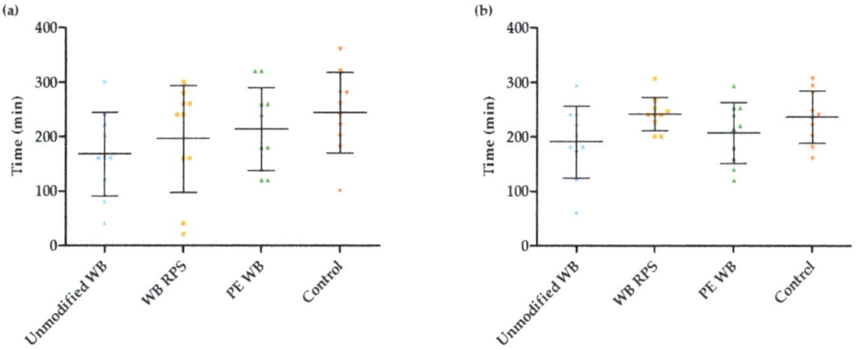

Figure 5. Wheat bran (WB) supplementation did not affect the start of the fermentation based on the $^{13}CO_2$-breath excretion (**a**) nor ^{13}C-labeled short-chain fatty acids (SCFA) concentrations in plasma (**b**) (n = 10). The middle line represents the mean with the standard deviation (whiskers).

3.4. *Estimation of the Duration of the Fermentation in the Presence of Different WB Fractions*

The duration of the fermentation was considered as a measure for the efficiency of fermentation with shorter duration, indicating a more efficient fermentation. On average, fermentation continued for 486 ± 40.9 min. However, the duration of the fermentation was not different when unmodified WB, WB RPS, and PE WB were administered to the subjects, compared to the control condition (Wilcoxon signed rank test; $p_{WB} = 0.201$, $p_{WBRPS} = 0.236$, $p_{PEWB} = 0.878$) (Figure 6).

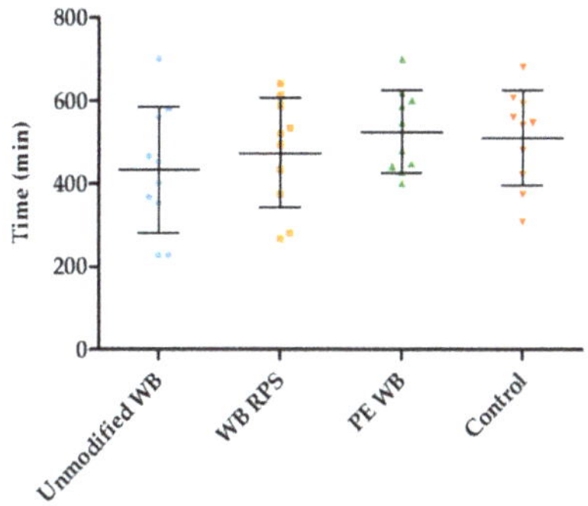

Figure 6. Wheat bran (WB) supplementation did not modify the duration of the fermentation (n = 10). The middle line represents the mean with the standard deviation (whiskers).

3.5. *^{13}C-SCFA Concentrations in Plasma Produced from the ^{13}C-Labeled Inulin*

Average concentrations of plasma ^{13}C-acetate, ^{13}C-propionate, and ^{13}C-butyrate originating from the colon, were presented as a function of time (Figure 7).

Influx of ^{13}C-acetate, ^{13}C-propionate, and ^{13}C-butyrate from the colon, reached a maximum value 360 ± 119 min after consuming the breakfast. Mean cumulative ^{13}C-SCFA concentrations

(n = 40) amounted to 18.5 ± 3.88 μmol·h·L^{-1} for acetate, 0.59 ± 0.17 μmol·h·L^{-1} for propionate, and 0.99 ± 0.3 μmol·h·L^{-1} for butyrate. However, cumulative ^{13}C-SCFA plasma concentrations were not different in the presence of any WB fraction, when compared to the control condition (Wilcoxon signed ranks test; Acetate: p_{WB} = 0.114, p_{WBRPS} = 0.878, p_{PEWB} = 0.721; Propionate: p_{WB} = 0.169, p_{WBRPS} = 0.646, p_{PEWB} = 0.139; Butyrate: p_{WB} = 0.169, p_{WBRPS} = 0.721, p_{PEWB} = 0.646; Total SCFA: p_{WB} = 0.074, p_{WBRPS} = 0.799, p_{PEWB} = 0.646) (Figure 8).

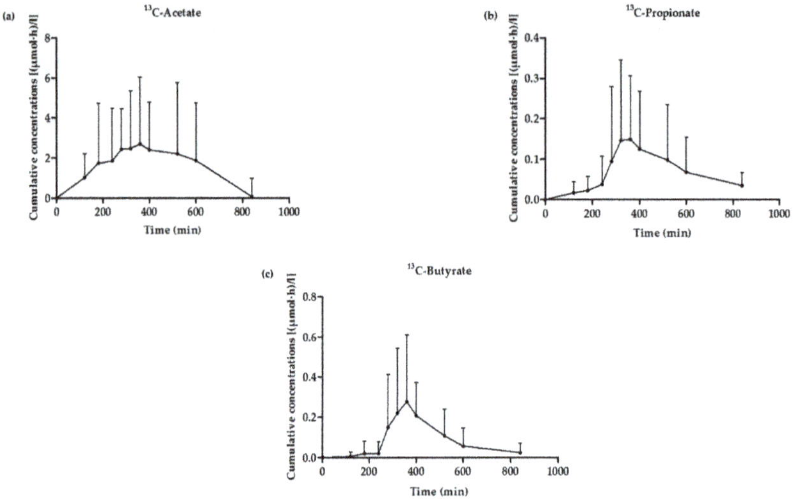

Figure 7. Average plasma concentrations of ^{13}C-acetate (**a**), ^{13}C-propionate (**b**) and ^{13}C-butyrate (**c**) originating from the colon as a function of time (n = 40).

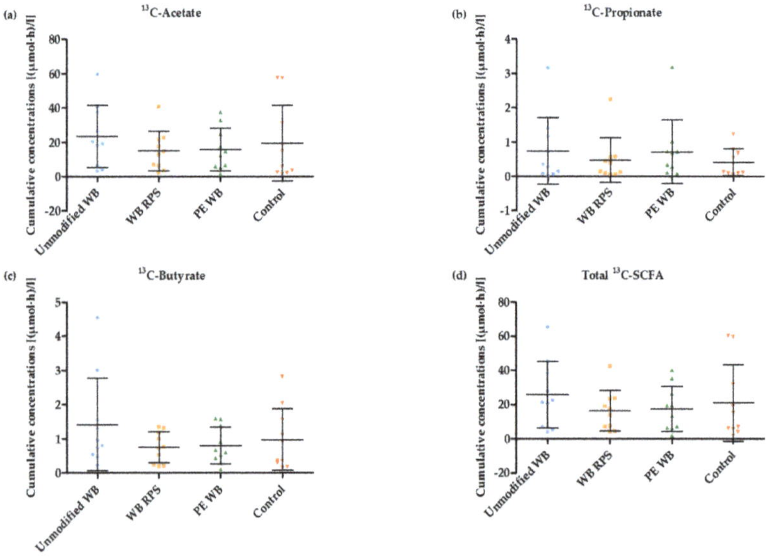

Figure 8. Wheat bran (WB) supplementation did not affect the cumulative ^{13}C-acetate (**a**), ^{13}C-propionate (**b**), ^{13}C-butyrate (**c**), total ^{13}C-SCFA (**d**) concentrations in plasma (n = 10). The middle line represents the mean with the standard deviation (whiskers).

3.6. Relative Proportion of Acetate, Propionate, and Butyrate after WB Supplementation

Stimulation of cross-feeding between colonic bacteria was evaluated by calculating the relative proportion of acetate, propionate, and butyrate for the different conditions. However, none of the WB fractions significantly influenced the relative proportion of acetate, propionate, and butyrate in the plasma, when compared to the control (Wilcoxon signed rank test; Acetate: $p_{WB} = 0.721$, $p_{WBRPS} = 0.959$, $p_{PEWB} = 0.575$; Propionate: $p_{WB} = 0.959$, $p_{WBRPS} = 0.445$, $p_{PEWB} = 0.959$; Butyrate: $p_{WB} = 0.575$, $p_{WBRPS} = 0.799$, $p_{PEWB} = 0.799$ (Figure 9).

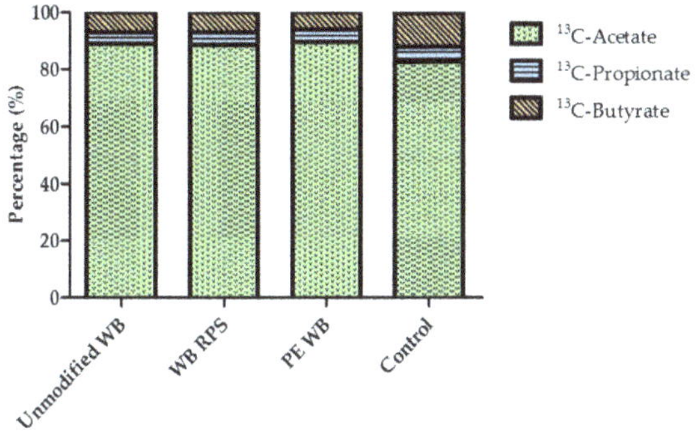

Figure 9. The proportions of ^{13}C-acetate, ^{13}C-propionate, and ^{13}C-butyrate in plasma were not affected by wheat bran (WB) (n = 10).

4. Discussion

Colonic production of SCFA from undigested carbohydrates has been increasingly recognized as a key process that contributes to both local gut and systemic health. The extent to which colonic-derived SCFA reach the systemic circulation may be an important parameter that determines the systemic health effects induced by dietary fiber consumption [25]. In the present study, we demonstrated that plasma SCFA are temporarily increased after consumption of a moderate dose of an easily fermentable carbohydrate.

The fact that we used uniformly stable isotope labeled inulin which, upon fermentation, resulted in the formation of labeled SCFA, allowed us to selectively quantify in plasma those SCFA originating from the inulin fermentation in the colon and to exclude confounders, like SCFA that were present in the colon at the start of the test days, SCFA that might have been produced due to partial fermentation of the WB fractions, or SCFA that have been endogenously produced. For example, plasma acetate is also produced from fatty acid oxidation and amino acid metabolism [28], and during ketogenesis in the mitochondria of the hepatocytes [29]. Colonic fermentation of ^{13}C-inulin contributed to increased plasma ^{13}C-SCFA concentrations for about 8 h, with maximal concentrations 6 h after consumption of the carbohydrate. It needs to be mentioned that the peak SCFA concentrations depend on the transit time of the substrates through the gastrointestinal tract, which is, apart from host factors, determined by the composition and caloric load of the breakfast meal and may vary with another test meal. Nevertheless, the results suggest that sustained increased plasma levels of SCFA might be obtained by three administrations of a considerable dose of an easily fermentable carbohydrate, evenly spread over a 24-h period. Furthermore, experiments which evaluate the health benefits of fermentable carbohydrates or prebiotics that are attributed to systemic SCFA, should preferably be performed in a time window between 6 and 10 h after administration of the carbohydrate.

To investigate whether insoluble particles could stimulate the fermentation of other carbohydrates in the colon, we used WB fractions that differed in tissue composition and particle size. Although reduction of particle size does not alter the composition of the WB fraction, it clearly modifies the physical properties of the WB. Destruction of cell walls during milling increases the specific surface area and the accessibility of intracellular cell components to degrading enzymes and, in this way, augments the fermentability of the WB fractions. In contrast, PE WB has been stripped of any fermentable material and mainly contains highly cross-linked dietary fiber that is hardly fermentable. We hypothesized that PE WB might facilitate fermentation by providing a platform on which bacteria can adhere, resulting in a more efficient exchange of microbial nutrients and metabolites between different types of bacteria; so-called cross-feeding. RPS WB may act in the same way, but has the additional advantage of being partly fermentable. If we would compare PE WB with a dinner table to which the bacteria draw up, WB RPS would be a dinner table filled with nutrients. Hence, we expected WB RPS to be more efficient in stimulating carbohydrate fermentation and cross-feeding.

Several factors may explain why WB did not stimulate the fermentation of inulin. First, inulin is an easily and rapidly fermentable substrate for colonic bacteria. It is possible that the fermentation proceeds so efficiently in baseline conditions that no room is left for improvement by the additional administration of WB platforms. Future studies may be performed with less rapidly fermentable carbohydrates, such as arabinoxylanoligosaccharides (AXOS). These oligosaccharides consist of a xylose backbone that is substituted with arabinose residues. By varying the degree of polymerization (DP) and the degree of substitution (DS), the rate of fermentation can be modulated. Unfortunately, ^{13}C-labeled AXOS derivatives are not commercially available. Second, the appearance of $^{13}CO_2$ in the breath and of ^{13}C-SCFA in the plasma, consistently occurred before arrival of the test meal in the colon, indicated by the appearance of $^{14}CO_2$ in the breath, suggesting that the fermentation of inulin had already started in the terminal ileum, where the bacterial density rapidly increases [30]. We used native inulin, which is a mixture of oligo- and polysaccharides, with a DP varying from 3 to 70 and an average DP of 25. The presence of short fructo-oligosaccharides most likely explains the early fermentation, as fermentation of short oligosaccharides proceeds more easily than that of longer chains [31]. Indeed, studies that use the increase in breath hydrogen excretion after administration of inulin as a marker of OCTT [26,32,33], generally use Raftiline HP® (Beneo, Mannheim, Germany) as the substrate, which only contains the long chains of inulin. This, at least in part, physical disconnection between the site of fermentation (terminal ileum) and main location of bacteria (colon), might hamper stimulation of the carbohydrate fermentation by bacteria adhered to the WB fractions.

Finally, repeated administration, rather than a single dose of WB, might have been more efficient for inducing a more efficient bacterial ecosystem. Nevertheless, in vitro incubation of human fecal samples with insoluble WB, showed that within 24 h (no earlier time point was tested) WB was already colonized by subsets of bacteria, suggesting a rapid colonization of insoluble particles [19]. Few studies have evaluated the impact of insoluble particles on SCFA production in vivo. Administration of resistant starch (RS) to pigs for two weeks resulted in increased cecal concentrations of butyrate, whereas combined administration of RS and WB resulted in increased butyrate concentrations in the more distal parts of the colon and in feces, suggesting that the addition of WB distally shifted fermentation [34]. These results could not be explained by partial fermentation of WB, as WB alone did not significantly increase butyrate concentrations. Also in humans, a diet supplemented with WB and RS for three weeks resulted in higher fecal proportions of butyrate and lower propionate proportions than WB alone, whereas fecal SCFA concentrations after the WB diet were not different from the values recorded during the control diet [35]. These observations support our hypothesis of improved carbohydrate fermentation due to the colonization of WB particles. However, alternative mechanisms also need to be considered. Increased fecal SCFA may also be due to the fact that WB accelerates whole gut transit time [36]. Indeed, both in vitro fermentation studies and human studies, indicate that SCFA production is increased with short transit time, and that longer transit times are associated with a shift from carbohydrate to protein fermentation [37–39]. It is important to note that fecal SCFA concentrations are the net result of production and absorption, and are difficult to relate to plasma SCFA.

Finally, we observed large inter- and intra-individual variations in plasma SCFA concentrations, which may have hampered detection of subtle changes in plasma SCFA due to WB intervention. Such large variations have also been reported in previous studies measuring SCFA [40–42] and may be due to variability in intestinal microbiota composition, colonic SCFA absorption and metabolism, and SCFA metabolism in the liver.

5. Conclusions

In this study, we showed that fermentation of a readily fermentable substrate results in increased plasma SCFA for about 8 h, suggesting that a sustained increase in plasma SCFA concentrations can be achieved when a moderate dose of fermentable carbohydrate is administered three times per day. Nevertheless, the addition of a single dose of different WB fractions did not further increase either the fermentation of the readily fermentable inulin, or cross-feeding between gut bacteria.

Acknowledgments: This research was conducted in the framework of an SBO-IWT project entitled "BRANDING: Cereal bran-based dispersions for gut health" and is supported by the "Vlaams Agentschap Innoveren en Ondernemen" (Vlaio, former IWT or "Agentschap voor Innovatie door Wetenschap en Technologie").

Author Contributions: L.D. and K.V. conceived and designed the experiments and wrote the paper; L.D., A.L. and G.V. performed the experiments and analyzed the data; J.V. and C.M.C. provided the wheat bran fractions and contributed to the revision of the manuscript.

Conflicts of Interest: The authors declare no conflict of interest.

References

1. Den Besten, G.; van Eunen, K.; Groen, A.K.; Venema, K.; Reijngoud, D.J.; Bakker, B.M. The role of short-chain fatty acids in the interplay between diet, gut microbiota, and host energy metabolism. *J. Lipid Res.* **2013**, *54*, 2325–2340. [CrossRef] [PubMed]
2. Macfarlane, G.T.; Macfarlane, S. Bacteria, colonic fermentation, and gastrointestinal health. *J. AOAC Int.* **2012**, *95*, 50–60. [CrossRef] [PubMed]
3. Hamer, H.M.; Jonkers, D.; Venema, K.; Vanhoutvin, S.; Troost, F.J.; Brummer, R.J. Review article: The role of butyrate on colonic function. *Aliment. Pharmacol. Ther.* **2008**, *27*, 104–119. [CrossRef] [PubMed]
4. Macfarlane, G.T.; Macfarlane, S. Fermentation in the human large intestine: Its physiologic consequences and the potential contribution of prebiotics. *J. Clin. Gastroenterol.* **2011**, *45*, S120–S127. [CrossRef] [PubMed]
5. Canfora, E.E.; Jocken, J.W.; Blaak, E.E. Short-chain fatty acids in control of body weight and insulin sensitivity. *Nat. Rev. Endocrinol.* **2015**, *11*, 577–591. [CrossRef] [PubMed]
6. Hong, Y.H.; Nishimura, Y.; Hishikawa, D.; Tsuzuki, H.; Miyahara, H.; Gotoh, C.; Choi, K.C.; Feng, D.D.; Chen, C.; Lee, H.G.; et al. Acetate and propionate short chain fatty acids stimulate adipogenesis via GPCR43. *Endocrinology* **2005**, *146*, 5092–5099. [CrossRef] [PubMed]
7. Park, J.; Kim, M.; Kang, S.G.; Jannasch, A.H.; Cooper, B.; Patterson, J.; Kim, C.H. Short-chain fatty acids induce both effector and regulatory T cells by suppression of histone deacetylases and regulation of the mtor-s6k pathway. *Mucosal. Immunol.* **2015**, *8*, 80–93. [CrossRef] [PubMed]
8. Smith, P.M.; Howitt, M.R.; Panikov, N.; Michaud, M.; Gallini, C.A.; Bohlooly, Y.M.; Glickman, J.N.; Garrett, W.S. The microbial metabolites, short-chain fatty acids, regulate colonic Treg cell homeostasis. *Science* **2013**, *341*, 569–573. [CrossRef] [PubMed]
9. Floch, M.H.; Hong-Curtiss, J. Probiotics and functional foods in gastrointestinal disorders. *Curr. Treat. Opt. Gastroenterol.* **2002**, *5*, 311–321. [CrossRef]
10. Marteau, P. Butyrate-producing bacteria as pharmabiotics for inflammatory bowel disease. *Gut* **2013**, *62*, 1673. [CrossRef] [PubMed]
11. Eeckhaut, V.; Ducatelle, R.; Sas, B.; Vermeire, S.; Van Immerseel, F. Progress towards butyrate-producing pharmabiotics: Butyricicoccus pullicaecorum capsule and efficacy in TNBS models in comparison with therapeutics. *Gut* **2014**, *63*, 367. [CrossRef] [PubMed]
12. Eeckhaut, V.; Machiels, K.; Perrier, C.; Romero, C.; Maes, S.; Flahou, B.; Steppe, M.; Haesebrouck, F.; Sas, B.; Ducatelle, R.; et al. Butyricicoccus pullicaecorum in inflammatory bowel disease. *Gut* **2013**, *62*, 1745–1752. [CrossRef] [PubMed]

13. Miquel, S.; Martin, R.; Rossi, O.; Bermudez-Humaran, L.G.; Chatel, J.M.; Sokol, H.; Thomas, M.; Wells, J.M.; Langella, P. Faecalibacterium prausnitzii and human intestinal health. *Curr. Opin. Microbiol.* **2013**, *16*, 255–261. [CrossRef] [PubMed]
14. Gibson, G.; Scott, K.; Rastal, R.A.; Kieran, M.T.; Hotchkiss, A.; Dubert-Ferrandon, A.; Gareau, M.; Eileen, M.F.; Saulnier, D.; Loh, G.; et al. Dietary prebiotics: Current status and new definition. *Food Sci. Technol. Bull.* **2010**, *7*, 1–19. [CrossRef]
15. Velázquez, M.; Davies, C.; Marett, R.; Slavin, J.L.; Feirtag, J.M. Effect of oligosaccharides and fibre substitutes on short-chain fatty acid production by human faecal microflora. *Anaerobe* **2000**, *6*, 87–92. [CrossRef]
16. Brouns, F.; Kettlitz, B.; Arrigoni, E. Resistant starch and "the butyrate revolution". *Trends Food Sci. Technol.* **2002**, *13*, 251–261. [CrossRef]
17. Moens, F.; Weckx, S.; De Vuyst, L. Bifidobacterial inulin-type fructan degradation capacity determines cross-feeding interactions between bifidobacteria and faecalibacterium prausnitzii. *Int. J. Food Microbiol.* **2016**, *231*, 76–85. [CrossRef] [PubMed]
18. Riviere, A.; Gagnon, M.; Weckx, S.; Roy, D.; De Vuyst, L. Mutual cross-feeding interactions between bifidobacterium longum subsp. Longum NCC2705 and eubacterium rectale ATCC 33656 explain the bifidogenic and butyrogenic effects of arabinoxylan oligosaccharides. *Appl. Environ. Microbiol.* **2015**, *81*, 7767–7781. [CrossRef] [PubMed]
19. Leitch, E.C.; Walker, A.W.; Duncan, S.H.; Holtrop, G.; Flint, H.J. Selective colonization of insoluble substrates by human faecal bacteria. *Environ. Microbiol.* **2007**, *9*, 667–679. [CrossRef] [PubMed]
20. Courtin, C.M.; Van den Broeck, H.; Delcour, J.A. Determination of reducing end sugar residues in oligo- and polysaccharides by gas-liquid chromatography. *J. Chromatogr. A* **2000**, *866*, 97–104. [CrossRef]
21. Gerits, L.R.; Pareyt, B.; Delcour, J.A. Single run hplc separation coupled to evaporative light scattering detection unravels wheat flour endogenous lipid redistribution during bread dough making. *LWT-Food Sci. Technol.* **2013**, *53*, 426–433. [CrossRef]
22. Jacobs, P.J.; Hemdane, S.; Dornez, E.; Delcour, J.A.; Courtin, C.M. Study of hydration properties of wheat bran as a function of particle size. *Food Chem.* **2015**, *179*, 296–304. [CrossRef] [PubMed]
23. Swennen, K.; Courtin, C.M.; Lindemans, G.C.J.E.; Delcour, J.A. Large-scale production and characterisation of wheat bran arabinoxylooligosaccharides. *J. Sci. Food Agric.* **2006**, *86*, 1722–1731. [CrossRef]
24. Urbaniak, G.U.; Plous, S. Research Randomizer. Available online: http://www.randomizer.org (accessed on 10 January 2015).
25. Boets, E.; Deroover, L.; Houben, E.; Vermeulen, K.; Gomand, S.V.; Delcour, J.A.; Verbeke, K. Quantification of in vivo colonic short chain fatty acid production from inulin. *Nutrients* **2015**, *7*, 8916–8929. [CrossRef] [PubMed]
26. Verbeke, K.; de Preter, V.; Geboes, K.; Daems, T.; van den Mooter, G.; Evenepoel, P.; Rutgeerts, P. In vivo evaluation of a colonic delivery system using isotope techniques. *Aliment. Pharmacol. Ther.* **2005**, *21*, 187–194. [CrossRef] [PubMed]
27. Zhao, G.; Liu, J.F.; Nyman, M.; Jonsson, J.A. Determination of short-chain fatty acids in serum by hollow fiber supported liquid membrane extraction coupled with gas chromatography. *J. Chromatogr. B Anal. Technol. Biomed. Life Sci.* **2007**, *846*, 202–208. [CrossRef] [PubMed]
28. Layden, B.T.; Angueira, A.R.; Brodsky, M.; Durai, V.; Lowe, W.L., Jr. Short chain fatty acids and their receptors: New metabolic targets. *Transl. Res.* **2013**, *161*, 131–140. [CrossRef] [PubMed]
29. Yamashita, H.; Kaneyuki, T.; Tagawa, K. Production of acetate in the liver and its utilization in peripheral tissues. *Biochim. Biophys. Acta* **2001**, *1532*, 79–87. [CrossRef]
30. Sartor, R.B. Microbial influences in inflammatory bowel diseases. *Gastroenterology* **2008**, *134*, 577–594. [CrossRef] [PubMed]
31. Van der Meulen, R.; Makras, L.; Verbrugghe, K.; Adriany, T.; De Vuyst, L. In vitro kinetic analysis of oligofructose consumption by *Bacteroides* and *Bifidobacterium* spp. Indicates different degradation mechanisms. *Appl. Environ. Microbiol.* **2006**, *72*, 1006–1012. [CrossRef] [PubMed]
32. Geboes, K.P.; Luypaerts, A.; Rutgeerts, P.; Verbeke, K. Inulin is an ideal substrate for a hydrogen breath test to measure the orocaecal transit time. *Aliment. Pharmacol. Ther.* **2003**, *18*, 721–729. [CrossRef] [PubMed]
33. Schneider, A.R.; Jepp, K.; Murczynski, L.; Biniek, U.; Stein, J. The inulin hydrogen breath test accurately reflects orocaecal transit time. *Eur. J. Clin. Investig.* **2007**, *37*, 802–807. [CrossRef] [PubMed]

34. Govers, M.J.; Gannon, N.J.; Dunshea, F.R.; Gibson, P.R.; Muir, J.G. Wheat bran affects the site of fermentation of resistant starch and luminal indexes related to colon cancer risk: A study in pigs. *Gut* **1999**, *45*, 840–847. [CrossRef] [PubMed]
35. Muir, J.G.; Yeow, E.G.; Keogh, J.; Pizzey, C.; Bird, A.R.; Sharpe, K.; O'Dea, K.; Macrae, F.A. Combining wheat bran with resistant starch has more beneficial effects on fecal indexes than does wheat bran alone. *Am. J. Clin. Nutr.* **2004**, *79*, 1020–1028. [PubMed]
36. De Vries, J.; Miller, P.E.; Verbeke, K. Effects of cereal fiber on bowel function: A systematic review of intervention trials. *World J. Gastroenterol.* **2015**, *21*, 8952–8963. [CrossRef] [PubMed]
37. Lewis, S.J.; Heaton, K.W. Increasing butyrate concentration in the distal colon by accelerating intestinal transit. *Gut* **1997**, *41*, 245–251. [CrossRef] [PubMed]
38. Macfarlane, G.T.; Macfarlane, S.; Gibson, G.R. Validation of a three-stage compound continuous culture system for investigating the effect of retention time on the ecology and metabolism of bacteria in the human colon. *Microb. Ecol.* **1998**, *35*, 180–187. [CrossRef] [PubMed]
39. Roager, H.M.; Hansen, L.B.; Bahl, M.I.; Frandsen, H.L.; Carvalho, V.; Gobel, R.J.; Dalgaard, M.D.; Plichta, D.R.; Sparholt, M.H.; Vestergaard, H.; et al. Colonic transit time is related to bacterial metabolism and mucosal turnover in the gut. *Nat. Microbiol.* **2016**, *1*, 16093. [CrossRef] [PubMed]
40. Bloemen, J.G.; Venema, K.; van de Poll, M.C.; Olde Damink, S.W.; Buurman, W.A.; Dejong, C.H. Short chain fatty acids exchange across the gut and liver in humans measured at surgery. *Clin. Nutr.* **2009**, *28*, 657–661. [CrossRef] [PubMed]
41. Boets, E.; Gomand, S.V.; Deroover, L.; Preston, T.; Vermeulen, K.; De Preter, V.; Hamer, H.; Van den Mooter, G.; De Vuyst, L.; Courtin, C.M.; et al. Systemic availability and metabolism of colonic-derived short-chain fatty acids in healthy subjects—A stable isotope study. *J. Physiol.* **2017**, *595*, 541–555. [CrossRef] [PubMed]
42. Peters, S.G.; Pomare, E.W.; Fisher, C.A. Portal and peripheral blood short chain fatty acid concentrations after caecal lactulose instillation at surgery. *Gut* **1992**, *33*, 1249–1252. [CrossRef] [PubMed]

nutrients

MDPI

Commentary

Toward a Personalized Approach in Prebiotics Research

Moul Dey

Department of Health and Nutritional Sciences, Box 2203, South Dakota State University, Brookings, SD 57007, USA; Moul.Dey@sdstate.edu; Tel.: +1-605-688-4050

Received: 14 December 2016; Accepted: 20 January 2017; Published: 26 January 2017

Abstract: Recent characterization of the human microbiome and its influences on health have led to dramatic conceptual shifts in dietary bioactives research. Prebiotic foods that include many dietary fibers and resistant starches are perceived as beneficial for maintaining a healthy gut microbiota. This article brings forward some current perspectives in prebiotic research to discuss why reporting of individual variations in response to interventions will be important to discern suitability of prebiotics as a disease prevention tool.

Keywords: prebiotics; disease prevention; dietary bioactives; resistant starch type 4; intervention response variability

---

The ancient Greek physician Hippocrates perceived food as the key player in the maintenance of health, not just as a fuel to run the human body. Since then, scientists have probed deeper into the role of diet in nutrient absorption and bodily function. In the late 1800s, scientists began isolating microorganisms from different parts of the human body including from the digestive tract. Some of these organisms were considered harmful and others beneficial. However, the concept of the human microbiome and its critical role in human health and diseases is more recent, emerging in the 21st century after the advent of next generation sequencing. Mapping microbiome diversity has unlocked many mysteries—but also triggered new questions. The answers to many such questions still elude us, including a very basic but pressing question, "what diet is ideal for a healthy gut microbiome?" It remains unknown if there is an ideal gut microbiome that can be considered "healthy", nor do we know of one ideal diet that can positively manipulate the microbiome of people of all ages across the globe. Furthermore, a plethora of contradictory research findings on what dietary component may or may not be healthy frequently confuse the public. Not too long ago, dietary fat used to be our worst enemy. With time, that spot was taken over by dietary sugars. Another example is soy, with its many known health benefits and a host of negative side effects [1]. While the reasons behind contradictory nutritional research are multi-faceted, one contributing factor may be researchers designing studies like modern medical research that predominantly aims for disease-specific diagnostic and therapeutic avenues. Scientists prioritize collective outcomes with high statistical significance. While these benchmarks are a sign of a successful clinical trial, individual responses to the dietary treatment are often ignored. For example, recently Zeevi et al. reported widespread and high interpersonal variability in post-prandial glucose response among healthy participants to common dietary components [2]. It is possible that researchers in dietary intervention studies frequently encounter similar variations, but they are under-reported.

Prebiotics are selectively fermented dietary ingredients such as resistant starches and some dietary fibers that change the composition and/or activity of the gastrointestinal microbiota, thus conferring benefits to the host's health [3]. While this newer type of functional food is increasingly popular, a recent systematic review of six prebiotic trials published before 6 November 2015 suggests that more randomized controlled trials are needed to support their clinical use [4]. More recently our group reported a microbiome signature in response to a resistant starch type 4 (RS4)-enriched diet in individuals with metabolic syndrome (NCT01887964, [5]). It was concluded that RS4 has prebiotic effects with a potential for metabolic disease prevention. This double-blind and placebo-controlled study is among a small number of prebiotic intervention studies conducted under a free-living setting reporting statistically significant changes across microbial composition and abundance, fecal short chain fatty acid levels, and host immunometabolic functions in response to RS4 consumption. More frequently, intervention studies end up being inconclusive or lack statistical power due to wide variability in responses among participants, particularly when conducted within natural living conditions [6]. Interestingly in our study, although statistical significance across most endpoints was observed, response variability was commonplace for bacterial abundance and metabolites as well as clinical endpoints in the host. Relative to average Americans, the study population (Hutterites living in eastern South Dakota) was more genetically homogeneous and had fewer differences in daily lifestyle due to their communal style of living. Their variability in microbiome response, however, came as little surprise. In earlier reports, microbiota varied both in steady state conditions and in response to diet, aging, and other lifestyle changes [7–9]. Quite possibly, a deeper mechanistic investigation on how RS4 functions at the molecular level may shed some light on such response variations in the future. However, here the author focusses on one other question that emerges from all of this: will it benefit the scientific community in the long run if such side observations of response variability are routinely reported? Is it possible that we are missing out on information that may hold the key to unlocking some of the mysteries of diet and the microbiome interactions by not reporting individual responses to dietary interventions? Currently, there is little enthusiasm from both scientists and publishers to report such information, as data without statistical significance would rarely contribute to the conclusions drawn from the work. The viewpoint is illustrated in Figure 1. We observed increases in *Ruminococcus lactaris* and *Eubacterium oxidoreducens* in the RS4 group compared to baseline and post-CF (control group, CF) [5]. The most common format for reporting such data is mean % change or fold change along with the *p*-value. Less frequently, individual data points with column means and associated descriptive statistical information are shown (Figure 1B,C). Collective data presentation formats, such as the one shown in Figure 1A, are less helpful in revealing the distinct nature of the two datasets.

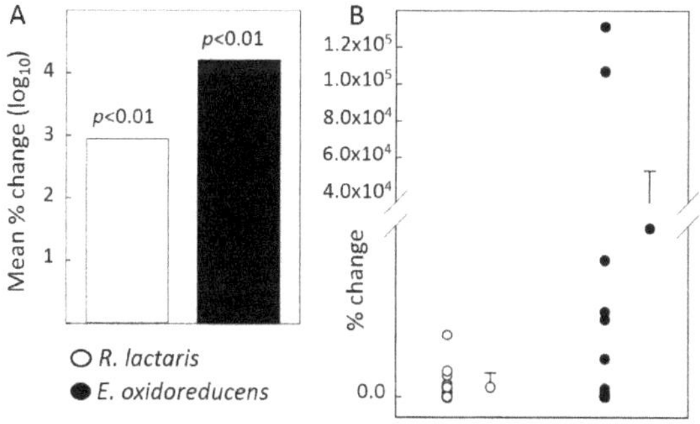

C

	R. lactaris	*E. oxidoreducens*
Sample size	19.0	19.0
Mean % change from baseline	901.5	15736.7
Std deviation	1378.9	37234.9
Std error	316.4	8542.3
C.I. of mean	664.6	17946.7
Range of change	5858.8	131,000.0
Maximum effect	5800.0	131,000.0
Minimum effect	-58.8 (decreased)	0.0
Median	437.5	135.7

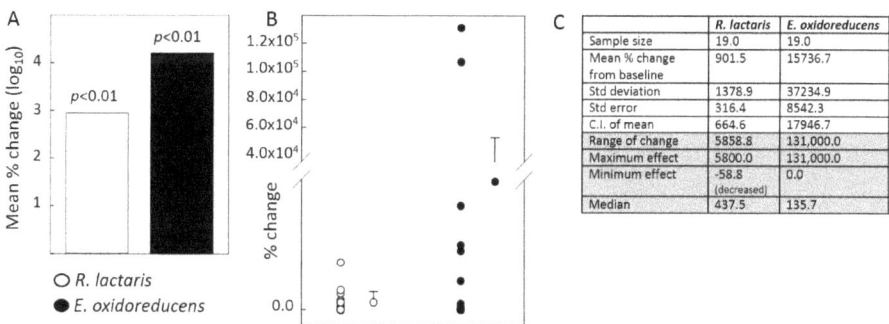

Figure 1. Data presentation formats. (**A**) Relative abundance of two bacterial species before and after RS4 treatment shown as mean % change ($\log_{10}$) with corresponding *p* values; (**B**) Percent change from before intervention of the same two bacterial species shown as individual data points with means and standard deviations on the side; (**C**) Descriptive statistical information from the two data sets presented in A and B. The information presented in the last four rows are less frequently reported in clinical trial publications.

Assessing disease risk in susceptible populations remains one major objective of personalized or precision nutrition, allowing for stratifications of subpopulations in a manner that improves the accuracy and cost-effectiveness of interventions and follow-ups. In addition, early prognosis and/or diagnosis may facilitate prophylactic treatment that would otherwise be unsuitable for a larger population. In this context, Zeevi et al. has proposed a machine-learning algorithm approach that integrates multiple features based on a preexisting large cohort data set to predict, for example, glycemic response to real-life meals [2]. While they have reported feasibility, cost-effectiveness of such an approach has not been determined. It must be taken into consideration that no one outcome alone, such as glycemic response, determines the overall health outcome of an individual. For example, being able to predict glycemic response may attenuate the risk of type 2 diabetes, but will not help with the prognosis of hyperlipidemia, heart disease, or cancer. Therefore, many large-scale endeavors, such as those reported by Zeevi et al., will be necessary to predict multiple clinical end-points or intermediate biomarkers before personalized overall health risk determination followed by preventive intervention is possible. For similar reasons, personalized microbiome profiling, while deemed promising as a tool for disease risk stratification, is not ready for translation to a clinical setting. It is only proposed that a predictive microbiome modeling system with more sophisticated readouts integrating multiple aspects of gut microbiota (composition, abundance, metagenomics, meta-transcriptomic, metabolomics, etc.) should be incorporated [10]. In addition, microbiome-based biomarkers for personalized prognostic, diagnostic, and treatment may vary by geographic locations, lifestyle, and many other factors. Therefore, while personalized microbiome profiling may be useful for predicting and mitigating disease, it will take a huge scientific undertaking before it is ready for the clinical setting.

In the past few decades, there has been a surge in metabolic diseases that affect quality of life and pose a substantial medical and economic burden on society. There is a growing interest in preventive measures to modify the risk of metabolic diseases, with diet proposed as a major player in public health promotion. Decades of generalized nutritional recommendations do not seem to be mitigating the metabolic health crisis, although at present there is no alternate to an overall healthy diet and regular physical activity recommendation for long-term health maintenance. Mounting evidence suggests a more personalized approach is required for health promotion through disease prevention and that such personalization cannot entirely rely on human genomic variations in case of complex metabolic diseases. Even taking into account the huge undertaking discussed above, current knowledge about the microbiome suggests that integrating microbiome profiling into patient care will likely allow for a faster, more accurate, and less invasive clinical decision-making processes. In this context, prebiotics will be critical components of personally tailored dietary interventions aimed at altering the microbiome to a more beneficial configuration for disease prevention. While the benefits of dietary fibers, many of which have prebiotic properties, are well-known, their mechanisms of action mostly remain a mystery. Without the knowledge of structure-function relationships between various prebiotics and microbial species as well as further consideration of the bilateral relationship of the microbiome and the host, personalized and effective use of prebiotics for disease prevention will be difficult. Large-scale characterization of the nutrition-microbiome-host metabolism axis will help delineate the integration of prebiotics in personalized diets for prevention of multi-factorial metabolic diseases. One caveat toward such effort is that disease prevention trials typically focus on intermediate outcomes because long-term follow-up of a large enough population, that will both adhere to the intervention as well as provide sufficient statistical power to detect differences, is technically difficult and prohibitively expensive. Regrettably, intermediate outcome measures do not always reflect the true preventive potential of an intervention as reported from the Look AHEAD (Action for Health in Diabetes) trial [11].

Looking to the future, it will be critical to consider the collective effects that are statistically significant, as well as individual response variations, for harnessing the many potential health benefits of prebiotics. Encouraging the scientific community to report variations observed in clinical trials, even if such observations may not meaningfully contribute to the main conclusions of the current study, will be important. Such data may be presented in formats that allow more holistic visualization of study results, including but not limited to, effect sizes, percentile ranking, minimum and maximum values, outliers, means, and medians. A recent commentary in Nature Methods discussed similar data presentation approaches in lieu of sample-to-sample variability and irreproducibility of scientific data, particularly in biomedical disciplines [12]. In addition to that, the author believes, this may also provide an opportunity to build on the vast repertoire of individual response variations that may not otherwise be possible for any one research study to capture. How such data may precisely inform clinical study designs and/or results in the future will depend on effective systematic reviews and meta-analysis outcome from the growing body of such data sets. Nevertheless, the author is hopeful that the information generated will facilitate better predictability of microbial and/or host-physiological response behavior in the direction of early prognosis and prevention.

Acknowledgments: The author's laboratory is currently supported by USDA National Institute of Food and Agriculture Hatch grant [1004817] as well as state and industry grants. No funding was directly utilized toward preparation of this manuscript.

Conflicts of Interest: The author declares no conflict of interest.

References

1. Messina, M. Soy and Health Update: Evaluation of the Clinical and Epidemiologic Literature. *Nutrients* **2016**, *8*, 754. [CrossRef] [PubMed]
2. Zeevi, D.; Korem, T.; Zmora, N.; Israeli, D.; Rothschild, D.; Weinberger, A.; Ben-Yacov, O.; Lador, D.; Avnit-Sagi, T.; Lotan-Pompan, M.; et al. Personalized Nutrition by Prediction of Glycemic Responses. *Cell* **2015**, *163*, 1079–1094. [CrossRef] [PubMed]
3. Roberfroid, M.; Gibson, G.R.; Hoyles, L.; McCartney, A.L.; Rastall, R.; Rowland, I.; Wolvers, D.; Watzl, B.; Szajewska, H.; Stahl, B.; et al. Prebiotic effects: Metabolic and health benefits. *Br. J. Nutr.* **2010**, *104*, S1–S63. [CrossRef] [PubMed]
4. Fernandes, R.; do Rosario, V.A.; Mocellin, M.C.; Kuntz, M.G.; Trindade, E.B. Effects of inulin-type fructans, galacto-oligosaccharides and related synbiotics on inflammatory markers in adult patients with overweight or obesity: A systematic review. *Clin. Nutr.* **2016**. [CrossRef] [PubMed]
5. Upadhyaya, B.; McCormack, L.; Fardin-Kia, A.R.; Juenemann, R.; Clapper, J.; Specker, B.; Dey, M. Impact of dietary resistant starch type 4 on human gut microbiota and immunometabolic functions. *Sci. Rep.* **2016**, *6*, 28797. [CrossRef] [PubMed]
6. Satija, A.; Yu, E.; Willett, W.C.; Hu, F.B. Understanding nutritional epidemiology and its role in policy. *Adv. Nutr.* **2015**, *6*, 5–18. [CrossRef] [PubMed]
7. Eckburg, P.B.; Bik, E.M.; Bernstein, C.N.; Purdom, E.; Dethlefsen, L.; Sargent, M.; Gill, S.R.; Nelson, K.E.; Relman, D.A. Diversity of the Human Intestinal Microbial Flora. *Science* **2005**, *308*, 1635–1638. [CrossRef] [PubMed]
8. Claesson, M.J.; Jeffery, I.B.; Conde, S.; Power, S.E.; O'Connor, E.M.; Cusack, S.; Harris, H.M.; Coakley, M.; Lakshminarayanan, B.; O'Sullivan, O.; et al. Gut microbiota composition correlates with diet and health in the elderly. *Nature* **2012**, *488*, 178–184. [CrossRef] [PubMed]
9. Carmody, R.N.; Gerber, G.K.; Luevano, J.M., Jr.; Gatti, D.M.; Somes, L.; Svenson, K.L.; Turnbaugh, P.J. Diet dominates host genotype in shaping the murine gut microbiota. *Cell Host Microbe* **2015**, *17*, 72–84. [CrossRef] [PubMed]
10. Zmora, N.; Zeevi, D.; Korem, T.; Segal, E.; Elinav, E. Taking it Personally: Personalized Utilization of the Human Microbiome in Health and Disease. *Cell Host Microbe* **2016**, *19*, 12–20. [CrossRef] [PubMed]
11. Look, A.R.G.; Wing, R.R.; Bolin, P.; Brancati, F.L.; Bray, G.A.; Clark, J.M.; Coday, M.; Crow, R.S.; Curtis, J.M.; Egan, C.M.; et al. Cardiovascular effects of intensive lifestyle intervention in type 2 diabetes. *N. Engl. J. Med.* **2013**, *369*, 145–154.
12. Halsey, L.G.; Curran-Everett, D.; Vowler, S.L.; Drummond, G.B. The fickle *p* value generates irreproducible results. *Nat. Methods* **2015**, *12*, 179–185. [CrossRef] [PubMed]

nutrients

MDPI

Article

Dietary Fiber and the Human Gut Microbiota: Application of Evidence Mapping Methodology

Caleigh M. Sawicki [1,2], Kara A. Livingston [1], Martin Obin [3], Susan B. Roberts [4], Mei Chung [5] and Nicola M. McKeown [1,2,*]

1 Nutritional Epidemiology, Jean Mayer USDA Human Nutrition Research Center on Aging at Tufts University, Boston, MA 02111, USA; caleigh.sawicki@tufts.edu (C.M.S.); kara.livingston@tufts.edu (K.A.L.)
2 Friedman School of Nutrition Science and Policy, Tufts University, Boston, MA 02111, USA
3 Nutrition & Genomics Laboratory, Jean Mayer USDA Human Nutrition Research Center on Aging at Tufts University, Boston, MA 02111, USA; martin.obin@tufts.edu
4 Energy Metabolism Laboratory, Jean Mayer USDA Human Nutrition Research Center on Aging at Tufts University, Boston, MA 02111, USA; susan.roberts@tufts.edu
5 Nutrition/Infection Unit, Department of Public Health and Community Medicine, Tufts University School of Medicine, Boston, MA 02111, USA; Mei_Chun.Chung@tufts.edu
* Correspondence: nicola.mckeown@tufts.edu; Tel.: +1-617-556-3008

Received: 15 December 2016; Accepted: 4 February 2017; Published: 10 February 2017

Abstract: Interest is rapidly growing around the role of the human gut microbiota in facilitating beneficial health effects associated with consumption of dietary fiber. An evidence map of current research activity in this area was created using a newly developed database of dietary fiber intervention studies in humans to identify studies with the following broad outcomes: (1) modulation of colonic microflora; and/or (2) colonic fermentation/short-chain fatty acid concentration. Study design characteristics, fiber exposures, and outcome categories were summarized. A sub-analysis described oligosaccharides and bacterial composition in greater detail. One hundred eighty-eight relevant studies were identified. The fiber categories represented by the most studies were oligosaccharides (20%), resistant starch (16%), and chemically synthesized fibers (15%). Short-chain fatty acid concentration (47%) and bacterial composition (88%) were the most frequently studied outcomes. Whole-diet interventions, measures of bacterial activity, and studies in metabolically at-risk subjects were identified as potential gaps in the evidence. This evidence map efficiently captured the variability in characteristics of expanding research on dietary fiber, gut microbiota, and physiological health benefits, and identified areas that may benefit from further research. We hope that this evidence map will provide a resource for researchers to direct new intervention studies and meta-analyses.

Keywords: dietary fiber; gut microbiota; evidence map; colonic fermentation; oligosaccharides; resistant starch; cereal fiber; *Bifidobacteria*; *Lactobacilli*

1. Introduction

According to the 2009 Codex Alimentarius definition of dietary fiber, which aims to unify the definition among all countries, dietary fiber includes all carbohydrate polymers of three or more monomeric units that resist digestion in the small intestine [1,2]. A further stipulation of this definition is that isolated or chemically synthesized fibers need to show a physiological health benefit. Epidemiological evidence consistently shows that higher intake of dietary fiber is associated with a reduced risk of chronic diseases, such as cardiovascular disease (CVD), type 2 diabetes, and cancer [3]. However, new research is interested in the role of the gut microbiota with respect to observed beneficial effects [4,5].

Research on the human gut microbiota, sometimes referred to as the "forgotten organ" [6], has exponentially increased over the past decade with recent advances in technology. There has been growing evidence that the microbiota not only produces metabolites that can influence host physiology, but these metabolites also play an integral role in the host immune system and metabolism through a complex array of chemical interactions and signaling pathways [7–9]. These interactions can greatly impact host health and risk of disease [7,10], and the microbiota have been linked to numerous diseases such as irritable bowel syndrome (IBS), asthma, allergy, metabolic syndrome, diabetes, obesity, cardiovascular disease, and colorectal cancer [11].

A number of factors can cause the composition of the microbiota to shift, including changes in diet [10]. Consumption of dietary fiber has been shown to influence the gut microbiota by altering bacterial fermentation, colony size, and species composition [12]. Non-digestible carbohydrates are the primary energy source for most gut microbes and, therefore, can directly impact those species that heavily depend on that substrate [13]. There can also be indirect impacts through cross-feeding, where some types of microbes depend on the by-products, or metabolites, of other types of microbes [14,15]. In addition to substrate availability, the magnitude and diversity of the microbiota are also greatly influenced by other aspects of the gut environment, including pH, host secretions, and transit time [11,12,16–19]. While certain dietary components play an important role in the gut environment, products of microbial fermentation can also have an influence [10,20]. For example, consumption of fermentable dietary fiber will provide substrates for microbial activity but will also increase the concentrations of fermentation products, such as short-chain fatty acids (SCFAs). A buildup of SCFAs subsequently lowers the colonic pH, which can then have dramatic effects on the composition of the microbiota [16,20,21]. Therefore, the relationship between diet, the gut microbiota, microbial activity, and gut physiology is complex.

The distribution of different strains or species of bacteria within the gut will determine the metabolic profile of the microbiota, which could have potential physiologic effects on health [10]. SCFAs, such as butyrate, acetate, and propionate produced by the fermentation of dietary fibers, may play a role in energy homeostasis, immune function, and host-microbe signaling [7,22,23], and prevention of diseases, such as bowel disease, colon cancer, and metabolic syndrome [20,24–26]. Therefore, fiber-induced modulation of the gut microbiota has gained interest for its potential impact on health and disease [27]. However, it is not well understood how and to what extent these changes may happen in a predictable way [28]. The first step toward answering these questions is to gather and summarize the current literature on dietary fiber and the gut microbiota, which can be done effectively using evidence mapping.

Evidence mapping is a new technique being applied in nutritional epidemiology to review and characterize the published research on a broad topic of interest, allowing for the identification of gaps and prioritizing new research questions [29–31]. Evidence maps may be considered as the first few steps in a systematic review but are generally more comprehensive in the scope of the research question [31,32]. Instead of a specific, targeted question, an evidence map aims to determine the research "landscape" of the topic area. Evidence mapping can provide a context for systematic reviews and meta-analyses by presenting a wide range of study designs and methods being utilized in the area of interest [29]. While systematic reviews are the method of choice for synthesizing study results, evidence mapping is a more efficient methodology for visualizing the evidence and is a particularly useful technique in fast-paced or rapidly growing areas of research, such as the human gut microbiota.

Our objective was to describe existing research on dietary fiber intake and the gut microbiota. Through the creation of an evidence map, we identify potential gaps in the research and highlight areas where new hypotheses may be addressed in future studies. Furthermore, we extended our evidence mapping to summarize broad study findings in a focused area regarding the effects of the oligosaccharide interventions on the gut microbial composition. In doing so, we demonstrate how this evidence map can be used as a platform to build on the existing evidence by answering the following two questions: (1) Can we identify specific gut microbial species that are modulated by dietary fiber? (2) Is there evidence that modulation of the gut microbiota is correlated with fermentation or physiological effects on host health?

2. Materials and Methods

Evidence mapping involves three major steps: (1) clearly defining a topic area and setting criteria around the questions of interest; (2) systematically searching for and selecting relevant studies based on pre-defined criteria, such as study design and outcomes of interest and, thereby, creating a "map" of available evidence; and (3) reporting on study characteristics and the extent of existing research [30–32].

To develop the dietary fiber and human gut microbiota evidence map, we utilized a newly developed Dietary Fiber Database (Version 3.0), containing data on published dietary fiber interventions [33]. The database, housed in the Systematic Review Data Repository (SRDR) [34], contains descriptive data extracted from dietary fiber intervention studies that were identified by a systematic literature search. It includes all human studies published from 1946 to May 2016 that examined the effect of dietary fiber on at least one of nine pre-defined physiological health outcomes. For the complete list of the inclusion/exclusion criteria, including the nine health outcomes, refer to Supplementary Materials Table S1.

The database includes two specific outcomes related to the gut microbiota: (1) modulation of colonic microflora; and (2) colonic fermentation/short-chain fatty acid concentration. Keywords used to identify these specific outcomes in the development of the database are provided in the Supplementary Methods. Our evidence map is comprised of all publications in the database reporting on at least one of these two outcomes.

Descriptive analyses were performed to examine the range of study designs, fiber interventions, and types of outcomes examined. Because evidence mapping is meant to capture the wider landscape of evidence and is, therefore, more inclusive and less homogenous than is usually required for a meta-analysis, results are specifically not represented. Due to the large variety of fiber interventions identified, fiber intervention exposures were grouped into categories according to structure or source, depending on how they were described in the original publication. If the same fiber intervention was given at different doses within the same study, that fiber type was only counted once for that study.

Microbiota outcomes identified by the database were examined in more detail and were re-classified into three categories: (1) fermentation, which included measures of SCFAs, breath markers (such as H_2 and CH_4), bacterial enzyme activity and metabolites, bile acid metabolism, and fiber digestibility (measured by fecal recovery); (2) bacterial composition, which included relative or absolute bacterial counts; and (3) colonic and fecal pH.

Weighted scatter plots were used to visualize the available evidence on different fiber types by outcome groups and sample size. Each bubble in the plot represents a single publication with the size of the bubble corresponding to the study sample size. Publications may be represented more than once throughout the plot if multiple fiber interventions or outcomes were reported but are not repeated within any single cross-sectional area.

To further explore the information captured in this evidence map, we isolated publications on the top most reported fiber type, oligosaccharides. We examined oligosaccharides in relation to bacterial composition and extracted more detailed information on the study characteristics, bacterial strains and/or species identified in the publication and the direction of change in strain/species frequency (increased, decreased, or remained the same) in response to the fiber intervention.

3. Results

A total of 188 distinct studies with at least one outcome related to the gut microbiota were identified in the Dietary Fiber Database (Version 3.0). The study design and population characteristics of these studies are summarized in Table 1.

Table 1. Study Design Characteristics.

Characteristic, *n* (% of Studies)	Total	Top Three Fiber Types		
		Oligosaccharides	Resistant Starch	Chemically Synthesized
n	188	38	30	28
Design				
Randomized, parallel	54 (29%)	14 (37%)	3 (10%)	10 (36%)
Randomized, crossover	127 (67%)	24 (63%)	27 (3%)	16 (57%)
Randomized, combined parallel and crossover	2 (1%)	0 (0%)	0 (0%)	1 (4%)
Non-Randomized	2 (1%)	0 (0%)	0 (0%)	0 (0%)
Unspecified Randomization	3 (2%)	0 (0%)	0 (0%)	1 (4%)
Sample size				
Less than 10	19 (10%)	1 (3%)	6 (20%)	2 (7%)
10 to 49	145 (77%)	29 (76%)	23 (77%)	23 (82%)
50 to 100	20 (11%)	6 (16%)	0 (0%)	2 (7%)
More than 100	4 (2%)	2 (5%)	1 (3%)	1 (4%)
Duration				
Acute (<1 week)	36 (19%)	4 (11%)	9 (30%)	6 (21%)
1–4 weeks	126 (67%)	26 (68%)	21 (70%)	20 (71%)
1–6 months	25 (13%)	8 (21%)	0 (0%)	2 (7%)
More than 6 months	1 (1%)	0 (0%)	0 (0%)	0 (0%)
Diet type				
Acute	36 (19%)	4 (11%)	9 (30%)	6 (21%)
Isocaloric/Maintenance	115 (61%)	26 (68%)	17 (57%)	12 (43%)
Weight Loss	2 (1%)	0 (0%)	0 (0%)	0 (0%)
Other/Unspecified	35 (19%)	8 (21%)	4 (13%)	10 (36%)
Age				
Adults (≥17 years *)	185 (98%)	37 (97%)	30 (100%)	27 (96%)
Adolescents (12–17 years)	1 (1%)	0 (0%)	0 (0%)	1 (4%)
Children (3–11 years)	2 (1%)	1 (3%)	0 (0%)	0 (0%)
Baseline Health				
Healthy	153 (81%)	34 (89%)	26 (87%)	27 (96%)
Overweight or Obese	7 (4%)	1 (3%)	0 (0%)	1 (4%)
Diabetic	1 (1%)	0 (0%)	0 (0%)	0 (0%)
Metabolically at Risk	8 (4%)	1 (3%)	2 (7%)	0 (0%)
Hyperlipidemia	6 (3%)	1 (3%)	1 (3%)	0 (0%)
GI/Digestive Issues	6 (3%)	0 (0%)	0 (0%)	0 (0%)
Other	7 (4%)	1 (1%)	1 (3%)	0 (0%)
Region				
Asia	6 (3%)	2 (5%)	1 (3%)	3 (11%)
Australia/New Zealand	16 (8%)	1 (3%)	7 (23%)	1 (4%)
Europe	114 (61%)	31 (81%)	17 (57%)	12 (43%)
North America	51 (27%)	4 (11%)	5 (17%)	12 (43%)
South America	1 (1%)	0 (0%)	0 (0%)	0 (0%)

* Only one study had an age range of 17–61 years, all other studies in adults included subjects ≥18 years.

The majority (96%) were randomized, controlled studies, with only two studies not randomized, and three studies with unknown randomization. The majority of studies used a crossover design compared to a parallel design (67% randomized, crossover; 29% randomized, parallel; and 1% combination of crossover and parallel designs). The size of the study samples ranged from 4 to 435 subjects, but the majority of studies (87%) had fewer than 50 subjects. Few studies (14%) had an intervention duration exceeding four weeks. Most (67%) lasted 1–4 weeks, and 19% were acute feeding interventions, which usually consisted of a single test meal. The subjects were described as healthy in the majority of studies (81%). Fewer studies involved subjects that were overweight or obese (4%), diabetic (1%), hyperlipidemic (3%), had metabolic syndrome or "at-risk" for metabolic syndrome (4%), digestive issues (3%), or risk factors for developing colon cancer (2%).

Within the 188 studies, 47 different fiber types were captured. These fiber interventions fell into 11 different categories, as detailed in Table 2.

Table 2. Fiber types (total studies = 188), 324 unique exposures.

Group	Studies (%)	Fiber Types	*n*
Oligosaccharide	38 (20%)	Fructooligosaccharide	22
		Galactooligosaccharide	11
		Arabinoxylan-oligosaccharides	6
		Xylo-oligosaccharide	2
		Soybean oligosaccharides	1
Resistant Starch	30 (16%)	Resistant starch type 1	1
		Resistant starch type 2 [a]	20
		Resistant starch type 3	11
		Resistant Starch, mixed or unspecified	4
Chemically synthesized	28 (15%)	Polydextrose	12
		Dextrin [g]	9
		Soluble corn fiber	7
		PolyGlycopleX (PGX)	2
		Resistant starch type 4	2
		Microcrystalline cellulose	1
		Solubilized potato polysaccharide	1
		Pullulan	1
		Butyrylated high amylose maize starch	1
Inulin	25 (13%)	Inulin	18
		Oligofructose-enriched inulin (OF-IN)	7
Bran	24 (13%)	Wheat Bran	12
		Oat Bran	9
		Corn bran	2
		Barley bran	1
		Rye Bran	1
		Bran	2
Cereal fiber	21 (11%)	Cereal fiber, wheat [b]	9
		Cereal fiber, barley [c]	8
		Cereal fiber, oat [d]	4
		Cereal fiber, rye [e]	4
		Cereal fiber [f]	3
Fruit/Vegetable/Plant fibers	15 (8%)	Vegetable fiber	6
		Lupin Kernel Fiber	3
		Sugar cane fiber	2
		Sugar Beet fiber	1
		Bean fiber	1
		Citrus fiber	2
		Fruit fiber	1
Combination	13 (7%)	Combination/Mixture	13
Gums and Mucilages	10 (5%)	Gums [h]	7
		Psyllium [i]	6
Other non-starch polysaccharides	9 (5%)	Pectin	4
		Cellulose	3
		Hemicellulose [j]	3
		Beta-glucan, barley	1
		Polysaccharide, non-starch	1
High fiber diet	4 (2%)	Dietary fiber	4

More specific fiber types described include [a] high-amylose maize starch; [b] whole-grain wheat; [c] barley flour, barley kernels; [d] oat kernels; [e] whole-grain rye, rye kernels; [f] whole-grain, mixture, or unspecified cereal fiber; [g] wheat dextrin, resistant dextrin, resistant maltodextrin, soluble fiber dextrin; [h] guar gum, gum arabic; [i] ispaghula, Metamucil; [j] arabinogalactan, xylans, glucomannan.

The fibers most frequently studied were oligosaccharides (20% of studies), resistant starch (16%), and chemically synthesized fibers (15%), followed closely by inulin (13%), bran (13%) and cereal fiber (11%). The study design characteristics for studies examining the top three fibers are also presented in Table 1. Notably, resistant starch had a higher proportion of studies with a sample size of fewer than 10 subjects, while oligosaccharides were more often examined in studies of much larger sample sizes and longer duration.

Table 3 reports the frequency and percentage of three major microbiota outcomes: bacterial composition (47% of studies), colonic/fecal pH (32%), and fermentation (76%). Fermentation is further broken down by the specific measurement used to determine the degree of fermentation. SCFA concentration (52%) and breath gas excretion (27%) were the most commonly measured markers of fermentation, but others included bacterial enzyme activity, bile acid metabolism, and fecal starch recovery.

Table 3. Microbiota outcomes (total studies = 188).

Outcome Group	Studies (%)
Fermentation	142 (76%)
SCFA concentration	98 (52%)
Breath gas excretion	50 (27%)
Bacterial enzyme activity	18 (10%)
Bile acids	15 (8%)
Fecal fiber/starch recovery	13 (7%)
Bacterial composition	88 (47%)
Colonic/fecal pH	60 (32%)

Figure 1 is a weighted scatter plot of the microbiota outcomes by fiber group. It provides a visual representation summarizing the research activity in this field. For example, while SCFA concentration and bacterial composition are studied often, fewer and less sizeable studies measure breath gas excretion and other markers of fermentation. Specific gaps in the research are readily identified. Notably, we can see that there are currently no published studies examining the effect of a high fiber whole-diet intervention on bacterial composition of the microbiota. This plot also shows active areas of interest. We can see, for example, that a large number of relatively larger studies have been published on bacterial composition and oligosaccharide interventions.

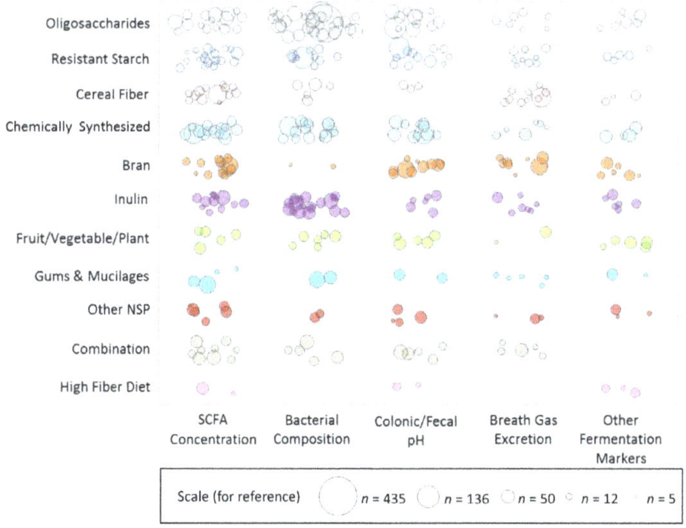

Figure 1. Weighted scatter plot of microbiota outcomes by fiber group. Each bubble in the plot represents a single publication with the size of the bubble corresponding to the study sample size. Studies may be represented more than once throughout the plot if multiple fiber interventions or outcomes were reported but are not repeated within any single cross-sectional area. Note that the outcome effect is not represented in this graphic, i.e., this does not reflect the effect of the fiber on the outcome.

Figure 2 is a weighted scatter plot displaying the other physiological health outcomes captured in this evidence map. Not surprisingly, gastrointestinal (GI) health, which includes measures of fecal bulking, laxation, and transit time, is very frequently studied along with the gut microbiota, but there is less evidence on satiety, adiposity, and blood pressure. There is also just one study published so far examining bone health in the context of dietary fiber and the gut microbiota, a very new emerging area of interest. Supplementary Materials Figures S1 and S2 present weighted scatter plots similar to those in Figure 2, restricted by study duration. The acute studies (Figure S1) exclusively examine the short-term fermentation response by measuring SCFA concentration and/or breath gas excretion, most frequently in cereal fibers, whereas studies of greater duration (Figure S2) examine more outcomes in a larger array of fiber types. Notably, however, there are no longer duration (>4 weeks) studies on resistant starch.

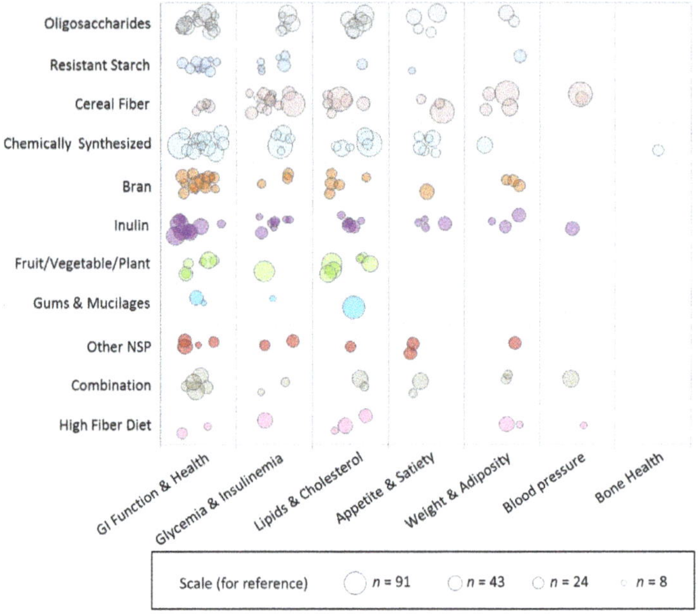

Figure 2. Weighted scatter plot of other physiological health outcomes by fiber group. Each bubble in the plot represents a single publication with the size of the bubble corresponding to the study sample size. Studies may be represented more than once throughout the plot if multiple fiber interventions or outcomes were reported but are not repeated within any single cross-sectional area. Note that the outcome effect is not represented in this graphic, i.e., this does not reflect the effect of the fiber on the outcome.

We extended our evidence mapping of the fiber–microbiota research landscape by examining one of the most active areas in more detail: oligosaccharide interventions and bacterial composition. There were 26 studies (from 25 publications) on this topic. Three of the studies utilized a dose of antibiotics to specifically examine the use of oligosaccharides to assist recolonization of the gut, and, for comparison purposes, we excluded these from this sub-analysis. Details of the remaining 23 studies are shown in Table 4. Studies were published between 1996 and 2015, and all were randomized controlled trials (9 parallel, 14 crossovers). Intervention durations ranged from 1 to 12 weeks, and sample size ranged from 15 to 136 (mean of 46) subjects. Notably, only one study recruited subjects that were overweight with metabolic syndrome, and one study recruited subjects that were overweight, while all the other studies reported on healthy subjects. Most studies had a similar age range, but there was one study in children and one specifically in older adults.

Among these 23 studies, there are 26 fiber interventions: eight fructooligosaccharides (FOS), nine galactooligosaccharides (GOS), six arabinoxylan-oligosaccharides (AX-OS), two xylo-oligosaccharide (XOS), and one soybean oligosaccharide. All but one study found a bifidogenic effect of oligosaccharides, with doses as small as 1.4 g/day (XOS) and a range of treatment forms, including tablets, beverages, and whole foods. Many studies also examined oligosaccharide impacts on *Lactobacilli* or *Lactobacillus–Enterococcus* frequency, with 19 studies reporting no effect, three reporting a positive effect, and one reporting a negative effect. Few publications reported decreases in bacterial strains/species, but among those that did, it was most often *Bacteroides*, with four studies finding a significant decrease in response to a GOS intervention. However, two intervention studies found no effect of GOS on *Bacteroides*, five interventions using other oligosaccharides also found no effect, and one XOS intervention found a significant increase in *Baceroides fragilis*. There were a number of other strains/species reported; however, it is important to note that some studies used targeted culturing techniques, whereas others used DNA sequencing to attempt to identify all species present.

Table 5 summarizes the other physiological outcomes examined within these studies. Ten out of the 26 interventions also significantly increased markers of fermentation, but only one intervention had a significant effect on fecal bulking, and only two had significant effects on transit time. Of the other physiologic outcomes examined in these studies, most were related to GI health. Only a few studies measured lipids, glucose, or insulin, and of those that did, only one study found a significant effect on total cholesterol and insulin.

Table 4. Characteristics of oligosaccharide interventions and direction of evidence on bacteria composition.

Reference	n	Design	Duration	Age, Mean (Range)	% Male	BL Health	BMI, Mean (Range)	Fiber Type (g/Day)	Form	Control	Method	Bacterial Composition Reported Measures
[35]	20	RCT, P, DB	12 days	(22–39)	50	Healthy	NR	FOS (12.5)	NR (3 oral doses)	Saccharose placebo	Stool (whole), Wilkins-Chalgren agar, Beerens' medium	↑ *Bifidobacteria* NS Total anaerobes
[36]	40	RCT, P	7 days	29.6 (18–47)	45	Healthy	NR	FOS (2.5, 5, 10, 20)	Powder	Saccharose powder	Stool (whole), Wilkins-Chalgren, Beeren's medium	↑ *Bifidobacteria* (at doses 5–20 g) NS Total anaerobes
[37]	15	RCT, C, DB	3 weeks	NR	~47	Healthy	NR	FOS (2.5)	Biscuits	Matched biscuits without FOS	Stool (partial), PCR-DGGE (denaturing gradient gel electrophoresis), fluorescent in situ hybridization (FISH)	NS *Bifidobacteria* NS Lactobaccilli NS Lactose-fermenting enterobacteria NS Total enterobacteria NS Enterococci
								GOS (2.5)	Biscuits			NS *Bifidobacteria* NS *Lactobaccilli* NS Lactose-fermenting enterobacteria NS Total enterobacteria NS *Enterococci*
[38]	136	RCT, P, DB	7 days	~30 (~18–54)	~41	Healthy	NR	FOS (2.5, 5.0, 7.5, 10)	NR (2 oral doses)	Sucrose and fully digestible maltodextrin placebo	Stool (partial), Wilkins-Chalgren agar. Beerens's medium, Bacteroides Bile Esculin agar, Lactobacillus agar, MRS agar, and McConkey agar	↑ *Bifidobacteria* NS Total anaerobes NS *Lactobacillus* NS *Baceroides* NS *Enterobacteria*
								GOS (2.5, 5.0, 7.5, 10)	NR (2 oral doses)			↑ *Bifidobacteria* NS Total anaerobes NS *Lactobacillus* NS *Baceroides* NS *Enterobacteria*
								SB-OS (2.5, 5.0, 7.5, 10)	NR (2 oral doses)			↑ *Bifidobacteria* NS Total anaerobes NS *Lactobacillus* NS *Baceroides* NS *Enterobacteria*
[39]	39	RCT, P, DB	30 days	60.4	0	Healthy	NR	FOS (7)	Cereal bars and gelified milk	Matched cereal bars and gelified milk without FOS	Stool (partial), temperature-gradient gel electrophoresis (TTGE), FISH	↑ *Bifidobacterium* spp. ↑ Bifidobacterium Animalis and related species NS Bacteroides and relatives NS Clostridium coccoides-Eubacterium rectale cluster NS Faecalibacterium prausnitzi subgroup NS Lactobacillus-Enterocococcus group NS Atopobium group

Table 4. *Cont.*

Reference	*n*	Design	Duration	Age, Mean (Range)	% Male	BL Health	BMI, Mean (Range)	Fiber Type (g/Day)	Form	Control	Method	Bacterial Composition Reported Measures
[40]	34	RCT, C, DB	2 weeks	27.7	100	Healthy	23.2	FOS (20)	Beverage (lemonade)	Matched lemonade with sucrose placebo	Stool (whole), RT-qPCR	↑ *Bifidobacteria* ↑ *Lactobacilli* NS *E. coli*
[41]	40	RCT, P	7 days	29	~45	Healthy	NR	FOS (2.5, 5.0, 7.5, 10)	Tablet	Sucrose and fully digestible maltodextrin placebo	Stool (partial), Wilkins-Chalgren agar, Beerens' medium, MRS agar, BBE agar, McConkey agar	↑ *Bifidobacteria* (all doses) ↑ Total Anaerobes (10 g only) NS *Lactobacilli* NS *Bacteroides* NS *Enterobacteria*
[42]	30	RCT, C, DB	7 days	36.3 (21–59)	~40	Healthy	NR	GOS (3.6, 7)	Powder, mixed with water	Matched sucrose placebo powder	Stool (whole), FISH	↑ *Bifidobacterium* ↑ Clostridium perfringens-histolyticum subgroup (3.6 g only) NS *Lactobacillus-Enterococcus* spp. NS Bacteroides-prevotella
	29			32.5 (19–55)	~45	Healthy	NR	GOS (7)	Powder, mixed with water	Matched powder without GOS		↑ *Bifidobacterium* ↓ Bacteroides-prevotella NS *Lactobacillus-Enterococcus* spp. NS Clostridium perfringens-histolyticum subgroup
[43]	44	RCT, C, DB	10 weeks	69.3 (64–79)	~36	Healthy	(22–31)	GOS (5.5)	Powder, mixed with water	Matched maltodextrin placebo	Stool (partial), FISH	↑ Bifidobacterium spp. ↑ *Lactobacillus-Enterococcus* spp. ↑ Clostridium coccoides-Eubacterium rectale group ↓ *Bacteroides* spp. ↓ Clostridium histolyticum group ↓ *Escherchia coli* ↓ *Desulfovibrio* spp.
[44]	64	RCT, P, DB	30 days	33 (22–51)	~41	Healthy	NR	FOS (5)	Powder, used to prepare a jelly	Commercial dessert (jelly, lemon flavored)	Stool (partial), Beerens' agar, Chromocult Coliform agar, Slanetz and Bartley medium, Rogosa agar, Wilkins-Chalgren anaerobe agar with 5% (v/v) defibrinated horse blood and G-N anaerobe selective supplement (OXOID), Perfringens agar with D-cycloserine.	↑ *Bifidobacterium* spp. ↓ Total coliforms ↓ *Escherichia coli* NS Total aerobes NS *Enterococcus* spp. NS Total anaerobes NS *Bacteroides* spp. NS *Lactobacillus* spp. NS *Clostridium perfringens*

Table 4. *Cont.*

Reference	*n*	Design	Duration	Age, Mean (Range)	% Male	BL Health	BMI, Mean (Range)	Fiber Type (g/Day)	Form	Control	Method	Bacterial Composition Reported Measures
[45]	20	RCT, C	3 weeks	24	30	Healthy	20.9	AX-OS (10)	Beverage (orange juice drink)	Matched maltodextrin placebo beverage	Stool (partial), real-time PCR, real-time PCR TaqMan, real-time PCR SYBR Green technology	↑ *Bifidobacteria* ↑ *Bifidobacterium adolescentis* ↓ *Lactobacilli* NS Total bacteria NS Roseburia-Eubacterium rectale NS *Enterobacteria*
[46]	39	RCT, C, DB	3 weeks	58.9 (50–81)	~46	Healthy	26.1 (19.7–38.4)	GOS (~8)	Beverage (orange juice drink)	Matched placebo beverage	Stool (partial), quantitative PCR, FISH	↑ *Bifidobacterium* ↓ *Bacteroides* NS *Total bacteria* NS *Lactobacillus* NS *Escherichia coli* NS Eubacterium rectales group NS Clostridium histolyticum group
[47]	60	RCT, P, DB	4 weeks	~20 (18–24)	~43	Healthy	~21.3	X-OS (5)	Beverage (orange juice drink)	Matched wheat maltodextrin placebo beverage	Stool (partial), quantitative PCR	↑ *Bifidobacterium* NS *Lactobacillus* NS *Peptostreptococcus* NS *Clostridium* NS *Firmicutes* NS *Bacteroidetes* NS Faecalibacterium prausnitzii NS *Roseburia* spp.
[48]	27	RCT, C, DB	3 weeks	25	~37	Healthy	20.9	AX-OS (2.14)	Wheat/rye bread	Matched wheat/rye or refined wheat bread, no AX-OS	Stool (partial), FISH	↑ *Bifidobacterium* NS Total bacteria NS Lactobacillus NS Lactobacillus rods NS Enterobacteriaceae NS *Clostridium* histolyticym/lituburiense
[49]	63	RCT, C, DB	3 weeks	42	~52	Healthy	23.3	AX-OS (2.4, 8)	Beverage (non-carbonated soft drink)	Placebo beverage with 0.25 g tricalcium phosphate, no AX-OS	Stool (partial), FISH, 4′-6-diamidino-2-phenylindole (DAPI)	↑ Bifidobacterium (8 g only) NS Total bacteria NS Lactobacilli NS Faecalibacterium prausnitzii NS Clostridium histolyticum-lituseburense NS Roseburia-Eubacterium rectale
[50]	40	RCT, C, DB	21 days	31.4 (18–55)	50	Healthy	23.3 (18.5–30.0)	AX-OS (2.2)	Wheat/rye bread	Matched wheat/rye bread without AX-OS	Stool (whole), FISH	↑ *Bifidobacterium* spp. ↑ *Escherichia coli* ↑ *Lactobacillus-Enterococcus* ↑ Total bacteria ↑ Bacteroides NS Clostridium histolyticum group NS Atopobium-Coriobacterium group NS Eubacterium rectale group NS Roseburia-Eubacteria NS Faecalibacterium prausnitzii cluster

Table 4. *Cont.*

Reference	*n*	Design	Duration	Age, Mean (Range)	% Male	BL Health	BMI, Mean (Range)	Fiber Type (g/Day)	Form	Control	Method	Bacterial Composition Reported Measures
[51]	65	RCT, C, DB	21 days	53.1 (18–75)	46	Healthy	27.8 (18.5–35.0)	AX-OS (2.2, 4.8)	Wheat-based ready-to-eat cereal	Wheat-based ready-to-eat cereal without AXOS	Stool (partial), FISH	↑ Bifidobacterium (4.8 g only, significant dose trend) NS Total bacteria NS *Lactobacillus* spp. NS Bacertoides NS Clostridium coccoides NS Roseburia intestinalis-Eubacterium rectale group NS Faecalibacterium prausnitzii NS Clostridium clusters I and II
[52]	48	RCT, C, DB	12 weeks	~44.6	36	OW, metabolic syndrome	~31.4	GOS (5.5)	Powder, mixed with water	Maltodextrin placebo	Stool (partial), FISH	↑ *Bifidobacteria* ↓ *Bacteroides* spp. ↓ *Clostridium histolyticum* group ↓ *Desulfovibrio* spp. NS Total bacteria NS *Lactobacillus-Enterococcus* spp. NS Clostridium coccoides-Eubacterium rectale group NS Atopobium cluster NS Eubacterium cylindroides NS Eubacterium hallii NS Beta-proteobacteria NS Clostridium cluster IX NS Faecalibacterium prausnizii cluster
[53]	28	RCT, C, DB	3 weeks	9.8 (8–12)	64	Healthy	NR	AX-OS (5.0)	Beverage	Placebo beverage with 0.25 g tricalcium phosphate, no AX-OS	Stool (partial), FISH	↑ Bifidobacteria NS Clostridium histolyticum/lituseburense NS Faecalibacterium prausnitzii NS Lactobacillus/Enterococcus NS Roseburia/Eubacterium rectale NS Total bacteria
[54]	32	RCT, P, DB	8 weeks	~32.4 (21–49)	~34.4	Healthy	~24.6	XOS (1.4, 2.8)	Tablet	Maltodextrin placebo	Stool (partial), 16 rRNA gene sequencing, pyrosequencing	↑ Bifidobacterium ↑ Total anaerobic flora ↑ Bacteroides fragilis (2.8 g only) ↑ Faecalibacterium (2.8 g only) ↑ Akkermansia (2.8 g only) ↓ Enterobacteriaceae (placebo only) NS Lactobacillus NS Clostridium NS Clustering
[55]	44	RCT, P, DB	14 d	~37 (18–60)	50	OW	~26.5 (25–28)	GOS (12.0)	Beverage (oolong tea)	Matched beverage with glucose	Stool, real-time quantitative PCR	↑ Bifidobacteria NS Total bacteria

Table 4. *Cont.*

Reference	*n*	Design	Duration	Age, Mean (Range)	% Male	BL Health	BMI, Mean (Range)	Fiber Type (g/Day)	Form	Control	Method	Bacterial Composition Reported Measures
[56]	40	RCT, C, DB	10 weeks	70 (65–80)	38	Healthy	NR	GOS (5.5)	Powder, mixed with water	Maltodextrin placebo	Stool (partial), FISH	↑ *Bifidobacterium* spp. ↑ *Bacteroides* spp. NS Atopobium cluster NS Clostridium coccoides/*E. rectale* NS Clostridium histolyticum group NS *Desulfovibrio* spp. NS *Escherichia coli* NS *Lactobacillus/Enterococcus* spp. NS Faecalibacterium prausnitzii NS Roseburia/Eubacterium rectale NS Total bacteria

Abbreviations: AX-OS, arabinoxylan-oligosaccharides; BL, baseline; C, crossover; DB, double-blind; FOS, fructooligosaccharides; GOS, galactooligosaccharides; MS, metabolic syndrome; NR, not reported; NS, no significant change; OW, overweight; P, parallel; RCT, randomized controlled trial; SB-OS, soybean oligosaccharides; X-OS, xylo-oligosaccharides; ~denotes a value that was calculated or estimated from the data available in the publication; ↑ significantly increased; ↓ significantly decreased.

Table 5. Other outcomes reported in oligosaccharide interventions reporting on bacterial composition.

Reference	Fiber Type	Evidence of Fermentation	Evidence of Fecal Bulking	Evidence of Changes in Transit Time	Evidence of Other Changes in Host Physiology
[35]	FOS	S	NS	–	S: GI symptoms (mild bloating) NS: Fecal pH
[36]	FOS	NS	–	–	S: GI symptoms (excess flatus) NS: Fecal pH
[37]	FOS	S	–	–	NS: GI symptoms
	GOS	S	–	–	NS: GI symptoms
[38]	FOS	–	–	NS	NS: GI symptoms, fecal pH
	GOS	–	–	NS	NS: GI symptoms, fecal pH
	SB-OS	–	–	NS	NS: GI symptoms, fecal pH
[39]	FOS	–	–	–	–
[40]	FOS	S	S	–	S: GI symptoms (flatulence and intestinal bloating) NS: fecal water pH
[41]	FOS	–	–	–	S: GI symptoms NS: fecal pH
[42]	GOS	–	–	–	–
	GOS	–	–	–	–
[43]	GOS	–	–	–	NS: Total and HDL cholesterol [#]
[44]	FOS	–	–	–	S: GI symptoms
[45]	AX-OS	–	NS	–	NS: Total, LDL, and HDL cholesterol [#]
[46]	GOS	–	–	–	NS: GI symptoms, stool consistency [#]
[47]	X-OS	S	–	–	NS: Stool consistency [#]
[48]	AX-OS	S	–	S	NS: Stool consistency [#]
[49]	AX-OS	S	–	NS	NS: Total energy intake, total and LDL cholesterol [#], stool consistency
[50]	AX-OS	S	–	–	–
[51]	AX-OS	S	NS	NS	NS: LDL cholesterol [#], fasting insulin and glucose, stool consistency
[52]	GOS	–	–	–	S: Total cholesterol and insulin NS: LDL, and HDL cholesterol, triglycerides, or fasting glucose
[53]	AX-OS	S	–	NS	NS: GI symptoms
[54]	X-OS	NS	–	NS	NS: Fecal pH, GI symptoms
[55]	GOS	–	NS	S	S: Satiety, total energy intake NS: Weight/Adiposity
[56]	GOS	S	NS	NS	–

Abbreviations: AX-OS, arabinoxylan-oligosaccharides; FOS, fructooligosaccharides; GOS, galactooligosaccharides; NS, no statistically significant health benefit was observed; S, a significant effect was observed; SB-OS, soybean oligosaccharides; X-OS, xylo-oligosaccharides; [#] No significant effect of intervention, but the effect was in a direction opposite to providing a health benefit.

4. Discussion

Observational/epidemiologic evidence shows that diets higher in fiber are associated with reduced risk of certain chronic diseases, such as heart disease, diabetes, and obesity [3,57], and these may be related to the effect of dietary fiber on the gut microbiota [4,5]. However, the present evidence map reveals that there is insufficient data from well-controlled dietary fiber interventions that study the gut microbiota in relation to intermediate risk factors of cardiometabolic disease or in relation to chronic conditions such as obesity. In fact, we found little evidence on the intersection of dietary fiber, the microbiota, and adiposity. Much of the current literature has shown positive effects of dietary fiber on gut function or beneficial bacterial species, or positive effects of dietary fiber on specific health outcomes, but few seem to be directly measuring these outcomes together, to provide evidence of a dietary fiber-modulated gut microbiota and health outcome [58,59].

Over the last 25 years, there has been a rapid increase in interest on dietary fiber and the microbiota, particularly with respect to prebiotics, such as oligosaccharides and inulin, as well as chemically synthesized fibers such as Polydextrose (PDX), soluble corn fiber, and PolyGlycopleX (PGX). From this map, we can see that the most actively researched fibers are oligosaccharides, resistant starch, and chemically synthesized fibers, followed closely by inulin, bran, and cereal fiber (Table 2), and the most common measures of the gut microbiota are SCFA concentration and bacterial composition (Table 3). The fiber and outcome most frequently studied together were oligosaccharides and bacterial composition, and we, therefore, examined these studies in more detail in summarizing our evidence map.

Oligosaccharides are short-chain saccharide polymers, generally made up of 3–10 carbohydrate monomers [60,61], and are known for their prebiotic activity. Prebiotics are defined as non-digestible foods that, when metabolized, alter the composition and/or activity of the microbiota in a such a way that promotes the health of the host [4,62,63]. Randomized controlled trials have consistently shown that oligosaccharides, and FOS in particular, increase *Bifidobacterium* (Table 4), a genus of oligosaccharide fermenting gut bacteria that may be beneficial to human health [64–66]. Despite the considerable number of studies showing this bifidogenic effect, few have actually examined direct relationships of this modulation of the gut microbiota to other physiological health outcomes. In our sub-analysis on oligosaccharides, we found that only five [43,45,51–53] of the 26 oligosaccharide interventions measuring bacterial composition also measured changes in lipids, and only two [51,52] measured glucose and insulin response. Additionally, only one study [52] found a small statistically significant beneficial effect on total cholesterol and insulin, while the rest found no beneficial effect. These findings are consistent with reviews by McRorie et al. [67–70], which conclude that clinical evidence does not support a link between soluble, non-viscous, readily fermentable fibers (such as oligosaccharides) and physiological health benefits on cholesterol, glycemic control, or laxation. Rather, these benefits are attributed to the physical properties of soluble, viscous/gel-forming fibers that are not readily fermented (such as beta glucan and raw guar gum).

However, readily-fermented fiber types, such as oligosaccharides and resistant starch, may have other important physiologic effects via the metabolites produced from microbial fermentation. The most studied products of fermentation are SCFAs, mainly butyrate, propionate, and acetate [25]. Up to 95% of SCFAs are absorbed by the colonocytes of the large intestine [20], and recent evidence has shown that they may play a role in health and prevention of disease, such as bowel disease, colon cancer, and metabolic syndrome [20,24–26]. SCFAs have been shown to affect gut health, immune function, energy metabolism, stimulation of the sympathetic nervous system, and serotonin release [4,7,20].

This evidence map also highlights areas where evidence is lacking. For instance, high-fiber diet interventions, where total dietary fiber was increased from a variety of sources, have the least number of publications. As more emphasis is put on the importance of dietary patterns rather than individual foods or food components [71], more whole-diet intervention studies need to be conducted to understand how these relationships among diet, the gut microbiota, and health work in the context of a whole diet. With respect to microbiota outcomes, fewer studies have measured bacterial enzyme activity, which may be more important than simply measuring changes in the bacterial composition because some strains or species may alter their function, and, therefore, their metabolites, in response to changes in the gut environment rather than their absolute number. Well-controlled human intervention trials incorporating "next generation" metagenomics, meta-transcriptomics and metabolomics will be vital to further understanding these changes in microbial activity. In addition, the microbiota composition or activity may be altered in people with chronic diseases such as obesity [58], and future research should consider whether diet may have differential effects depending on underlying health status. Based on this evidence map, the majority of fiber research on the gut microbiota was conducted in healthy adults (81%).

The definition of fiber has been a moving target, and fibers, being one of the most heterogeneous groups of associated molecules, have been categorized in many different contexts, including by source, structure, or physical properties (solubility, fermentability, etc.). Further, fibers may be delivered/consumed as isolated supplements, but they are more often consumed intact in whole foods (such as in raw fruits and vegetables), or in processed foods (including processes such as cooking, milling, and baking). The food matrix is important to consider because other components of the food, such as phytochemicals, may provide synergistic effects [72,73], and the degree of processing can alter the structure and physical attributes of the fiber [70]. All of these factors contribute to the type and extent of microbial utilization [28]. Therefore, it is important for future studies to describe the dietary fiber intervention in as much detail as possible, and, where applicable, define the characteristics of the fibers being studied.

Creating an updatable evidence map of microbiota-related outcomes allows researchers to obtain a more global view of the research landscape, including its history, current trajectory, and specific areas or research questions lacking data or consensus. Since the Dietary Fiber Database used for this evidence map captures literature going back to 1946, it is important to note that the literature in the database often represents evolving knowledge about particular fiber types. This is both a strength and limitation of the database and the evidence mapping process overall, and it highlights the importance of reviewing the totality of available evidence. For instance, bran is well represented in the evidence map, and although the effect of bran on the microbiota was of interest in earlier publications, it is now well-established that insoluble bran is not very readily fermented and may have less of an effect on the microbiota. Instead, interest has shifted toward more fermentable fibers such as the prebiotics and chemically synthesized fibers.

Unlike systematic reviews, which generally address a narrower, focused question with extensive quality analysis and risk of bias assessment, the primary goal of evidence mapping is to identify patterns and provide a broader context within which systematic reviews may occur. As such, in Tables 4 and 5, we did not provide information on effect size of the significance, as this information was not reported in the published fiber database [33]. Furthermore, because of the complex nature of dietary fiber and the size of the literature on dietary fiber, the database which this evidence map is based on has some inherent limitations, which are detailed in a separate publication [33]. Notably, the database was limited to publications in PubMed, and studies were only included if there was a well-defined dietary fiber intervention with a concurrent control. Further, because this database was designed to specifically capture certain health outcomes, other publications of interest to microbiota research may not be represented.

A major strength of this evidence map is that it is a cost effective way of summarizing the data on dietary fiber and the gut microbiota. For instance, the data presented in Tables 4 and 5 may be used to guide future work, such as a meta-analysis, which would provide more specific information to quantify statistical significance. We were able to use a previously created database in order to efficiently identify potentially relevant literature. Although we closely reviewed the subset of relevant literature identified via the database, we saved significant resources in conducting initial, broad searches which would inevitably yield a large amount of irrelevant literature to screen through. The result is a'useful platform to visualize the current evidence, which can be used to summarize the volume of existing research, generate new hypotheses, direct systematic reviews and meta-analyses, and can be continually updated.

5. Conclusions

In conclusion, this evidence map summarizes the existing literature on dietary fiber interventions and the human gut microbiota. This is a rapidly growing area of interest, but well-controlled human interventions are needed to support the associations being seen in animal and observational studies. We hope that this evidence map will provide a resource for researchers to direct new intervention studies and meta-analyses.

Supplementary Materials: The following are available online at http://www.mdpi.com/2072-6643/9/2/125/s1, Table S1: Inclusion/Exclusion Criteria. Supplementary Methods. Figure S1: Acute studies: weighted scatter plot of other microbiota outcomes by fiber group presents weighted scatter. The acute studies exclusively examine the short-term fermentation response by measuring SCFA concentration and/or breath gas excretion, most frequently in cereal fibers. Figure S2: Longer duration studies: weighted scatter plot of other microbiota outcomes by fiber group. Studies of greater duration examine more outcomes in a larger array of fiber types. Notably, however, there are no longer duration (>4 weeks) studies on resistant starch.

Acknowledgments: Funding support provided by a research grant from the International Life Science Institute, North America Branch, Technical Committee on Carbohydrates and from the USDA Agricultural Research Service (agreement 58-1950-0-014). We acknowledge Katherine Rancaño for her assistance with the tables.

Author Contributions: N.M.M. and M.C. designed research; C.M.S. and K.A.L. conducted research; M.C., S.B.R. and M.O. provided expertise on the following areas: evidence mapping methodology, dietary fibers, and gut microbiota; C.M.S. and K.A.L. analyzed data; C.M.S. and N.M.M. wrote paper; and N.M.M. had primary responsibility for final content. All authors have read and approved the final manuscript.

Conflicts of Interest: N.M.M. is supported in part by a research grant from the General Mills Bell Institute of Health and Nutrition and an unrestricted gift from Proctor and Gamble. C.M.S., K.A.L., M.O., S.B.R. and M.C. declare no conflicts of interest.

References

1. Codex Alimentarius Commission. *Codex Alimentarius Commission Report of the 30th Session of the Codex Committee on Nutrition and Foods for Special Dietary Uses*; Codex Alimentarius Commission: Cape Town, South Africa, 2008.
2. Jones, J.M. CODEX-aligned dietary fiber definitions help to bridge the "fiber gap". *Nutr. J.* **2014**, *13*, 34. [CrossRef] [PubMed]
3. Dahl, W.J.; Stewart, M.L. Position of the Academy of Nutrition and Dietetics: Health implications of dietary fiber. *J. Acad. Nutr. Diet.* **2015**, *115*, 1861–1870. [CrossRef] [PubMed]
4. Slavin, J. Fiber and prebiotics: Mechanisms and health benefits. *Nutrients* **2013**, *5*, 1417–1435. [CrossRef] [PubMed]
5. Conlon, M.A.; Bird, A.R. The impact of diet and lifestyle on gut microbiota and human health. *Nutrients* **2014**, *7*, 17–44. [CrossRef] [PubMed]
6. O'Hara, A.M.; Shanahan, F. The gut flora as a forgotten organ. *EMBO Rep.* **2006**, *7*, 688–693. [CrossRef] [PubMed]
7. Nicholson, J.K.; Holmes, E.; Kinross, J.; Burcelin, R.; Gibson, G.; Jia, W.; Pettersson, S. Host-gut microbiota metabolic interactions. *Science* **2012**, *336*, 1262–1267. [CrossRef] [PubMed]
8. Hooper, L.V.; Littman, D.R.; Macpherson, A.J. Interactions between the microbiota and the immune system. *Science* **2012**, *336*, 1268–1273. [CrossRef] [PubMed]
9. Clemente, J.C.; Ursell, L.K.; Parfrey, L.W.; Knight, R. The impact of the gut microbiota on human health: An integrative view. *Cell* **2012**, *148*, 1258–1270. [CrossRef] [PubMed]
10. Flint, H.J.; Duncan, S.H.; Scott, K.P.; Louis, P. Links between diet, gut microbiota composition and gut metabolism. *Proc. Nutr. Soc.* **2015**, *74*, 13–22. [CrossRef] [PubMed]
11. Blumberg, R.; Powrie, F. Microbiota, disease, and back to health: A metastable journey. *Sci. Transl. Med.* **2012**, *4*, 137rv7. [CrossRef] [PubMed]
12. Flint, H.J. The impact of nutrition on the human microbiome. *Nutr. Rev.* **2012**, *70* (Suppl. 1), S10–S13. [CrossRef] [PubMed]

13. David, L.A.; Maurice, C.F.; Carmody, R.N.; Gootenberg, D.B.; Button, J.E.; Wolfe, B.E.; Ling, A.V.; Devlin, A.S.; Varma, Y.; Fischbach, M.A.; et al. Diet rapidly and reproducibly alters the human gut microbiome. *Nature* **2014**, *505*, 559–563. [CrossRef] [PubMed]
14. Belenguer, A.; Duncan, S.H.; Calder, A.G.; Holtrop, G.; Louis, P.; Lobley, G.E.; Flint, H.J. Two routes of metabolic cross-feeding between *Bifidobacterium adolescentis* and butyrate-producing anaerobes from the human gut. *Appl. Environ. Microbiol.* **2006**, *72*, 3593–3599. [CrossRef] [PubMed]
15. Falony, G.; Vlachou, A.; Verbrugghe, K.; De Vuyst, L. Cross-feeding between *Bifidobacterium longum* BB536 and acetate-converting, butyrate-producing colon bacteria during growth on oligofructose. *Appl. Environ. Microbiol.* **2006**, *72*, 7835–7841. [CrossRef] [PubMed]
16. El Oufir, L.; Flourié, B.; Bruley des Varannes, S.; Barry, J.L.; Cloarec, D.; Bornet, F.; Galmiche, J.P. Relations between transit time, fermentation products, and hydrogen consuming flora in healthy humans. *Gut* **1996**, *38*, 870–877. [CrossRef] [PubMed]
17. Stephen, A.M.; Wiggins, H.S.; Cummings, J.H. Effect of changing transit time on colonic microbial metabolism in man. *Gut* **1987**, *28*, 601–609. [CrossRef] [PubMed]
18. Lewis, S.J.; Heaton, K.W. Increasing butyrate concentration in the distal colon by accelerating intestinal transit. *Gut* **1997**, *41*, 245–251. [CrossRef] [PubMed]
19. Graf, D.; Di Cagno, R.; Fåk, F.; Flint, H.J.; Nyman, M.; Saarela, M.; Watzl, B. Contribution of diet to the composition of the human gut microbiota. *Microb. Ecol. Health Dis.* **2015**, *26*, 26164. [CrossRef] [PubMed]
20. Den Besten, G.; van Eunen, K.; Groen, A.K.; Venema, K.; Reijngoud, D.-J.; Bakker, B.M. The role of short-chain fatty acids in the interplay between diet, gut microbiota, and host energy metabolism. *J. Lipid Res.* **2013**, *54*, 2325–2340. [CrossRef] [PubMed]
21. Duncan, S.H.; Louis, P.; Thomson, J.M.; Flint, H.J. The role of pH in determining the species composition of the human colonic microbiota. *Environ. Microbiol.* **2009**, *11*, 2112–2122. [CrossRef] [PubMed]
22. Samuel, B.S.; Shaito, A.; Motoike, T.; Rey, F.E.; Backhed, F.; Manchester, J.K.; Hammer, R.E.; Williams, S.C.; Crowley, J.; Yanagisawa, M.; et al. Effects of the gut microbiota on host adiposity are modulated by the short-chain fatty-acid binding G protein-coupled receptor, Gpr41. *Proc. Natl. Acad. Sci. USA* **2008**, *105*, 16767–16772. [CrossRef] [PubMed]
23. Wong, J.M.W.; de Souza, R.; Kendall, C.W.C.; Emam, A.; Jenkins, D.J.A. Colonic health: Fermentation and short chain fatty acids. *J. Clin. Gastroenterol.* **2006**, *40*, 235–243. [CrossRef] [PubMed]
24. Tan, J.; McKenzie, C.; Potamitis, M.; Thorburn, A.N.; Mackay, C.R.; Macia, L. The role of short-chain fatty acids in health and disease. *Adv. Immunol.* **2014**, *121*, 91–119. [PubMed]
25. Birt, D.F.; Boylston, T.; Hendrich, S.; Jane, J.-L.; Hollis, J.; Li, L.; McClelland, J.; Moore, S.; Phillips, G.J.; Rowling, M.; et al. Resistant starch: Promise for improving human health. *Adv. Nutr. Int. Rev. J.* **2013**, *4*, 587–601. [CrossRef] [PubMed]
26. Hamer, H.M.; Jonkers, D.; Venema, K.; Vanhoutvin, S.; Troost, F.J.; Brummer, R.-J. Review article: The role of butyrate on colonic function. *Aliment. Pharmacol. Ther.* **2008**, *27*, 104–119. [CrossRef] [PubMed]
27. Flint, H.J.; Scott, K.P.; Louis, P.; Duncan, S.H. The role of the gut microbiota in nutrition and health. *Nat. Rev. Gastroenterol. Hepatol.* **2012**, *9*, 577–589. [CrossRef] [PubMed]
28. Hamaker, B.R.; Tuncil, Y.E. A perspective on the complexity of dietary fiber structures and their potential effect on the gut microbiota. *J. Mol. Biol.* **2014**, *426*, 3838–3850. [CrossRef] [PubMed]
29. Althuis, M.D.; Weed, D.L. Evidence mapping: Methodologic foundations and application to intervention and observational research on sugar-sweetened beverages and health outcomes. *Am. J. Clin. Nutr.* **2013**, *98*, 755–768. [CrossRef] [PubMed]
30. Bragge, P.; Clavisi, O.; Turner, T.; Tavender, E.; Collie, A.; Gruen, R.L. The global evidence mapping initiative: Scoping research in broad topic areas. *BMC Med. Res. Methodol.* **2011**, *11*, 92. [CrossRef] [PubMed]
31. Hetrick, S.E.; Parker, A.G.; Callahan, P.; Purcell, R. Evidence mapping: Illustrating an emerging methodology to improve evidence-based practice in youth mental health. *J. Eval. Clin. Pract.* **2010**, *16*, 1025–1030. [CrossRef] [PubMed]
32. Wang, D.D.; Shams-White, M.; Bright, O.J.M.; Parrott, J.S.; Chung, M. Creating a literature database of low-calorie sweeteners and health studies: Evidence mapping. *BMC Med. Res. Methodol.* **2016**, *16*, 1. [CrossRef] [PubMed]

33. Livingston, K.A.; Chung, M.; Sawicki, C.M.; Lyle, B.J.; Wang, D.D.; Roberts, S.B.; McKeown, N.M. Development of a publicly available, comprehensive database of fiber and health outcomes: Rationale and methods. *PLoS ONE* **2016**, *11*, e0156961. [CrossRef] [PubMed]
34. McKeown, N.M.; Chung, M.; Livingston, K.A.; Sawicki, C.M.; Wang, D.D.; Blakeley, C.; Jia, Y.; Baruch, N.; Karlsen, M.; Brown, C. Project: Diet-Related Fibers and Human Health Outcomes, Version 1 (Retired Version). Available online: http://srdr.ahrq.gov/projects/564 (accessed on 7 September 2015).
35. Bouhnik, Y.; Flourié, B.; Riottot, M.; Bisetti, N.; Gailing, M.F.; Guibert, A.; Bornet, F.; Rambaud, J.C. Effects of fructo-oligosaccharides ingestion on fecal bifidobacteria and selected metabolic indexes of colon carcinogenesis in healthy humans. *Nutr. Cancer* **1996**, *26*, 21–29. [CrossRef] [PubMed]
36. Bouhnik, Y.; Vahedi, K.; Achour, L.; Attar, A.; Salfati, J.; Pochart, P.; Marteau, P.; Flourié, B.; Bornet, F.; Rambaud, J.C. Short-chain fructo-oligosaccharide administration dose-dependently increases fecal bifidobacteria in healthy humans. *J. Nutr.* **1999**, *129*, 113–116. [PubMed]
37. Tannock, G.W.; Munro, K.; Bibiloni, R.; Simon, M.A.; Hargreaves, P.; Gopal, P.; Harmsen, H.; Welling, G. Impact of consumption of oligosaccharide-containing biscuits on the fecal microbiota of humans. *Appl. Environ. Microbiol.* **2004**, *70*, 2129–2136. [CrossRef] [PubMed]
38. Bouhnik, Y.; Raskine, L.; Simoneau, G.; Vicaut, E.; Neut, C.; Flourié, B.; Brouns, F.; Bornet, F.R. The capacity of nondigestible carbohydrates to stimulate fecal bifidobacteria in healthy humans: A double-blind, randomized, placebo-controlled, parallel-group, dose-response relation study. *Am. J. Clin. Nutr.* **2004**, *80*, 1658–1664. [PubMed]
39. Clavel, T.; Fallani, M.; Lepage, P.; Levenez, F.; Mathey, J.; Rochet, V.; Sérézat, M.; Sutren, M.; Henderson, G.; Bennetau-Pelissero, C.; et al. Isoflavones and functional foods alter the dominant intestinal microbiota in postmenopausal women. *J. Nutr.* **2005**, *135*, 2786–2792. [PubMed]
40. Ten Bruggencate, S.J.M.; Bovee-Oudenhoven, I.M.J.; Lettink-Wissink, M.L.G.; Katan, M.B.; van der Meer, R. Dietary fructooligosaccharides affect intestinal barrier function in healthy men. *J. Nutr.* **2006**, *136*, 70–74. [PubMed]
41. Bouhnik, Y.; Raskine, L.; Simoneau, G.; Paineau, D.; Bornet, F. The capacity of short-chain fructo-oligosaccharides to stimulate faecal bifidobacteria: A dose-response relationship study in healthy humans. *Nutr. J.* **2006**, *5*, 8. [CrossRef] [PubMed]
42. Depeint, F.; Tzortzis, G.; Vulevic, J.; I'anson, K.; Gibson, G.R. Prebiotic evaluation of a novel galactooligosaccharide mixture produced by the enzymatic activity of *Bifidobacterium bifidum* NCIMB 41171, in healthy humans: A randomized, double-blind, crossover, placebo-controlled intervention study. *Am. J. Clin. Nutr.* **2008**, *87*, 785–791. [PubMed]
43. Vulevic, J.; Drakoularakou, A.; Yaqoob, P.; Tzortzis, G.; Gibson, G.R. Modulation of the fecal microflora profile and immune function by a novel trans-galactooligosaccharide mixture (B-GOS) in healthy elderly volunteers. *Am. J. Clin. Nutr.* **2008**, *88*, 1438–1446. [PubMed]
44. Mitsou, E.K.; Turunen, K.; Anapliotis, P.; Zisi, D.; Spiliotis, V.; Kyriacou, A. Impact of a jelly containing short-chain fructo-oligosaccharides and *Sideritis euboea* extract on human faecal microbiota. *Int. J. Food Microbiol.* **2009**, *135*, 112–117. [CrossRef] [PubMed]
45. Cloetens, L.; Broekaert, W.F.; Delaedt, Y.; Ollevier, F.; Courtin, C.M.; Delcour, J.A.; Rutgeerts, P.; Verbeke, K. Tolerance of arabinoxylan-oligosaccharides and their prebiotic activity in healthy subjects: A randomised, placebo-controlled cross-over study. *Br. J. Nutr.* **2010**, *103*, 703–713. [CrossRef] [PubMed]
46. Walton, G.E.; van den Heuvel, E.G.H.M.; Kosters, M.H.W.; Rastall, R.A.; Tuohy, K.M.; Gibson, G.R. A randomised crossover study investigating the effects of galacto-oligosaccharides on the faecal microbiota in men and women over 50 years of age. *Br. J. Nutr.* **2012**, *107*, 1466–1475. [CrossRef] [PubMed]
47. Lecerf, J.-M.; Dépeint, F.; Clerc, E.; Dugenet, Y.; Niamba, C.N.; Rhazi, L.; Cayzeele, A.; Abdelnour, G.; Jaruga, A.; Younes, H.; et al. Xylo-oligosaccharide (XOS) in combination with inulin modulates both the intestinal environment and immune status in healthy subjects, while XOS alone only shows prebiotic properties. *Br. J. Nutr.* **2012**, *108*, 1847–1858. [CrossRef] [PubMed]
48. Damen, B.; Cloetens, L.; Broekaert, W.F.; François, I.; Lescroart, O.; Trogh, I.; Arnaut, F.; Welling, G.W.; Wijffels, J.; Delcour, J.A.; et al. Consumption of breads containing in situ-produced arabinoxylan oligosaccharides alters gastrointestinal effects in healthy volunteers. *J. Nutr.* **2012**, *142*, 470–477. [CrossRef] [PubMed]

49. François, I.E.J.A.; Lescroart, O.; Veraverbeke, W.S.; Marzorati, M.; Possemiers, S.; Evenepoel, P.; Hamer, H.; Houben, E.; Windey, K.; Welling, G.W.; et al. Effects of a wheat bran extract containing arabinoxylan oligosaccharides on gastrointestinal health parameters in healthy adult human volunteers: A double-blind, randomised, placebo-controlled, cross-over trial. *Br. J. Nutr.* **2012**, *108*, 2229–2242. [CrossRef] [PubMed]
50. Walton, G.E.; Lu, C.; Trogh, I.; Arnaut, F.; Gibson, G.R. A randomised, double-blind, placebo controlled cross-over study to determine the gastrointestinal effects of consumption of arabinoxylan-oligosaccharides enriched bread in healthy volunteers. *Nutr. J.* **2012**, *11*, 36. [CrossRef] [PubMed]
51. Maki, K.C.; Gibson, G.R.; Dickmann, R.S.; Kendall, C.W.C.; Chen, C.-Y.O.; Costabile, A.; Comelli, E.M.; McKay, D.L.; Almeida, N.G.; Jenkins, D.; et al. Digestive and physiologic effects of a wheat bran extract, arabino-xylan-oligosaccharide, in breakfast cereal. *Nutrition* **2012**, *28*, 1115–1121. [CrossRef] [PubMed]
52. Vulevic, J.; Juric, A.; Tzortzis, G.; Gibson, G.R. A mixture of trans-galactooligosaccharides reduces markers of metabolic syndrome and modulates the fecal microbiota and immune function of overweight adults. *J. Nutr.* **2013**, *143*, 324–331. [CrossRef] [PubMed]
53. François, I.E.J.A.; Lescroart, O.; Veraverbeke, W.S.; Marzorati, M.; Possemiers, S.; Hamer, H.; Windey, K.; Welling, G.W.; Delcour, J.A.; Courtin, C.M.; et al. Effects of wheat bran extract containing arabinoxylan oligosaccharides on gastrointestinal parameters in healthy preadolescent children. *J. Pediatr. Gastroenterol. Nutr.* **2014**, *58*, 647–653. [CrossRef] [PubMed]
54. Finegold, S.M.; Li, Z.; Summanen, P.H.; Downes, J.; Thames, G.; Corbett, K.; Dowd, S.; Krak, M.; Heber, D. Xylooligosaccharide increases bifidobacteria but not lactobacilli in human gut microbiota. *Food Funct.* **2014**, *5*, 436–445. [CrossRef] [PubMed]
55. Morel, F.B.; Dai, Q.; Ni, J.; Thomas, D.; Parnet, P.; Fança-Berthon, P. α-Galacto-oligosaccharides dose-dependently reduce appetite and decrease inflammation in overweight adults. *J. Nutr.* **2015**, *145*, 2052–2059. [CrossRef] [PubMed]
56. Vulevic, J.; Juric, A.; Walton, G.E.; Claus, S.P.; Tzortzis, G.; Toward, R.E.; Gibson, G.R. Influence of galacto-oligosaccharide mixture (B-GOS) on gut microbiota, immune parameters and metabonomics in elderly persons. *Br. J. Nutr.* **2015**, *114*, 586–595. [CrossRef] [PubMed]
57. Hur, I.Y.; Reicks, M. Relationship between whole-grain intake, chronic disease risk indicators, and weight status among adolescents in the National Health and Nutrition Examination Survey, 1999–2004. *J. Acad. Nutr. Diet.* **2012**, *112*, 46–55. [CrossRef] [PubMed]
58. Ley, R.E.; Bäckhed, F.; Turnbaugh, P.; Lozupone, C.A.; Knight, R.D.; Gordon, J.I. Obesity alters gut microbial ecology. *Proc. Natl. Acad. Sci. USA* **2005**, *102*, 11070–11075. [CrossRef] [PubMed]
59. Kalliomäki, M.; Collado, M.C.; Salminen, S.; Isolauri, E. Early differences in fecal microbiota composition in children may predict overweight. *Am. J. Clin. Nutr.* **2008**, *87*, 534–538. [PubMed]
60. Carbohydrates in Human Nutrition. *Report of a Joint FAO/WHO Expert Consultation*; Food and Agriculture Organization, World Health Organization (FAO/WHO): Rome, Italy, 1997; pp. 1–140.
61. American Association of Cereal Chemists (AACC). The Definition of Dietary Fiber. Report of the Dietary Fiber Definition Committee to the Board of Directors of the American Association of Cereal Chemists. *Cereal Foods World* **2001**, *46*, 112–126.
62. Valcheva, R.; Dieleman, L.A. Prebiotics: Definition and protective mechanisms. *Best Pract. Res. Clin. Gastroenterol.* **2016**, *30*, 27–37. [CrossRef] [PubMed]
63. Bindels, L.B.; Delzenne, N.M.; Cani, P.D.; Walter, J. Towards a more comprehensive concept for prebiotics. *Nat. Rev. Gastroenterol. Hepatol.* **2015**, *12*, 303–310. [CrossRef] [PubMed]
64. Cummings, J.H.; Antoine, J.-M.; Azpiroz, F.; Bourdet-Sicard, R.; Brandtzaeg, P.; Calder, P.C.; Gibson, G.R.; Guarner, F.; Isolauri, E.; Pannemans, D.; et al. PASSCLAIM—Gut health and immunity. *Eur. J. Nutr.* **2004**, *43* (Suppl. 2), II118–II173. [CrossRef] [PubMed]
65. Meyer, D. Inunlin, gut microbes, and health. In *Dietary Fiber and Health*; Cho, S.S., Almeida, N., Eds.; CRC Press Taylor & Francis Group: Boca Raton, FL, USA, 2012; pp. 169–183.
66. Tojo, R.; Suárez, A.; Clemente, M.G.; de los Reyes-Gavilán, C.G.; Margolles, A.; Gueimonde, M.; Ruas-Madiedo, P. Intestinal microbiota in health and disease: Role of bifidobacteria in gut homeostasis. *World J. Gastroenterol.* **2014**, *20*, 15163–15176. [CrossRef] [PubMed]
67. McRorie, J.W. Evidence-based approach to fiber supplements and clinically meaningful health benefits, part 1: What to look for and how to recommend an effective fiber therapy. *Nutr. Today* **2015**, *50*, 82–89. [CrossRef] [PubMed]

68. McRorie, J.W. Evidence-based approach to fiber supplements and clinically meaningful health benefits, part 2: What to look for and how to recommend an effective fiber therapy. *Nutr. Today* **2015**, *50*, 90–97. [CrossRef] [PubMed]
69. Mcrorie, J.W.; Fahey, G.C. A review of gastrointestinal physiology and the mechanisms underlying the health benefits of dietary fiber: Matching an effective fiber with specific patient needs. *Clin. Nurs. Stud.* **2013**, *1*, 82–92. [CrossRef]
70. McRorie, J.W.; McKeown, N.M. Understanding the physics of functional fibers in the gastrointestinal tract: An evidence-based approach to resolving enduring misconceptions about insoluble and soluble fiber. *J. Acad. Nutr. Diet.* **2017**, *17*, 251–264. [CrossRef] [PubMed]
71. 2015–2020 Dietary Guidelines—Health.gov. Available online: https://health.gov/dietaryguidelines/2015/guidelines/ (accessed on 15 December 2016).
72. Okarter, N.; Liu, R.H. Health benefits of whole grain phytochemicals. *Crit. Rev. Food Sci. Nutr.* **2010**, *50*, 193–208. [CrossRef] [PubMed]
73. Vitaglione, P.; Mennella, I.; Ferracane, R.; Rivellese, A.A.; Giacco, R.; Ercolini, D.; Gibbons, S.M.; La Storia, A.; Gilbert, J.A.; Jonnalagadda, S.; et al. Whole-grain wheat consumption reduces inflammation in a randomized controlled trial on overweight and obese subjects with unhealthy dietary and lifestyle behaviors: Role of polyphenols bound to cereal dietary fiber. *Am. J. Clin. Nutr.* **2015**, *101*, 251–261. [CrossRef] [PubMed]

nutrients

MDPI

Article

Whole Grains Contribute Only a Small Proportion of Dietary Fiber to the U.S. Diet

Sibylle Kranz [1,*], Kevin W. Dodd [2], Wen Yen Juan [3], LuAnn K. Johnson [4] and Lisa Jahns [4]

1 Department of Kinesiology, University of Virginia, Charlottesville, VA 22904, USA
2 National Cancer Institute, Bethesda, MD 20892, USA; doddk@mail.nih.gov
3 Nutrition Assessment and Evaluation, Office of Nutrition and Food Labeling, Center for Food and Applied Nutrition, United States Food and Drug Administration, College Park, MD 20740, USA; wenyen.juan@fda.hhs.gov
4 United States Department of Agriculture, Agricultural Research Service, Grand Forks Human Nutrition Research Center, Grand Forks, ND 58203, USA; luann.johnson@ars.usda.gov (L.K.J.); lisa.jahns@ars.usda.gov (L.J.)
* Correspondence: sibylle.kranz@virginia.edu; Tel.: +1-434-924-7904

Received: 14 December 2016; Accepted: 14 February 2017; Published: 17 February 2017

Abstract: Dietary fiber (DF), found in whole fruits, vegetables, and whole grains (WG), is considered a nutrient of concern in the US diet and increased consumption is recommended. The present study was designed to highlight this critical importance of the difference between WG, high-fiber WG, and sources of fiber that are not from WG. The study is based on the two-day diets reported consumed by the nationally representative sample of Americans participating in What We Eat In America, the dietary component of the National Health and Nutrition Examination Survey from 2003–2010. Foods consumed were classified into tertiles of DF and WG and the contribution of fiber by differing levels of WG content were examined. Foods containing high amounts of WG and DF only contributed about 7% of total fiber intake. Overall, grain-based foods contributed 54.5% of all DF consumed. Approximately 39% of DF came from grain foods that contained no WG, rather these foods contained refined grains, which contain only small amounts of DF but are consumed in large quantities. All WG-containing foods combined contributed a total of 15.3% of DF in the American diet. Thus, public health messaging needs to be changed to specifically encourage consumption of WG foods with high levels of DF to address both recommendations.

Keywords: whole grain intake; dietary fiber; nutrition monitoring; Dietary Guidelines for Americans; healthy diet; sources of dietary fiber

---

1. Introduction

1.1. Dietary Fiber

Dietary fiber (DF), which occurs in whole fruits, vegetables, and whole grains (WG), is considered a nutrient of concern in the US diet and increased consumption is recommended. [1] In the UK, recommendations are 30 g/day for adults [2]. The recommended DF intake in the US is at least 14 g of fiber per 1000 kcal of total energy consumed, which translates to roughly 19 g per day for children 1–3 years old to between 25–35 g per day for adults [3]. Although intake increased slightly among some Americans over a 10-year period [4], fiber intake is low in the American diet with less than 3% of the population meeting recommendations [5,6]; most Americans consume very low amounts [7]. As fiber intake is inversely associated with body weight [8–12], cardiovascular disease (CVD) risk factors [13–15], some cancers, and potentially type 2 diabetes and other chronic diseases [16,17], it is important to increase consumption to improve population health. The greatest source of fiber in the diet is vegetables (22%), followed by mixed dishes (12%), yeast breads (12%), and fruits (11%) [4].

1.2. Whole Grains

One of the sources of dietary fiber, WG, has also been associated with decreased risks of obesity, type 2 diabetes, and CVD [18–20]. The World Health Organization recommends consuming WG as part of a healthy diet [21]. Many countries and organizations also have recommendations for WG intake, although intake guidelines vary substantially [22]. WG were first introduced as a food group for recommended intake in the Dietary Guidelines for Americans (DGA) 2005 and have been maintained as part of the USDA Healthy US-Style Food Patterns as a food group to be recommended in the 2015–2020 DGA [23,24]. The 2015–2020 DGA provides food-based guidance and recommends that Americans consume at least one-half of their daily suggested total grains as WG, which is equivalent to at least 3 oz. equivalents per day for many individuals consuming more than 1600 calories per day. However, nationally representative intake data suggest that only 2%–7% of Americans meet this recommendation [25,26]. The greatest sources of WG in the diet of adults are yeast breads (27%), ready-to-eat (RTE) cereals (23%), and pastas, cooked cereal and rice (21%) [4]. However, those food sources are not generally 100% WG. The American diet does not include many foods that are 100% WG, but rather foods that contain some small proportion of WG, such as breads, cereals, or pastry made with some WG flour. The US Food and Drug Administration classification of WG is limited to those products which retain all of the main biological components of the grain (germ, endosperm, and bran) in the same relative proportion as in the intact grain [27], which is not necessary related to the amount of dietary fiber. Therefore, the "whole grain"-containing foods recommended by the DGA encompass a wide variety of foods, ranging from those with proportionally low to those with very high amounts of dietary fiber, depending upon the type of grain.

1.3. Significance

DGA recommendations focus on increasing the consumption of WG [28,29] to half of all consumed grains, however, due to the large variation of dietary fiber content in WG foods (g/100 g), it is important to differentiate between high fiber and low fiber WG foods. The present study was designed to highlight this critical importance of the difference between WG, high-fiber WG, and sources of fiber that are not from WG. A previous analysis using the 2009–2010 National Health and Nutrition Examination Survey (NHANES) found that fiber consumption was related to WG consumption [30]; however, the sample was small (only one NHANES wave), which limited the amounts of food that were included in the analysis. Due to the high number of foods in the US food supply that use the words "whole grain" in several locations on food packaging for marketing purposes, a timely research question is: "what are the food sources of DF consumed by the American population, and what proportion of dietary fiber is contributed by WG?" To answer this question, we pooled data from 8 years of NHANES surveys in the US, from 2003–2004 to 2009–2010 and examined the relationships between WG foods and DF from these foods.

2. Materials and Methods

2.1. Data Set

The study is based on the two-day diets reported consumed by the nationally representative sample of Americans participating in What We Eat In America (WWEIA), the dietary component of NHANES, and is reflected in oz. equivalent of the MyPlate "whole grains" food group [31]. NHANES is a nationally representative, cross-sectional survey of the non-institutionalized civilian U.S. population and is conducted by the National Center for Health Statistics, Centers for Diseases Control and Prevention. Details of both WWEIA and NHANES can be found elsewhere [32]. In short, participants completed two interviewer-assisted 24-h recalls; day one recalls were administered in-person and day two recalls were conducted over the phone. Primary caregivers reported proxy intake for children less than six years old and assisted children ages 6–11 years; individuals age 12 and older self-reported their previous day's food intake. All dietary interviews were conducted by trained interviewers using the U.S. Department of Agriculture's Automated Multiple-Pass Method [33].

For this study, total grain, WG, and DF intakes were estimated using day one dietary intake data collected from 34,391 individuals aged 2 years and older participating in the WWEIA, NHANES 2003–2004, 2005–2006, 2007–2008, and 2009–2010 continuing surveys.

WG were defined as grains that include the entire grain kernel—the bran, germ, and endosperm. WG values were obtained for all reported foods in all survey years using the MyPyramid Equivalents Database (MPED), 2.0 for USDA Survey Food Codes, 2003–2004 (MPED 2.0) and the Center for Nutrition Policy and Promotion Addendum to MPED 2.0 [34,35]. At the time of analysis, the new MPED including the Equivalents database for NHANES 2009–2010 was not available, thus the authors generated a proxy food list to identify the food codes containing WG. Since only a small proportion of Americans meet the WG or the DF dietary guidance, consumption patterns were not based on the intake level of the individuals but conducted on the food level, to help explain why so many Americans have insufficient amounts of WG and DF in their diets. Foods containing WG were categorized as described below. Dietary fiber intake values were obtained from the USDA Food and Nutrition Database for Dietary Studies (FNDDS) version 2.0 and version 4.1 [36].

2.2. Study Variables

Four categories of dietary fiber density food (no, low, medium, or high dietary fiber) and five categories of WG food (not a grain food, a grain food with no WG, a grain food with low amounts of WG, a grain food with medium amounts of WG, and a grain food with high amounts of WG) were established. The dietary fiber and WG categories "low, medium, and high" were established based on unweighted tertiles of dietary fiber density (g/100 g of food) and of WG density (oz. equivalents /100 g of food) of all food codes in the FNDDS that were reported consumed at least once in day one dietary intake data. As this research focuses on WG and fiber intake, foods not containing grains were not included in analysis beyond the description of their contribution to total fiber intake.

To maintain the nationally representative character of the data, the calculation of the proportion of foods consumed in each of the fiber (low, medium, high) and WG (no grains, no WG, low WG, medium WG, and high WG) categories in the total population and the male and female population of 2–18 years old and 19–85 years old were computed using survey sample weights. All analyses were performed using SAS, version 9.3 (SAS Institute, Cary, NC, USA). It is important to point out that this analysis was conducted to identify the foods available to the consumer based on their WG and DF content and their contribution to average usual intake, not to any particular individual's dietary intake. This approach was chosen to highlight the complexity of access to high-fiber foods in the US food supply.

3. Results

The number of survey respondents and their socio-economic characteristics are reflected in Table 1. Approximately 50% of the sample were males, more individuals were Non-Hispanic white and more had higher than high school education, which is reflective of the US census data. The educational levels of individuals 18 years and younger are not reported here, as they are likely still in school and their terminal degrees are not known. A greater proportion of younger individuals was from low-income families while the majority of the adult population was from medium or high income households.

Table 1. Characteristics of study population, 2003–2010.

Participant Characteristic	Children 2–18		Adults 19 & Older	
	Males	Females	Males	Females
Unweighted sample size (*N*)	6775	6646	10,181	10,789
Gender (%)	50.7	49.3	47.9	52.1
Race-ethnicity (%)				
Non-Hispanic white	30.9	29.3	34.0	36.8
Non-Hispanic black	7.0	7.4	5.1	6.3
Mexican American	9.5	9.1	6.1	6.1
Other	3.3	3.4	2.6	2.8
Poverty Income Ratio (PIR) (%)				
<1.3	15.5	16.4	9.0	12.0
1.3–1.84	5.8	5.4	4.6	5.8
1.85–3.4	12.8	11.4	11.5	12.5
>3.4	17.1	15.7	22.8	21.8
Education (%)				
No high school diploma	N/A	N/A	8.9	9.8
High school graduate	N/A	N/A	12.3	13.0
More than high school	N/A	N/A	26.6	29.2

All foods analyzed were reported as consumed by the population. As shown in Table 2, foods containing high amounts of WG and DF only contributed about 7% of total fiber intake. Overall, all grain-based foods consumed only contributed 54.5% of all DF consumed—the remaining 45.5% of DF was supplied from non-grain foods. Approximately 39% of DF came from grain foods that contained no WG, rather these foods contained refined grains, which contain only small amounts of DF but are consumed in large quantities. All WG-containing foods combined contributed a total of 15.3% of DF in the American diet.

Table 2. Percent of whole grain and fiber consumed by tertiles of WG (oz. equivalents/100 g food) and dietary fiber (g/100 g food) in diets of Americans ages 2–85 years, 2003–2010.

Whole Grain (Tertiles)	Fiber (Tertiles)	WG %	Fiber %	% Reporting
High WG (WG $\geq$ 1.33)	High Fiber (DF $\geq$ 1.7)	50.4	6.6	7.9
Medium WG (0.71 < WG < 1.33)	High Fiber (DF $\geq$ 1.7)	29.9	4.7	7.9
	Medium Fiber (0.9 < DF < 1.7)	10.5	0.8	1.1
	Low Fiber (0 < DF $\leq$ 0.9)	0.2	0.01	0.02
Low WG (0 < WG $\leq$ 0.71)	High Fiber (DF $\geq$ 1.7)	8.1	3.0	6.8
	Medium Fiber (0.9 < DF < 1.7)	0.1	0.1	0.2
	Low Fiber (0 < DF $\leq$ 0.9)	0.9	0.1	0.6
No WG	Any Fiber (DF > 0)	0.0	39.2	33.1
Total		100.0	54.5	

The distribution of total DF contributed by each of the five WG categories is reflected in Figure 1. The distribution did not differ between the total population and the age and gender subgroups, thus, results from the subgroups are not included but are available upon request. As the pie charts show, low DF consumers obtained approximatly 2/3 of their daily average DF from food sources that were not grains. The proportional contribution of non-grains decreased with increasing level of total DF in the diet, in that the high DF diets were characterized by having only approximately 35% from non-grain food sources but approximately 25% were from medium or high WG foods.

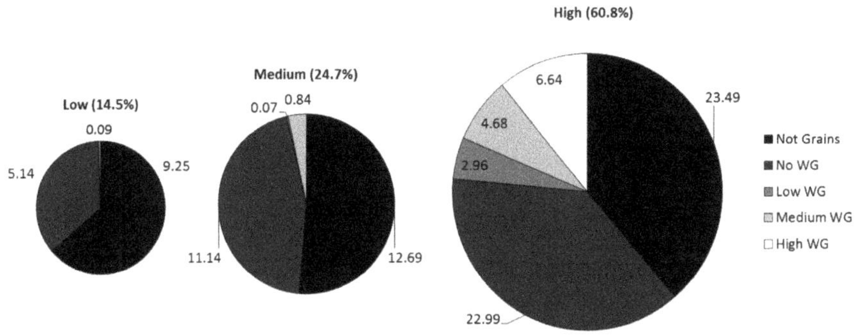

Figure 1. Percent of total dietary fiber intake provided by low, medium, and high fiber foods (defined by g fiber/100 g food) in the diets of Americans ages 2–85 years old.

4. Discussion

Sixty percent of Americans report trying to consume more fiber and WG; however, 35% believe that they are already getting enough WG [37]. Recent discussions on venues to improve the American diet have concluded that while WG foods are a good source of several essential nutrients and should be continued to be emphasized as part of a healthy diet, efforts to improve DF intake will fail if they are based solely on the recommendation to increase WG foods [38]. Therefore, such efforts should specifically encourage the consumption of high-fiber foods, including high-fiber WG foods such as multigrain bread, popcorn, or high-fiber ready-to-eat cereal.

Results from the present study are in concordance with these findings. Data indicate that the WG foods consumed by Americans contribute very little to total DF intake. Estimates show that more than three-fourths of DF consumed by adults and children were provided by foods that are not grains or are refined grains but do not contain WG. It is noteworthy to point out that the proportion of DF from WG products might be higher if individuals would consume the recommended amount of WG. However, since only a very small proportion of the American population falls into that category, no generalizable models to predict potential DF from WG foods can be established [28,38].

In previous research, we showed that the majority of DF in children's diets was provided by high consumption of low-fiber foods, and that healthy-weight children were more likely to consume high-fiber foods than overweight/obese children [39]. Thus, in an effort to address overweight/obesity in American children the relationship between WG and DF has to be clarified to motivate the population to seek foods that are high in DF and WG. Currently, this differentiation is not clear, which is due in part to the fact that WG consumption is encouraged by the DGA in terms of "servings of WG-containing foods" while the recommendation for DF expressed in the DRI as 14 g/1000 kcal consumed is not as widely distributed. DF consumers had diets that were disproportionately high in non-grain or non-WG foods; only a very small proportion of the fiber consumed originated from low WG food. In the medium and high DF diets, however, the diversity of the sources of fiber increased and included at least some amounts of medium or high WG foods. One could assume that even low DF consumers would have some portion of the DF they consume from medium or high WG foods but the data indicate individuals with low DF select an intake pattern in which those foods are avoided. Future research is needed to understand (a) if consumers are aware that their diets are low in DF and (b) the factors leading to this pattern of low WG and low DF diets. Once this information has been generated, potential intervention points to move consumers to a diet that contains at least some medium and high WG foods can be developed and implemented.

It is noteworthy to point out that some of the consumer's misconceptions about their DF intake are likely based on the use of two different metrics: front-of package labeling about the food being a "good" source of WG, while food's content of DF can be labeled using the CODEX definitions for nutrient claims ("high" in fiber (must contain 6 g DF/100 g of food, or 3 g DF per 100 kcal from the food, or 20% of dietary reference values delivered in one serving). To eliminate this confusion, packages would have to be labeled with two statements: one concerning the level of WG in the product and another to address the amount of DF in the food.

As all studies based on the NHANES, this study too has several limitations. First, our analysis was based on self-reported dietary intake records, which may include biased reporting and may not be reflective of the rapidly changing U.S. food supply. Many more high-fiber foods may be available in the American food supply but if they were not reported by the participants of NHANES, they were not included in this analysis. Our approach, therefore, may well underestimate the number of high WG, high-fiber foods in the marketplace. Also, the food industry has responded to the recommendation to consume more dietary fiber by reformulating food products and adding WG, fiber, or both. Currently it is not possible to differentiate between naturally occurring fibers and fiber added to products, such as wheat bran added to breads. Furthermore, the food supply now also includes different, new, types of fiber, which are found in foods in varying proportions and which may have disparate health effects.

Despite the limitations, the strengths of this study include the large, nationally representative sample and the use of four NHANES waves, which increases the variety and number of foods included in the analysis. Also, unlike other researchers who categorize consumers by their level of WG or DF intake, we focused on a food-based analysis to help explain the high proportion of Americans not meeting the intake guidelines. Although this effort requires the establishing of a different set of cut points, it allows the data-driven analysis, thus enhancing our understanding of the population intake patterns. In this particular instance, the methodology specifically developed for this project to optimally estimate WG and DF intake sources moves the field beyond other studies, which were limited by describing intakes in pre-established groups of people who meet or fail to meet the intake recommendations [40]. Based on the study presented here, public health efforts to change the intake behavior of those who do not meet the WG and DF intake recommendations can be developed.

5. Conclusions

The Dietary Guidelines for Americans include the recommendation to consume at least 50% of grains from WG and the DRI stipulate that a healthy diet contain 14 g of DF per 1000 kcal consumed. Most Americans don't meet either recommendation. The data presented here show that the WG products consumed by Americans are very low in dietary fiber, thus, public health messaging needs to be changed to encourage consumption of WG foods with high levels of DF to address both recommendations.

Acknowledgments: Financial support was provided by the USDA/Agricultural Research Service, (USDA 3062-51000-051-00D) and The Kellogg Citizenship Fund.

Author Contributions: S.K. conceived of this study and led all analysis and the writing of publications and presentation materials, L.J. and W.J. significantly contributed to the conceptualization of the design, K.D. led the statistical analysis, and L.K.J. conducted all programming involved in this study. All authors have read and agreed to the final version of this manuscript.

Conflicts of Interest: The authors declare no conflict of interest. The funding sponsors had no role in the design of the study; in the collection, analyses, or interpretation of data; in the writing of the manuscript, and in the decision to publish the results.

References

1. U.S. Department of Health and Human Services; U.S. Department of Agriculture. *2015–2020 Dietary Guidelines for Americans*, 8th ed.2015. Available online: https://health.gov/dietaryguidelines/2015/guidelines/ (accessed on 13 December 2016).
2. NHS. How to Get More Fibre into Your Diet. Available online: http://www.nhs.uk/Livewell/Goodfood/Pages/how-to-get-more-fibre-into-your-diet.aspx/ (accessed on 13 January 2017).

3. Institute of Medicine of the National Academy of Sciences. *Dietary Reference Intakes for Energy, Carbohydrate, Fiber, Fat, Fatty Acids, Cholesterol, Protein, and Amino Acids (Macronutrients)*; National Academy Press: Washington, DC, USA, 2002.
4. McGill, C.; Fulgoni, V.L., III; Devareddy, L. Ten-year trends in fiber and whole grain intakes and food sources for the United States population: National Health and Nutrition Examination Survey 2001–2010. *Nutrients* **2015**, *7*, 1119. [CrossRef] [PubMed]
5. Keast, D.R.; Fulgoni, V.L.; Nicklas, T.A.; O'Neil, C.E. Food sources of energy and nutrients among children in the United States: National Health and Nutrition Examination Survey 2003–2006. *Nutrients* **2013**, *5*, 283–301. [CrossRef] [PubMed]
6. O'Neil, C.E.; Keast, D.R.; Fulgoni, V.L.; Nicklas, T.A. Food sources of energy and nutrients among adults in the US: NHANES 2003–2006. *Nutrients* **2012**, *4*, 2097–2120. [CrossRef] [PubMed]
7. Lin, B.H.; Yen, S.T. The U.S. Grain Consumption Landscape: Who Eats Grain, in What Form, Where, and How Much? Economic Research Report Number 50. United States Department of Agriculture, Department of Economic Research Service, 2007–2011. Available online: http://purl.umn.edu/55967 (accessed on 13 December 2016).
8. Gropper, S.S.; Acosta, P.B. The therapeutic effect of fiber in treating obesity. *J. Am. Coll. Nutr.* **1987**, *6*, 533–535. [CrossRef] [PubMed]
9. Johnson, L.; Mander, A.P.; Jones, L.R.; Emmett, P.M.; Jebb, S.A. Energy-dense, low-fiber, high-fat dietary pattern is associated with increased fatness in childhood. *Am. J. Clin. Nutr.* **2008**, *87*, 846–854. [PubMed]
10. Slavin, J.L. Dietary fiber and body weight. *Nutrition* **2005**, *21*, 411–418. [CrossRef] [PubMed]
11. Howarth, N.C.; Huang, T.T.; Roberts, S.B.; McCrory, M.A. Dietary fiber and fat are associated with excess weight in young and middle-aged US adults. *J. Am. Diet. Assoc.* **2005**, *105*, 1365–1372. [CrossRef] [PubMed]
12. Du, H.; van der, A.D.; Boshuizen, H.C.; Forouhi, N.G.; Wareham, N.J.; Halkjaer, J.; Tjonneland, A.; Overvad, K.; Jakobsen, M.U.; Boeing, H.; et al. Dietary fiber and subsequent changes in body weight and waist circumference in European men and women. *Am. J. Clin. Nutr.* **2010**, *91*, 329–336. [CrossRef] [PubMed]
13. Overby, N.C.; Sonestedt, E.; Laaksonen, D.E.; Birgisdottir, B.E. Dietary fiber and the glycemic index: A background paper for the Nordic nutrition recommendations 2012. *Food. Nutr. Res.* **2013**, *57*. [CrossRef] [PubMed]
14. Johansson-Persson, A.; Ulmius, M.; Cloetens, L.; Karhu, T.; Herzig, K.H.; Onning, G. A high intake of dietary fiber influences C-reactive protein and fibrinogen, but not glucose and lipid metabolism, in mildly hypercholesterolemic subjects. *Eur. J. Nutr.* **2014**, *53*, 39–48. [CrossRef] [PubMed]
15. Slavin, J. Fiber and prebiotics: Mechanisms and health benefits. *Nutrients* **2013**, *5*, 1417–1435. [CrossRef] [PubMed]
16. Kranz, S.; Brauchla, M.; Slavin, J.L.; Miller, K.B. What do we know about dietary fiber intake in children and health? The effects of fiber intake on constipation, obesity, and diabetes in children. *Adv. Nutr.* **2012**, *3*, 47–53. [CrossRef] [PubMed]
17. Kaczmarczyk, M.M.; Miller, M.J.; Freund, G.G. The health benefits of dietary fiber: Beyond the usual suspects of type 2 diabetes mellitus, cardiovascular disease and colon cancer. *Metabolism* **2012**, *61*, 1058–1066. [CrossRef] [PubMed]
18. Anderson, J.W.; Baird, P.; Davis, R.H., Jr.; Ferreri, S.; Knudtson, M.; Koraym, A.; Waters, V.; Williams, C.L. Health benefits of dietary fiber. *Nutr. Rev.* **2009**, *67*, 188–205. [CrossRef] [PubMed]
19. Jonnalagadda, S.S.; Harnack, L.; Hai Liu, R.; McKeown, N.; Seal, C.; Liu, S.; Fahey, G.C. Putting the whole grain puzzle together: Health benefits associated with whole grains—Summary of American society for nutrition 2010 satellite symposium. *J. Nutr.* **2011**, *141*, 1011S–1022S. [CrossRef] [PubMed]
20. Cho, S.S.; Qi, L.; Fahey, G.C.; Klurfeld, D.M. Consumption of cereal fiber, mixtures of whole grain and bran, and whole grains and risk reduction in type 2 diabetes, obesity, and cardiovascular disease. *Am. J. Clin. Nutr.* **2013**, *98*, 594–619. [CrossRef] [PubMed]
21. World Health Organization. Healthy Diet Fact Sheet n°394. Available online: http://www.who.int/mediacentre/factsheets/fs394/en/ (accessed on 13 January 2017).
22. Oldways Trust. Whole Grain Guidelines Worldwide. Available online: http://wholegrainscouncil.org/whole-grains-101/how-much-enough/whole-grain-guidelines-worldwide (accessed on 13 January 2017).

23. U.S. Department of Health and Human Services; U.S. Department of Agriculture. *Dietary Guidelines for Americans 2005*. Available online: https://www.cnpp.usda.gov/dietary-guidelines-2005 (accessed on 13 December 2016).
24. U.S. Department of Agriculture; U.S. Department of Health and Human Services. Dietary Guidelines for Americans 2010. Available online: https://www.cnpp.usda.gov/dietary-guidelines-2010 (accessed on 13 December 2016).
25. Krebs-Smith, S.M.; Guenther, P.M.; Subar, A.F.; Kirkpatrick, S.I.; Dodd, K.W. Americans do not meet federal dietary recommendations. *J. Nutr.* **2010**, *140*, 1832–1838. [CrossRef] [PubMed]
26. O'Neil, C.E.; Nicklas, T.A.; Zanovec, M.; Cho, S. Whole-grain consumption is associated with diet quality and nutrient intake in adults: The National Health and Nutrition Examination Survey, 1999–2004. *J. Am. Diet. Assoc.* **2010**, *110*, 1461–1468. [CrossRef] [PubMed]
27. Food and Drug Administration. *Draft Guideline: Whole Grains Label Statements, Guidance for Industry and FDA Staff*; Food and Drug Administration: College Park, MD, USA, 2006.
28. Clemens, R.; Kranz, S.; Mobley, A.R.; Nicklas, T.A.; Raimondi, M.P.; Rodriguez, J.C.; Slavin, J.L.; Warshaw, H. Filling America's fiber intake gap: Summary of a roundtable to probe realistic solutions with a focus on grain-based foods. *J. Nutr.* **2012**, *142*, 1390s–1401s. [CrossRef] [PubMed]
29. Nicklas, T.A.; O'Neil, C.E.; Liska, D.J.; Almeida, N.G.; Fulgoni, V.L., III. Modeling dietary fiber intakes in US adults: Implications for public policy. *Food Nutr. Sci.* **2011**, *2*, 925–931. [CrossRef]
30. Reicks, M.; Jonnalagadda, S.; Albertson, A.M.; Joshi, N. Total dietary fiber intakes in the US population are related to whole grain consumption: Results from the national health and nutrition examination survey 2009 to 2010. *Nutr. Res.* **2014**, *34*, 226–234. [CrossRef] [PubMed]
31. U.S. Department of Agriculture. ChooseMyPlate.gov. Available online: https://www.choosemyplate.gov/ (accessed on 13 December 2016).
32. Centers for Disease Control and Prevention; National Center for Health Statistics. National Health and Nutrition Examination Survey (NHANES). Available online: https://www.cdc.gov/nchs/nhanes/ (accessed on 13 December 2016).
33. Moshfegh, A.J.; Rhodes, D.G.; Baer, D.J.; Murayi, T.; Clemens, J.C.; Rumpler, W.V.; Paul, D.R.; Sebastian, R.S.; Kuczynski, K.J.; Ingwersen, L.A.; et al. The US Department of Agriculture Automated Multiple-Pass Method reduces bias in the collection of energy intakes. *Am. J. Clin. Nutr.* **2008**, *88*, 324–332. [PubMed]
34. Bowman, S.A.; Friday, J.E.; Moshfegh, A. MyPyramid Equivalents Database, 2.0 for USDA Survey Foods 2003–2004. Available online: https://www.ars.usda.gov/northeast-area/beltsville-md/beltsville-human-nutrition-research-center/food-surveys-research-group/docs/mped-databases-for-downloading/ (accessed on 26 February 2017).
35. Center for Nutrition Policy and Promotion. CNPP 03-04 Fruit Database. Available online: https://www.cnpp.usda.gov/healthy-eating-index-support-files-03-04 (accessed on 16 February 2017).
36. Food and Nutrient Database for Dietary Studies. Available online: https://www.ars.usda.gov/northeast-area/beltsville-md/beltsville-human-nutrition-research-center/food-surveys-research-group/docs/fndds/ (accessed on 16 February 2017).
37. International Food Information Council. 2016 Food and Health Survey. Available online: http://www.foodinsight.org/sites/default/files/2016-Food-and-Health-Survey-Report_%20FINAL_0.pdf (accessed on 13 December 2016).
38. Mobley, A.R.; Slavin, J.L.; Hornick, B.A. The future of grain foods recommendations in dietary guidance. *J. Nutr.* **2013**, *143*, 1527S–1532S. [CrossRef] [PubMed]
39. Brauchla, M.; Juan, W.; Story, J.; Kranz, S. Sources of dietary fiber and the association of fiber intake with childhood obesity risk (in 2–18 years old) and diabetes risk of adolescents 12–18 years old: NHANES 2003–2006. *J. Nutr. Metab.* **2012**, *2012*. [CrossRef] [PubMed]
40. Hur, I.Y.; Reicks, M. Relationship between whole-grain intake, chronic disease risk indicators, and weight status among adolescents in the National Health and Nutrition Examination Survey, 1999–2004. *J. Am. Diet. Assoc.* **2012**, *112*, 46–55. [CrossRef] [PubMed]